Essentials of Neurosurgic
Anesthesia & Critical Car

D1434158

Ansgar M. Brambrink · Jeffrey R. Kirsch

Editors

Essentials of Neurosurgical Anesthesia & Critical Care

Strategies for Prevention, Early Detection, and Successful Management of Perioperative Complications

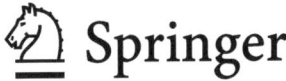 Springer

Editors

Ansgar M. Brambrink, MD, PhD
Professor, Department of Anesthesiology
and Perioperative Medicine
Oregon Health and Science University
School of Medicine
Portland, Oregon 97239
USA

Jeffrey R. Kirsch, MD
Professor and Chair, Department of
Anesthesiology and Perioperative Medicine
Oregon Health and Science University
School of Medicine
Portland, Oregon 97239
USA

ISBN 978-0-387-09561-5   e-ISBN 978-0-387-09562-2
DOI 10.1007/978-0-387-09562-2
Springer New York Dordrecht Heidelberg London

Library of Congress Control Number: 2011941433

Printed on acid-free paper

Springer is part of Springer Science+Business Media (www.springer.com)

To our families:
Petra, Jan, Phillip, Helen and Lucas (AB)
and
Robin, Jodi, Alan and Ricki (JK)
Thank you for your patience, love, and
understanding.

Foreword

Caring for acutely ill neurosurgical patients is a difficult business. The illnesses are serious and the stakes are high, particularly in the perioperative period. Further complicating matters is that damage to the central nervous system almost invariably leads either directly or indirectly to dysfunction in multiple organ systems. *Essentials of Neurosurgical Anesthesia and Critical Care* recognizes this complexity and comes at it not from the narrow perspective of a particular specialty but from the standpoint of what the patient needs. The result is a multi-disciplinary, problem-driven, solution-oriented compendium that will appeal to first-line healthcare providers who care for acutely ill neurosurgical patients, whether they be physicians, trainees, physician assistants, or perioperative or advanced practice nurses.

The editors are experienced and respected neuroanesthesiologists and neurocritical care physicians, and they have recruited an impressive group of authors from the fields of neurosurgery, anesthesiology, neurology, critical care, and nursing to contribute expertise. No handbook is a substitute for a full-length textbook or the reading of original research in the field, and this handbook is no exception. But, when the rubber meets the road at the patient's bedside, prevention, detection, and action trump theory. The guidance provided in these pages is informed by theory and science but is distilled by experts in the field and presented in a practical, accessible format that will help the provider anticipate problems and develop an informed and reasonable action plan when complications do arise. For the neurosurgical patient in the perioperative period or neurocritical care unit, that is the essence of good care. That is what this Handbook is about.

Boston, Massachusetts   Gregory Crosby, MD

Preface

Today, treatment decisions are expected to be evidence-based, and the pursuit of excellence in clinical practice is an essential element for achieving success in the current health care environment.

Perioperative care of patients with central nervous system diseases is evolving rapidly as increasing numbers of operative interventional techniques and strategies are developed. Physicians, nurses, nurse practitioners and physician assistants treat patients throughout the immediate perioperative period, including during diagnostic procedures and interventional radiology procedures, and frequently participate in critical care treatment for this patient population.

We believe that the broad spectrum of neuroanesthesiology and neurocritical care providers should have a clear understanding of (1) the disease process including pathophysiology, specific diagnostics, and treatment options, (2) the concepts and relevant details of the available neurosurgical interventions, techniques, and (3) means necessary to provide safe and comfortable anesthesia and perioperative care for these patients.

This handbook, entitled *Essentials of Neurosurgical Anesthesia & Critical Care*, is intended to serve as a quick reference guide for those involved in the perioperative care of neurosurgical patients. It is not meant to substitute for a full-length textbook in this field.

Our handbook focuses on day-to-day clinical practice and supports the first-line healthcare provider by anticipating problems and complications in neurosurgical anesthesia and critical care and suggesting solutions and appropriate management. All chapters are dedicated to a single area of concern and designed to walk the reader from the problem to the solution, using a structured algorithmic approach. In addition, each chapter summarizes key knowledge for the practitioner in the field, as necessary, and tables and illustrations are included for quick and easy reference. At the end of each chapter, the most important elements are highlighted for the reader, and references for further reading are provided.

Our handbook is perceived and edited out of the strong belief that perioperative medicine is a true multi-specialty discipline and that patient care is best delivered with a genuine collaborative approach. Therefore, we hope that this handbook will be useful for all healthcare providers involved in the perioperative treatment of neurosurgical patients including trainees in anesthesiology and neurosurgical critical care as well as faculty members in both fields, physician assistants, nurse practitioners, nurse anesthetists, and perioperative nurses.

We believe the handbook format is best because it allows the clinician to have immediate access to solutions to problems in the operating room, post-anesthesia care unit, intensive care unit, or wherever they may occur. Even if the practitioner has the best reference on their office shelf, it is not helpful when acute problems occur at the bedside. This handbook, however, will be portable to every place of practice and will make it easy for the practitioner to identify or quickly review several good solutions for a given problem at anytime.

We have been fortunate that several international leaders in the fields agreed to contribute to our project, and we are convinced that clinicians in both private practice and academic medicine will benefit from the concise information provided from multiple institutions from around the world.

We hope that this book may help to improve further the safety and comfort of our patients who unfortunately have to undergo risky procedures to receive relief from diseases affecting the central nervous system.

Portland, OR, USA   Ansgar M. Brambrink, MD, PhD
July 2011   Jeffrey R. Kirsch, MD

Acknowledgment

The Editors express their tremendous appreciation to Kathy Gage who has supported this project through the entire process from initial conceptualization, through the correspondence between authors, editors, and publisher, to the meticulous tracing of all contributions in their various stages of completion and who has provided editorial support where needed.

Contents

Contributors

Kenneth Abbey, MD, JD Department of Anesthesiology and Perioperative Medicine, Oregon Health & Science University, Portland, OR, USA

Osama Ahmed, MD Department of Neurosurgery, Louisiana State University Health Sciences Center Shreveport, Shreveport, LA, USA

Chinwe Ajuba-Iwuji, MD Department of Anesthesiology and Critical Care Medicine, Johns Hopkins University School of Medicine, Baltimore, MD, USA

Chloe Allen-Maycock, MD Department of Anesthesiology, Legacy Salmon Creek Medical Center, PeaceHealth Southwest Medical Center, Vancouver, WA, USA

Inger Aliason, MD Departments of Anesthesiology, The University of Oklahoma College of Medicine, Oklahoma City, OK, USA

John H. Arnold, MD Departments of Anaesthesia, Perioperative and Pain Medicine, and Respiratory Care/ECMO/Biomedical Engineering, Children's Hospital Boston, Harvard Medical School, Boston, MA, USA

Syed Arshad, MD Department of Neurosurgery, Kaiser Sacramento Medical Center, University of California, San Francisco, Sacramento, CA, USA

Joshua H. Atkins, MD, PhD Departments of Anesthesiology and Critical Care, and Otorhinolaryrgology, Head & Neck Surgery, Perelman School of Medicine at the University of Pennsylvania, Philadelphia, PA, USA

Michael Aziz, MD Department of Anesthesiology and Perioperative Medicine, Oregon Health & Science University, Portland, OR, USA

Stanley L. Barnwell, MD, PhD Department of Neurological Surgery and Dotter Interventional Institute, Oregon Health & Science University, Portland, OR, USA

Paul Bascom, MD, FACP Department of Hematology and Oncology, Oregon Health & Science University, Portland, OR, USA

Sarice Bassin, MD Southwest Medical Group Neurology Associates, PeaceHealth Southwest Medical Center, Vancouver, WA, USA

Verna L. Baughman, MD Departments of Anesthesiology and Neurosurgery, University of Illinois Medical Center, Chicago, IL, USA

Audrée A. Bendo, MD Department of Anesthesiology, State University of New York Downstate Medical Center, Brooklyn, NY, USA

Walter van den Bergh, MD, PhD Department of Intensive Care, Academic Medical Center, Amsterdam, The Netherlands

Michael Bernhard, MD Emergency Department/Emergency Admission Unit, University Hospital of Leipzig, Leipzig, Germany

Thomas Bleck, MD, FCCM Departments of Neurosurgery and Anesthesiology, Rush University Medical Center, Chicago, IL, USA

Marc J. Bloom, MD, PhD Department of Anesthesiology, New York University School of Medicine, Langone Medical Center, New York, NY, USA

Meghan Bost, MD Anesthesia Associates of Medford, Medford, OR, USA

Bernd W. Böttiger, MD, DEAA, FESC, FERC Department of Anesthesiology and Intensive Care Medicine, University of Cologne School of Medicine, Cologne, Germany

Carrie C. Bowman, MS, CRNA Department of Anesthesiology, Georgetown University School of Medicine, Washington, DC, USA

Ansgar M. Brambrink, MD, PhD Departments of Anesthesiology and Perioperative Medicine, Neurology and Neurologic Surgery, Oregon Health & Science University, Portland, OR, USA

Evgeni Brotfain, MD Department of Anesthesiology and Intensive Care, Soroka University Medical Center, Ben-Gurion University of the Negev, Beer-Sheva, Israel

Guillermo Bugedo, MD Department of Intensive Care Medicine, Faculty of Medicine, Pontificia Universidad Catolica de Chile, Santiago, Chile

Kim J. Burchiel, MD Department of Neurological Surgery, Oregon Health & Science University, Portland, OR, USA

Christoph S. Burkhart, MD Department of Anaesthesia and Intensive Care Medicine, University of Basel, Basel, Switzerland

Luis Castillo, MD Department of Intensive Care Medicine, Faculty of Medicine, Pontificia Universidad Catolica de Chile, Santiago, Chile

Matthew T.V. Chan, MBBS, FANZCA, FHKCA, FHKAM Department of Anaesthesia and Intensive Care, The Chinese University of Hong Kong, Shatin, NT, Hong Kong SAR

Daniel J. Cole, MD Department of Anesthesiology, Mayo Clinic, Scottsdale, AZ, USA

Richard C. Corry, MB, ChB, FRCA Department of Anaesthesia, Royal Victoria Hospital, Belfast, UK

Olaf L. Cremer, MD, PhD Department of Intensive Care Medicine, University Medical Center Utrecht, Utrecht, The Netherlands

Edward Crosby, MD, FRCPC Department of Anaesthesia, University of Ottawa, Ottawa, ON, Canada

Martin H. Dauber, MD Department of Anesthesia and Critical Care, The University of Chicago Medical Center, Chicago, Illinois, USA

Alejandro E. Delfino, MD Department of Anesthesia, Escuela de Medicina, Pontificia Universidad Católica de Chile, Santiago, Chile

Jayant Deshpande, MD, MPH Departments of Pediatrics and Anesthesiology, Arkansas Children's Hospital, University of Arkansas for Medical Sciences, Little Rock, AR, USA

Nina Deutsch, MD Department of Anesthesiology and Pain Medicine, Children's National Medical Center, Washington, DC, USA

Judith Dinsmore, MBBS, FRCA Department of Anaesthesia and Intensive Care Medicine, St. George's University Hospital Trust, London, UK

Justin P. Dodge, MD Department of Radiology, Landstuhl Regional Medical Center, Landstuhl, RP, Germeny

Shuji Dohi, MD, PhD Emeritus of Gifu University, Department of Anesthesiology and Pain Medicine, Gifu University Graduate School of Medicine, Gifu, Japan

Karen B. Domino, MD, MPH Department of Anesthesiology and Pain Medicine, University of Washington School of Medicine, Seattle, WA, USA

Andrea M. Dower, BSc, MD, FRCPC Department of Anesthesia, McMaster University, Hamilton, ON, Canada

Doortje C. Engel, MD, PhD, MBA Department of Neurosurgery, Cantonal Hospital St. Gallen, St. Gallen, Switzerland

Kristin Engelhand, MD, PhD Department of Anesthesiology, University Medical Center, Johannes Gutenberg University, Mainz, Germany

Miko Enomoto, MD Department of Anesthesiology and Perioperative Medicine, Oregon Health & Science University, Portland, OR, USA

Kirstin M. Erickson, MD Department of Anesthesiology, Mayo Clinic, Rochester, MN, USA

Peter A. Farling, MB, BCh, FRCA Department of Anaesthesia, Royal Victoria Hospital, Belfast, UK

Tacson Fernandez, MBBS, FCARCSI, FIPP, DPM Department of Anaesthetics and Pain Medicine, Imperial College Hospitals Healthcare NHS Trust, London, UK

Jeremy D. Fields, MD Departments of Neurology and Dotter Interventional Institute, Oregon Health & Science University, Portland, OR, USA

Stuart Friess, MD Department of Anesthesiology and Critical Care Medicine, The Children's Hospital of Philadelphia, Philadelphia, PA, USA

E. Paige Gerbic, MD Columbia Anesthesia Group, Vancouver, WA, USA

Heike Gries, MD, PhD Department of Anesthesiology and Perioperative Medicine, Oregon Health & Science University, Portland, OR, USA

Lori E. Guidone, PA-C Department of Neurological Surgical, Oregon Health & Science University, Portland, OR, USA

Amy E. Guthrie, MSN, CNS, ACHPN Department of Oregon Health & Science University, Portland, OR, USA

Casey H. Halpern, MD Department of Neurosurgery, Hospital of the University of Pennsylvania, Philadelphia, PA, USA

Ola Harrskog, MD, DEAA Department of Anesthesiology and Perioperative Medicine, Oregon Health & Science University, Portland, OR, USA

Mark Helfaer, MD Departments of Anesthesiology and Critical Care, Pediatrics, and Nursing, Perelman School of Medicine at the University of Pennsylvania, Philadelphia, PA, USA

James G. Hilliard, MS, CRNA Department of Anesthesiology and Perioperative Medicine, Oregon Health & Science University, Portland, OR, USA

Nicholas Hirsch, FRCA, FRCP, FFICM Department of Neuroanesthesia, National Hospital for Neurology and Neurosurgery, London, UK

Yulia Ivashkov, MD Department of Anesthesiology and Pain Medicine, University of Washington, Seattle, WA, USA

Leslie C. Jameson, MD Department of Anesthesiology, University of Colorado at Denver School of Medicine, Aurora, CO, USA

Daniel J. Janik, MD Department of Anesthesiology, University of Colorado at Denver School of Medicine, Aurora, CO, USA

Jan-Peter A. H. Jantzen, MD, PhD, DEAA Department of Anaesthesiology, Intensive Care Medicine and Pain Management, Academic Teaching Hospital Hannover Nordstadt, Hannover, Germany

W. Scott Jellish, MD, PhD Department of Anesthesiology, Loyola University Medical Center, Stritch School of Medicine, Maywood, IL, USA

Zeev N. Kain, MD Department of Anesthesiology & Perioperative Care, University of California, Irvine Medical Center, Orange, CA, USA

Patricia K.Y. Kan, MBBS, FANZCA, FHKCA, FHKAM Department of Anaesthesia and Intensive Care, The Chinese University of Hong Kong, Shatin, NT, Hong Kong SAR

Christopher Karsanac, MD Department of Anesthesiology, Vanderbilt University Medical Center, Nashville, TN, USA

Masahiko Kawaguchi Department of Anesthesiology, Nara Medical University, Kashihara, Nara, Japan

Todd J. Kilbaugh, MD Department of Anesthesiology and Critical Care Medicine, The Children's Hospital of Philadelphia, Philadelphia, PA, USA

Jeffrey R. Kirsch, MD Department of Anesthesiology and Perioperative Medicine, Oregon Health & Science University, Portland, OR, USA

Jürgen Knapp, MD Department of Anesthesiology, University of Heidelberg, Heidelberg, Germany

Jeffrey Koh, MD Department of Anesthesiology and Perioperative Medicine, Oregon Health & Science University, Portland, OR, USA

Lawrence Lai, MD Department of Anesthesiology, The State University of New York Downstate Medical Center, Brooklyn, NY, USA

Kirk Lalwani, MD, FRCA, MCR Department of Anesthesiology and Perioperative Medicine, Oregon Health & Science University, Portland, OR, USA

Arthur M. Lam, MD, FRCPC Department of Neuroanesthesia and Neurocritical Care, Swedish Neuroscience Institute, Seattle, WA, USA

Gregory J. Latham, MD Department of Anesthesiology and Pain Medicine, Seattle Children's Hospital, Seattle, WA, USA

Chanhung Z. Lee, MD, PhD Department of Anesthesia and Perioperative Care, University of California, San Francisco School of Medicine, San Francisco, CA, USA

Chris C. Lee, MD, PhD Department of Anesthesiology, Washington University School of Medicine in St. Louis, St. Louis, MO, USA

Lorri Lee, MD Department of Anesthesiology and Pain Medicine, University of Washington School of Medicine, Seattle, WA, USA

Mitchell Y. Lee, MD Department of Anesthesiology, New York University School of Medicine, New York, NY, USA

Akiva Leibowitz, MD Department of Anesthesiology and Critical Care, Soroka University Medical Center, Ben Gurion-University of the Negev, Beer-Sheva, Israel

Min Li, MD Department of Anesthesiology, Peking University Third Hospital, Peking University Health Science Center, Beijing, China

Pamela A. Lipsett, MD, FACS, FCCM Department of Surgery, Johns Hopkins University School of Medicine, Baltimore, MD, USA

Kenneth C. Liu, MD Departments of Neurological Surgery and Radiology, University of Virginia Health System, Charlottesville, VA, USA

Philip E. Lund, MD Department of Anesthesiology, Kaiser Sunnyside Medical center, Clackamas, OR, USA

Andrew Maas, MD Department of Neurosurgery, University Hospital Antwerp, Edegem, Belgium

Elizabeth M. Macri, MD Neurocritical Care, Presbyterian Hospital, Albuquerque, NM, USA

Pirjo Manninen, MD, FRCPC University of Toronto, Toronto Western Hospital University, Health Network, Toronto, Ontario, Canada

Edward M. Manno, MD FCCM, FAAN, FAHA Department of Neurology and Neurological Surgery, Cerebrovascular Center, Cleveland Clinic, Cleveland, OH, USA

Lynn D. Martin, MD, MBA Department of Anesthesiology and Pain Medicine Seattle Children's Hospital, University of Washington, Seattle, WA, USA

Timothy W. Martin, MD, MBA Department of Anesthesiology, Arkansas Children's Hospital, UAMS College of Medicine, Little Rock, AR, USA

Basil Matta, MD, FRCA Department of Emergency and Perioperative Care, Cambridge University Hospitals, Cambridge, UK

Craig D. McClain, MD, MPH Department of Anesthesiology, Perioperative and Pain Medicine, Children's Hospital Boston, Boston, MA, USA

Michael L. McManus, MD, MPH Department of Anesthesiology, Perioperative and Pain Medicine, Children's Hospital Boston, Harvard Medical School, Boston, MA, USA

Lingzhong Meng, MD Department of Anesthesiology & Perioperative Care, University of California, Irvine Medical Center, Orange, CA, USA

Andrew H. Milby, MD Department of Orthopaedic Surgery, University of Pennsylvania School of Medicine, Philadelphia, PA, USA

Paul D. Mongan, MD Department of Anesthesiology, University of Colorado at Denver School of Medicine, Aurora, CO, USA

Laurel E. Moore, MD Department of Anesthesiology, University of Michigan Medical School, Ann Arbor, MI, USA

Debra E. Morrison, MD Department of Anesthesiology and Perioperative Care, University of California, Irvine Medical Center, Orange, California, USA

Wibke Müller-Forell, MD, PhD Institute for Neuroradiology, University Medical Center Johannes Gutenberg University, Mainz, Germany

Hernán R. Muñoz, MD, MSc Department of Anesthesia, Escuela de Medicina, Pontificia Universidad Católica de Chile, Santiago, Chile

David Murray, MD Department of Anesthesiology, Washington University School of Medicine in St. Louis, St. Louis, MO, USA

Mary Newton, MBBS, FRCA The National Hospital for Neurology and Neurosurgery, London, UK

Carl Helge Nielsen, MD Department of Anesthesiology, Washington University School of Medicine, St. Louis, MO, USA

Dolores B. Njoku, MD Departments of Anesthesiology and Critical Care Medicine, Pediatrics and Pathology, Johns Hopkins University School of Medicine, Baltimore, MD, USA

Andrea Orfanakis, MD Department of Anesthesiology and Perioperative Medicine, Oregon Health & Science University, Portland, OR, USA

Murat Oztaskin, BA, RA Dotter Interventional Institute, Oregon Health & Science University, Portland, OR, USA

Chanannait Paisansathan, MD Department of Anesthesiology, University of Illinois at Chicago, Chicago, IL, USA

Amit Prakash, MD, FRCA Department of Anesthesia, Toronto Western Hospital, Toronto, ON, Canada

Tariq Parray, MD Department of Anesthesiology Arkansas Children's Hospital, University of Arkansas for Medical Sciences, Little Rock, Arkansas, USA

Patricia Harper Petrozza, MD Department of Anesthesiology, Wake Forest Baptist Medical Center, Winston Salem, NC, USA

Sadeq A. Quraishi, MD, MHA Department of Anaesthesia, Harvard Medical School, Boston, MA, USA

Sally E. Rampersad, MB, FRCA Department of Anesthesiology and Pain Medicine, Settle Children's Hospital, University of Washington, Seattle, WA, USA

Debra A. Reeves, RN, BS, BSN Division of Perioperative Services,
Oregon Health & Science University, Portland, OR, USA

Denise H. Rhoney, Pharm.D, FCCP, FCCM Department of Pharmacy Practice,
Wayne State University, Eugene Applebaum College of Pharmacy
and Health Sciences, Detroit, MI, USA

Robert Hugo Richardson, MD Departments of Pulmonary and Critical Care
Medicine, General Medicine and Geriatrics, Oregon Health & Science University,
Portland, OR, USA

Claudia Robertson, MD Department of Neurosurgery, Baylor College
of Medicine, Houston, TX, USA

Abraham Rosenbaum, MD Department of Anesthesiology and Perioperative
Care, University of California, Irvine Medical Center, Orange, CA, USA

Allison Kinder Ross, MD Departments of Anesthesiology and
Pediatrics, Duke University School of Medicine, Durham, NC, USA

Steven Roth, MD Department of Anesthesia and Critical Care,
The University of Chicago Pritzker School of Medicine, Chicago, IL, USA

Peter Rothwell, MD Department of Clinical Neuroscience, John Radcliffe
Hospital, Oxford, UK

Neil E. Roundy, MD Department of Neurological Surgery,
Oregon Health & Science University, Portland, OR, USA

Irene Rozet, MD Department of Anesthesiology and Pain Medicine, University
of Washington and VA Puget Sound Health Care System, Seattle, WA, USA

Renata Rusa, MD Department of Anesthesiology and Perioperative Medicine,
Oregon Health & Science University, Portland, OR, USA

Susan Ryan, PhD, MD Department of Anesthesia and Perioperative Care,
University of California, San Francisco, San Francisco, CA, USA

R. Alexander Schlichter, MD Department of Anesthesiology and Critical Care,
University of Pennsylvania School of Medicine,
Philadelphia, PA, USA

Martin Schott, MD Department of Anesthesiology, Intensive Care and Pain
Management, Academic Teaching Hospital Hannover Nordstadt, Hannover, Germany

Ursula Schulz, MD, D.Phil Nuffield Department of Neurosciences,
University of Oxford, Oxford, UK

James M. Schuster, MD, PhD Department of Neurosurgery,
University of Pennsylvania School of Medicine, Philadelphia, PA, USA

Valerie Sera, MD Professor of Anesthesiology and Perioperative Medicine,
Oregon Health & Science University, Portland, OR, USA

Donald Shaffner, MD Department of Anesthesiology and Critical Care Medicine, Johns Hopkins The Medical Institutions, Baltimore, MD, USA

Robert E. Shangraw, MD, PhD Department of Anesthesiology and Perioperative Medicine, Oregon Health & Science University, Portland, OR, USA

Punita Sharma, MD Department of Anesthesiology and Critical Care Medicine, Johns Hopkins Medicine Bayview Medical Center, Baltimore, MD, USA

Yoram Shapira, MD, PhD Department of Anesthesiology and Critical Care, Soroka University Medical Center, Ben-Gurion University of the Negev, Beer-Sheva, Israel

Frederick Sieber, MD Department of Anesthesiology and Critical Care Medicine, The Johns Hopkins Medicine Bayview Medical Center, Baltimore, MD, USA

Tod B. Sloan, MD, MBA, PhD Department of Anesthesiology, The University of Colorado Denver School of Medicine, Aurora, CO, USA

Edward R. Smith, MD Department of Neurosurgery, Children's Hospital Boston, Harvard Medical School, Boston, MA, USA

Martin Smith, MBBS, FRCA, FFICM Department of Neurocritical Care, National Hospital for Neurology and Neurosurgery, University College London Hospitals, Queen Square, London, UK

Mary Denise Smith, RN, MSN, CNS Departments of Internal Medicine and Palliative Medicine, Oregon Health & Sciences University, Portland, OR, USA

Martin Soehle, MD, PhD, DESA Department of Anaesthesiology and Intensive Care Medicine, University of Bonn, Bonn, Germany

Sulpicio G. Soriano, MD, FAAP Department of Anaesthesia, Harvard Child Hospital, Boston, MA, USA

Michael J. Souter, MB, ChB, FRCA Department of Anesthesiology and Pain Medicine and Department of Neurological Surgery, University of Washington School of Medicine, Seattle, WA, USA

Luzius A. Steiner, MD, PhD Department of Anaesthesia, University Hospital Center and University of Lausanne, Lausanne, Switzerland

Stephan P. Strebel, MD Department of Anaesthesia, University Clinics of Basel, and University Hospital Center and University of Lausanne, Switzerland

Mary K. Sturaitis, MD Departments of Anesthesiology and Neurosurgery, Rush University Medical Center, Chicago, IL, USA

José I. Suarez, MD Department of Neurology, Baylor College of Medicine, Houston, TX, USA

Dieter Suhr, MD Department of Anesthesiology, International Neuroscience Institute (INI), Hannover, Germany

Pekka Talke, MD Department of Anesthesia and Perioperative Care, University of California, San Francisco, San Francisco, CA, USA

Rene Tempelhoff, MD Department of Anesthesiology, Washington University School of Medicine, St. Louis, MO, USA

Concezione Tommasino, MD Department of Anesthesiology and Intensive Care, University of Milan, H San Paolo Medical School, Milan, Italy

Kamila Vagnerova, MD Department of Anesthesiology and Perioperative Medicine, Oregon Health & Science University, Portland, OR, USA

Panayiotis N. Varelas, MD, PhD Departments of Neurology & Neurosurgery, Henry Ford Hospital, Detroit, MI, USA

Monica S. Vavilala, MD Departments of Anesthesiology and Pain Medicine and Neurological Surgery, Radiology, University of Washington and Harborview Injury Prevention and Research Center, Harborview Medical Center, Seattle, WA, USA

Gerhard K. Wolf, MD Department of Anesthesiology, Perioperative and Pain Medicine, Children's Hospital Boston, Harvard Medical School, Boston, MA, USA

Jeffrey Yoder, MD Saint Anthony's Hospital, Denver, CO, USA

William L. Young, MD Departments of Anesthesia and Perioperative Care, Neurological Surgery and Neurology, University of California, San Francisco, CA, USA

Liping Zhang, MD Department of Anesthesiology, Peking University Health Science Center, Beijing, China

Alexander Zlotnik, MD, PhD Department of Anesthesiology and Critical Care, Soroka University Medical Center, Ben Gurion-University of the Negev, Beer-Sheva, Israel

Part I
Basics of Neuroanesthesia Care

Chapter 1
The Adult Central Nervous System: Anatomy and Physiology

Punita Sharma and Frederick Sieber

Overview

The human brain consists of three basic subdivisions – the cerebral hemispheres, the brain stem, and the cerebellum. Speech is represented by two main areas – Broca's area in the inferior frontal lobe (expressive speech) and the Wernicke's area in the temporoparietal cortex (interpretation of language) (Fig. 1.1). Language localization is found in 96% of population in the left. The basal ganglia are a collection of nuclei deep in the white matter of cerebral cortex and contain the substantia nigra. A decrease in function of the dopaminergic neurons located in the substantia nigra causes Parkinson's disease. The cerebral hemispheres are connected together medially by the corpus callosum. The limbic areas of the brain include the hypothalamus, amygdala, hippocampus, and limbic cortex. Optic nerve (second) leaves the retina of the eye and travels to the optic chiasm, located just below and in front of the pituitary gland. In the optic chiasm, the optic nerve fibers arising from the nasal half of each retina cross over to the other side; but the nerve fibers originating in the temporal retina do not cross over. The nerve fibers become the optic tract, the optic radiation and reach the visual cortex in the occipital lobe of the cerebrum.

The brainstem is located at the juncture of the cerebrum and the spinal column. It consists of the midbrain, pons, and the medulla oblongata. Two cranial nerves are associated with the midbrain, the oculomotor (3rd) which emerges from the interpeduncular fossa and the trochlear (4th) cranial nerves which emerges from the dorsal

P. Sharma, MD (✉)
Department of Anesthesiology, and Critical Care Medicine, Johns Hopkins
Medicine Bayview Medical Center, Baltimore, MD, USA
e-mail: punitatripathi@hotmail.com

F. Sieber, MD
Department of Anesthesiology and Critical Care Medicine, The Johns Hopkins Medicine
Bayview Medical Center, Baltimore, MD, USA

A.M. Brambrink and J.R. Kirsch (eds.), *Essentials of Neurosurgical
Anesthesia & Critical Care*, DOI 10.1007/978-0-387-09562-2_1,
© Springer Science+Business Media, LLC 2012

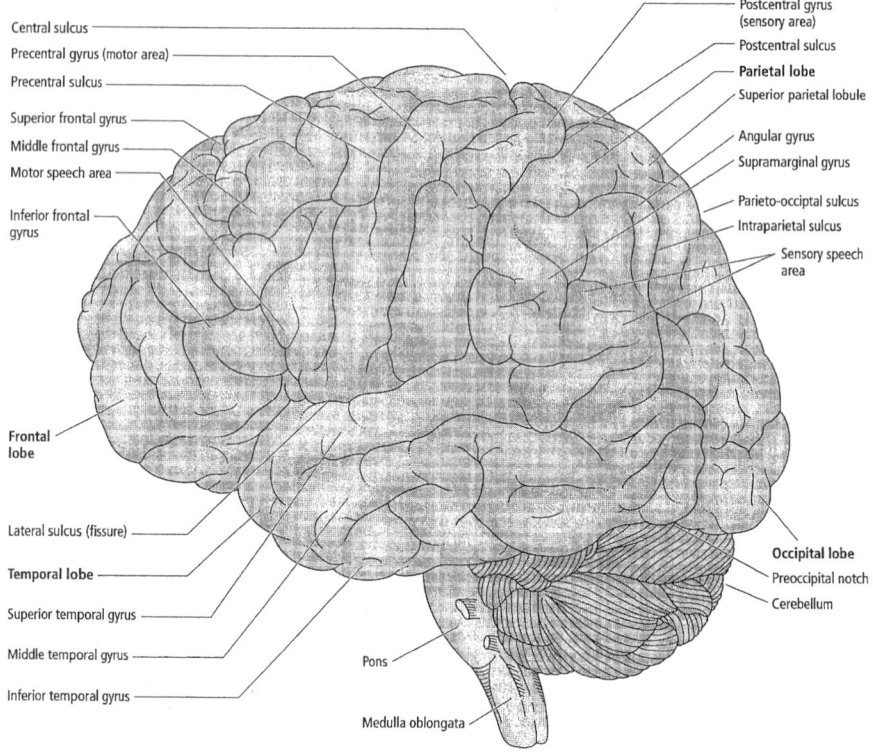

Central sulcus

Precentral gyrus (motor area)

Precentral sulcus

Superior frontal gyrus

Middle frontal gyrus

Motor speech area

Inferior frontal gyrus

Frontal lobe

Lateral sulcus (fissure)

Temporal lobe

Superior temporal gyrus

Middle temporal gyrus

Inferior temporal gyrus

Postcentral gyrus (sensory area)

Postcentral sulcus

Parietal lobe

Superior parietal lobule

Angular gyrus

Supramarginal gyrus

Parieto-occipital sulcus

Intraparietal sulcus

Sensory speech area

Occipital lobe

Preoccipital notch

Cerebellum

Pons

Medulla oblongata

Fig. 1.1 Lateral surface of the brain

surface of the brain stem. The cranial nerves associated with the pons are the trigeminal (5th), abducens (6th), facial (7th), and the two components of the auditory (8th). The 5th cranial nerve passes through the rostral part of the middle cerebellar peduncle. The 6th lies on the floor of the fourth ventricle is partially encircled by the 7th cranial nerve and emerges from the ventral surface of the brain stem at the junction between the pons and medulla. The 7th and 8th cranial nerve emerge from the lateral surface of the pons at the cerebellopontine angle. The red nucleus is a structure in the rostral midbrain involved in motor coordination. It is less important in its motor functions for humans than in many other mammals because, in humans, the corticospinal tract is dominant. The reticular formation is composed of a number of diffuse nuclei in the medulla, pons, and midbrain. The ascending reticular formation is also called the reticular activating system (RAS) and is responsible for the sleep–wake cycle. The descending reticular formation is involved in posture, equilibrium, and motor movement. It is also responsible for autonomic nervous system activity (vasomotor center), and stimulation of different portions of this center causes either a rise in blood pressure and tachycardia (pressor area) or a fall in blood pressure and bradycardia (depressor area). Medulla is the most caudal part of the brain stem.

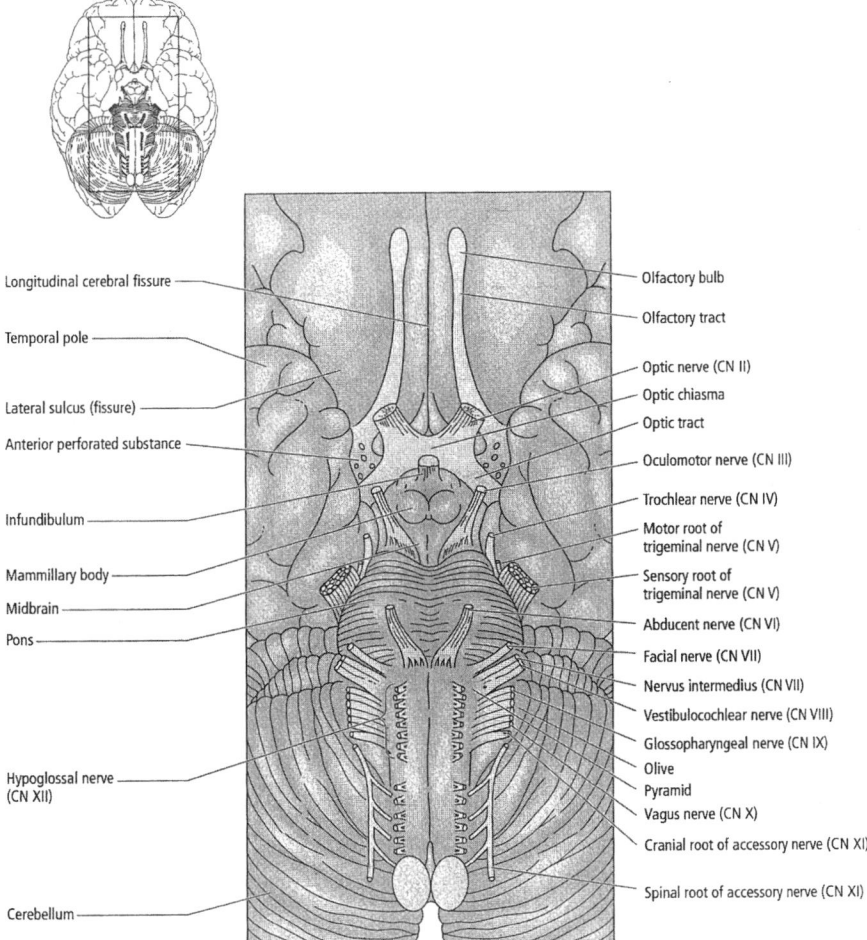

Longitudinal cerebral fissure

Temporal pole

Lateral sulcus (fissure)

Anterior perforated substance

Infundibulum

Mammillary body

Midbrain

Pons

Hypoglossal nerve
(CN XII)

Cerebellum

Olfactory bulb

Olfactory tract

Optic nerve (CN II)

Optic chiasma

Optic tract

Oculomotor nerve (CN III)

Trochlear nerve (CN IV)

Motor root of
trigeminal nerve (CN V)

Sensory root of
trigeminal nerve (CN V)

Abducent nerve (CN VI)

Facial nerve (CN VII)

Nervus intermedius (CN VII)

Vestibulocochlear nerve (CN VIII)

Glossopharyngeal nerve (CN IX)

Olive

Pyramid

Vagus nerve (CN X)

Cranial root of accessory nerve (CN XI)

Spinal root of accessory nerve (CN XI)

Fig. 1.2 Cranial nerves at the base of brain

The cranial nerves associated with the medulla are the glossopharyngeal nerve (9th), vagus (10th), accessory (11th), and the hypoglossal (12th) (Fig. 1.2).

The cerebellum is a trilobed structure, lying posterior to the pons and medulla oblongata and inferior to the occipital lobes of the cerebral hemispheres, that is responsible for the regulation and coordination of complex voluntary muscular movement as well as the maintenance of posture and balance. In contrast to the neocortex, cerebellar lesions produce ipsilateral disturbances.

The skull consists of the anterior, middle, and the posterior cranial fossa. Anterior cranial fossa accommodates the anterior lobe of brain. Middle cranial fossa contains the two temporal lobes, the parietal and part of the occipital lobe of brain. The posterior cranial fossa is part of the intracranial cavity located between the foramen magnum and

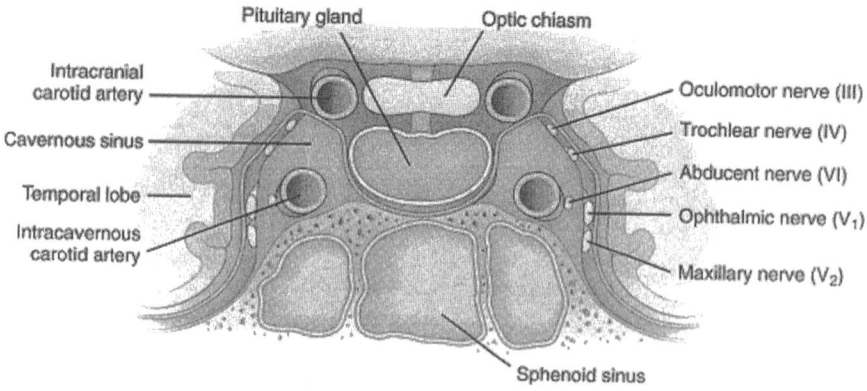

Fig. 1.3 Anatomical structure of cavernous sinus

tentorium cerebri. It contains part of the occipital lobe, brainstem, and cerebellum. The brain is covered by the dural membranes which enclose the venous sinuses.

The cavernous sinuses are paired, venous structures located on either side of the sella turcica (Fig. 1.3). They contain the carotid artery, its sympathetic plexus, and the third, fourth, and sixth cranial nerves. In addition, the ophthalmic branch and occasionally the maxillary branch of the fifth nerve traverse the cavernous sinus. The nerves pass through the wall of the sinus, while the carotid artery passes through the sinus itself. The pituitary gland is located inside the sella turcica, a round bony cavity that is separated from the sphenoid sinuses by a thin bone, the floor of the sella, which forms part of the roof of the sphenoid sinuses.

The Circle of Willis provides the blood supply to the cerebrum. It is formed by the two internal carotid arteries, which are responsible for 80% blood supply to the brain, and the vertebral artery, which is responsible for about 20% blood supply to the brain. The internal carotids and vertebral arteries anastomose together at the base of the brain. The Circle of Willis is associated with frequent anatomical variations, and a complete Circle of Willis is found only in 50% of the population. The anterior and middle cerebral arteries, which originate from the Circle of Willis, form the anterior circulation and supply the forebrain. Each gives rise to branches that supply the cortex and branches that penetrate the basal surface of the brain, supplying deep structures such as the basal ganglia, thalamus, and internal capsule. The lenticulostriate arteries arise from the middle cerebral artery and supply the basal ganglia and thalamus. The posterior circulation of the brain supplies the posterior cortex, the midbrain, and the brainstem and comprises arterial branches arising from the posterior cerebral, basilar, and vertebral arteries. Midline arteries supply medial structures; lateral arteries supply the lateral brainstem; and dorsal–lateral arteries supply dorsal–lateral brainstem structures and the cerebellum (Fig. 1.4).

Most of the blood in the brain can be found in its venous system. Blood is drained into superficial and deep cerebral veins and veins of the posterior fossa. The superficial veins drain the surface of the brain cortex and lie within the cortical sulci. The deep cerebral veins drain the white matter, basal ganglia, diencephalon, cerebellum,

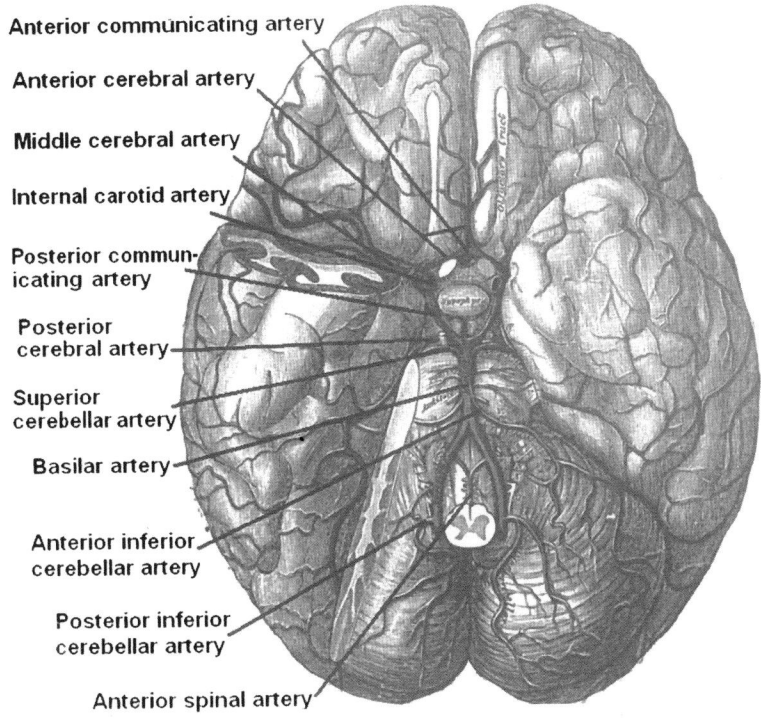

Anterior communicating artery

Anterior cerebral artery

Middle cerebral artery

Internal carotid artery

Posterior communicating artery

Posterior cerebral artery

Superior cerebellar artery

Basilar artery

Anterior inferior cerebellar artery

Posterior inferior cerebellar artery

Anterior spinal artery

Fig. 1.4 Arterial supply of the brain

and brainstem. The deep veins join to form the great cerebral vein. The veins of posterior fossa drain blood from the cerebellar tonsils and the posteroinferior cerebellar hemispheres. In addition, the diploic veins drain the blood between layers of bone in the skull. Emissary veins connect the veins near the surface of the skull to the diploic veins and venous sinuses. All the blood is drained into the meningeal sinuses, which mainly drain into the internal jugular vein. Usually, the right jugular vein is the dominant one, receiving most of the blood from the brain. The veins and sinuses of the brain lack valves. Pressure of drainage vessels in the neck is directly transmitted to intracranial venous structures (Fig. 1.5).

The vertebral column is composed of 33 vertebrae. Each vertebra is composed of a vertebral body, neural arch, pedicle, and a lamina (Fig. 1.6). The two lamina join together posteriorly to form the spinous process. The ligaments stabilizing the vertebral column from exterior to interior are the supraspinous, interspinous, ligamentum flavum, posterior longitudinal, and anterior longitudinal ligaments (Fig. 1.7). The ligaments provide flexibility without allowing excessive movement which could damage the cord. The human spine is also affected by aging. The intervertebral disks become drier, more fibrous and less resilient.

The spinal cord is a long cylindrical structure covered by membranes which lies in the vertebral canal. The spinal cord is the continuation of the medulla. It extends

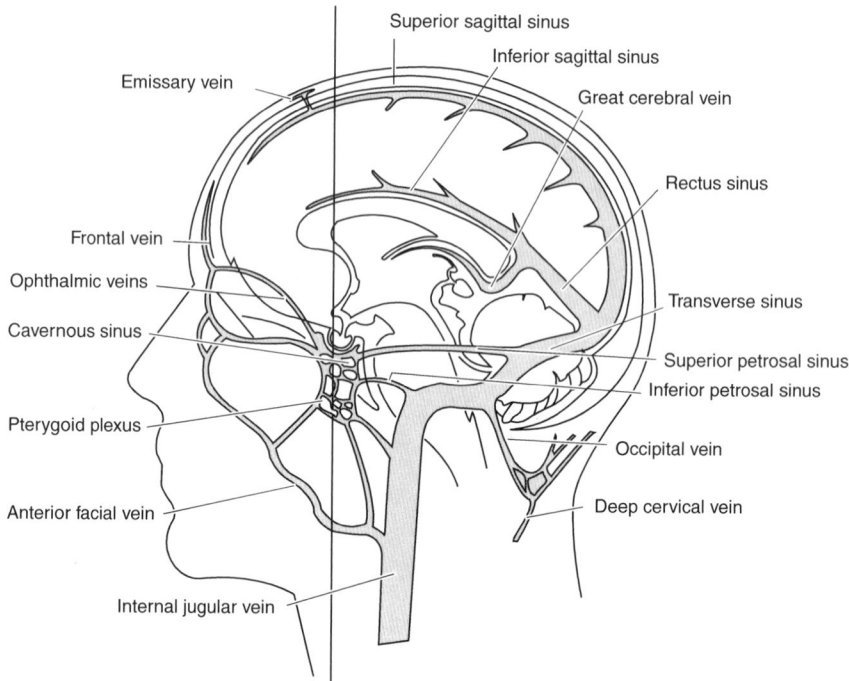

Fig. 1.5 Venous drainage of the brain

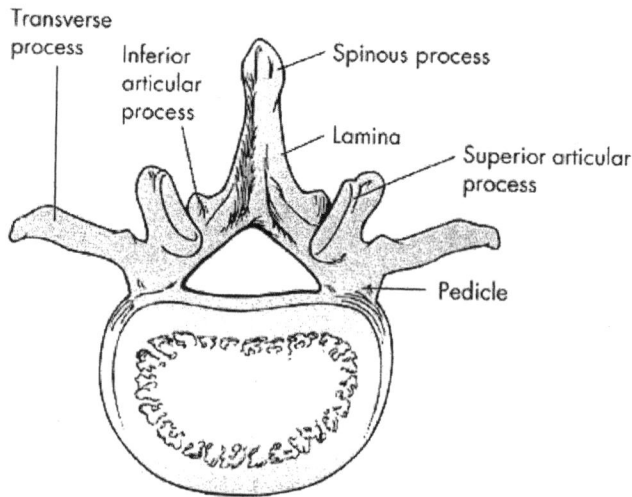

Fig. 1.6 Lumbar vertebra

Fig. 1.7 Ligaments
supporting the vertebrae

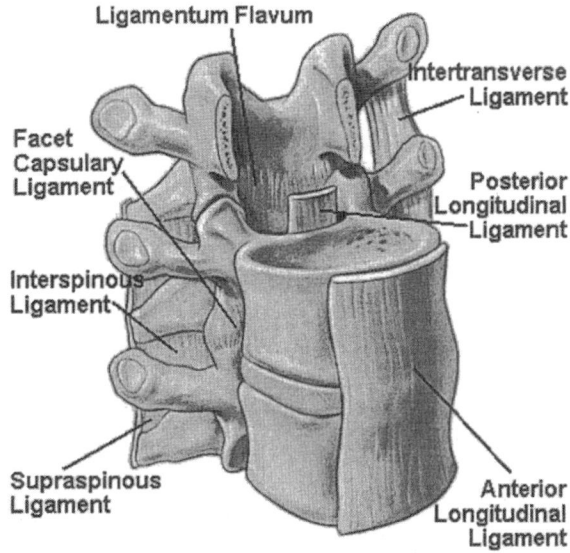

from the foramen magnum to the lower border of first lumbar vertebral. It has two
enlargements, cervical and lumbosacral, corresponding to the innervation of the
upper and lower extremities. It ends in the conus medullaris. The anterior portion of
the spinal cord contains the motor tracts, while the posterior cord contains the sensory tracts. The mean spinal cord blood flow in the cervical and lumbar segments is
40% higher than the thoracic segment. The watershed area of the spinal cord blood
flow is the mid-thoracic region. The spinal cord receives its blood supply principally
from three longitudinal vessels. The single anterior spinal artery is formed by the
two vertebral arteries which supply the anterior 75% of the cord and the two posterior spinal arteries formed by the posterior inferior cerebellar artery and supply the
posterior 25% of the cord (Fig. 1.8). The anterior and posterior arteries alone can
only supply enough blood to maintain the upper cervical segments of the spinal
cord. The blood supply to the lower levels of the spinal cord is provided by the
radicular arteries which anastamose with the anterior and posterior spinal arteries.
The artery of Adamkiewicz, a major radicular artery located in lower thoracic or
upper lumbar region, provides most of the blood supply to the lower cords.
Autoregulation maintains spinal cord blood flow by altering vascular resistance in
response to changes in the mean arterial blood pressure (MAP).

  The ascending spinal tracts are contained in the posterior column of the spinal
cord and terminate in the medulla. They are sensory in nature. After decussation in
the medulla, the second-order neurons form an ascending bundle and terminate in
the thalamus from where they reach the post-central gyrus via third-order neurons
(Fig. 1.9). The descending tract, called the corticospinal tract, is motor in nature.
Corticospinal tract fibers originate in the cerebral cortex in the precentral gyrus and
90% decussate at the level of the medulla. Lesions above the medullary decussation

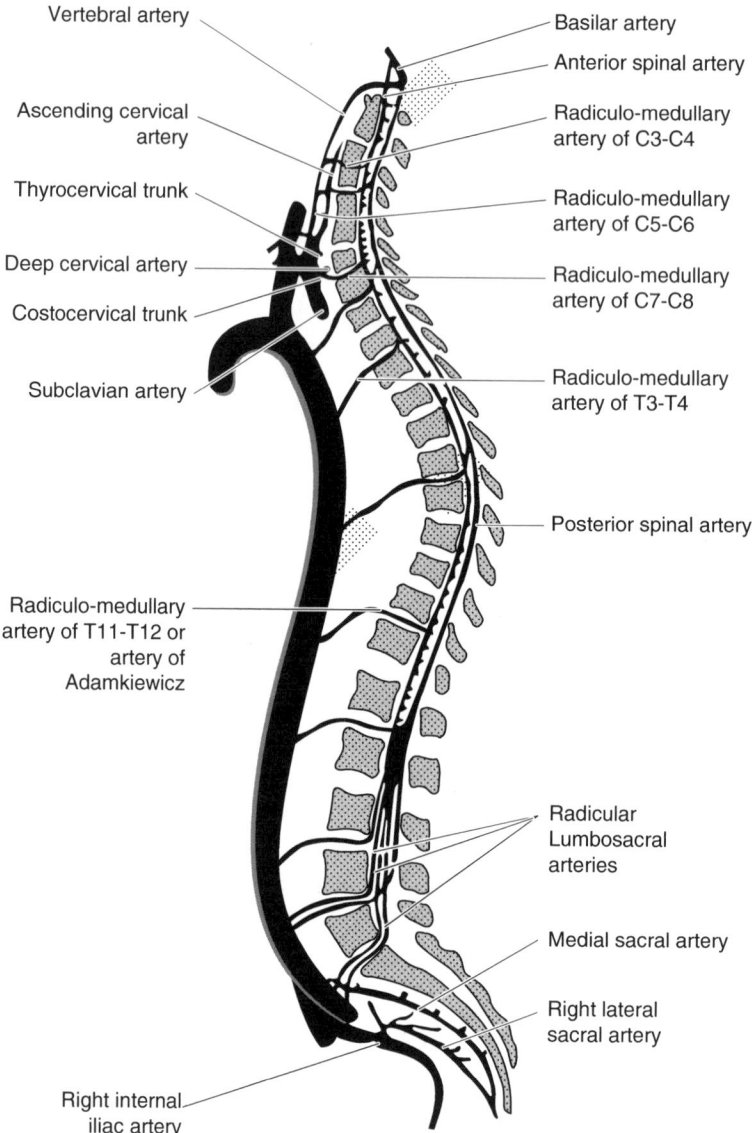

Vertebral artery

Ascending cervical
artery

Thyrocervical trunk

Deep cervical artery

Costocervical trunk

Subclavian artery

Radiculo-medullary
artery of T11-T12 or
artery of
Adamkiewicz

Basilar artery

Anterior spinal artery

Radiculo-medullary
artery of C3-C4

Radiculo-medullary
artery of C5-C6

Radiculo-medullary
artery of C7-C8

Radiculo-medullary
artery of T3-T4

Posterior spinal artery

Radicular
Lumbosacral
arteries

Medial sacral artery

Right lateral
sacral artery

Right internal
iliac artery

Fig. 1.8 Blood supply of the spinal cord

cause contralateral paralysis and those below medullary decussation cause ipsilateral paralysis (Fig. 1.10).

The ventricular system of the brain is composed of two lateral ventricles and two midline ventricles called the third and fourth ventricles which contain the cerebrospinal fluid (CSF). The chambers are connected to allow the flow of CSF between

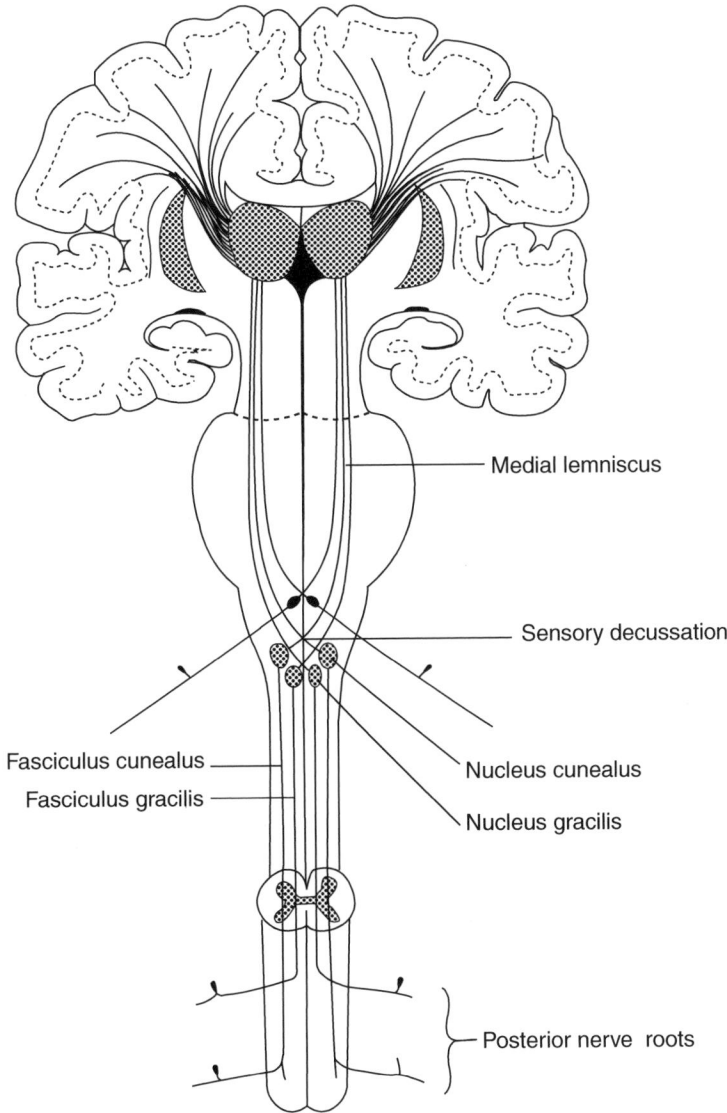

Medial lemniscus

Sensory decussation

Fasciculus cunealus

Fasciculus gracilis

Nucleus cunealus

Nucleus gracilis

Posterior nerve roots

Fig. 1.9 Sensory pathway

two lateral ventricles to the third ventricles through the Foramen of Monroe. This then communicates through the aqueduct of Sylvius (Mesencephalic aqueduct) to the fourth ventricle (Fig. 1.11). The CSF flows out into the subarachnoid spaces of the brain and the spinal cord through the medial foramen of Magendie and lateral foramen of Luschka. The chambers of the ventricular system are lined with ependymal cells and are continuous with the central canal enclosed within the spinal cord. CSF is a dynamic medium, which is produced and absorbed constantly, and functions as

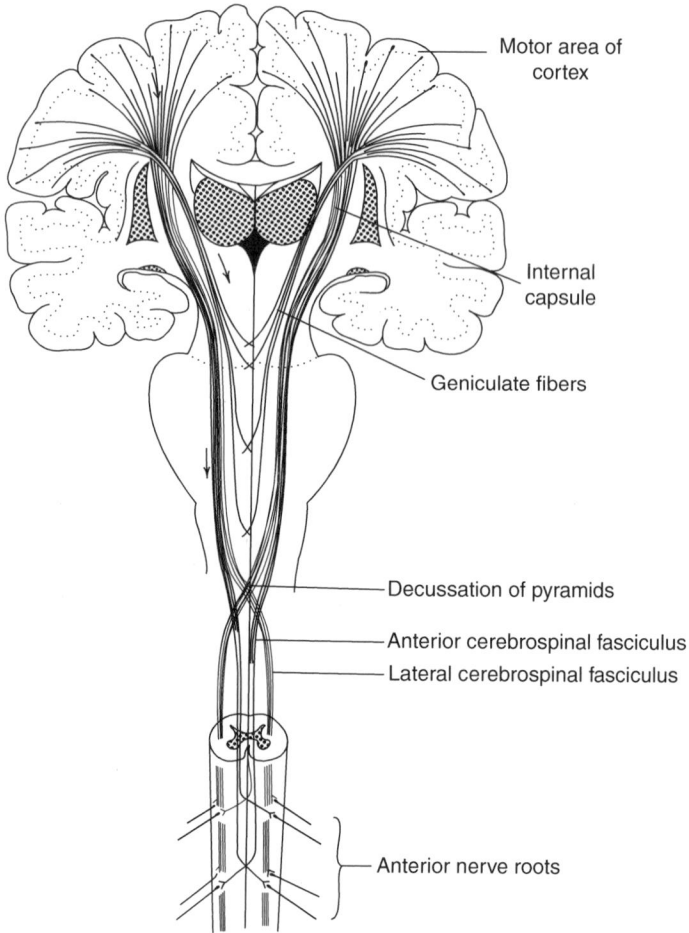

Fig. 1.10 Motor pathway (corticospinal tract)

the brain's drainage system. Under normal circumstances, a human being produces approximately 0.35 ml/min (500 ml/day) of CSF. The total volume of CSF at a given time is 150 ml, which means that the CSF is replaced approximately four times a day. The majority of CSF is formed in the choroid plexus of the lateral ventricles by filtration of plasma through fenestrated capillaries and also by the active transport of water and dissolved substances through the epithelial cells of the blood–CSF barrier. CSF may also be formed by the lymph-like drainage of the brain's extracellular fluid. Reabsorption of CSF takes place mostly in the arachnoid villi and granulations into the circulation. The mechanism behind the CSF reabsorption is the difference between the CSF pressure and venous pressure. CSF formation is reduced by decreased blood flow through the choroid, hypothermia, increased serum osmolarity, and increased ICP. The main compensatory mechanism for an increase

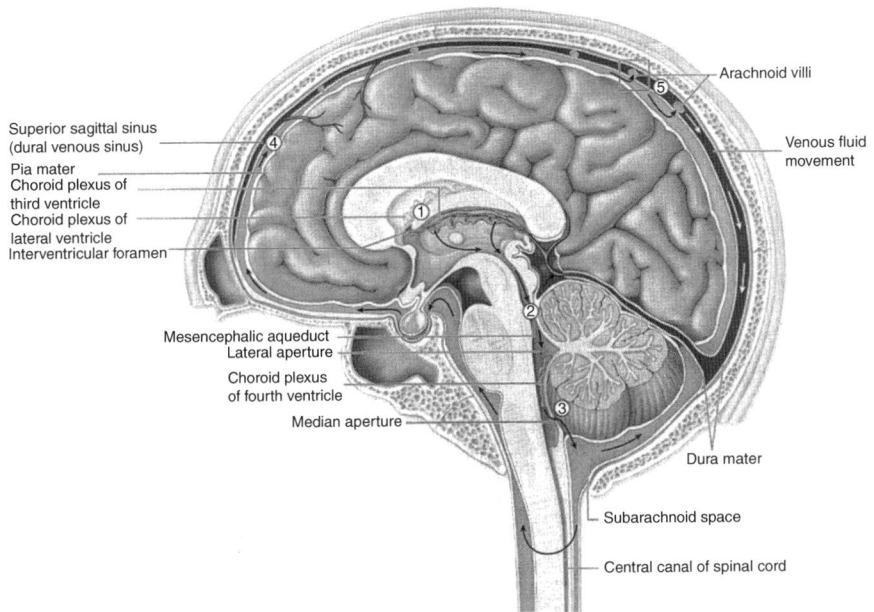

Fig. 1.11 Circulation of cerebrospinal fluid. (1) CSF formation, (2) circulation of CSF in the ventricle, (3) CSF flow into subarachnoid space, (4) CSF circulation around the brain, and (5) absorption into circulation

in CSF volume includes displacement of CSF from cranial to spinal compartment, increase in CSF absorption, decrease in CSF production, and a decrease in cerebral blood volume (mainly venous).

The blood–brain barrier (BBB) isolates the brain from the plasma and is formed by the interaction of capillary endothelial cells with astrocytes in the brain. Water, gases, glucose, and lipophilic substances are freely permeable through the BBB. Proteins and polar substances are poorly permeable through the BBB. The brain is protected from the circulating toxins by the BBB.

The brain tissue has a high energy requirement and is responsible for about 20% of total body oxygen consumption. The cerebral metabolic rate, expressed as oxygen consumption ($CMRO_2$), averages 3.5 ml/100 g/min in adults. $CMRO_2$ is greatest in the gray matter of the cerebral cortex. Brain oxygen consumption supports two major functions – basic cellular maintenance (45%) and nerve impulse generation and transmission (55%). Glucose is the main substrate for energy production in the brain.

Normal cerebral blood flow (CBF) varies with the metabolic activity. Blood flow in gray matter is about 80 ml/100 g/min and in white matter is 20 ml/100 g/min. The average CBF is about 50 ml/100 g/min. There is coupling between the CBF and $CMRO_2$. The precise mechanism responsible for this coupling has not been identified, but it has been suggested that local by-products of metabolism (K+, H+, lactate, adenosine) are responsible for this coupling. Nitric oxide, a potent vasodilator has also been suggested to play a role. Glial processes may serve as a conduit for the coupling.

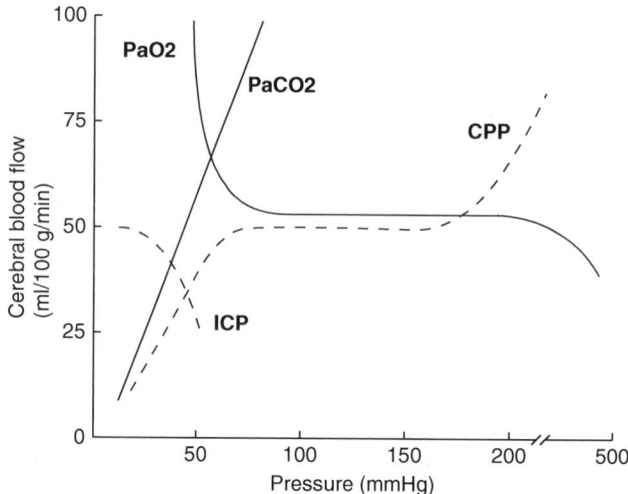

Fig. 1.12 Autoregulation of cerebral blood flow (CPP curve). Perfusion is increased in the setting of hypoxia or hypercarbia

Cerebral autoregulation maintains CBF relatively constant between cerebral perfusion pressures of 50 and 150 mmHg (Fig. 1.12). The mechanism of autoregulation is not understood but is probably due to myogenic and metabolic factors. Cerebral perfusion pressure (CPP) is calculated by subtraction of intracranial pressure (ICP) from mean arterial pressure, CPP = MAP − ICP.

The cranial vault is a rigid structure with fixed total volume, consisting of brain (80%), blood (12%), and CSF (8%). An increase in one component must be offset by an equivalent decrease in another to prevent a rise in the ICP. Intracranial compliance is measured by change in ICP in response to a change in intracranial volume ($\Delta V/\Delta P$). Intracranial elastance ($\Delta P/\Delta V$) is high because a small change in intracranial volume, ΔV, can cause a large change in ICP, ΔP. The pressure–volume relationship between ICP, volume of CSF, blood, and brain tissue, and CPP is known as the Monro-Kellie hypothesis (Fig. 1.13).

Anatomical changes that occur in the brain during normal aging are reduction in brain weight and volume with ventriculomegaly and sulcal expansion. The white matter volume of the cerebrum, cerebellum, corpus callosum, and pons remains fairly intact across all ages. Global CBF decreases about 10–20% because there is less brain mass to perfuse as we age.

Implications for the Neurosurgical Patient

Brain anatomy is important in identifying the different non-silent areas of the brain with respect to the surgical procedure being performed and helps to prevent devastating deficits. For instance, awake craniotomy or cortical mapping may be performed

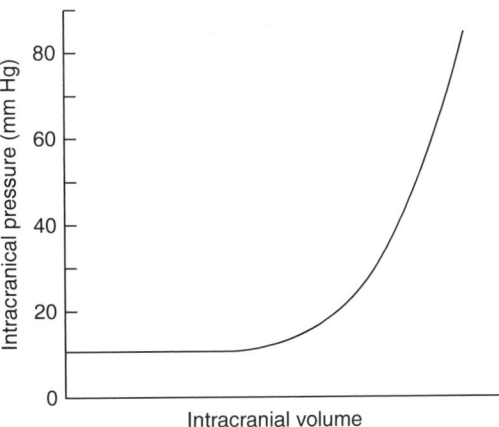

Fig. 1.13 Intracranial compliance curve – initial change in volume causes a slight rise in ICP; further increase causes a marked rise in ICP

when tumors or epileptic foci are close to cortical areas for speech or motor function or temporal structures critical to short-term memory. The Wada test determines the dominant lobe for suitability of temporal lobectomy. Deep brain stimulation of the globus pallidus interna or subthalamic nucleus improves many features of advanced Parkinson's disease. In addition, surgical approach and intraoperative events have anatomical implications. A frontotemporal craniotomy is used to approach anterior circulation aneurysms. Aneurysms originating from the posterior circulation require a subtemporal exposure, suboccipital exposure or a combined subtemporal, and suboccipital exposure. Brain stem stimulation can cause ventricular and supraventricular arrhythmias. Profound arterial hypertension can result from stimulation of the fifth cranial nerve. Significant bradycardia and escape rhythms can be caused from the stimulation of vagus nerve. Arterial hypotension can result from pontine or medullary compression. Brain stem lesions may result in abnormal breathing patterns.

Cranial nerve injury is a significant risk in surgery of the cerebellopontine angle and brain stem; therefore, intraoperative stimulation, monitoring and recording of electromyographic potential of cranial nerve with motor component is utilized to preserve the integrity of these nerves. Direct injury to portions of the RAS located within the pons, midbrain, or diencephalon (hypothalamus and thalamus) produces unconsciousness. Locked-in syndrome occurs with focal injury to the ventral pons and is often associated with basilar artery stroke. It results in patients who are quadriplegic, nonverbal, but awake and alert as the RAS is spared and volitional eye blinking is preserved.

The signs of corticospinal pathway dysfunction include initial weakness, followed by flaccid paralysis and then decorticate rigidity. Extensor (Babinski) toe response indicates acute or chronic injury of the corticospinal tracts in the brain and spinal cord. A Hoffman's response, which is the upper extremity equivalent of a Babinski response, can also provide additive lateralizing information. When damage involves subcortical structures (basal ganglia), decerebrate rigidity occurs.

Basal ganglia damage may also lead to athetoid or choreiform movements. The absence of vestibuloocular and oculocephalic reflex suggests brainstem damage in the pons between the vestibular nuclei (CN VIII) and oculomotor (CN III) and abducens (CN VI) nuclei, which control lateral eye movements. Flexor posturing (decorticate) indicates brain dysfunction above the level of the red nucleus in the midbrain (the area which mediates flexor response). Extensor posturing (decerebrate) indicates brainstem dysfunction below the level of the red nucleus. A hemispheric injury presents with contralateral hyporeflexia. Patients with acute spinal cord shock are hyporeflexive below the level of involvement (Table 1.1).

During spinal surgery, evoked potential monitoring may be used to evaluate spinal cord integrity. Sensory evoked potentials (SEP) evaluate the functional integrity of the ascending sensory pathways, mostly ending in the somatosensory cortex. Motor evoked potentials (MEP) test the functional integrity of the corticospinal tracts, which mainly originate in the motor cortex. The wake up test is also utilized to document the anterior motor component of the spinal cord (anterior column).

CBF is linearly related to $PaCO_2$ from 20 to 70 mmHg, when the autoregulation is intact. Hypocapnia causes cerebral vasoconstriction. Hypercapnea causes vasodilatation and increases the CBF. This change is mainly dependent on the pH alteration in the extracellular fluid of the brain. Change in PaO_2 from 60 to over 300 mmHg has little influence on CBF (Fig. 1.12). Hematocrit alters blood viscosity and affects blood flow; a low hematocrit increases blood flow by decreasing viscosity. Hypothermia decreases neuronal metabolism and reduces CBF, whereas hyperthermia has the opposite effect. $CMRO_2$ decreases by 6–7% for each reduction in 1°C.

Increased ICP may occur through one of several mechanisms: increase in CSF volume (due to blockage in CSF circulation or absorption), increase in brain tissue volume (tumor or edema), or increase in cerebral blood volume (intracranial bleed or vasodilatation). Communicating hydrocephalus occurs when the obstruction is at the point of CSF absorption (arachnoid granulation) and herniation is less likely to occur. In noncommunicating hydrocephalus, obstruction occurs within the ventricular system and herniation syndrome may be seen. Once there is a critical increase in ICP, brain herniation may occur. Ventriculostomy may be performed to decrease ICP in such cases. If drainage of CSF is performed via lumbar puncture in the presence of increased ICP, there is a risk of brain stem herniation through the foramen magnum. Aging increases intracranial CSF volume due to cerebral atrophy and creates nonpathological low-pressure hydrocephalus.

Concerns and Risks

Spinal cord lesions above C 3 lead to diaphragmatic paralysis, and the patient is totally ventilator dependent. This is because the phrenic nerve, which is the principal nerve supply of the diaphragm, is formed by C 3, 4, and 5 nerve roots. Acute spinal cord injury at the level of C 6 presents as spinal shock from a total loss of

Table 1.1 Diagnosis of cranial nerve damage in ICU

Cranial nerve	Test cranial nerve	Cerebral lobe affected	Presentation
Cranial nerve 1 (Olfactory nerve)	Not practical in ICU	Frontal lobe, pituitary tumor, anterior cranial fossa fracture	Loss of sense of smell (anosmia)
Cranial nerve 2 (Optic nerve)	Limited in unconscious patient	Distal to optic chiasm Lesion pressing on optic chiasm Lesion proximal to chiasm	Monocular blindness Bitemporal hemianopia Homonymous hemianopia
Cranial nerve 3 (Oculomotor nerve)	Pupillary exam	Uncal and temporal lobe herniation	Ptosis, divergent squint, pupillary dilatation, loss of accommodation, and light reflexes
Cranial nerve 4, 5, 6 (Trochlear, Trigeminal, Abducent)	Lightly poking the patient's cheeks with a sharp object or stimulating the nasal cavity with a cotton swab (CN V)	Cavernous sinus lesion, injury to base of skull	Loss of corneal reflex 5 (corneal damage), convergent squint 6
Cranial nerve 7 (Facial)	Facial movement	Large cerebellopontine tumors	Muscles of face, anterior two-thirds of tongue
Cranial nerve 8 (Auditory)		Cerebellopontine tumors, acoustic neuromas	Unilateral deafness
Cranial nerve 9, 10 (Glossopharyngeal, Vagus)	Gag reflex by tongue blade or suction catheter	Posterior third of tongue and pharynx	Absence of gag reflex (increased risk of aspiration), nasal speech, vocal cord paralysis 10
Cranial nerve 11 (Accessory)	Limited	Central branch arising from the medullary nuclei and spinal accessory branch arising in the first five to six cervical spinal segments from the lateral portion of the ventral horn	Central branch supplies the larynx and spinal accessory to trapezius and sternocleidomastoid – inability to shrug
Cranial nerve 12 (hypoglossal)	Limited in unconscious patient	Muscle of tongue, damaged during carotid surgery	Aspiration

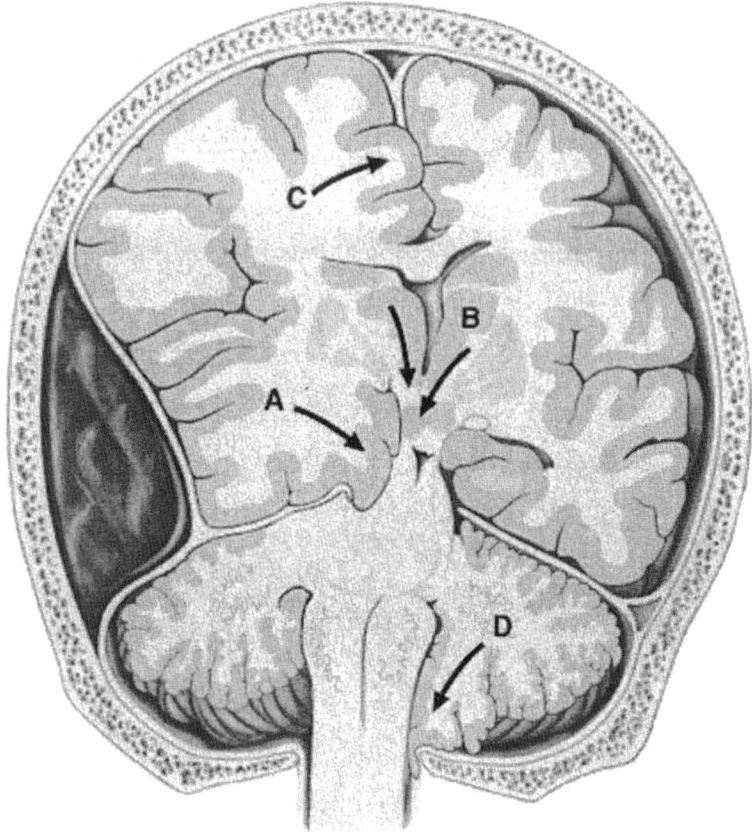

Fig. 1.14 Potential sites of brain herniation (A) uncal, (B) central, (C) subfalcine, (D) tonsillar. Transcalvarial is not shown in this figure

impulses from the higher centers. Epidural hematoma (EDH) is a traumatic accumulation of blood between the inner table of the skull and the stripped-off dural membrane. EDHs are usually arterial in origin with 70–80% located in the temporoparietal region where skull fractures cross the path of the middle meningeal artery or its dural branches. Expanding high-volume EDHs can produce a midline shift and subfalcine herniation of the brain resulting in compression of cerebral tissue and impingement on the third cranial nerve. This results in ipsilateral pupillary dilation and contralateral hemiparesis or extensor motor response. On the other hand, subdural hematomas are generally the result of venous bleeding of bridging veins (between the cortex and venous sinuses).

The brain is vulnerable to ischemic injury because of its high oxygen consumption and near-total dependence on aerobic glucose metabolism. Prolonged reduction

Table 1.2 Herniation syndromes and its clinical manifestations

Herniation of uncus of temporal lobe	Supratentorial	Pressure on ipsilateral occulomotor nerve, posterior cerebral arteries and cerebral peduncle-pupillary abnormalities, contralateral hemiplegia, possible ipsilateral medial occipital lobe infarction
Central herniation (midline structure)	Supratentorial	Downward movement of diencephalon through tentorial notch against immobile basilar artery may cause brain stem hemorrhage
Subfalcine (when the brain is pushed into the opposite half of the cranium under the falx cerebri)	Supratentorial	Cingulate gyrus injury, ischemia in anterior cerebral artery distribution
Tonsillar herniation	Supra or infratentorial	A rapid and fatal event unless it is recognized immediately and treated; the cerebral tonsil descends through the foramen magnum leading to the compression of brain stem and respiratory arrest; rarely posterior fossa mass pushing the posterior fossa contents through the tentorium cerebelli into the supratentorial compartment
Transcalvarial herniation	Supra or infratentorial	Any area beneath a defect in the skull

of CBF below 20–25 ml/100 g/min is associated with cerebral impairment (slowing of EEG), between 15 and 20 ml/100 g/min produces a flat EEG, while values below 10 ml/100 g/min are associated with irreversible structural brain damage. Autoregulation is impaired by hypoxia, ischemia, hypercapnia, trauma, and certain anesthetic agents. A rightward shift in the autoregulatory curve occurs with chronic hypertension and sympathetic activation (shock or stress). A leftward shift occurs in hypoxia, hypercarbia, and vasodialators. When CPP exceeds the upper limit of autoregulation, the BBB may be disrupted, leading to cerebral edema.

Any increase in ICP is initially well compensated; however, once the compliance is exhausted a small increase in volume causes an exponential rise in ICP leading to herniation (see Fig. 1.14). Herniation syndromes (Table 1.2) can be reversible if treated immediately and effectively and are encountered when the pressure in one compartment of the brain results in extrusion of the contents into an adjacent compartment with accompanying mechanical damage. Depressed level of consciousness with dilated pupils is the first clinical sign of a herniation syndrome and is usually accompanied by a Cushing response (elevation in the systolic blood pressure with accompanying bradycardia).

Key Points

- In the corticospinal tract, lesions above the medullary decussation cause contralateral paralysis and those below medullary decussation cause ipsilateral paralysis.
- Brain anatomy is important in identifying the different non-silent areas of the brain with respect to the surgical procedure being performed and helps to prevent devastating deficits.
- Cranial nerve injury is a significant risk in surgery of the cerebellopontine angle and brain stem.
- Lumbar puncture for drainage of CSF is performed below the L1 vertebra to prevent damage to the spinal cord. Most spinal cord injuries occur at the mid-cervical or thoracolumbar region. The watershed area of the spinal cord blood flow is the mid-thoracic region.
- CBF is linearly related to $PaCO_2$ from 20 to 70 mmHg when the autoregulation is intact. Hypocapnia causes cerebral vasoconstriction and can lead to brain ischemia. Hypercapnea causes vasodilatation and increases the CBF.
- Increased ICP may occur through one of several mechanisms: increase in CSF volume (due to blockage in CSF circulation or absorption), increase in brain tissue volume (tumor or edema), or increase in cerebral blood volume (intracranial bleed or vasodilatation).
- The brain is vulnerable to ischemic injury because of its high oxygen consumption and near-total dependence on aerobic glucose metabolism.
- Any increase in ICP is initially well compensated; however, once the compliance is exhausted, a small increase in volume causes an exponential rise in ICP leading to herniation.

Suggested Reading

Bendo AA, Kass IS, Hartung J, Cottrell JE. Anesthesia for neurosurgery. In: Barash PG, Cullen BF, Stoelting RK, editors. Clinical anesthesia. 5th ed. Philadelphia: Lippincott Williams & Wilkins; 2006. p. 746–89.

Cottrell JE, Smith DS. Anesthesia and neurosurgery. 4th ed. St Louis: Mosby; 2001.

Drummond JC, Patel PM. Neurosurgical anesthesia. In: Miller's anesthesia. 6th ed. Philadelphia: Elsevier, Churchill Livingstone; 2005. p. 2127–73.

Newfield P, Cottrell JE, editors. Handbook of neuroanesthesia. 4th ed. Philadelphia: Lippincott Williams & Wilkins; 2006.

Patel PM, Drummond JC. Cerebral physiology and effects of anesthetics and techniques. In: Miller's anesthesia. 6th ed. Philadelphia: Elsevier, Churchill Livingstone; 2005. p. 813–57.

Chapter 2
Neuroendocrine Physiology: Fundamentals and Common Syndromes

Joshua H. Atkins

Introduction

Hormonal signaling systems are critical to basic homeostatic functions. They support the control of volume status, blood pressure, cellular metabolism, and intracellular signaling. The hypothalamic–pituitary–adrenal (HPA) axis, in particular, comprises systems to regulate sodium and water balance, steroid hormone production, glucose metabolism, and thyroid function. Each hormonal system is controlled via negative and positive feedback loops. In addition, activity levels are affected by intersystem modulation. These feedback mechanisms, with the goal of immediate homeostatsis, often cloud hormonal measurement and diagnosis in the critically ill patient. Any kind of intracranial pathology and, in particular, traumatic brain injury (TBI), stroke, or cerebral hemorrhage disequilibrate the HPA axis. This frequently results in deleterious clinical sequelae. In addition, endocrine disorders unrelated to neuropathology have significant impact on neurophysiology. Thus, dysfunction of the HPA axis must be recognized and carefully managed during the perioperative period.

J.H. Atkins, MD, PhD (✉)
Departments of Anesthesiology and Critical Care, and Otorhinolaryrgology,
Head & Neck Surgery, Perelman School of Medicine at the University of
Pennsylvania, Philadelphia, PA, USA
e-mail: atkinsj@uphs.upenn.edu

A.M. Brambrink and J.R. Kirsch (eds.), *Essentials of Neurosurgical
Anesthesia & Critical Care*, DOI 10.1007/978-0-387-09562-2_2,
© Springer Science+Business Media, LLC 2012

Overview

Sodium and Water Balance

The extracellular fluid volume reflects total body sodium. Under healthy physiologic conditions, the plasma sodium concentration reflects total body water. The plasma osmolality is sensed by the hypothalamus and tightly regulated. Abnormalities of serum Na^+ are common in the neurosurgical and neurotrauma setting. Hypo- or hypernatremia frequently stems from aggressive perioperative volume resuscitation (e.g., following trauma, hemorrhage, or in the context of cerebral vasospasm). Dysfunction of the hypothalamus, pituitary, or adrenal glands is a common secondary cause for sodium or water imbalance.

Antidiuretic Hormone (Arginine Vasopressin, Desmopressin [Synthetic])

Antidiuretic hormone (ADH) is produced in the hypothalamus, and it is stored and secreted by the posterior pituitary in response to (1) increased plasma osmolality as detected in the hypothalamus; (2) decreased plasma volume as detected by peripheral and central baroreceptors; (3) general stress, pain, or increased ICP; and (4) a decrease in plasma angiotensin.

Circulating ADH induces an increase in free water absorption in renal collecting ducts (receptor: V2 GPCR), release of CRH/ACTH (receptor: V1b GPCR in hypothalamus), blood pressure (receptor: V1a), and release of atrial natriuretic peptide (ANP).

Natriuretic Peptides

Natriuretic peptides [e.g., ANP, BNP, C-type natriuretic peptide (CNP)] are released by the cardiac atria and by the hypothalamus in response to increased intravascular volume (atrial wall tension) and increased ICP. Natriuretic peptides increase renal sodium excretion and vascular permeability. Natriuretic peptides also antagonize ADH effects as well as angiotensin II effects. Natriuretic peptides, *produced in the brain*, modulate systemic effects of circulating ANP (which does not cross the blood–brain barrier) via receptors in the hypothalamus (e.g., decrease H_2O and salt appetite), and they decrease sympathetic tone via actions on the brainstem. Brain ANP can effect localized increases in cerebral blood flow and decreased CSF production and is actively transported out of the brain across the blood brain barrier. Plasma BNP levels may increase as a result of subarachnoid hemorrhage and contribute to hypovolemia and be a marker of associated cardiac dysfunction. (Taub

Table 2.1 Diagnostic criteria for SIADH

• Volume status? euvolemia or mild hypervolemia
• Urine output? low urine output (as low as 500 mL/d)
• Urine osmolality? concentrated urine (>800 mOsm/L)
• Plasma osmolality? ↓plasma osmolality (us. <280 mOsm/L) ↓Na⁺
• Consider or exclude CSW (see below and table)

Neurocritical Care 2011) Elevated BNP levels may be associated with cerebral ischemia from multiple etiologies, including vasospasm, after SAH. Overall, little is known about the role and the clinical significance of CNP.

Implications for the Neurosurgical Patient

Sodium and Water Balance

Derangements of water and sodium in the neurosurgical population, especially acute changes, are concerning for possible clinical sequelae that include: cerebral edema, altered mental status, seizure, or coma, increased ICP, cerebral hypoperfusion, cerebral vasospasm, and bridging vein rupture with associated subdural hemorrhage.

Frequently, the clinician is alerted by an abnormal serum sodium concentration, which triggers a thorough workup. Complete evaluation must take into consideration the multiple causes of altered serum sodium concentrations, and these must be evaluated in the final differential diagnosis.

Hyponatremia (<135 mEq/L)

A lower than normal serum sodium concentration reflects excess of free water (fluid overload) or an improper sodium loss. Clinical symptoms usually manifest with an acute drop of serum sodium concentration to lower than 125 mEq/L and include muscle weakness, cerebral edema, lethargy, confusion, seizures, and coma. Hyponatremia that develops over many days and continues chronically can be tolerated for quite some time without major signs or symptoms. The main hormonal mediators leading to hyponatremia are ADH (classical symptom complex called syndrome of inappropriate ADH release: SIADH) and ANP (atrial natriuretic protein; causing increased natriuresis). The differential diagnosis of hyponatremia includes SIADH, cerebral salt wasting syndrome (CSW) and dilutional state (volume overload and hyperprotein state). Hyponatremia is also found with Addison's disease because of reduced production of aldosterone, an adrenal hormone that acts to increase reabsorption of sodium in the kidney tubules. Ultimately, a careful assessment of the fluid/volume status will guide diagnosis and management. The total sodium deficit may be estimated via the formula: $0.5–0.6 \times (\text{wt. in kg}) \times (\text{goal-measured Na}^+)$.

Table 2.2 Treatment of SIADH

---

o Goal to correct Na⁺ levels gradually

o Normal saline with free water restriction usually adequate

o Loop diuretics (cause net free water loss)

o Correct deficit gradually

   ▪ 10 mEq/L over 24 h; or 1–2 mEq/L in first hour in symptomatic patients

   ▪ 3% Hypertonic saline to correct severe Na⁺ deficit

o Tolvaptan (SamscaR) - renal ADH receptor antagonist (15mg-60mg PO daily)

o Demeclocycline (1–2 mg PO/d) blocks renal action of ADH

   ▪ Side-effect profile similar to tetracyclines

   ▪ May be nephrotoxic

Syndrome of Inappropriate Secretion of ADH

SIADH is an umbrella classification for the clinical presentation of hyponatremia with euvolemia or mild hypervolemia (Table 2.1). SIADH is a common diagnosis after TBI, brain surgery, and in association with intrinsic neuropathology. In addition, there are many other confounding etiologies. The hallmark laboratory finding of SIADH is a continued secretion of ADH despite decreased plasma osmolality. However, elevated serum ADH concentration is not specific for SIADH. Elevated ADH levels have also been reported in the context of opioid treatment, general anesthesia, perioperative stress response, brain tumors, and CSW. ADH levels are also increased in the treatment phase of DI.

Treatment of hyponatremia must be accomplished gradually (Table 2.2), as too rapid correction may result in permanent structural injury in the brainstem (e.g., central pontine myelinolysis). In addition, hyperchloremic metabolic acidosis is a common finding when the primary treatment for hyponatremia involves administration of saline. To avoid this concern, many clinicians administer sodium as a mixture of chloride and acetate salts.

Cerebral Salt Wasting Syndrome

CSW is a diagnosis of exclusion that presents as hyponatremia (secondary to renal sodium loss) with hypovolemia and maintained or elevated urine output. Unfortunately, there is no simple assessment method available to determine the intravascular volume status of a patient. The central venous pressure (CVP) may be useful for a trend. Serial cardiac echo examinations also help to assess intravascular volume, but require significant expertise and are expensive to perform. Systolic pressure variation (SPV) as measured by the pulse oximetry plethysmograph or arterial line wave form is helpful to assess volume status in patients receiving positive pressure ventilation. CSW may be particularly common in subarachnoid hemorrhage. Likely, CSW develops secondary to the derangement of neurohumeral signals which results in increased ANP levels and decreased renal sympathetic input (Tables 2.3 and 2.4).

Table 2.3 Diagnostic criteria for CSW

Likely present if criteria for SIADH are met *but*
1. Patient demonstrates ↓↓Na⁺ with trial of fluid restriction
   - Fluid restriction may be deleterious in some patients (e.g., SAH)
2. Clinical indicators of hypovolemia
   - Decreased skin turgor, ↓ serial body weights, hypotension (esp. orthostasis), low CVP
3. Other markers (serum BUN, uric acid, ANP, ADH) are nonspecific and not clinically useful
4. Measurement of urine Na⁺ excretion and urine osmolality may support the diagnosis but is seldom of practical clinical utility
   - Often complicated in the neuro setting by diuretics, mannitol, or stress response ↑ in ADH

Table 2.4 Treatment of CSW

5. 0.9% Saline resuscitation corrects Na⁺ in many cases
6. Enteral salts if clinically feasible (calculate mEq/day) typically 1–2 g PO TIDaily
7. Consider hypertonic saline if inadequate response or need for more rapid initial correction (i.e. severely symptomatic hyponatremia)
8. Consider fludrocortisone in refractory cases 0.1–0.2 mg PO daily
   - Hypokalemia and hypertension are possible side effects of fludrocortisone
9. Monitor sodium levels and fluid balance closely

Hypernatremia (>145 mEq/L)

Severe elevation of Na⁺ serum levels (>160 mEq/L) is associated with increased mortality in neuro ICU patients. Symptoms include change in mental status, seizures, myoclonus/hyperreflexia, and nystagmus. Acute hypernatremia may also result in structural, permanent injury in the brainstem (e.g., central pontine myelinolysis). In addition, patients may show signs of intravascular volume depletion, cerebral hypoperfusion, and/or cerebral vasospasm. Intravascular hypernatremia will cause water to move from brain cells, resulting in decreased brain volume, which carries the risk of disruption of bridging veins and subsequent subdural hematoma. Hypernatremia can be caused by central or nephrogenic diabetes insipidus (DI) or can be iatrogenic, secondary to aggressive saline infusion. Less likely, it develops with overly aggressive diuresis. Hypernatremia can also be seen with mineralocorticoid excess, as is observed with Conn's syndrome or Cushing's syndrome (accompanied by a reduction in serum potassium levels). It is important to differentiate between central DI and nephrogenic DI. Central DI is caused by an interruption of hypothalamic signaling (anatomic and ischemic), with subsequent reduction in ADH secretion from the posterior pituitary (e.g., after TBI, tumor resection, vasospasm of anterior circulation, brain death). Nephrogenic DI is characterized by lack of renal response to serum ADH associated with critical illness, antibiotics, contrast, or renal insult.

Common symptoms for both central and nephrogenic DI are hypernatremia, hyperosmolality, and dilute polyuria. Central DI presents with severely reduced urine osmolatity: <200 mOsm/L versus 200–500 mOsm/L with nephrogenic DI. Table 2.5 lists diagnostic criteria for DI, and Table 2.6 list strategies for initial management of DI.

Table 2.5 Diagnostic criteria for DI

- Classic triphasic response (which can confuse later interpretation of SIADH/hyponatremia) evolves over days:
  - o Polyuria (often >1 L/h) and hypernatramia followed by reduced urine output (presumed to be secondary to ADH release from dying cells) and hyponatremia, and finally resolution or permanence of DI
- Frequently transient or permanent (without associated phases)
- Commonly presents > 12 h after surgery
- Rarely presents intraoperatively:
  - o Intraoperative presentation (phase 1) is associate with hypovolemia
  - o ↓Plasma volume may ↑ risk of venous air embolism during surgery
- Differentiate polyuria vs. diuresis associated with fluid resuscitation or osmotic/pharmacologic diuresis:
  - o Response of Na⁺ and urine output to fluid restriction (unless contraindicated)
  - o No increased UOsm (30 mOsm/L) within hours of fluid restriction → Central DI
  - o Hyperosmolar serum

Table 2.6 Initial management of DI

- o Fluid restriction for diagnosis
- o Volume/free water replacement (0.9% or 0.45% saline)
- o Synthetic desmopressin for central diabetes insipidus
  - ▪ IV (5–50 mcg/day)
  - ▪ Give intranasally in non-critically ill patients
- o Timed urine volumes, serum Na⁺ and urine osmolality/specific gravity guide therapy
- o Correct gradually over days to avoid rebound cerebral edema

Concerns and Risks

Sodium and Water Balance

The use of diuretic and osmotic agents or hypervolemic therapy with saline will invariably complicate the clinical assessment of sodium derangements. A careful assessment of overall volume status is critical in determining diagnosis and treatment plan. For example, treatment should be fluid replacement in patients who have water deficit versus fluid restriction in patients thought to have SIADH, while fluid and sodium administration would be the best treatment for patients with CSW. In contrast, volume restriction in a patient with CSW, for example, would further worsen volume deficit and hyponatremia, especially in the context of vasospasm and impending cerebral ischemia following subarachnoid hemorrhage. Also, aggressive treatment of hyponatremia can lead to over-correction (i.e., hypernatremia) and an associated demyelination syndrome, while aggressive treatment of hypernatremia may result in cerebral edema due to organic intracerebral osmoles that exist in brain.

Key Points
Sodium and Water Balance (Table 2.7)

- Always consider Na$^+$ abnormality in setting of pituitary tumor/intracranial surgery, hypothalamic injury, TBI, seizure, treatment for cerebral vasospasm/stroke, or acute/chronic change in mental status.
- Na$^+$ derangements may simply be related to fluid management (e.g., hypervolemic therapy, hypertonic saline, diuretics, or normal saline with stress-elevated ADH).
- Clinical picture more helpful than diagnostic testing in diagnosis.
- Other endocrine disease (adrenal, thyroid) must be considered.
- If increased Na$^+$ consider DI or over-resuscitation with saline.
- If decreased Na$^+$ consider SIADH or CSW.
- Correct abnormalities gradually with frequent measurement and monitoring.

Overview

Steroid Hormone Physiology

Cortisol is the primary glucocorticoid hormone of clinical relevance. It is secreted by the zona fasciculata of the adrenal gland in response to adrenocorticotropic hormone (ACTH). ACTH, in turn, is secreted by the pituitary in response to corticotropin-releasing hormone (CRH) produced by the hypothalamus. Cortisol is key to the regulation of energy metabolism, electrolyte homeostasis, and immune function. It interacts with nuclear receptors found throughout the body including the brain. The secretion of cortisol is tightly regulated along the HPA axis. Dysregulation at any point of the HPA axis will result in excess or deficiency of cortisol with marked clinical consequences. The basal daily cortisol requirement ranges between 15 and 25 mg hydrocortisone (8 mg/m^2/d; conversions: prednisone $= 0.25 \times$ hydrocortisone; dexamethasone $= 0.04 \times$ hydrocortisone). Cortisol production is subject to diurnal variation as well as modulation from a host of physiologic factors. Measurement of random cortisol levels is rarely useful in clin-

Table 2.7 Features of Common Na$^+$ derangements

Central DI	CSW	SIADH
Serum Na+ >145 mEq/L	Serum Na + <135 mEq/L	Serum Na + <135 mEq/L
PE suggests hypovolemia	PE suggests hypovolemia	PE = euvolemia/hypervolemia
	↑Na$^+$ with saline admin	↓Na with saline admin
1° Defect in water handling	1° Defect in Na$^+$ handling	1° Defect in water handling
↑Serum osmolality	↓Serum osmolality	↓Serum osmolality
Low urine Osm	High urine osm	High urine osm
IV Desmopressin	↓Na with fluid restriction	↑Na with fluid restriction
	Oral salt tablets	HTS if severe ↓Na$^+$
	HTS if severe ↓Na$^+$	Oral tolvaptan

Table 2.8 Pathophysiology of primary adrenal insufficiency (Addison's disease)

- Absence of glucocorticoid and mineralocorticoid function
- $\downarrow$ [Na$^+$]$_p$, $\uparrow$[K$^+$]$_p$ (absent aldosterone effects)
- Primary clinical issue: hypotension/hypovolemia/shock
- May lead to cerebral hypoperfusion and cerebral ischemia
- Diagnose by total plasma cortisol levels and CRH levels
- Hyperpigmentation 2° $\uparrow$ pituitary secretion of ACTH precursor $\rightarrow$ $\uparrow\alpha$-MSH

ical assessment of the HPA axis although AM cortisol levels may be useful in conjunction with other tests and the clinical presentation. It should be noted that although dexamethasone is a commonly prescribed steroid in clinical medicine, it has no mineralocorticoid activity. In addition, it is important to recognize that cortisol requirements increase as much as five times basal requirements under physiologic stress (e.g., infection, shock, and surgery). Inadequate steroid administration during stress will result in hemodynamic instability (primarily hypotension), hypoglycemia, hyponatremia and hyperkalemia. However, for most surgeries, "stress-dosing" of steroids for patients on chronic steroid supplementation is no longer routine. Stress steroid dosing is not based on strong supportive evidence. Current evidence supports maintenance dosing (i.e. the usual daily dose) on the day of surgery with additional intravenous supplementation with hydrocortisone supplementation, if overt hypotension presents in the perio-operative period. Laboratory testing using cortisol levels or ACTH stimulation tests does not appear to be helpful in the majority of patients.

Aldosterone is the primary mineralocorticoid of clinical concern. Mineralocorticoid activity is central to the maintenance of effective plasma volume via the renin–angiotensin–aldosterone axis. Aldosterone is secreted by the adrenal cortex in response to many physiologic events (e.g., hypotension, hypovolemia, and acidosis), in response to the production of ACTH, and in response to release of adrenoglomerulotropin from the pineal gland. Aldosterone acts to promote sodium and water reuptake and potassium secretion from the glomerulo-filtrate in the kidney. In addition, CNS aldosterone receptors contribute to the modulation of fluid balance. Fludrocortisone (Fluorinef) is the only available therapeutic drug that approximates the aldosterone activity.

Adrenal Insufficiency

Frequently, patients with adrenal insufficiency remain free of clinical signs and symptoms during normal daily activities. Those who develop a chronic disease develop nonspecific symptoms such as lethargy, muscle weakness, dizziness, syncope, and diarrhea or constipation. However, adrenal insufficiency may present as acute crisis secondary to infection, physiologic stress (trauma and major surgery), or abrupt withdrawal of steroid supplementation. Adrenal insufficiency should always be considered in the setting of refractory hypotension/shock. Pathophysiology of primary adrenal insufficiency is described in Table 2.8.

Table 2.9 Causes of secondary adrenal insufficiency

- Inadequate production of hypothalamic CRH or pituitary ACTH
  - Pituitary irradiation/surgery/compression/infarction
  - Pituitary ischemia (Sheehan's, stroke)
  - Pituitary hemorrhage
    - Brain imaging may aid diagnosis (MRI)
    - Presentation includes headache/visual symptoms
    - Sudden onset
  - Craniopharyngioma resection
- Suppression of HPA by exogenous steroids
- Inadequate ramp-up of cortisol production in response to physiologic stress
  - Critical illness, major surgery, trauma
  - Common subclinical presentation
- May present intraoperatively or in ICU as refractory hypotension
- Iatrogenic due to etomidate use for anesthesia or sedation. Etomidate inhibits 11-beta-hydroxylase needed for cortisol synthesis

Table 2.10 Diagnosis of adrenal insufficiency

- Clinical suspicion based on history presentation; response to empiric therapy. In many groups (and especially in acute illness) the tests below lack sensitivity
- ↓ Random plasma cortisol levels; or no ↑ levels in the presence of physiologic stress
- CRH, ACTH, insulin stimulation tests
  - Decreased cortisol production 30/60 min after IV ACTH c/w diagnosis
  - CRH stim. test differentiates pituitary and hypothalamic disease
  - Insulin tolerance test
    - Hypoglycemia after 0.1 U IV insulin
    - If HPA normal accompanied by ↑ serum cortisol
- Differentiate from Addison's
  - Absence of hyperpigmentation
  - Absence of signs of mineralocorticoid deficiency (normal K^+)

Addison's Disease

Primary adrenal insufficiency is commonly caused by autoimmune or infectious processes, cancer, adrenal infarction, or adrenalectomy. It is associated with inadequate production of both glucocorticoid and mineralocorticoid hormones, which then require pharmacologic replacement (e.g., hydrocortisone and fludrocortisone).

Secondary Adrenal Insufficiency

If adrenal insufficiency develops in the absence of intrinsic adrenal pathology, the symptom complex is called "secondary adrenal insufficiency." A multitude of causes can lead to secondary adrenal insufficiency and are summarized in Table 2.9. Tables 2.10 and 2.11 describe diagnostic criteria and treatment options for adrenal insufficiency, respectively.

Table 2.11 Treatment of adrenal insufficiency

- Treat empirically in cases of high clinical suspicion
- Hydrocortisone 150–300 mg IV per day approximates a physiologic stress dose
- Supplemental steroids must be tapered to avoid recrudescence
- Fludrocortisone (0.05–0.2 mg/d) provides mineralocorticoid replacement
  - ○ Only necessary in Addison's management
  - ○ Hydrocortisone (20 mg) approximates 0.05 mg fludrocortisone
  - ○ In secondary adrenal insufficiency
- Assess for cause of acute insufficiency

Table 2.12 Causes, diagnosis, and treatment of Cushing's syndrome/disease

Causes

- Cushing's disease: primary pituitary overproduction of ACTH
- Cushing's syndrome: associated with increase in cortisol from other origin other than pituitary ACTH excess
- Exogenous corticosteroids (e.g., treatment for perifocal brain edema, autoimmune disease, Addison's disease)
- Oversecretion of cortisol in adrenal glands OR primary ACTH secreting tumor (e.g., small-cell lung cancer)

Diagnosis

- Plasma cortisol and ACTH levels
- Urine cortisol levels
- Dexamethasone suppression test
- Pituitary imaging (MRI) and petrosal ACTH sampling

Treatment

- Surgery, pulse radiotherapy, and medical pharmacotherapy with dopamine agonists (bromocriptine) and direct cortisol synthesis inhibitors (ketoconazole, metyrapone)

Cushing's Disease and Syndrome

Cushing's syndrome results from an overproduction of ACTH in the pituitary, which results in overproduction of cortisol by adrenal glands (Cushing's disease). Excess cortisol can also be due to primary overproduction in the adrenal glands or from overproduction of ACTH by paraneoplastic tissue (observed in patients with small cell lung cancer) (Table 2.12). Most commonly, the Cushing's-like syndrome is due to excessive glucocorticoid administration in the treatment of edema surrounding brain tumors, asthma, arthritis, or for immune suppression in the setting of organ transplantation. The syndrome is characterized by hyperglycemia, insulin resistance, and metabolic syndrome; blood pressure elevation, central obesity, and dyslipidemia.

Implications for the Neurosurgical Patient

Steroid Hormone Derangements

Increased plasma cortisol levels (e.g., with Cushing's disease, exogenous steroid therapy) are associated with significant clinical problems. For example, patients are likely to develop a metabolic syndrome with glucose intolerance. Excessively increased blood glucose levels are associated with increased morbidity after TBI and stroke, increased diuresis followed potentially by hypovolemia and systemic hypotension. Hyperglycemia is also associated with increased infection risk.

Patients with Cushing's disease may present with mass effect in their brain, if associated with enlarging pituitary adenoma. Overall, patients with elevated cortisol may present with hypertension (intravascular volume excess), obesity, and difficulty with venous access or airway management, impaired cognition, memory, and muscle strength, which may confuse neurologic assessment. Therapeutic application of exogenous steroids should be guided by great caution. Some patients treated with exogenous hydrocortisone may, in fact, show an enhanced response to vasopressors/catecholamines, which can be used favorably in the context of circulatory compromise or shock.

Decreased plasma cortisol levels (e.g., with Addison's disease or secondary adrenal insufficiency) expose the critically ill neurosurgical patient to the risk of severe complications. These include: (1) systemic hypotension with decreased CPP, (2) hyponatremia with associated effects (see above section), (3) decreased mental status, (4) hypoglycemia, (5) fever with increased cerebral metabolic rate, and (6) diminished response to catecholamines/vasopressors.

Concerns and Risks

Of particular concern in the neurocritical care patient population are missed diagnosis of adrenal insufficiency, inadequate supplementation of steroids in the perioperative period and uncontrolled hyperglycemia associated with increased plasma cortisol levels from endogenous or exogenous sources. The use of etomidate for induction or sedation of anesthesia is a risk factor for secondary adrenal insufficiency in patients with poor physiologic reserve.

Key Points
Steroid Physiology

- Cortisol requirements significantly increase with physiologic stress
- Accurate assessment of adrenal axis in critical illness is very challenging
  - Normal levels may be misleading in diagnosis
  - Serum cortisol is highly protein bound
- Free (active) levels fluctuate with stress–response and critical illness
- Adrenal insufficiency should always be considered with shock in setting of critical illness
  - Benefits of empiric therapy may outweigh risks

Overview

Thyroid Hormone

Thyroid hormone is produced by thyroid gland in response to thyroid stimulating hormone (TSH) released by the anterior pituitary and thyroid releasing hormone (TRH) in the hypothalamus. Thyroid hormone is present in the serum as T3, T4, and rT3, where free (not protein bound) T3 is the active form of the hormone. Levels of free T3 are dependent on a variety of factors, including protein binding that can be dramatically impacted by critical illness. Careful analysis of the clinical presentation with an emphasis on specific syndromes and thyroid ultrasonagraphy are useful in diagnosis. Disruption of thyroid hormone levels lead either to hypothyroidsm (not enough T3) or hyperthyroidism (excess T3). Tables 2.13 and 2.14 summarize the pathophysiologic characteristics of the two states. Table 2.15 lists the therapeutic interventions in case of a hyperthyroid crisis ("thyroid storm"). Table 2.16 summarizes the implications for the neurosurgical patient.

Table 2.13 Pathophysiology of hypothyroidism

- Primary hypothyroidism
  - Decreased production of thyroid hormone by the thyroid gland
  - Commonly subclinical
  - Often associated with adrenocortical insufficiency
  - Laboratory studies typically indicate elevated TSH (>4 mIU/mL) and low free T4 and total T3
  - Thyroid disease secondary to CNS pathology may present with ↓, nl. or ↑ TSH
  - Laboratory values (esp. TSH) may be influenced by critical illness
- Secondary hypothyroidism
  - Associated with neurologic disease, particularly if the process involves the pituitary or hypothalamus
    - ↓TSH or ↓TRH
  - Also common during chronic treatment with amiodarone

Table 2.14 Pathophysiology of hyperthyroidism

- Elevated thyroid activity most commonly associated with
  - Graves' disease due to the activation of the thyrotropin receptor by autoantibodies
  - Toxic ademona/multinodular goiter
- Laboratory values: depressed TSH; elevated free T4 level
- TSH may be elevated in pituitary adenoma
- Acute thyrotoxicosis transforms into life-threatening *thyroid storm* during acute physiologic stress: anesthesia, surgery, trauma, infection, exogenous iodine bolus
- Thyroid storm presents with:
  - Hyperthermia (fever/sweating)
  - Increased carbon dioxide production/metabolic rate
  - Arrhythmia, especially atrial fibrillation
  - Seizure/coma
  - Severe hypertension advancing to CHF and shock

Table 2.15 Management of thyroid storm

1. Acetaminophen and active cooling if indicated
2. Beta-blockade for control of tachycardia (propanolol if no pulm contraindications)
3. Intravenous hydrocortisone (100–150 mg IV q8h)
4. Methimazole (rectal, oral, IV) or propythiouracil (PO, rectal)
5. Potassium or sodium iodide (4–6 drops PO q6h)

Table 2.16 Implications for the neurosurgical patient: Thyroid function

- *Hypothyroidism* (especially severe or late; rarely in subclinical)
  - Goiter with airway compromise (PE, symptomatology, CT)
    - ↑ tongue size can occur
  - Preoperative hypovolemia (induction hypotension)
  - Nonspecific ECG changes (esp. low voltage and T-waves)
    - May also evidence amyloid-related conduction abnormalities
  - Decreased gastric emptying (aspiration risks)
  - Impaired ventilatory response to hypoxia or hypercapnea
  - Weakness of accessory muscles (respiratory function)
  - Possible decreased hemostasis
  - Decreased BMR with hypothermia
  - Depressed myocardial contractility
  - Delayed emergence
  - Opioid sensitivity
  - Associated hypoglycemia, anemia, SIADH
  - Myxedema coma
    - Decreased mental status, hypothermia, non-pitting LE edema
    - Very elevated TSH, extremely low T3, T4
  - No effect on MAC of potent agents or nitrous oxide
- *Hyperthyroidism*
  - Goiter (as above)
  - Fever with increased cerebral metabolic rate
  - Hypercapnia with increased cerebral blood flow/volume
  - Cardiac arrhythmias – especially atrial fibrillation
  - Cardiomyopathy with clinical heart failure syndrome
  - Changed in mental status with seizures or coma in thyroid storm
  - Neurologic features: visual symptoms, muscle weakness, tremor
  - Possible hypercortisolism 2° to accelerated metabolism of steroids
  - Hyperglycemia

Concerns and Risks

Thyroid Function

Advanced hypothyroidism may manifest in the perioperative period with neurologic symptoms, respiratory failure, or delayed emergence that may confound postoperative assessment. Thus, hypothyroid patients presenting for surgery should be adequately treated with thyroid hormone if possible before their operation. Similarly, hyperthyroidism must be treated, if at all possible, prior to surgery, because malignant hyperthyroidism and the associated hypermetabolic state carries the risk for deleterious cardiovascular and neurologic complications during the perioperative period.

Key Points
Thyroid Function

- Thyroid dysfunction can be difficult to assess in setting of physiologic stress response and critical illness
- Clinical hyperthyroidism can advance to life-threatening thyrotoxicosis in the perioperative setting
  - Suppress hyperthyroid state prior to OR unless surgery is emergent
- Depressed thyroid function should be normalized before elective surgery

---

Overview

Additional Neuroendocrine Systems

Pheochromocytoma

Pheochromocytoma is a metabolically active neuroendocrine tumor of chromaffin cells commonly found in the adrenal glands, although these tumors can be found in other sites. A high suspicion of pheochromocytoma should be raised in neurosurgical patients with a history of neurofibromatosis type I, Von Hippel-Lindau disease, multiple endocrine neoplasia type II, and familial carotid body tumors. Routine screening is recommended prior to elective surgery in these patients and should also be given consideration for patients with severe hypertension of unknown etiology, especially in the 30–40 year age group, Presenting symptoms may also include headache, excessive truncal sweating, palpitations, or panic attacks. These tumors secrete norepinephrine, and sometimes epinephrine, resulting in hemodynamic instability such as paroxysmal swings in blood pressure and, most frequently, severe hypertension. The release of catecholamines is triggered by physiologic stress or physical manipulation of the lesion.

The standard diagnostic tests are measurement of plasma-free metanephrines (high specificity) and 24-h urine metanephrines (high sensitivity). The clonidine suppression test is sometimes employed. Physiologic tests are complemented by sensitive imaging modalities, including MRI and scintigraphy.

The masses can go undiagnosed, then manifest as exaggerated autonomic responses during anesthesia for unrelated surgical procedures. In the untreated patient with pheochromocytoma, desensitization of beta-receptors may occur and be associated with decreased response to exogenously administered catecholamines. Significant volume depletion also occurs in the setting of chronically elevated sympathetic tone. As a result of these derangements, cardiovascular collapse may occur during induction and maintenance of general anesthesia.

In patients with known pheochromocytoma, preoperative antagonism of catecholamine effects (usually over weeks preceding surgery) is essential. Therapy should start with a peripheral alpha-1 antagonist such as phenoxybenzamine, followed by the addition of beta-antagonists. Beta-selective antagonists should not be administered before alpha blockade, as negative inotropy in the setting of unopposed alpha-receptor-mediated vasoconstriction can result in acute ventricular dysfunction. Furthermore, beta-blockade alone is contraindicated because it does not prevent and can actually augment effects of catecholamines at alpha-adrenoreceptors. Finally, the addition of the catecholamine synthesis inhibitor alpha-methyl-p-tyrosine (AMPT) 10–14 days prior to surgery is current standard of care, as it decreases the requirement for peripheral adrenergic blockade resulting in greatly improved perioperative hemodynamic stability. Preoperative volume repletion is clearly beneficial. Adequate preoperative preparation may be demonstrated by controlled hypertension, minimal orthostasis, and minimal ectopy on heart rhythm monitoring on the day of surgery.

Intraoperative management consists of IV infusion of titratable antihypertensives, which may include alpha- and beta-blockers as well as direct vasodilators. Administration of indirectly acting vasopressors, such as ephedrine, may have unpredictable effects and is best avoided. If the surgical plan includes tumor excision (or clamping of veins draining the mass), dramatic hypotension should be anticipated shortly thereafter due to the loss of catecholamines in a patient aggressively alpha-blocked. The plan for anesthesia should, therefore, include invasive arterial monitoring, with preparation for post-excision resuscitation, hemodynamic support, and cortisol supplementation (if adrenal).

Growth Hormone/Acromegaly

Growth hormone is secreted by the anterior pituitary gland and is a diffuse regulator of cellular metabolism. The hormone stimulates production of insulin-like growth factor I, serum levels of which may be diagnostic for the disorder. Growth hormone excess, commonly due to a hyperactive pituitary macroadenoma, is common in neurosurgical patients presenting for pituitary surgery.

Acromegaly from growth hormone excess has important anesthetic considerations. These include: (1) potential for a difficult airway (including postoperative airway obstruction) due to diffuse soft-tissue enlargement, laryngeal calcification, recurrent laryngeal nerve involvement, and severe sleep apnea; (2) cardiac dysfunction including conduction abnormalities, cardiomyopathy, microvascular disease, and severe hypertension; (3) associated abnormalities of other hormones of the HPA axis with attendant derangements; (4) challenging intravenous access due to diffuse skin thickening; (5) and possible increase risk of positioning related nerve injury due to pre-existing nerve compression or entrapmemt in fascial compartments.

Frequently, surgical excision of a pituitary adenoma is performed via a transphenoidal approach under general endotracheal anesthesia. Special attention is necessary in airway management. This includes consideration regarding the impact of anesthetic agents (esp. benzodiazepines and opioids) on postoperative respiratory function. Preoperative cardiac assessment including ECG and echocardiography should be strongly considered. Electrolytes should also be checked prior to surgery and serially after resection in the intensive care unit (see diabetes insipidus above).

Pineal Gland

The pineal gland is a neuroendocrine structure situated midline in the subarachnoid space below the third ventricle with no blood–brain barrier (BBB). Its physiologic function is the secretion of melatonin, which is synthesized from serotonin. Melatonin is involved in the neurohumoral modulation of human sleep/wake cycles as well as pubescence. Currently, melatonin neurochemistry is an area of research interest. Adrenogloumerulotropin produced by the pineal gland is one of the triggers of aldosterone secretion. Tumors of the pineal gland may present for resection. Symptoms may include abnormal pubescence, gaze palsy, and increased ICP (due to obstructive of the cerebral aqueduct by the tumor). Respective operations may require the sitting position during surgery.

Insulin

Insulin is a peptide hormone secreted by the β-cells of the pancreas. It modulates glucose metabolism via a variety of receptors and signaling pathways. In certain disease states (e.g. metabolic syndrome (DM), infection, critical illness, and shock), the physiologic effects of insulin are decreased. Insulin exerts anti-inflammatory properties that may improve perioperative neurologic outcome. Glucose management using insulin for neurosurgical patients remains a controversial topic of high clinical interest. Optimal target ranges for glucose in the neurosurgical patient have not been determined. There is general agreement that severe hyperglycemia is both a marker of injury severity and clinically deleterious in most settings. This is counter-balanced by concern of neurologic injury from hypoglycemia that frequently accompanies tight control regimens. In most cases a plasma glucose level greater than 150 mg/dL should be treated.

Key Points
Additional Neuroendocrine Systems

- Pheochromocytoma is a metabolically active neuroendocrine tumor associated with episodic severe hypertension
  - Suspect based on associated syndrome (neurofibromatosis I, MEN II, Von Hippel-Lindau) or symptoms
  - Diagnosis: plasma-free and urine metanephrines
  - Optimal perioperative management requires preoperative therapy with anti-catecholaminergic agents
- Acromegaly results from growth hormone excess
  - Tissue changes associated with growth hormone excess predispose patients to difficult airway management, and cardiomyopathy
- Insulin is a primary regulatory hormone of glucose metabolism
  - Insulin action is frequently impaired during physiologic stress or injury resulting in hyperglycemia
  - Hyperglycemia (>200 mg/dL is deleterious in patients with neurologic injury
  - Treatment of hyperglycemia should target a moderate reduction to avoid the significant risks of plasma or cerebral hypoglycemia

Suggested Reading

Adler S. Disorders of body water homeostasis in critical illness. Endocrinol Metab Clin N Am. 2006;35:873–94.

Atkins JH, Smith DS. A review of perioperative glucose control in the neurosurgical population. J Diabet Sci Technol. 2009;3(6):1352–64.

Bouillon R. Acute Adrenal Insufficiency. Endocrinol Metab Clin N Am. 2006;35:767–75.

Langouche L, Van den Berghe G. The dynamic neuroendocrine response to critical illness. Endocrinol Metab Clin N Am. 2006;35:771–91.

Loh JA, Verbalis JG. Disorders of sodium and water metabolism associated with pituitary disease. Endocrinol Metab Clin N Am. 2008;37:213–34.

Nayak B, Burman K. Thyrotoxicosis and thyroid storm. Endocrinol Metab Clin N Am. 2006;35:663–86.

Sterns RH, Silver SM. Cerebral salt wasting syndrome versus SIADH: What difference? J Am Soc Nephrol. 2008;19:194–6.

Chapter 3
Cerebral Edema: Pathophysiology and Principles of Management

Andrea Orfanakis

Overview

Edema, while often benign elsewhere in the body, is almost always of clinical significance when it occurs within the cranial vault. Unlike nearly every other tissue area, the cranium is uniquely intolerant to any change in mass, no matter how insignificant that change may be. The classical thinking of the inhabitants of the cranium and the resultant pressure created by their presence is defined by the Monroe-Kellie Doctrine. Tissue cells, blood, and cerebrospinal fluid (CSF) maintain a consistent presence within the cranium and spinal cord areas. When any single component increases, the other two have a limited capacity to shift into accessory spaces so as to avoid a rise in intracranial pressure. Once that capacity to buffer is reached, elastance is limited, and very small increases in volume produce an exponential rise in pressure (Fig. 3.1). It is at this point in the elastance curve that the risk of herniation and/or excessive decrease in cerebral perfusion pressure becomes a real threat.

Implications for the Neurosurgical Patient

Cerebral edema is a common comorbidity in the neurosurgical patient with intracranial pathology. The anesthesiologist will encounter patients with every degree of disease, from local edema surrounding a tumor in an elective surgical case to a level one admission to the operating theater for malignant intracranial hypertension with impending herniation syndrome. Understanding the therapies available will allow the anesthesiologist to optimize each patient for the full perioperative period. Opioids

A. Orfanakis, MD (✉)
Department of Anesthesiology and Perioperative Medicine, Oregon Health & Science University, Portland, OR, USA
e-mail: orfanaka@ohsu.edu

A.M. Brambrink and J.R. Kirsch (eds.), *Essentials of Neurosurgical Anesthesia & Critical Care*, DOI 10.1007/978-0-387-09562-2_3,
© Springer Science+Business Media, LLC 2012

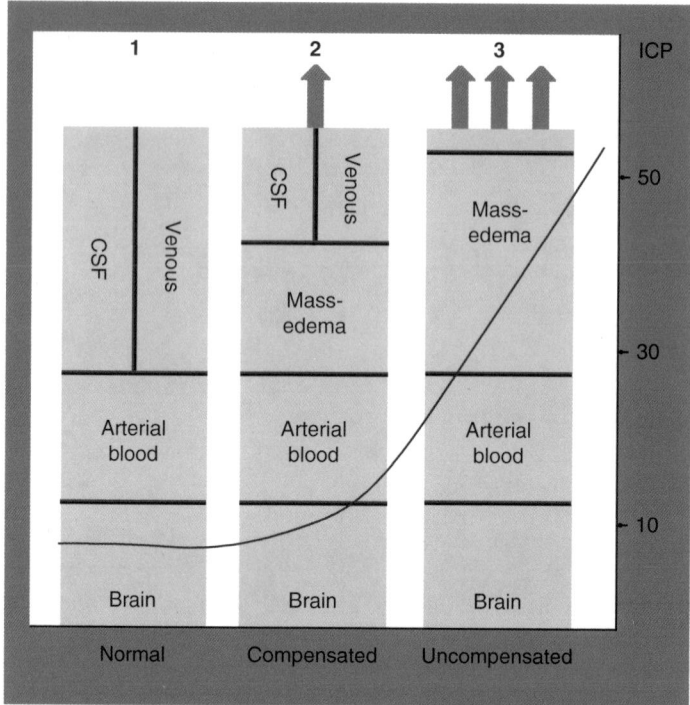

Fig. 3.1 The relationship between intracranial pressure and cerebral volume (CSF, blood, brain tissue) as expressed by the Monroe-Kellie Doctrine during both compensated and uncompensated states. Reproduced from Pediatric Health 2009; 3(6):533–541 with permission of Future Medicine Ltd

and anxiolytics in the preoperative area, or in any patient spontaneously breathing, while appropriate, should only be used very carefully, with concern for increasing $PaCO_2$ and subsequent intracranial vasodilatation and a consecutive rise in intracranial pressure in addition to the loss of the neurologic exam. These same concerns will be present upon emergence from anesthesia. The decision to extubate the trachea must take into account the patient's ability to trigger respirations at an appropriate carbon dioxide level. For this reason, continuous $EtCO_2$ monitoring is recommended. During anesthesia induction, tracheal intubation and positioning attention should be paid to avoid cough, ventilator dysynchrony, and periods of apnea. When positioning, the head and neck should ideally be midline (little to no rotation) and without towels or dressings which could compromise venous drainage of the neck. Head elevation, for instance, via reversed Trendelenburg's position, should be considered to further improve venous outflow. Intraoperatively, if hyperosmolar therapy is employed to "relax" the brain to optimize surgical approach or respond to brain edema, plasma sodium, and osmolarity should be checked regularly, particularly in longer cases. If rapid correction of cerebral edema is warranted, such as in acute herniation syndromes, immediate hyperventilation, so as to lower

Table 3.1 Cerebral edema subtypes

Category	Clinical disease state
Vasogenic	Inflammatory state (meningitis e.g.)
	High altitude cerebral edema
	Encephalopathy of HELLP
	Traumatic brain injury
	Intracranial hemorrhage
	Venous sinus thrombosis
	Hypertension
	Ischemia
	Tumor
	PRESS
Cytotoxic	Intracerebral hemorrhage
	Venous sinus thrombosis
	Traumatic brain injury
	Toxin exposure
	Ischemia
	Reyes syndrome
Interstitial	Hydrocephalus
	Transependymal edema
Osmotic	Acute hepatic failure
	Diabetic ketoacidosis encephalopathy
	Hemodialysis encephalopathy

$PaCO_2$, combined with rapid administration of hyperosmolar solutions is the most acutely responsive strategy. Hyperventilation will only demonstrate efficacy for several hours, as the brain will eventually readjust its autoregulatory thresholds. Also, sudden swings in the opposite (hypercapneic) direction can produce equally rapid increases in intracranial pressure and should be avoided. Upon transport to the PACU or ICU, the same care that was given to maintenance of $PaCO_2$, head and neck positioning (including avoiding restrictive dressings or endotracheal tube circumferential tape), and avoidance of cough or emesis should be continued.

Pathophysiology

Four descriptive subtypes of cerebral edema, namely cytotoxic, vasogenic, osmotic, and interstitial, have been defined, though rarely is only one present clinically. Complex pathophysiologic processes are at play during cerebral injury, and, though the above divisions may be overly simplistic, discussing these "subtypes" is a useful means with which to plan effective treatment strategies so as to minimize secondary injury (Table 3.1).

Cytotoxic edema refers to swelling of critical cellular elements following an insult associated with energy demand and substrate mismatch. This type of edema is not limited in that it can affect both gray and white matter. Cytotoxic edema occurs when metabolically active cells are depleted of their energy (ATP) stores resulting in profound breakdown of key cellular functions, as, for example, the maintenance and restoration of cell membrane functionality and organized neurotransmitter release. The former results in rapid ion currents via respective ion channels and the latter in an excessive neurotransmitter release (e.g., glutamate) into the interstitial spaces resulting in further stimulation of ion channel conduction. Both ion flux and transmitter release potentiate each other which is deleterious in the context of exhausted energy levels. Excessive ion currents, in particular sodium and calcium, influx into the cells and cause respective volumes of water to enter the cell, thus resulting in rapid development of cellular edema ultimately leading to the destruction of cellular integrity. If the brain areas are immediately reperfused, affected cell groups may eventually replenish their energy production and reestablish their electrolyte balance. In contrast, cells in continuously underperfused areas, which are still partially intact and survived the immediate catastrophic ion influx, are at risk of a subsequent insult via multiple intracelluar pathways triggered largely by excessive intracellular calcium levels: the active elimination of calcium to the outside of the cell results in a trade of sodium ions to the interior. This trade contributes to the significant osmotic gradient, pulling water into the cell further fueling cellular edema formation. Calcium is a critical element for the activation of a multitude of intracellular mechanisms including signaling cascade and protein synthesis. Excess calcium causes further disruption of intracellular functions and ultimately can lead to the activation of cell death programs resulting in apoptotic cell death. Above-mentioned events result in the activation of the inflammatory cascade wherein inflammatory intermediaries begin their assault on cellular elements. When the cell membranes of both neurons and endothelial cells are under attack by the cytokine and arachidonic acid cascades, the result is disruption of the blood–brain barrier. Chemokines signal for the involvement of white cells leading to the release of reactive oxygen species, nitric oxide-free radicals, and proteases. Once the cell membrane is violated, the cellular integrity of the brain cells is ultimately lost, and the damage is irreversible, causing "cytotoxic" brain edema (Fig. 3.2). This type of brain edema frequently blends with vasogenic edema (see below), as the endothelial cells become affected, and is typical of an ischemic stroke. Other causes of cytotoxic edema include trauma and toxin exposure.

Vasogenic edema results from damage to capillaries caused by attack on tight junction integrity and basal laminar structure by proteases and free radicals. Vasogenic edema can occur in traumatic brain injury, tumor, ischemia, and inflammatory conditions, such as meningitis, owing to capillary leak. Hypertensive encephalopathy syndromes such as PRES (posterior reversible encephalopathy syndrome) or hepatic encephalopathy of HELLP (hemolysis, elevated liver enzymes, low platelets) are two other etiologies of vasogenic edema. Once the capillary is damaged, the blood–brain barrier is violated, and proteins and blood products can leak into brain parenchyma. As noted above, neutrophils from the invading blood can activate inflammatory cascades which lead to permanent cellular damage. Additionally, this leak of proteins

Fig. 3.2 Hemispheric
cytotoxic brain edema 72 h
after large middle cerebral
artery ischemic stroke and
decompressive
hemicraniectomy. Note the
loss of gray white
differentiation and fungating
appearance of brain tissue
exiting the cranial vault

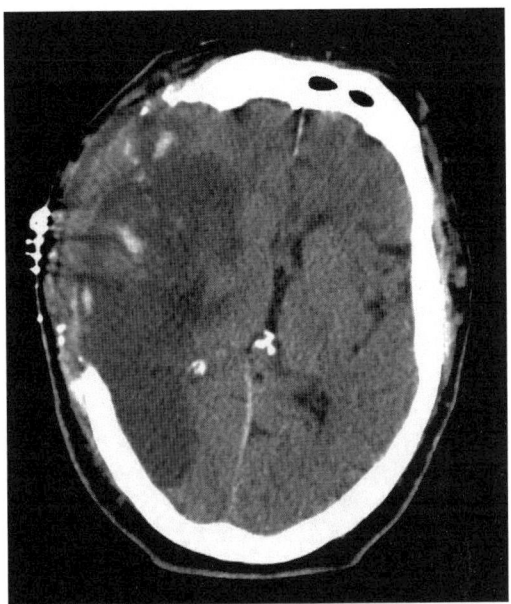

Fig. 3.3 Vasogenic edema
surrounding well-demarcated
brain tumor

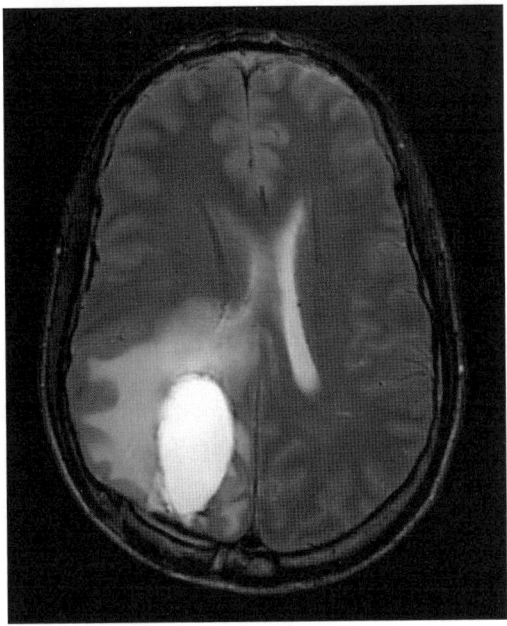

can offset the carefully controlled osmotic gradient within the brain and lead to an
increase in free water movement into the interstitial spaces. Vasogenic edema typically affects white matter only (Fig. 3.3). As the cellular structure is largely maintained, vasogenic edema can be highly responsive to osmotherapy and steroids.

Interstitial edema refers to inadequate cerebral spinal fluid absorption and resultant hydrocephalus. Medical therapy for this class of edema has questionable benefit. While diuretics such as acetazolimide and furosemide can decrease CSF production, the effect on intracranial pressure and outcomes is inconsistent and weakly supported. Surgical therapy or placement of an intraventricular catheter is a more definitive therapy for this variety of cerebral edema.

In addition to the three above-mentioned types, *osmotically driven cerebral edema* loosely describes a group of disorders whose pathophysiology involves acute changes in osmolarity. Acute hepatic failure, as can be seen for instance following acetaminophen toxicity, can lead to extensive and difficult to treat cerebral edema. The exact mechanism of this insult is poorly understood. Hyperosmolar states, where blood osmolality is corrected rapidly, can lead to shifts of fluid into cerebral cells. Both hemodialysis encephalopathy and diabetic ketoacidosis are two such examples. Hemodialysis encephalopathy can be seen following first time initiation of hemodialysis and should be a concern in patients presenting with Blood Urea Nitrogen above 50 mg/dL. Aggressive first time dialysis should be avoided in such cases. Diabetic patients presenting in acute ketotic acidosis are similarly at risk when rapidly corrected.

Concerns and Risks

Cerebral edema is a moderately manageable pathologic state. Key elements of management include continuous neurologic monitoring, avoidance of both hypoosmolar and hyponatremic states, and maintenance of cerebral perfusion throughout.

Monitoring

The cornerstone of cerebral monitoring is frequent, repeated neurologic examination. Subtle changes can be detected by an experienced examiner and may be the earliest indication of clinically significant cerebral edema. When a patient is unable to be frequently examined, due to low level of alertness, sedation or neuromuscular paralysis, serial neuroimaging may be warranted. Direct ICP monitoring can be useful in appropriate situations. Intraventricular catheters are most commonly employed as they provide accurate continuous pressure measurement as well as the option to drain CSF as a therapeutic means in the setting of hydrocephalus or malignant intracranial hypertension. Risks associated with intraventricular catheters include, but are not limited to, bleeding upon placement, infection, clotting of the catheter, and assumed risk associated with withholding anticoagulation. The fiberoptic intraparenchymal monitor is a useful second option for monitoring intracranial hypertension. Certain risks are lower with this device, such as injury upon placement, bleeding, and infection. The main drawback is the inability to drain CSF.

Table 3.2 Therapeutic options in cerebral edema

Therapy	Clinical state	Dose/duration	Associated risks
Hyperventilation	Acute crisis or impending herniation	Temporizing measure only $PaCO_2$ 28–32	Vasoconstriction leading to ischemia
Head position	All states	Continuous	
Mannitol	Acute crisis, herniation, interstitial, cytotoxic, osmotic edema	Bolus 0.5–1 g/kg Redose 0.25–0.5 mg/kg Q6h goal serum osmolality 310–320	Electrolyte disturbances, rebound edema associated with rapid withdrawal; concern for worsening midline shift in large hemispheric lesions
Hypertonic saline	Acute crisis, herniation, interstitial, osmotic, cytotoxic, and vasogenic edema	Multiple formulations available. Impending herniation 30 ml of Bolus 23.4% rapidly Maintenance of hypernatremia `3% with goal plasma sodium 145–155 mEq/L	Rebound edema associated with withdrawal Damage to peripheral vessels Volume overload
Steroids	Vasogenic edema surrounding tumor	Dexamethasone 4–6 mg Q4–6 h	No role in ischemia, trauma, hemorrhage
Pharmacologic coma	Salvage therapy from any pathology	Pentobarbital 10 mg/kg bolus, 1–4 mg/kg/h (Alternative propofol)	Infection Lack of neurologic exam Hypotension, cardiac depression Prolonged half life
Intraventricular catheter	Intracranial hypertension, hydrocephalus	Continuous	Infection
Hemicraniectomy	Refractory intracranial hypertension Large hemispheric stroke	Within 0–48 h	Surgical risks

Treatment

Treatment of cerebral edema is approached in a stepwise fashion from least invasive to most (Table 3.2). The nonpharmacologic options should be initiated in all patients. Raising the head of the bed at least 30° and maintaining a midline position without neck rotation helps to optimize venous drainage from the brain. Obstructed venous drainage results in increased ICP and a reduced arterial perfusion. If a definitive airway has been placed, hyperventilation is a reasonable option for treatment in the very short term. Vasoconstriction associated with decreased arterial CO_2 levels is a useful rescue technique, but the effectiveness will be lost in 6–8 h as the brain resets its acid/base equilibrium. However, an arterial PCO_2 28–32 should be the aim, as lower partial pressures can lead to excessive vasoconstriction and ischemia. Just as the vasoconstrictive effects of a low arterial PCO_2 are rapid, a sudden rise in arterial PCO_2 can produce equally rapid vasodilatation. It is, therefore, important to carefully follow the $PaCO_2$ in patients whose $PaCO_2$ has recently been lowered. This is of particular importance in the postoperative care unit or in any head injury patient who is spontaneously breathing and receiving narcotics.

Steroids serve a therapeutic role in the treatment of vasogenic edema associated with tumors. Their use in ischemic brain injury is unsupported and in traumatic brain injury may prove deleterious.

Osmotherapy theoretically aims to maximize intravascular oncotic pressures, thereby producing a gradient down which both intracellular and extracellular brain water may move into the vasculature and exit the cranial vault. Any osmotic agent, therefore, is only of utility if it can remain largely within the cerebral vessel and does not cross the blood–brain barrier. Where the blood-brain barrier is disrupted, an osmotic agent could potentially enter the interstitial spaces and lead to rebound cerebral edema. Mannitol, a six carbon sugar alcohol, is the most well-studied osmotic therapeutic in cerebral edema. Mannitol is typically packaged in a 20% solution and can be administered in 0.25–1 g/kg boluses in acute cerebral edema. Larger doses have been studied, and their effectiveness has been outweighed by the resultant electrolyte imbalances. Mannitol will produce a profound osmotic diuresis, and electrolytes and serum osmolality should be checked regularly. A hyperosmolar state on the order of 310–320 mOsm/L should be the target. Higher osmolarity is appropriate in certain situations but should be attempted with caution. Mannitol has been extensively studied for its extraosmotic properties, which include increases in blood volume and decrease in blood viscosity leading to improved cerebral blood flow, antioxidant properties, decrease in CSF production, and inhibition of apoptosis. Mannitol will have a greater effect on cells within the uninjured hemisphere and could, therefore, theoretically lead to worsening midline shift.

Hypertonic saline has become increasingly more popular in the last 30 years as a resuscitative fluid in brain injury. Hypertonic saline is supplied in a variety of concentrations, the most common being 3, 7.5, and 23.4%. Unless an emergency situation warrants peripheral administration, hypertonics should be transfused through central venous access. For acute resuscitative efforts, 30 ml of 23.4% or 250 ml of 3% have been successfully administered as a rapid bolus dose, typically followed by an infusion of low-concentrated hypertonic solution (frequently 3% sodium preparations) to maintain a hypernatremic state. The goal is serum sodium of 145–155 mEg/L in most cases. Certain instances may warrant slightly higher serum sodium concentrations but should once again be approached with extreme caution. Large infusions of chloride ion can produce a hyperchloremic metabolic acidosis. For continuous infusion, a 50:50 mix of sodium chloride with sodium acetate is preferable. Similar to the use of mannitol, withdrawal of hypertonic saline should be approached systematically and with care. Initial therapy calls for hypernatremia for

24–72 h followed by a slow taper of the infusion while monitoring level of edema, serum sodium concentration, and neurologic exam. A slow taper to normonatremia over a period of days is ideal, and hyponatremia, or acute decreases in sodium more than 2–3 mEq/L per day, should be avoided. Extraosmotic properties of hypertonic saline include increased tissue oxygen delivery, decreased CSF production, and increased CSF resorption. Preliminary laboratory data also suggests possible neurohumoral and anti-inflammatory properties may exist. Finally, loop diuretics such as furosemide are sometimes used, but their utility is controversial and not recommended by all authors. Aggressive diuresis can lead to decreases in cardiac output and cerebral perfusion pressure. Furosemide is an excellent agent for use in the diuresis of free water, and, if that loss can be replaced with hypertonic saline solution concomitantly, then dehydration may be avoided and hypernatremia achieved more quickly.

When the above therapies prove ineffective, more aggressive approaches aimed at salvage of brain tissue may be employed as a last resort. Pharmacologic coma is one such option; the goal here being to reduce neuronal activity which in turn will reduce cerebral metabolic rate of oxygen or $CMRO_2$. Cerebral blood flow is coupled directly to cerebral metabolic rate and will also decrease under pharmacologic coma. Barbiturates are the drugs of choice for instituting a pharmacologic coma. Pentobarbital coma is initiated with a bolus dose of 5–10 mg/kg followed by an infusion rate of 1–4 mg/kg/h titrate to goal reduction in intracranial pressure less than 20 mmHg. Complications of barbiturate coma include cardiac depression, increased infection risk, and long half life which could delay the time to return of reasonably assessable neurologic function. Propofol, a shorter acting hypnotic, is a second option.

Unremitting intracranial hypertension despite the aforementioned therapies is a possible candidate for hemicraniectomy with duraplasty. Hemicraniectomy, performed within the first 48 h, has demonstrated improvement in both morbidity and mortality in the large ischemic stroke population. For this therapy to be effective, it needs to be completed within 48 h and ideally sooner.

Key Points

- Cerebral edema is by definition a pathologic state
- Four subtypes of cerebral edema exist, and their correct diagnosis can appropriately direct therapy
- Monitoring, particularly the neurologic exam, is the key to early detection of clinically significant cerebral edema and thereby prevention of secondary injury
- Therapy for cerebral edema should be approached in a stepwise fashion, employing least invasive measures first
- Upon termination of any therapeutic measure, slow taper as opposed to sudden withdrawal is the recommended course

Suggested Reading

Bardutzky J, Schwab S. Antiedema therapy in ischemic stroke. Stroke. 2007;38(11):3084–94.

Bradley WG. Neurology in clinical practice. 5th ed. Philadelphia, PA: Butterworth Heinemann Elsevier; 2008. p. 1694–708.

Brouns R, De Deyn PP. Neurological complications in renal failure: a review. Clin Neurol Neurosurg. 2004;107(1):1–16.

Hofmeijer J, Kappelle LJ, Algra A, Amelink GJ, van Gijn J, van der Worp HB, et al. Surgical decompression for space-occupying cerebral infarction (the Hemicraniectomy After Middle Cerebral Artery infarction with Life-threatening Edema Trial [HAMLET]): a multicentre, open, randomised trial. Lancet Neurol. 2009;8(4):326–33.

Kahle KT, Simard JM, Staley KJ, Nahed BV, Jones PS, Sun D. Molecular mechanisms of ischemic cerebral edema: role of electroneutral ion transport. Physiology (Bethesda). 2009;24:257–65.

Kramer DJ, Canabal JM, Arasi LC. Application of intensive care medicine principles in the management of the acute liver failure patient. Liver Transpl. 2008;14 Suppl 2:S85–9.

Qureshi AI, Suarez JI. Use of hypertonic saline solutions in treatment of cerebral edema and intracranial hypertension. Crit Care Med. 2000;28(9):3301–13.

Chapter 4
Management of Fluids, Electrolytes, and Blood Products in Neurosurgical Patients

Renata Rusa and Sadeq A. Quraishi

Overview

- The major fluid compartments of the body are the intracellular compartment and the extracellular compartment, which is subdivided into intravascular and interstitial spaces.
- The volume of the individual compartments may change in a disease state or as the body adapts to environmental stress.
- In peripheral tissues, the primary determinant of fluid movement across capillaries (i.e., between the intravascular and interstitial spaces) is the oncotic gradient produced by large plasma proteins such as albumin.
- Unlike the peripheral tissues, the brain and spinal cord are isolated from the intravascular compartment by the blood–brain barrier.
- The primary determinant of water movement across the intact blood–brain barrier is the osmotic pressure gradient produced by osmotically active particles including plasma sodium and other electrolytes.
- Intravenous infusion of solutions hyperosmolar to plasma (e.g., 3% sodium chloride, mannitol) will lead to a decrease in brain water content and intracranial pressure (ICP). Administration of excess free water (e.g., hypoosmolar or dextrose-containing electrolyte-free solutions) will lead to increased brain water content and ICP.
- Osmotically active particles as well as plasma proteins may "leak" into the cerebral tissue where the blood–brain barrier has been disrupted and thus contribute to worsening cerebral edema in such regions.

R. Rusa, MD (✉)
Department of Anesthesiology and Perioperative Medicine, Oregon Health &
Science University, Portland, OR, USA
e-mail: rusar@ohsu.edu

S. Quraishi, MD, MHA
Department of Anaesthesia, Harvard Medical School, Boston, MA, USA

A.M. Brambrink and J.R. Kirsch (eds.), *Essentials of Neurosurgical Anesthesia & Critical Care*, DOI 10.1007/978-0-387-09562-2_4,
© Springer Science+Business Media, LLC 2012

- Intravenous administration of hyperosmolar solutions results in a decrease in water content in brain where blood brain barrier is intact to make room for the injured brain.

Implications for the Neurosurgical Patient

Perioperative fluid management in neurosurgical patients poses special challenges.

- The presence and treatment of elevated ICP, surgical bleeding, and a variety of pathophysiological derangements associated with neurologic injury may lead to significant hypovolemia, electrolyte abnormalities, anemia, and coagulopathy.

Care must be taken to:

- Maintain hemodynamic stability, optimal cerebral perfusion pressure, and oxygen delivery to the CNS tissue and
- Minimize the impact of fluid resuscitation on the development or exacerbation of cerebral edema.

The goals of fluid resuscitation are (see Tables 4.1–4.5):

- Restore intravascular volume and cerebral perfusion pressure and
- Achieve a slightly hyperosmolar state.

The clinician can choose from a variety of intravenous fluids including crystalloid, hypertonic saline, colloid, and blood products as dictated by the clinical scenario. The typical initial fluid choice for an elective craniotomy is a combination of Lactated Ringer's and 0.9% saline (Table 4.6).

Table 4.1 Commonly used IV solutions

Commonly used intravenous solutions	Osmolarity (mOsm/L)
Plasma osmolarity	270–295
Crystalloid	
Lactated Ringer's	273
0.9% Normal saline	308
D5 Lactated Ringer's	525
20% Mannitol	1,098
3% Hypertonic saline (HS)	1,026
Colloids	
6% Hetastarch	310
Pentastarch	326
6% Dextran (70)	300
5% Albumin	300
25% Albumin	1,500
HS colloid mixture	
7.5% HS 6% Dextran[a]	2,568

[a]Available in Europe

Table 4.2 Common causes of hyponatremia

Dilution
Excess water intake
Administration of hypoosmolar fluids
Use of diuretics
Mannitol, thiazides
Adrenal insufficiency
Hypothyroidism
Hyperglycemia
Cerebral salt wasting syndrome
Common in subarachnoid hemorrhage
Associated with hypovolemia
SIADH
CNS disorders
Chronic infections
Medications, e.g., carbamazepine
Organ failure
Cirrhosis, congestive heart failure, nephrotic syndrome
Associated with hypervolemia

SIADH syndrome of inappropriate antidiuretic hormone secretion

Table 4.3 Common causes of hypernatremia

Dehydration
Diabetes insipidus
Use of hypertonic saline

Table 4.4 Common causes of hypokalemia

Combined use of osmotic and loop diuretics
Hypomagnesemia
Intracellular potassium shift secondary to
Hyperventilation
Insulin infusion

Table 4.5 Considerations for assessing intravascular volume

History
Preoperative fasting and insensible losses
Presence of hemorrhage
Use of diuretics
Use of hyperosmotic intravenous contrast
Physical exam
Vital signs: presence of fever, tachycardia, hypotension
Orthostatic tachycardia and hypotension
Status of neck veins, skin turgor, mucous membranes
Oliguria
Pulmonary edema
Monitors
Trend in CVP or PAOP
Marked reduction in arterial pulse pressure or stroke volume with positive pressure ventilation signifying intravascular depletion

CVP central venous pressure, *PAOP* pulmonary artery occlusion pressure

Table 4.6 Indications for commonly used intravenous fluids and blood products

Indication	Fluid or blood product	Amount
Fluid maintenance	Lactated Ringer's	1:1 Crystalloid/fluid loss ratio; (usual rate: NS at 1.5 mL/kg/h)
Insensible and interstitial losses	0.9% Saline (normal saline, NS)	
Brain relaxation for exposure during craniotomy	20% Mannitol	0.25–2 g/kg
	3% Sodium chloride (hypertonic saline, HS)	5 mL/kg
Treatment of elevated ICP	20% Mannitol	0.25–2 g/kg
	3% Saline (HS)	200 mL
Replacement of blood loss	Lactated Ringer's, NS	3:1 Crystalloid/blood loss ratio
	Colloid	1:1 Colloid/blood loss ratio
	Hetastarch 6%	If used, limit to 20 mL/kg/24 h
	Red cells – ideally washed, leukoreduced, <15 days old	1 Unit should raise Hgb by 1 g/dL or Hct by 3%
Disseminated intravascular coagulation (DIC)		
Elevated INR, PTT	Fresh Frozen Plasma	Start at 10–15 mL/kg
Fibrinogen < 100 mg/dL	Cryoprecipitate	1 Pool (6 bags) raises fibrinogen by 45 mg/dL
Thrombocytopenia < 100,000 in a bleeding patient	Platelets pheresed	1 Bag (4 pooled units) raise platelets by 30,000/μL

Concerns and Risks (Table 4.7)

Anemia

- Has been associated with worse neurologic outcome in cardiopulmonary bypass surgery and with perioperative visual loss in prone spine surgery.
- The ideal hematocrit for optimizing cerebral blood flow and oxygen delivery in focal ischemia model is currently believed to be 30–34%. Higher hematocrit results in increased blood viscosity; hematocrit ≤ 25% results in decreased oxygen-carrying capacity.
- Normovolemic hemoglobin levels of 7–9 g/dL appear to be safe for the general ICU patient population.
- There is insufficient evidence to allow recommendations regarding:
  - The "safe" level of anemia for patients with neurologic injury; or
  - Whether correction of anemia by transfusing red cells has beneficial or detrimental effects on neurologic outcome.

Table 4.7 Concerns and risks of fluid management in neurosurgical patients

Under-resuscitation	Hypotension, inadequate cerebral perfusion pressure, secondary brain injury
Over-resuscitation	Exacerbation of cerebral edema
Hyponatremia	<120–125 mEq/L – change in mental status, seizures
Hypernatremia	>160–170 mEq/L – change in mental status, seizures
Lactated Ringer's	Hypoosmolar state, hyponatremia
0.9% Saline	Hyperchloremic metabolic acidosis
Dextrose solutions	Hypoosmolar state, hyperglycemia exacerbating cerebral injury
20% Mannitol	Hyponatremia
	Loss of bicarbonate – metabolic acidosis
	Excessive diuresis – intravascular volume depletion, electrolyte losses
	Rebound cerebral edema
	Hyperkalemia with high doses (2 g/kg)
Hypertonic saline	Hypernatremia
	Hyperchloremic metabolic acidosis
	Rebound cerebral edema when plasma sodium falls
	Tearing of cerebral veins – intracerebral hemorrhage
	Excessive diuresis – intravascular volume depletion, renal failure
	Central pontine myelinolysis – with rapid rise of plasma sodium from hyponatremic levels; malnourished and alcoholic patients at increased risk
	Sclerosis of veins
	Interference with coagulation and platelet aggregation
Synthetic colloids	Interference with coagulation, factor VIII complex; potential increased risk for intracranial hemorrhage
	No clear benefit compared with crystalloid as a resuscitative fluid
	Renal impairment
	Allergic reactions
	Pruritus
	Interference with blood cross-matching with dextran
Albumin	Expensive
	No clear benefit compared with crystalloid as a resuscitative fluid; potential harm in patients with traumatic brain injury

Transfusion of Blood Products

Current concerns regarding blood product transfusion in the developed world focus more on the immunomodulating effects of transfusion rather than transmission of infectious agents (Table 4.8). Transfusion-related acute lung injury (TRALI) is thought to be the leading cause of transfusion-related mortality.

Table 4.8 Examples of risks associated with transfusion of blood products

Risk	Risk per unit transfused
Infectious risks	
HIV	1:1.5–4.7 million
Hepatitis C	1: 1.9–3.1 million
Hepatitis B	1: 31,000–205,000
Hemolytic reactions	
Acute	1:13,000
Delayed	1:1,600
Alloimmunization	1:1,600
Immunosuppression	1:1
TRALI	1:5,000

Adapted in part from reference by Marik and Corwin 2008

Table 4.9 Special circumstances

Traumatic brain injury	Subarachnoid hemorrhage
Risk of coagulopathy and DIC	Electrolyte abnormalities
Multitrauma	Hypocalcemia, hypomagnesemia,
massive hemorrhage	Hypokalemia
dilutional coagulopathy	Hyponatremia
Neurogenic pulmonary edema	Cerebral Salt Wasting Syndrome
Hyponatremia	SIADH
Cerebral salt wasting syndrome	Avoid hypovolemia
SIADH	Vasospasm – therapeutic goal: hypervolemia

Special Circumstances (Table 4.9)

Key Points

- Fluid management goal is a euvolemic, slightly hyperosmolar state.
- Avoid hypoosmolar fluids and dextrose-containing solutions unless needed to treat hypoglycemia.
- Consider using hypertonic saline, unless contraindicated, to treat elevated ICP in a hypovolemic, hemodynamically unstable patient.
- In anemic patients with neurologic injury, there is insufficient evidence regarding transfusion thresholds. Do not use an arbitrary hemoglobin number; weigh risks of transfusion (e.g.,TRALI, immunosuppression) with benefits of oxygen delivery to injured CNS tissue.

Suggested Reading

Barron ME, Wilkes MM, Naviskis RJ. A systematic review of the comparative safety of colloids. Arch Surg. 2004;139:552–63.

Hare GM, Tsui AK, McLaren AT, et al. Anemia and cerebral outcomes: Many questions, fewer answers. Anesth Analg. 2008;107:1356–70.

Himmelseher S. Hypertonic saline solutions for treatment of intracranial hypertension. Cur Opin Anaesthesiol. 2007;20:414–26.

Madjdpour C, Spahn DR. Allogeneic red blood cell transfusions: Efficacy, risks, alternatives and indications. BJA. 2005;95:33–42.

Marik PE, Corwin HL. Efficacy of red blood cell transfusion in the critically ill: A systematic review of the literature. Crit Care Med. 2008;36:2667–74.

Patel PM, Drummond JC. Cerebral physiology and the effects of anesthetics and techniques. In: Miller RD et al., editors. Miller's anesthesia. 6th ed. Philadelphia: Elsevier; 2005. p. 817–8.

The American Thoracic Society Documents. Evidence-based colloid use in the critically ill: American thoracic society consensus statement. Am J Respir Crit Care Med. 2004;170:1247–59.

Chapter 5
Key Monitoring in Neuroanesthesia: Principles, Techniques, and Indications

Martin Smith

Overview

One of the primary roles of the neuroanesthesiologist is to maintain cerebral perfusion to meet the brain's metabolic demands and, under circumstances of reduced perfusion, to protect the brain. Since secondary cerebral insults can be systemic or cerebral in origin, monitoring techniques must include measurement of systemic and cerebral physiologic variables to guide optimization of cerebral hemodynamics and oxygenation. The spinal cord is at risk of injury during spine surgery, and monitoring can minimize these risks. Some neuromonitoring techniques are well established, whereas others are relatively new to clinical practice and their indications are still being evaluated (Table 5.1).

Implications for the Neurosurgical Patient

Monitoring Systemic Physiologic Variables

Monitoring systemic physiologic variables guides manipulation of blood pressure and arterial blood gases to optimize cerebral perfusion and oxygenation. Routine monitoring includes EKG, arterial oxygen saturation (pulse oximetry), arterial blood pressure, end-tidal carbon dioxide tension and temperature. Noninvasive blood pressure monitoring is appropriate for minor cases, but an invasive arterial catheter should be placed to allow beat-to-beat blood monitoring and arterial blood gas analysis during intracranial and complex spine surgery and in patients with

M. Smith, MBBS, FRCA, FFICM (✉)
Department of Neurocritical Care, National Hospital for Neurology and Neurosurgery,
University College London Hospitals, Queen Square, London, UK
e-mail: martin.smith@uclh.nhs.uk

A.M. Brambrink and J.R. Kirsch (eds.), *Essentials of Neurosurgical
Anesthesia & Critical Care*, DOI 10.1007/978-0-387-09562-2_5,
© Springer Science+Business Media, LLC 2012

Table 5.1 Applications of neuromonitoring techniques

Monitoring technique	Established intraoperative applications	Established neurointensive care applications	Invasive/noninvasive	Modalities monitored
Intracranial pressure	Yes	Yes	Invasive	• ICP • CPP • Pressure reactivity
Transcranial Doppler	Yes	Yes	Noninvasive	• Estimate of CBF • Cerebral vasospasm
Quantitative regional cerebral blood flow	No	No	Invasive	• Absolute regional CBF
Jugular venous oximetry	Yes	Yes	Invasive	• Global cerebral oxygenation • AVDO$_2$
Brain tissue oxygenation	No	Yes	Invasive	• Regional brain tissue oxygen tension
Near infrared spectroscopy	Yes	Research	Noninvasive	• Cerebral oxygenation • Cerebral hemodynamics
Cerebral microdialysis	No	Research	Invasive	• Cerebral cellular energy status • Brain tissue biochemistry
Electroencephalography	Yes	Yes	Noninvasive	• Seizure activity • Cerebral ischemia • Cortical mapping
Electromyography	Yes	Yes	Noninvasive	• Peripheral and cranial nerve damage
Somatosensory evoked potentials	Yes	Yes	Noninvasive	• Sensory pathways • Spinal cord posterior columns • Cerebral ischemia
Motor evoked potentials	Yes	No	Noninvasive	• Motor pathways • Spinal cord

ICP intracranial pressure, *CPP* cerebral perfusion pressure, *CBF* cerebral blood flow, *AVDO$_2$* arteriovenous oxygen content difference, *ECF* extracellular fluid, *LPR* lactate:pyruvate ration, *EMG* electromyogram

Table 5.2 Comparison of intracranial pressure monitoring devices

Method	Advantages	Disadvantages
Intraventricular catheter	• Gold standard measure of ICP • Measures global ICP • Allows therapeutic drainage of CSF • In vivo calibration possible	• Insertion may be difficult • Invasive • Risk of hematoma • Risk of ventriculitis
Microtransducer sensor	• Intraparenchymal/subdural placement • Low procedure complication rate • Low infection risk • Low zero drift over time	• No in vivo calibration • Measures local pressure
Epidural sensor	• Easy to insert • Dura not penetrated • Low infection risk	• Limited accuracy • Rarely used

significant comorbidities. Central venous pressure and cardiac output monitoring allow more accurate assessment of intravascular volume and guide titration of vasopressors and inotropes. These modalities should be considered in patients with neurogenic cardiovascular instability and when substantial blood loss is anticipated. Urine output and fluid balance should be monitored when large fluid shifts are likely, particularly if osmotic diuretics will be administered or in the presence of neurogenic fluid disturbances such as diabetes insipidus.

Monitoring the Central Nervous System

Intracranial Pressure

Different methods of monitoring intracranial pressure (ICP) are available (Table 5.2), but an intraventricular catheter or intraparenchymal, catheter-tip microtransducer system are most commonly used in clinical practice. ICP monitoring allows measurement and display of absolute ICP, calculation of cerebral perfusion pressure (CPP), identification of pathologic ICP waveforms, and derivation of indices describing cerebrovascular pressure reactivity. Although the indications for ICP monitoring after traumatic brain injury (TBI) are well established, other intraoperative indications are less clearly defined. However, perioperative ICP monitoring should be considered in patients with TBI, large brain tumors with mass effect, hydrocephalus, intracranial and subarachnoid hemorrhage, and in the presence of significant cerebral edema from whatever cause. Postoperative ICP monitoring after intracranial surgery is indicated in any patient who will remain sedated or if there is a risk of intracranial hypertension.

Cerebral Blood Flow

Transcranial Doppler ultrasonography (TCD) is a noninvasive technique that measures cerebral blood flow velocity (FV) from the Doppler shift caused by moving red blood cells in basal cerebral vessels. Changes in cerebral blood flow (CBF) can be estimated from changes in FV. TCD can be used to assess cerebral perfusion, carbon dioxide reactivity, and cerebral autoregulation. Reductions in FV correlate with cerebral ischemia and have been used as an indication for shunt placement during carotid endarterectomy. TCD identifies intraoperative emboli and can differentiate between air and particulate emboli. TCD is also widely used in the diagnosis and monitoring of cerebral vasospasm, which is confirmed when FV exceeds 120–140 cm/s or if the ratio between FV in the middle cerebral and internal carotid arteries (the Lindegaard ratio) exceeds 3.

Thermal diffusion flowmetry (TDF) provides a sensitive, real-time assessment of absolute regional CBF (rCBF). TDF catheters have recently become available for clinical use, and, although there are limited clinical data with this new technique, intraoperative rCBF monitoring might be useful where there is a risk of focal cerebral ischemia.

Cerebral Oxygenation

Assessment of perfusion alone is insufficient to identify potential cerebral ischemia because changes in CBF might be associated with appropriately coupled changes in metabolism. Cerebral oxygenation monitoring assesses the adequacy of cerebral perfusion by measuring the balance between cerebral oxygen delivery and utilization.

Jugular venous oxygen saturation (SjO_2), and estimation of the cerebral arteriovenous oxygen and lactate differences, are well-established methods of assessing the balance between global cerebral oxygen delivery and utilization. The jugular venous catheter must be correctly placed to minimize contamination from the extracranial circulation, which is minimal when the catheter tip lies level with the mastoid process above the lower border of the first cervical vertebra on a lateral cervical spine radiograph. SjO_2 accurately reflects *global* changes only if the dominant jugular bulb is cannulated, although in practice the right side is usually chosen. The complications and contraindications of SjO_2 monitoring are same as for the insertion of an internal jugular central venous line, though the incidence of thrombosis of the cannulated jugular vein has not been quantified. Intermittent samples aspirated from the catheter provide a "snapshot" of the brain's oxygenation and metabolic status, whereas fiberoptic catheters allow continuous monitoring and on-line display of SjO_2. Normal SjO_2 is 55–75%, and interpretation of SjO_2 changes is straightforward (Table 5.3). Because SjO_2 is a global flow-weighted measure, it is relatively insensitive to regional ischemia. Jugular venous desaturation may indicate cerebral hypoperfusion secondary to decreased CPP or hypocapnea-related reduction in CBF, and SjO_2 can be used to guide intraoperative blood pressure and ventilatory management. SjO_2 monitoring is widely used after TBI, and treatment of jugular

Table 5.3 Interpretation of changes in jugular venous oxygen saturation

Jugular venous saturation	Relative CBF and $CMRO_2$ changes	Causes
Normal SjO_2 (55–75%)	CBF and $CMRO_2$ balanced	
Low SjO_2 (<50%)	$\downarrow$CBF or $\uparrow CMRO_2$	$\downarrow$Blood pressure
		$\downarrow PaCO_2$
		Seizures
		Fever
		$\uparrow$ICP or $\downarrow$CPP
		Vasospasm
		Arterial hypoxia
High SjO_2 (>80%)	$\uparrow$CBF or $\downarrow CMRO_2$	Hyperemia
		Failure of oxygen utilization (mitochondrial failure)
		Hypothermia
		Sedation
		Arteriovenous shunting
		Brainstem death

SjO_2 jugular venous oxygen saturation, *CBF* cerebral blood flow, $CMRO_2$ cerebral metabolic rate for oxygen, $PaCO_2$ arterial carbon dioxide tension, *ICP* intracranial pressure, *CPP* cerebral perfusion pressure

venous desaturation may improve outcome. SjO_2 has also been used to guide therapeutic hyperventilation, but this is controversial because of its lack of sensitivity to regional ischemia.

Brain tissue oxygen partial pressure: Direct measurement of brain tissue oxygen tension ($PbrO_2$) is becoming established as the "gold standard" bedside measure of cerebral oxygenation. $PbrO_2$ catheters incorporate a gold polarographic (Clark-type) cell which reduces oxygen as it diffuses from the brain across a semipermeable membrane into the catheter, generating an electrical current that is proportional to the tissue oxygen tension. $PbrO_2$ is a *highly focal* measure allowing selective monitoring of critically perfused tissue. The $PbrO_2$ threshold for ischemia is < 10 mmHg. $PbrO_2$ monitoring has been most widely used in TBI where reduced $PbrO_2$ is associated with poor outcome. There is also preliminary evidence that therapy directed toward maintenance of $PbrO_2$, in addition to ICP and CPP, is associated with reduced mortality. $PbrO_2$ monitoring is likely to find varied intraoperative applications because it allows rapid detection of cerebral ischemia and the potential to manipulate systemic and intracranial variables before irreversible neuronal damage occurs. However, it takes around 1 h following insertion of the probe for $PbrO_2$ readings to stabilize, and this has obvious implications for intraoperative monitoring.

Near infrared spectroscopy (NIRS) is a noninvasive technique based on the transmission and absorption of near infrared light (700–1,000 nm) at multiple wavelengths as it passes through tissue. Oxygenated and deoxygenated hemoglobin have different and characteristic absorption spectra in the near infrared range, and cortical oxygenation and hemodynamic status can be determined by their relative absorption of near infrared light using transcranial reflectance spectroscopy. Clinical monitors usually incorporate an absolute measure of regional cerebral tissue oxygen saturation

(ScO$_2$), and this is a reliable and continuous measure of the balance between cerebral oxygen delivery and utilization. Using NIRS it is now also possible to measure changes in the concentration of oxidized cytochrome c oxidase (CCO), the terminal complex of the mitochondrial electron transfer chain responsible for over 95% of oxygen metabolism. NIRS-derived CCO offers the potential to assess cerebral mitochondrial redox state and cellular energy status. There has been an increase in the clinical experience with commercially available cerebral oximeters following some evidence that NIRS-guided brain protection protocols might lead to reduced neurologic complications and improved patient outcomes after cardiac surgery. NIRS is now used routinely in some centres to monitor cerebral oxygenation during carotid surgery where it offers advantages over established techniques, such as the electroencephalogram (EEG) and TCD, in terms of simplicity. However, it is currently impossible to specify an accurate NIRS-derived threshold that can be widely applied to guide shunt placement or detect cerebral ischemia during carotid surgery. There are no data to support the wider application of NIRS to monitor cerebral oxygenation during routine anesthesia and surgery and its application in brain injury is as yet undefined. Concerns remain over "contamination" of the NIRS signal from extracerebral sources, but modern techniques have relatively high sensitivity and specificity to intracranial changes. The clinical applications of NIRS techniques are currently limited, but technological developments offer the real potential for a single NIRS device to deliver simultaneous monitoring of cerebral oxygenation, hemodynamics, and cellular energy status over multiple regions of interest.

Metabolic Monitoring

Cerebral microdialysis (MD) allows bedside analysis of biochemical substances in brain tissue extracellular fluid (ECF). Normal values for commonly measured MD variables and their clinical relevance have been established (Table 5.4). Cerebral MD is able to monitor cerebral tissue hypoxia/ischemia and also cellular energy failure, and biochemical trends provide clinical information that can be used to guide treatment decisions. MD has been widely used on the neurointensive care unit to evaluate the adequacy of tissue perfusion and oxygenation, guide CPP management, and assess the physiologic response to therapy. MD has the potential to detect biochemical markers of ischemia before the development of clinical symptoms or changes in other monitoring modalities. The intraoperative indications for MD are not fully evaluated, but it might find a role in procedures that run the risk of regional hypoxia/ischemia. The temporal resolution of current MD techniques is likely to limit intraoperative applications, but on-line, real-time MD methods are being developed and have been tested in research settings during intracranial neurosurgery.

Electrophysiologic Monitoring

Electroencephalography: The electroencephalogram (EEG) is a voltage–time recording of spontaneous cortical electrical activity measured from electrodes placed

Table 5.4 Bedside biomarkers measured by cerebral microdialysis

Microdialysis variable	Normal values	Monitor of	Comments
Glucose	>1.5–2.0 mmol/L	• Cerebral glucose supply • Hypoxia/ischemia • Cerebral hyperglycolysis	Reduced brain ECF glucose associated with poor outcome after brain injury
Lactate:pyruvate ratio	<20–25	• Hypoxia/ischemia • Cellular redox state • Impairment of cellular metabolism	Increased LPR most reliable marker of hypoxia/ischemia Identifies cellular energy crisis
Glycerol	<100 µmol/L	• Hypoxia/ischemia • Cell death	Cell membrane degradation following cell death releases glycerol into brain ECF
Glutamate	<15–20 µmol/L	• Excitoxicity • Hypoxia/ischemia	Wide variability in glutamate levels makes interpretation difficult

ECF extracellular fluid, *LPR* lactate:pyruvate ratio

Table 5.5 Intraoperative electroencephalographic monitoring

Advantages
- Noninvasive
- Continuous, on-line monitoring
- Localized information
- Correlates with reductions in cerebral blood flow and oxygenation
- Identification of seizures
- Identification of cerebral ischemia

Disadvantages
- Trained neurophysiologoist required for interpretation
- Influenced by anesthetic agents
- Influenced by systemic physiologic changes, e.g., hypothermia
- Subject to artifacts from electrical and diathermy "noise"
- Insensitive to subcortical changes

at specific locations on the scalp. The electrical signal is amplified, filtered, and displayed in multiple channels (usually eight per hemisphere) to give a continuous EEG recording that is analyzed in terms of frequency, amplitude, and location. Interpretation of the EEG is complex, but several automated EEG processing systems are now available that allow interpretation by nonexperts. EEG techniques have been developed to monitor depth of anesthesia, but their indications and application are not unique to neurosurgical anesthesia and will not be considered here.

Reduction in CBF below 20 ml/100 g/min results in decrease in the frequency and amplitude of the EEG, which becomes flattened when CBF falls below 10 ml/100 g/min. Quantitative analysis of these changes has been used to monitor cerebral ischemia, although intraoperative EEG monitoring has limitations (Table 5.5). The

Table 5.6 Intraoperative indications for electrophysiologic monitoring

EEG	EMG	SSEP	MEP	BAEP	VEP
Depth of anesthesia monitoring	Acoustic neuroma surgery	Spinal deformity surgery	Spinal deformity surgery	V, VII and VIIIth nerve surgery	Pituitary and suprasellar lesions
Epilepsy surgery	Posterior fossa surgery	Intrinsic spinal cord lesions	Intrinsic spinal cord lesions	Posterior fossa lesions	Retro-orbital lesions
Carotid artery surgery	Spinal surgery	Parietal cortex lesions	Motor cortex lesions	Diagnosis of brainstem death	Occipital cortex lesions

EEG electroencephalography, *EMG* electromyography, *SSEP* somatosensory evoked potential, *MEP* motor evoked potential, *BAEP* brainstem auditory evoked potential, *VEP* visual evoked potential

electrocorticogram (ECoG) is the EEG measured directly from the cortical surface. This can be used to identify the site of an epileptogenic focus during epilepsy surgery, and after-discharges (that can precipitate seizures) during mapping of eloquent areas with electrical cortical stimulation during awake craniotomy. Nonconvulsive seizures and cortical spreading depolarization, which represents an inherent component of progressive cerebral metabolic failure, are common in patients with acute brain injury, and continuous EEG and ECoG monitoring are increasingly being used in "at risk" patients.

Electromyography (EMG) allows assessment of cranial and peripheral nerves via needle electrodes placed in or near specific muscles (Table 5.6). EMG activity is detected if the nerve innervating the muscle is touched or stretched during surgery, thereby alerting the neurosurgeon that the nerve is at risk of damage. Seventh nerve monitoring is widely used during acoustic neuroma surgery. Muscle relaxants are best avoided during EMG monitoring. However, they are utilized in some centers and the doses carefully adjusted to maintain two strong twitches during train-of-four monitoring. With clear communication between anesthesiology and neuromonitoring teams, using muscle relaxants in this way facilitates simultaneous EMG and somatosensory evoked potential (SSEP) monitoring in the same patient.

Evoked potentials (EP) are used during intracranial and spine surgery (Table 5.6) to identify reversible changes and allow intervention before permanent neurologic injury occurs. SSEPs monitor the integrity of sensory pathways, including peripheral nerves, and motor evoked potentials (MEP) the motor pathways. Cortical SSEPs are recorded from the cerebral cortex using scalp electrodes following electrical stimulation of a peripheral nerve and subcortical responses from electrodes placed adjacent to the upper cervical spine. MEPs are generated following transcranial stimulation of the motor cortex with a high-voltage electrical source and the evoked responses recorded as compound motor action potentials in peripheral muscles (myogenic MEPs), via epidural/intrathecal electrodes or via an electrode placed directly on the exposed spinal cord during surgery. MEPs are recorded following a

Table 5.7 Effects of anesthetic agents on evoked potentials and EMG

Agent	SSEP latency	SSEP amplitude	MEP amplitude	EMG
Volatile agents	+ + +	– – –	– – –	0
Nitrous oxide	+	– –	– –	0
Propofol	+ +	– –	– –	0
Barbiturates	+ +	– –	– –	0
Benzodiazepines	+	–	–	0
Opioids	±	±	±	0
Muscle relaxants	0	0	– –	Best avoided[a]

SSEP somatosensory evoked potential, *MEP* motor evoked potential
+ + + large increase, + + moderate increase, + mild increase, ± minimal effect, – – – large decrease,
– – moderate decrease, – mild decrease, 0 no effect
[a]Muscle relaxants utilized in some centers and the doses carefully adjusted to maintain two strong twitches during train-of-four monitoring

single, brief stimulation volley, whereas SSEPs require multiple stimulations and signal averaging.

Spinal cord injury may occur during spine surgery because of ischemia secondary to spinal distraction and disruption of perforating radicular vessels or because of direct trauma during placement of pedicle screws or resection of an intrinsic spinal cord lesion. Multimodal electrophysiologic monitoring, using SSEP, MEP, and EMG (from upper and/or lower limbs as appropriate), is recommended because no single method can sufficiently cover the complex functions of the spinal cord. MEPs are more sensitive to spinal cord ischemia than SEPs and correlate better with motor function after spine surgery. SSEPs and MEPs are sensitive to anesthetic agents (Table 5.7) and SSEPs additionally to physiologic changes, such as hypotension and alterations in $PaCO_2$. Total intravenous anesthesia techniques, with a high-dose opioid component, are recommended during SSEP and MEP monitoring.

Cortical SSEPs may also be used to monitor cerebral ischemia during intracranial and carotid endarterectomy surgery. Visual evoked potentials (VEP) monitor the visual pathways but are technically difficult and exquisitely sensitive to anesthetic agents. Lesions at different parts of the auditory pathway can be identified by changes in the amplitude or latency of one of the five waves that make up the complex brainstem auditory evoked potentials (BAEP). BAEPs are relatively resistant to anesthetic agents.

Concerns and Risks

Detecting and treating cerebral and spinal cord ischemia are key factors in the intraoperative management of the neurosurgical patient. Monitoring detects changes early so that the neuroanesthesiologist and neurosurgeon can intervene and minimize the risk of irreversible central nervous system damage and poor neurologic outcome.

Given the physiologic complexity of the brain and spinal cord, it is not surprising that a single variable or a single device is unable to provide adequate monitoring during surgery. Multimodality electrophysiologic monitoring during complex spine surgery is well-established and guides interventions that can minimize the risk of permanent neurologic injury. Although intracranial monitoring, including measures of cerebral perfusion, oxygenation and metabolic status, is recommended during the management of critically ill brain injured patients on the neurointensive care unit, many modalities are less suited to the operating room because of incompatibility or inadequate temporal resolution. Currently, every monitor of cerebral perfusion and oxygenation has its own specific shortcomings and none is a standard of care in the intraoperative period. However, technical advances are likely to lead to the development of monitors that allow noninvasive, continuous, multi-site measurement of cerebral hemodynamics, oxygenation, and metabolic status.

Key Points

- The neuroanesthesiologist plays a key role in protecting the brain and spinal cord from intraoperative ischemic injury by maintenance of brain and spinal cord perfusion and oxygenation.
- Multimodal monitoring techniques are established during complex spine surgery and guide interventions and prevent permanent neurologic injury.
- Multimodal systemic and cerebral monitoring techniques guide intraoperative management of blood pressure and arterial blood gases, particularly in patients at risk of secondary cerebral ischemia.
- Many cerebral monitoring techniques that are widely used during neurointensive care do not translate well into the operating room.
- The ideal intraoperative cerebral monitor would allow noninvasive, simultaneous measurement of cerebral oxygenation, hemodynamic, and metabolic status over multiple regions of interest.

Suggested Reading

Chan M, Gin T, Goh K. Interventional neurophysiologic monitoring. Curr Opin Anaesthesiol. 2004;17:389–96.

Nortje J, Gupta AK. The role of tissue oxygen monitoring in patients with acute brain injury. Br J Anaesth. 2006;97:95–106.

Schell RM, Cole DJ. Cerebral monitoring: jugular vein oximetry. Anesth Analg. 2000;90: 559–66.

Smith M. Monitoring intracranial pressure in traumatic brain injury. Anesth Analg. 2008;106: 240–8.

Tisdall M, Smith M. Cerebral microdialysis: research technique or clinical tool? Br J Anaesth. 2006;97:18–25.

Highton D, Elwell C, Smith M. Noninvasive cerebral oximetry: is there light at the end of the tunnel? Curr Opin Anaesthesiol. 2010;23:576–81.

Part II
Preoperative Concerns of the Neuroanesthesiologist

Chapter 6
Cardiovascular Risk and Instability: Evaluation, Management, and Triage

Philip E. Lund and Jeffrey R. Kirsch

Overview

The cardiovascular system interacts with the neurologic system on many levels. This has implications for disease states in both systems. Therefore, when treating patients with neurosurgical disease, the provider must consider and be prepared to address pathological changes and consequences of treatment in the cardiovascular system. In the USA alone, approximately one of five persons has been diagnosed with some form of cardiovascular disease; and 40% of these patients are 65 years of age or more. With the progressive increase in life expectancy in the 21st century, the percentage of patients with significant cardiovascular disease and a comorbid neurological condition is also expected to increase.

Implications for the Neurosurgical Patient

Signs of Myocardial Damage

Cardiac disease in the neurosurgical population increases the overall morbidity and mortality. In patients who have suffered a cerebrovascular accident (stroke), cardiac manifestations may include EKG changes, cardiac arrhythmias, myocardial injury, and dysfunction, as well as neurogenic pulmonary edema.

P.E. Lund, MD (✉)
Department of Anesthesiology, Kaiser Sunnyside Medical Center, Clackamas, OR, USA
e-mail: pel@philiplund.net

J.R. Kirsch, MD
Department of Anesthesiology and Perioperative Medicine, Oregon Health &
Science University, Portland, OR, USA

A.M. Brambrink and J.R. Kirsch (eds.), *Essentials of Neurosurgical Anesthesia & Critical Care*, DOI 10.1007/978-0-387-09562-2_6, © Springer Science+Business Media, LLC 2012

EKG changes are very common in stroke patients and occur in 49–100% of cases, with higher incidence in patients suffering from intracerebral or subarachnoid hemorrhage and lower incidence in patients with ischemic stroke. These changes consist of large inverted T waves, prolonged QT intervals, and large U waves, all observed primarily in the septal leads. This pattern has been considered distinctive of cerebrovascular accidents. Arrhythmias ranging from bradycardia to fatal ventricular fibrillation are also seen in the acute period following onset of stroke symptoms.

Elevation of troponins and echocardiographic changes consistent with myocardial ischemia may also exist in this group. These typically reversible (but significant) changes seen on echocardiography span the whole clinical spectrum from hypokinesis with normal cardiac index to low output cardiac failure. However, in a cohort of patients who sustained subarachnoid aneurysmal hemorrhage, no differences in mortality were found in patients demonstrating cardiac abnormalities vs. patients in the control group. This finding may be due to the lack of coronary artery disease in many of the patients who present with signs and symptoms of cardiac injury in connection with their neurological insult. Nonetheless, any serious cardiac manifestation is a potential risk factor for mortality and additional morbidity and should be treated to prevent further decline of cardiac function.

Hypothalamic stress following subarachnoid hemorrhage (increased intracranial pressure) leads to a massive release of catecholamines. This causes hypertension and increased cardiac work, which result in the cardiac sequelae. Despite these "sequelae", there is usually no permanent cardiac injury, and, therefore, no consistent association with EKG abnormalities, histological cardiac lesions, or serum markers of cardiac injury.

Neurosurgical Patients and Anticoagulation

Pharmacological and Physiological Risks for Bleeding. Patients with neurosurgical disorders are often older and, therefore, can have disease processes that require anticoagulation for management. These typically originate from the cardiovascular system and include atrial fibrillation, thromboembolism, or atherosclerotic manifestations like carotid artery disease.

Anticoagulant therapy can cause spontaneous bleeding. Listed below are several classes of pharmacological agents with representative drugs that can cause bleeding.

- Antiplatelet agents: Acetylsalicylic acid (ASA), clopidogrel (Plavix), and abciximab (Rheopro)
- Heparins: Unfractionated (no trade name, usually from pork intestine); low-molecular-weight heparins (LMWHs) – enoxiparin (Lovenox), dalteparin (Fragmin)
- Inhibitors of Vitamin K-dependent coagulation factors: Warfarin (Coumadin) with a half-life of 36–42 h

- Direct thrombin inhibitors: Lepirudin, bivalirudin, agatroban (all parenteral drugs)
- Fibrinolytic agents: Tissue-type plasminogen activator (tPA).

In addition to these pharmacological risks, patients may present with congenital clotting defects (e.g., Von Willebrand's disease, hemophilia). Further, patients with unrelated diseases may be prescribed pharmaceuticals with anticoagulant properties and/or have interactions with other drugs that act to change the patient's coagulation status (i.e., drug–drug, drug–food, and drug–genomic interactions). In addition, patients with severe liver disease may manifest increased bleeding tendency due to decreased synthetic function of the liver with reduced production of coagulation factors. Patients who have a malignancy may have antibodies to clotting factors and/ or to platelets or have a consumptive coagulopathy and present with excessive bleeding (in addition to their neurologic disease).

Assessing Coagulation Status. Coagulation status is most commonly determined by measuring the International Normalized Ratio (INR) of the prothrombin time (PT) test, which indicates function of vitamin K-dependent coagulation factors and the synthetic function of the liver. Fibrinogen levels can also be useful in assessing the coagulation status of the perioperative neurosurgical patient since fibrinogen is the main "building block" of clot. The activated partial thromboplastin time (APTT) test helps to assess the effectiveness of unfractionated heparin; and measuring Factor Xa levels helps to assess the effectiveness of LMWHs, although this test is not commonly used.

Unfortunately, it is somewhat difficult to get a quick evaluation of platelet function in patients on antiplatelet agents. A normal platelet count does not ensure normal platelet function. Lancet-induced bleeding time is also not a good predictor of platelet function. There are specialized tests to evaluate platelet function, but these are generally not readily available. Examples are flow cytometry, thromboelastography (TEG), and Sonoclot evaluations.

D-Dimer is a test that helps to assess the presence of a hypercoagulation state, which may be present in some stroke patients. There are two main types of stroke: ischemic (85% of all strokes) and hemorrhagic (15%). Ischemic stroke occurs when an obstruction in the arterial system causes ischemia in the brain. Hemorrhagic stroke occurs when a vessel ruptures and bleeds into the brain or into the subarachnoid space (when a large vessel ruptures). In hemorrhagic stroke patients, coagulation increases when fibrinogen is converted to fibrin to form a clot. This process yields fibrin degradation products, and a positive D-dimer test signals a high level of these products in the plasma. (It should be noted that D-dimer is a nonspecific test and may also be elevated following surgery, liver disease, heart disease, and cancer.)

Many more specialized tests are available and may be ordered by a hematologist when caring for a complicated patient. For a patient who requires reversal of anticoagulation, the general approach is to first elucidate the level of anticoagulation and define the mechanism of anticoagulation. Normally, all common coagulation tests (INR, APTT, CBC including platelet count, fibrinogen, and D-dimer) are performed simultaneously to expedite the diagnosis. In the acute patient, more advanced coagulation investigations may not be available in a timely manner, since more sophisticated blood tests require longer processing times.

Treating coagulation disorders. Treatment for coagulation defects in neurologically impaired patients targets specific deficiencies that persist after stopping anticoagulation therapy. For bleeding patients with platelet dysfunction, platelets should be transfused. This is also recommended for patients with a normal platelet count when platelet dysfunction is suspected. The target value for platelet count is 50,000 for patients scheduled for surgery or for patients with hemorrhage that could be life-threatening. The usual recommended dose is 1 U of platelets per 10 kg body weight. One unit of platelets will increase the platelet count by $5–10 \times 10^9$ per liter. (One unit of platelets is 5×10^{10} platelets in 50–70 mL plasma; typically, 5–10 U [random donor platelets] are pooled in one component bag for ease of administration. Apheresis platelets [from a single donor] may also be used and contain $3–5 \times 10^{11}$ platelets in 200–400 mL plasma, equivalent to 4–6 U of platelets. Platelet transfusion is also the treatment of choice for reversal of antiplatelet agents such as clopidogrel.

DDAVP at a dose of 0.3 µg/kg can also be tried to improve coagulation in patients on antiplatelet agents. DDAVP releases factor VIII and Von Willebrand factor and is a manufactured analog of vasopressin without its vasoconstrictive effects. However, like AVP, DDAVP causes antidiuresis and could be associated with congestive heart failure in patients with poor cardiac function. Therefore, smaller doses of DDAVP (e.g., 0.15 µg/kg) should be considered for elderly patients and patients with cardiovascular diseases.

Unfractionated heparin has an antidote in protamine. The usual dose is 1 mg protamine (IV) for each 100 U of heparin given. This dose is reduced by 50% (i.e., 0.5 mg protamine for each 100 U of heparin) at 60–120 min after heparin has been discontinued. The recommended rate of administration is 5 mg protamine per minute. Intravenous protamine can cause hypotension via histamine release as well as more severe reactions such as anaphylaxis and, very rarely, catastrophic pulmonary vasoconstriction (resulting in pulmonary hypertension and vascular collapse). In patients with significant neurologic disease, treatment of these protamine reactions should be primarily supportive, with standard approaches ranging from small boluses of intravenous fluid and intravenous ephedrine (or phenylephrine) to treat hypotension up to full treatment of anaphylaxis with intravenous fluids, epinephrine, anti-histamines, and possibly steroids and intubation, if indicated.

Subcutaneous heparin for prophylaxis of deep vein thrombosis (DVT) is usually not reversed. LMWHs, unfortunately, cannot be fully reversed by protamine. However, some authors recommend 1 mg of protamine (IV) for each milligram of enoxaparin administered over the previous 4–8 h. Anticoagulation by inhibitors of vitamin K-dependent pathways can be reversed by administering vitamin K, either intravenously (risk of anaphylaxis and hypotension) or subcutaneously. In non-life-threatening situations, the recommended dose of vitamin K is 1–2 mg. For life-threatening situations, the recommended dose is 10 mg vitamin K, which accelerates the onset of effect and also presents a higher risk of complication. The higher dose is also associated with some difficulty in subsequent titration of anticoagulation; however, in the case of brain hemorrhage, this becomes a secondary concern. Vitamin K should not be used as sole treatment to reverse anticoagulation because it takes hours to normalize INR. For immediate effect, fresh frozen plasma (FFP) should be infused at 15–20 mL/kg. However, administration of FFP increases the risk for anaphylaxis, blood-borne diseases (e.g., HIV, hepatitis), and fluid overload, with subsequent heart failure, because of the large amount of FFP that may be required to achieve the desired level of improved coagulation.

When clinicians have significant concern about the negative consequences of the large volume of fluid required when using FFP to improve coagulation, an alternate treatment option is to infuse prothrombin complex concentrates at doses based on weight and actual INR and INR goal. Typical doses are 15–50 U/kg. Factor IX concentrates can also be administered.

Recombinant-activated Factor VII is currently being investigated as a treatment for coagulopathy. The FDA indication for clinical administration of recombinant-activated Factor VII is bleeding associated with hemophilia and antibodies to Factors VIII or IX. A wide range of doses has been tested, but the typical dose is approximately 90 μg/kg. Off-label recombinant-activated Factor VII has been used in a variety of clinical bleeding scenarios, including neurosurgical bleeding, with varied results.

Fibrinolytic agents such as tPA can be reversed by 6–8U of platelets or cryoprecipitate (6–8 doses) that contains Factor VIII. No antidotes are known for bleeding due to the administration of direct thrombin inhibitors. Congenital clotting defects and bleeding are best managed with help from an experienced hematologist.

Hypertension and Neurosurgical Disease

Many neurosurgical disease states such as intracerebral hemorrhage, ischemic neurological injury, and carotid artery disease are affected by the blood pressure. Finding an optimal level of blood pressure depends on many factors including severity of chronic hypertension, patient age, and impairment of intracranial compliance (e.g., patients with elevated ICP). Blood pressure control may be particularly critical in patients with (or at risk for) hemorrhage in areas that place neurologic tissue at risk for further injury (e.g., brain or spinal cord).

For individual patients with neurologic injury, the optimal blood pressure range is often difficult to establish. Ideally, the blood pressure range would allow for optimal cerebral perfusion without placing the patient at risk for cerebral hemorrhage or edema. This can be difficult to demonstrate since CT and MRI – the usual scanning methods – are static exams and are impractical for providing information over time. More advanced studies such as PET scanning can give more insight but are not readily available. One study in stroke patients shows a U-shaped blood pressure curve with increased mortality for patients presenting with blood pressures greater than 220/111 or less than 100/61. Hypotension is rare in patients in the acute setting of stroke. When hypotension is observed in this population, potential etiologies include aortic dissection, dehydration, blood loss, sepsis, and decreased cardiac output.

If hypotension is noted, immediate steps should be taken to correct the hypotension and to identify and treat the underlying cause.

Hypertension is more commonly seen in the acute setting following stroke, and the possible etiologies include acute stress, pain, hypoxia, and increased ICP. For patients with intracerebral hemorrhage, the 2007 AHA/ASA guidelines suggest (class IIb evidence) only reducing blood pressure to approximately 160/90 (mean blood pressure 110 mmHg). First-line antihypertensives should be agents that are unlikely to inadvertently raise ICP (e.g., labetalol, nicardipine, esmolol, and enalapril). Significantly increased ICP can manifest as severe impairment following acute stroke, severe hypertension, bradycardia, decreased level of consciousness, and abnormal respirations (i.e., Cushing's reflex). Since these findings are often premorbid, it is critical that the clinician define the nature of the intracranial pathology and treat appropriately. Great caution must be used in administering direct vasodilators to control blood pressure (e.g., nipride and nitroglycerin) as these drugs may cause reduced cerebral perfusion and increased ICP with worsening of neurologic injury.

Cerebral Vasospasm

Following subarachnoid hemorrhage or severe head injury, many patients develop acute cerebral vasospasm causing cerebral ischemia. The current treatment principle is to keep the cerebral perfusion pressure (CPP) above 60–70 mmHg by managing the patient with fluids and vasopressors to ensure adequate perfusion. Following aneurysmal subarachnoid hemorrhage, many centers employ a strategy of pharmacologically induced hypertension and hypervolemia in hopes of facilitating improved cerebral perfusion. This treatment approach places the patient at risk for myocardial dysfunction (an imbalance between myocardial oxygen consumption and supply) and congestive heart failure.

Concerns and Risks

The EKG changes reflect myocardial processes caused by sympathetic stimulation associated with neurosurgical bleeding, even in patients with no organic ischemic cardiac disease. To ensure optimal oxygen delivery to the brain, support of circulation must be initiated when cardiac dysfunction leads to decreased cerebral oxygenation and perfusion. With appropriate hemodynamic monitoring (e.g., invasive arterial pressure, central venous pressure, and possibly pulmonary artery pressure) to guide therapy, standard treatment with inotropes may be necessary for low cardiac output states that have been confirmed by clinical exam and supporting investigations such as echocardiography. Anti-arrhythmics are indicated for hemodynamically significant arrhythmias. These treatments are started in all patients when indicated. A cardiac workup can then be performed to separate the patients with true underlying cardiac disease from patients with only temporary cardiovascular manifestations resulting from their acute neurological condition.

Anticoagulation therapies can worsen the outcome of the neurosurgical process and must often be discontinued after carefully weighing the risk/benefit ratio of continued anticoagulation vs. discontinuation. Patients are placed on anticoagulation treatment for a variety of reasons, and some indications may be weaker than others. For example, some biological cardiac valve prostheses may not need more aggressive anticoagulation than aspirin; on the other hand, cardiac stents require more intensive anticoagulation therapy, and discontinuation would place the patient at risk for catastrophic stent thrombosis – in BMS (bare metal stents) especially the first month and in DES (drug-eluding stents) especially the first year. These treatment decisions are best made in consultation with a cardiologist.

In acute ischemic strokes, acute lowering of the blood pressure may decrease the risk for hemorrhagic transformation (cerebral hemorrhage after an ischemic stroke) and cerebral edema; however, actively lowering the blood pressure can worsen neurological injury by increasing the ischemia in the penumbra (the zone of reversible ischemia surrounding the infarct) because of inadequate driving pressure through a stenosis. In contrast, a blood pressure that is too high can cause increased edema and increased bleeding, especially in patients with ruptured aneurysms or arteriovenous malformations who are at risk for rebleeding.

Consideration should be given to maintaining an adequate CPP, i.e., greater than 70 mmHg. CPP is the difference between mean arterial pressure and the downstream pressure, either the jugular venous pressure or the intracranial pressure, whichever is higher. For stable patients, noninvasive blood pressure monitoring is adequate; but in unstable patients who require continuous intravenous antihypertensives, and in deteriorating patients, an invasive arterial catheter should be considered to provide beat-to-beat monitoring and an easy way to measure metabolic status. Unfortunately, this metabolic information will only reflect the global status and not the focal values that would better guide therapy. For patients with cardiac disease, control of blood pressure is indicated to tip the myocardial oxygen balance in favor of reduced work and, therefore, lower the risk for ischemia.

Key Points

- Signs of myocardial damage without underlying cardiac disease can be present in patients with neurosurgical disease, and these manifestations must be evaluated and treated.
- Rapid and aggressive reversal of anticoagulation may be indicated in patients with critical bleeding in the central nervous system.
- Control of blood pressure is often necessary to mitigate the effects of hypertension on intracerebral hemorrhage. It reduces the risk for rebleeding in patients with hemorrhagic strokes and reduces the risks for cerebral edema and hemorrhagic transformation in patients with ischemic strokes.

Suggested Reading

Morgenstern LB, Hemphill JC 3rd, Anderson C, Becker K, Broderick JP, Connolly ES Jr, Greenberg SM, Huang JN, MacDonald RL, Messé SR, Mitchell PH, Selim M, Tamargo RJ. Guidelines for the management of spontaneous intracerebral hemorrhage: a guideline for healthcare professionals from the American Heart Association/American Stroke Association. American Heart Association Stroke Council and Council on Cardiovascular Nursing. Stroke. 2010;41(9): 2108–29.

Khaja AM. Acute ischemic stroke management: administration of thrombolytics, neuroprotectants, and general principles of medical management. Neurol Clin. 2008;26(4):943–61.

Kopelnik A, Zaroff JG. Neurocardiogenic injury in neurovascular disorders. Crit Care Clin. 2006;22(4):733–52.

Macmillan CS, Grant IS, Andrews PJ. Pulmonary and cardiac sequelae of subarachnoid haemorrhage: time for active management? Intensive Care Med. 2002;28(8):1012–23.

Powner DJ, Hartwell EA, Hoots WK. Counteracting the effects of anticoagulants and antiplatelet agents during neurosurgical emergencies. Neurosurgery 2005;57(5):823–31, discussion 823–31.

Chapter 7
Risk Assessment of Critical Carotid Stenosis Treatment: Suggestions for Perioperative Management

Elizabeth M. Macri

Overview

Carotid stenosis is typically caused by an atherosclerotic plaque that is most commonly found in the internal carotid artery at the point of bifurcation of the common carotid artery. It is classified as asymptomatic if there have been no ischemic events related to it, or symptomatic if there is a history of a stroke or transient ischemia attack (TIA). Carotid stenosis is evaluated by carotid ultrasound, magnetic resonance angiogram (MRA) with or without contrast, CT angiogram (CTA) or angiogram. MRA and ultrasound are typically screening tests, and CTA and/or angiogram are usually done before carotid endarterectomy (CEA) or carotid artery stenting (CAS) to accurately assess the degree of stenosis. Intervention is indicated for those with 70–99% stenosis but not for those with complete occlusion. It may be beneficial for those with 50–69% stenosis in centers known to have a very low surgical morbidity and mortality.

The decision to treat with CEA or CAS is dependent on a number of factors. Those who have early restenosis due to intimal hyperplasia following CEA and require another intervention may benefit from CAS instead. Those who are considered high risk may be better candidates for CAS than CEA. Factors that may make patients high risk include

- Severe cardiac disease
- Severe pulmonary disease
- Contralateral carotid occlusion
- History of neck surgery or neck radiation
- Contralateral laryngeal nerve palsy
- Recurrent stenosis after previous CEA
- Age >80

E.M. Macri, MD (✉)
Neurocritical Care, Presbyterian Hospital, Albuquerque, NM, USA
e-mail: elizabethmacri@yahoo.com

A.M. Brambrink and J.R. Kirsch (eds.), *Essentials of Neurosurgical Anesthesia & Critical Care*, DOI 10.1007/978-0-387-09562-2_7,
© Springer Science+Business Media, LLC 2012

Carotid endarterectomy: An arterial line is placed for intraoperative hemodynamic monitoring and should be maintained for the postoperative period. Fluid use in the neurosurgical patient is typically normal saline without dextrose or Ringer's Lactate.

The skin incision is either made bordering the sternocleidomastoid muscle or transversely over the jugular bulb. This is followed by dissection of overlying tissues away from the common carotid to above the bifurcation. The internal, common and external arteries are clamped sequentially, systemic heparin is given and the artery is then cut longitudinally. The plaque of interest is almost exclusively at the bifurcation and internal carotid artery origin. A vascular shunt may be placed at this time (see below). A dissection plane between the intima and media is made with removal of the plaque. The edges are tapered carefully to avoid leaving a gap that could result in a dissection after blood flow is restored. Repair of the artery may be primary, may involve a graft using the saphenous vein or an artificial patch such as Dacron or polytetrafluoroethylene (PTFE). The distal internal carotid is then unclamped, allowing retrograde flow of debris. The internal carotid artery is then reclamped and the common and external carotids are unclamped. This allows a flushing of debris away from the internal carotid.

Thrombin-soaked gel may be placed over the suture site, and, once hemostasis is achieved, the wound is closed with or without a drain.

Carotid artery stenting: An arterial line is placed for intraoperative hemodynamic monitoring and should be maintained for the postoperative period. Fluid use in the neurosurgical patient is typically normal saline without dextrose or Ringer's Lactate.

The femoral artery is accessed percutaneously followed by 5F short sheath placement. Heparin, 50–80 U/kg is then administered with a goal aPTT of 250–300. A guide wire is advanced to the innominate or left common carotid artery followed by catheter cannulation with subsequent DSA imaging of the distal arterial anatomy of interest. The guide wire is then navigated across the internal carotid lesion. A neuroprotective device in the form of a distal filter or balloon or proximal common and external carotid occlusive device is deployed prior to stent placement. In preparation for hemodynamic changes with carotid bulb expansion, atropine or glycopyrrolate should be ready as well as an IV vasopressor and antihypertensive. A stent or angioplasty balloon plus stent is advanced via catheter to the site of the lesion. The stent may be self-expanding or a balloon-assist device which is then deployed at the site of the lesion. The sheath is removed and the femoral artery is closed with the surgeon's preferred device.

Implications for the Neurosurgical Patient

Preoperative evaluation involves assessing cardiac function, degree of CNS involvement, if any, and degree of CNS reserve.

A thorough neurologic exam should be performed prior to surgery to provide an accurate clinical baseline. A preoperative computed tomography (CT) or magnetic resonance imaging (MRI) of the brain should be done in the symptomatic patient. This can assess the magnitude of the stroke, if any and exclude other CNS disorders that may cause focal neurologic symptoms, such as bleed or mass lesion.

Intracranial aneurysm: An intracranial aneurysm distal to the carotid artery is at risk of rupture secondary to hemodynamic changes during CEA. Clipping an aneurysm in a vascular territory fed by a carotid artery with significant stenosis is associated with a potential risk of ischemia. There is no clear consensus as to which should be treated first – the more symptomatic lesion is generally treated first.

Cardiac disease: Perioperative mortality associated with CEA is <0.5–3%, with a higher risk associated with nontertiary care centers. The major cause of mortality is cardiac events. A preoperative cardiac assessment is of paramount importance. In addition to chest X-ray and EKG, additional cardiac assessment should be performed, including exercise stress testing, dobutamine echocardiography, or dipyridamole imaging, or cardiac catheterization, if indicated.

Those with atherosclerotic disease of the carotid are at risk of atherosclerotic disease of other vessels, in addition to cardiac. A preoperative evaluation for abdominal aortic aneurysm and peripheral vascular disease should be performed.

Aspirin: Antiplatelet therapy with aspirin reduces the risk of stroke of any cause in patients undergoing CEA. Recommended dose is 81–325 mg daily. Consensus guidelines from the American Academy of Neurology (AAN) and the American College of Chest Physicians (ACCP) recommend starting aspirin prior to CEA and continuing indefinitely as long as there are no contraindications [e.g., GI bleeding, history of TTP (thrombotic thrombocytopenic purpura) or history of aspirin allergy]. Recommendation for carotid stenting is to initiate or continue aspirin therapy preoperatively and continue indefinitely postprocedure.

Clopidogrel: For carotid stent patients, clopidogrel should be continued or be started at 75 mg daily 7 days prior to the procedure. For those scheduled for the stenting within 7 days, a 300 mg loading dose should be used followed by 75 mg daily until 30 days after the procedure. Clopidogrel use in CEA patients is typically used for those who are aspirin-intolerant.

Statins have shown benefit in symptomatic patient preoperatively and may have benefit in asymptomatic patients. Discontinuation prior to surgery may result in a loss of this benefit. Perioperative use of statins may be of benefit.

Concerns and Risks

Complications Associated with Carotid Endarterectomy

- Carotid clamping with risk of ischemia

    - Preoperative assessment of risk
    - Intraoperative monitoring
    - Selective shunting

- Hemodynamic lability
- Reperfusion syndrome

- Postoperative stroke
- Local versus general anesthesia
- Postoperative hematoma
- Nerve damage

Complications Associated with Carotid Stenosis

- Stroke
- Reperfusion/hyperperfusion syndrome
- Hemodynamic lability
- Carotid stent fracture
- Restenosis
- Dissection

As mentioned previously, both procedures are associated with a cardiac risk. Possible independent risk factors for poor outcome (30 day mortality) following carotid intervention include: age ≥ 80, severe heart disease, severe lung disease, renal failure or insufficiency, diabetes, stroke as the indication for intervention, poor preoperative functional status, limited surgical access, prior cervical irradiation, prior ipsilateral CEA, contralateral carotid occlusion.

Possible independent risk factors for stroke within 30 days of surgery include intraoperative transfusion, baseline hemiplegia, shorter height (likely representing smaller artery size), and increased intraoperative anesthesia time.

Assessing risk/tolerance of carotid clamping: The internal carotid artery is clamped during CEA surgery, exposing the associated hemisphere to hypoperfusion. If there is a cerebrovascular reserve in the form of flow from collaterals, the patient may be able to tolerate this ischemia. Assessment of cerebrovascular reserve can be done using preoperative TCD or acetazolamide brain-perfusion testing.

Preoperative assessment of risk: TCD can be used preoperatively to measure the degree of decrease of MCA mean flow velocity when the internal carotid artery is compressed. Acetazolamide stress brain-perfusion SPECT or MRI perfusion with acetazolamide can be used in high-risk patients to assess vascular response and determine the need for intraoperative shunt.

Intraoperative monitoring: 80–85% of patients tolerate carotid artery clamping without suffering ischemic complications. Predicting those who are less likely to tolerate it well is part of preoperative management in the form of assessing vascular reserve capacity with good collateral flow via the circle of Willis. Establishing which patients will not tolerate carotid artery clamping may be performed in a number of ways intraoperatively.

- Frequent neurologic assessment in the patient having CEA with local anesthesia only.
- Continuous intraoperative EEG monitoring – with emergence of slow waves (delta/theta/disorganization) indicating the need for selective shunting.

• Measuring stump pressures may be performed – with high pressures (50–60 mmHg) indicating adequate collateral flow and low pressures indicating the need for shunt. The stump pressure is also referred to a "back pressure" and is the pressure distal to the carotid clamping which is typically measured invasively. There is little evidence to support the use of this variable.

Selective shunting: A shunt between the common carotid and the internal carotid distal to the surgical site. This is indicated for evidence of cerebral ischemia. There is an associated risk of intimal tear resulting in carotid dissection when normal flow is restored.

Labile blood pressure: Manipulation of the carotid bulb can cause hypertension or hypotension. Hypotension increases the risk of ischemic cerebral injury. Elevated blood pressure can occur with increased risk of bleeding if there is reperfusion injury as well as increased risk of surgical site tear or neck hematoma. Hemodynamic instability during carotid manipulation may be prevented by asking the surgeon to inject local anesthetic into the adventitia over the carotid bulb. Blood pressure is most labile for 12–24 h after surgery which warrants constant postoperative constant monitoring with an intra-arterial catheter.

Reperfusion syndrome: 1–3% of patient have reperfusion syndrome after CEA or 1.1% after carotid stenting, characterized by intracranial hemorrhage or seizures within the first 2 weeks. Although this typically occurs when MCA flow is 200–300% greater than preoperative rates, it can occur with an increase of as little as 20% and may therefore occur at "normal" systemic blood pressures because of altered autoregulation.

Reperfusion syndrome typically presents with a headache, worse when lying down, may present with seizures with a subsequent Todd's paralysis mimicking stroke and may have petechial or frank cerebral hemorrhage. Hemorrhage occurs in 0.5% of patients after a CEA, usually within the first 2 weeks.

Reperfusion syndrome should be evaluated with imaging studies such as a CT head or MRI. Perfusion weighted imaging (PWI) shows increased cerebral blood flow (CBF) in the hemisphere served by the postoperative carotid that is increased anywhere from 20 to 300% above the contralateral hemisphere. Transcranial Doppler (TCD) studies may not reveal increased middle cerebral artery velocities and their use to predict reperfusion syndrome has not been reliably substantiated.

Possible risks for reperfusion syndrome include greater than 80% preoperative stenosis, recent cerebral infarct, decreased cerebral vasoreactivity preoperatively and reduced preoperative CBF.

Minimizing the risk of reperfusion is best done by strict control of the blood pressure below a systolic blood pressure of 150. Aggressive control with nicardipine, labetolol, esmolol, or enalaprilat intravenously may be indicated. Avoid the use of vasodilators that may increase cerebral blood flow and intracranial pressure such as nitroglycerine, nitroprusside, and hydralazine. This tight blood pressure goal should be started as soon as blood flow is restored and maintained for 10–14 days after the procedure. Most labile blood pressure issues resolve within 24 h of surgery.

Hemorrhage should be managed with tight blood pressure control – systolic blood pressure <140, reversal of heparin if present and platelet transfusion if anti-platelets have been used.

Seizures due to reperfusion syndrome should be managed with antiepileptics such as phenytoin (Dilantin) – 20 mg/kg loading dose at 50 mg/min IV, or fosphenytoin (Cerebyx) – 20 mg/kg phenytoin equivalents (PE) loading dose at 150 mg/min IV.

Postoperative stroke: This may be assessed by portable ultrasound, angiography, or immediate return to the OR for suspected CEA site clotting. Early research has shown greater benefit from angiography with stenting versus repeat surgery for clot removal. Starting a heparin drip in these patients may be done immediately but a CT scan of the head would be justified to rule out intracranial hemorrhage.

Local versus general anesthesia: For CEA, local versus general anesthesia is generally the choice of the surgeon in consultation with the anesthesiologist and there has been no documented difference in mortality or 30-day risk of stroke between the two. If the patient is a poor general anesthesia candidate, regional anesthesia in the form of a superficial cervical plexus block may be performed. Local anesthesia with sedation is typically performed for carotid stenting and allows for an accurate intraprocedural neurologic exam.

Postoperative hematoma: Postoperative hematoma is more common in those on anticoagulation. There is also a greater risk of neck hematoma in those undergoing combined CEA and CABG. This is often managed conservatively but may require a return to the OR for surgical control of the bleeding source. Venous oozing may be managed with heparin reversal using protamine and careful direct pressure for several minutes. Rarely, a neck hematoma, following CEA, may result in airway obstruction. Under these circumstances, opening the wound at the bedside, prior to gaining definitive control in the OR, may be life saving.

Nerve damage: A number of nerves may be damaged during CEA surgery:

1. Vagus nerve – lies in the carotid sheath with the carotid artery and jugular vein and is at risk.
2. Recurrent laryngeal nerve – presents with unilateral vocal cord paralysis.
3. Facial nerve – marginal mandibular branch affecting lateral orbicularis oris muscle resulting in lower facial asymmetry.
4. Hypoglossal nerve – protrusion of tongue yields deviation toward side of injury.
5. Trigeminal nerve – with sensory loss in areas affected.
6. Ansa hypoglossus – innervates the strap muscles of the neck – may be sacrificed during surgery.
7. Sympathetic chain – causing ipsilateral Horner's syndrome.

Most cranial nerve injuries are temporary with only 0.5% of patients suffering from one at 4 months. The only risk factor for cranial nerve injury is surgery longer than 2 h.

Parotitis can occur secondary to manipulation during surgery, but this is uncommon.

Oxygen concentration: For CEA patients, oxygen concentration should be kept as low as possible while maintaining good oxygen saturation in patients who do not have an endotracheal tube or laryngeal mask airway to decrease the risk of intraoperative fire during a surgery that involves the use of electrocautery in the head or neck region.

Bilateral CEA: The risk of neck hematoma, laryngeal nerve damage and bilateral cerebral ischemia has led to the staged procedure with each CEA being performed a week or more apart.

Restenosis: This may be early (within 3 years) or late (greater than 3 years) and may warrant a repeat surgery. Early restenosis risk factors are age <65, female gender and smoking. Repeat surgery is associated with increased risk of stroke or death at 30 days compared to initial surgery. This risk is less if stenosis recurs within 2 years as this is most likely due to intimal hyperplasia, not plaque formation.

Acute or subacute restenosis can occur with 0.5–2% of carotid stents. Stenosis beyond 30 days is typically due to neointimal hyperplasia. Drug-eluting stents are rarely used for carotid stents and the use of bare metal stents warrants the use of aspirin indefinitely and of clopidogrel for a variable length of time postprocedure.

Key Points

- The highest risk of mortality in post-CEA patients is from cardiac causes. Investigation and medical optimization of these patients is crucial.
- Tight blood pressure control must be instituted as soon as flow is returned to the internal carotid artery during surgery and must be maintained for 1–14 days – the first 24 h are the most labile and the most critical.
- Patients are at risk for reperfusion injury with intracranial hemorrhage and seizures which must be treated with reversal of anticoagulation, platelets, tight blood pressure control and antiepileptics, as indicated.
- Close postoperative monitoring of hemodynamic and neurologic status in a critical care setting for at least the first 24 h is often indicated.

Suggested Readings

Adhiyaman V, Alexander S. Cerebral hyperperfusion syndrome following carotid endarterectomy. QJM. 2007;100(4):239–44.

Anderson CS, Huang Y, et al. Intensive blood pressure reduction in acute cerebral haemorrhage trial (INTERACT): a randomised pilot trial. Lancet Neurol. 2008;7(5):391–9.

Fisher JE, editor. Mastery of surgery. 5th ed. Philadelphia, PA: Lippincott Williams & Wilkins; 2007.

Hans J, Wilke II, Ellis JE, McKinsey JF. Carotid endarterectomy: perioperative and anesthetic considerations. J Cardiothorac Vasc Anesth. 1996;10(7):928–49.

Mulholland MW, Lillemoe KD, et al. Greenfield's surgery: scientific principles and practice. 4th ed. Philadelphia, PA: Lippincott Williams & Wilkins; 2006.

Chapter 8
Subarachnoid Hemorrhage: Risk Assessment and Perioperative Management

Chanhung Z. Lee, Pekka Talke, and Susan Ryan

Overview

Blood in the subarachnoid space is usually a result of a ruptured cerebral arterial aneurysm but also can be due to a ruptured arteriovenous malformation, tumor, embolic stroke, or trauma. In this chapter, we will focus on subarachnoid hemorrhage (SAH) from rupture of a cerebral aneurysm. An estimated 1–5% of adults harbor intracranial aneurysms. In the USA alone, each year there are at least 30,000 patients who have SAH due to rupture of a cerebral aneurysm.

Implications for the Neurosurgical Patients

The morbidity and mortality rates are very high in aneurysmal SAH patients. About 20% patients die before reaching a hospital, 25% die subsequently from the initial hemorrhage or its complications, and 20% die from rebleeding. Up to 50% of survivors will have long-term neurological deficits.

Institutional factors have been shown to influence the outcome after aneurysmal SAH. Treatment of a ruptured cerebral aneurysm consists of surgical clipping or endovascular coil embolization. Proper perioperative care is vital to facilitate therapeutic interventions and to reduce morbidity and mortality in this high-risk patient population. This chapter will focus on the management of aneurysmal SAH-related perioperative complications and concerns relating to neuroanesthesia.

C.Z. Lee, MD, PhD (✉) • P. Talke, MD • S. Ryan, MD, PhD
Department of Anesthesia and Perioperative Care, University of California, San Francisco
School of Medicine, San Francisco, CA, USA
e-mail: clee4@anesthesia.ucsf.edu

A.M. Brambrink and J.R. Kirsch (eds.), *Essentials of Neurosurgical
Anesthesia & Critical Care*, DOI 10.1007/978-0-387-09562-2_8,
© Springer Science+Business Media, LLC 2012

Concerns and Risks

Typical initial medical measures after aneurysmal SAH include mild sedation and analgesics for anxiety and headache, prevention of arterial blood pressure elevation, and avoidance of antiplatelet agents. Blood pressure frequently rises precipitously as a result of the initial intracranial hemorrhage, presumably as a result of acute elevation of intracranial pressure (e.g., Cushing response). Unbearable headache and anxiety may also be contributing factors. Placement of an intra-arterial catheter enables continuous blood pressure monitoring and helps to guide blood pressure management. It is reasonable to maintain systolic blood pressure below 150–160 mmHg. Beta-blockers and short-acting calcium channel blockers are commonly used to control hypertension. Coexisting intracranial hypertension may impair cerebral perfusion. Systemic hypotension, therefore, should be avoided.

Airway and Ventilation Management

Most patients with aneurysmal SAH will be intubated during the surgery or procedure in which the aneurysm is treated. However, earlier endotracheal intubation and mechanical ventilation may be required in some patients with significant decline of consciousness and in those experiencing seizures. In these patients, inability to protect the airway may lead to aspiration, often resulting in pneumonitis or pneumonia. Mechanical ventilation may also be needed in patients that have neurogenic or cardiogenic pulmonary edema. To keep the patient comfortable and easy to wake up for neurological exam, propofol or dexmedetomidine are good choices for sedation during mechanical ventilation.

Current goals of mechanical ventilation in SAH patients are to support adequate oxygenation and to maintain normocarbia. Both hypoventilation and hyperventilation should be avoided unless specifically indicated. Hypoventilation can lead to cerebral vasodilation and increase in intracranial pressure (ICP), while hyperventilation may cause vasoconstriction and worsen cerebral ischemia. Transmural pressure, defined as the difference between mean arterial pressure (MAP) and ICP, is an indication of aneurysm wall tension. Inadvertent hyperventilation may decrease ICP and, as a consequence, increase transmural pressure across the aneurysm; this can potentially lead to rerupture of the aneurysm. In the event of dangerously high ICP, transient hyperventilation may be indicated to reduce ICP. This should help to prevent global hypoperfusion while other more definitive interventions are considered.

Aneurysm Rerupture

Recurrence of aneurysmal hemorrhage is a major acute complication after SAH and carries significant catastrophic risks. The incidence of rebleeding from a ruptured aneurysm is around 30% in the first month following SAH, with the peak in the first 7 days. Rerupture is associated with a 60% mortality and poor outcome. Early treatment of the aneurysm reduces the risk of rebleeding.

Rebleeding from the cerebral aneurysm is a major intraoperative complication with incidence around 20%. Intraoperative rupture of the aneurysm results in high morbidity and mortality. Although intraoperative aneurysm rerupture is most commonly due to surgical manipulation of the aneurysm, prevention of aneurysm rerupture by aggressively limiting the degree and duration of systemic hypertension has been one of the major goals for the anesthesiologist. Maintaining a stable transmural pressure and adequate cerebral perfusion pressure should be central to anesthesia managements. Significant increase in MAP or decrease in ICP will increase transmural pressure, which may precipitate the rupture of the aneurysmal vessel wall.

A deep plane of anesthesia should be ensured to prevent acute increases in blood pressure during stressful events, such as laryngoscopy and endotracheal intubation, head pinning, tissue dissection, and dural opening. Careful and incremental administration of medications such as propofol and short-acting narcotics can be used for induction of anesthesia to ensure the stability of cerebral perfusion. Meticulous care is needed to control ventilation. In patients without intracranial hypertension, the goal is to keep the patient normocarbic, avoiding decreases in ICP before the dura is opened, while subsequent mild hyperventilation may be used to relax the brain to facilitate surgical explorations and to reduce the potential damage from tissue retraction. Generous application of local anesthetics can help to avoid acute cardiovascular effects secondary to head pinning and extradural tissue dissection.

During surgical clipping, maintaining adequate blood pressure is important to ensure adequate cerebral perfusion to reduce injury from ischemic insults. Intraoperatively, blood pressure is typically controlled to maintain cerebral perfusion pressure between 70–90 mmHg. Intraoperative hypotension may increase the risk for retractor-induced cerebral ischemia and injury. Transient induced hypotension may be infrequently requested by the surgeon immediately prior to clipping the aneurysm to allow for more secure placement of the permanent clip on the neck of the aneurysm. In addition, if intraoperative aneurysm rupture occurs, induced hypotension will decrease the rate of bleeding into the surgical field, thereby helping the surgeon gain better control. In contrast, induced hypertension may be needed to raise blood pressure above baseline levels to augment collateral blood flow if the surgeon applies temporary clipping of the feeding arteries to reduce the rupture risk of the aneurysm during surgical manipulation of the dome. Although use of temporary clips decrease the risk of rebleeding during surgical manipulation, this practice results in an area of cerebral ischemia, which can be minimized by the use of controlled hypertension. Blood pressure management can also be guided by intraoperative neurophysiological monitoring, such as somatosensory-evoked potential and motor-evoked potential monitoring. An extensive review of endovascular treatment of ruptured aneurysms is discussed elsewhere in this book.

Postoperative hypertension is not uncommon after aneurysm clipping. It should be treated cautiously using intermittent boluses of beta-blockers and/or intravenous infusions of short-acting vasodilators. Excessive hypertension may result in the formation of brain edema and a hematoma, while hypotension may increase the risk for cerebral ischemia secondary for postsurgical traction edema, perforator vessel occlusion, and regional cerebral vasospasm.

Elevation of Intracranial Pressure

Cerebral aneurysmal rupture can cause a sudden rise in ICP, which accounts for the sudden onset of a severe headache and transient loss of consciousness that occur in half of the patients with aneurysmal SAH. The development of acute hydrocephalus can also cause a rapid rise in ICP. Patients with increased ICP may develop stupor and coma. Increased ICP can be gradually lowered by use of osmotic diuretics (e.g., mannitol or hypertonic saline), and the placement of a ventriculostomy. Elevation of the head to 30° will improve venous outflow and thereby facilitate the control of ICP. Perioperatively, patients with intracranial hypertension can be slightly hyperventilated.

Subacute hydrocephalus may also increase ICP and can develop over days or weeks, presumably due to occlusion of arachnoid granulations. Subacute hydrocephalus can be associated with impaired mentation and should be differentiated from vasospasm-induced neurologic changes. Temporary external ventricular drain or permanent CSF diversion is recommended in symptomatic patients to treat subacute hydrocephalus.

Cardiac Complications

SAH-related various cardiac abnormalities are fairly common. 40 to 70% of SAH patients exhibit abnormal ECG tracings, ranging from ST segment changes, T-wave abnormalities, QT prolongation, new U waves to life-threatening arrhythmias. SAH initiated neurocardiogenic injury may result in myocardiac cell damage and ventricular dysfunction, which, in turn, are also associated with adverse neurological outcome. The degree of cardiac morbidity is often related to the severity of the SAH.

The mainstay of treatment should be supportive. Electrolyte abnormalities should be corrected. Drugs that can potentially prolong QT interval should be avoided. In the event of clinically significant cardiac arrhythmia and myocardial injury, an urgent cardiology consultation is recommended for further evaluation.

Vasospasm

Vasospasm refers to the narrowing of the cerebral arteries at the base of the brain following SAH, secondary to thickening of the blood vessel walls. It usually develops

3–14 days after the initial hemorrhage, with the prevalence as high as 30–70%. Vasospasm is a major threat to life in patients surviving the treatment after SAH. Signs of new onset of neurological deterioration from cerebral ischemia and/or infarction are usually the warning presentations of cerebral vasospasm. Diagnosis of cerebral vasospasm can be made with transcranial Doppler or cerebral angiography.

The goal for the management of cerebral vasospasm is to reduce the threat of ischemic neuronal damage by controlling intracranial pressure, decreasing metabolic rate of cerebral oxygen consumption, and improving cerebral blood flow. Early oral nimodipine therapy has been shown to reduce poor outcome related to SAH. Some evidence also points at a role for nicardipine, an intravenous calcium channel blocker, in reducing vasospasm and brain ischemia after SAH.

A mainstay in treatment for acute symptomatic vasospasm includes the combination of triple "H"s – hypertension (mainly after the aneurysm has been treated), hypervolemia, and hemodilution. The target for the treatment is to raise the systolic blood pressure 20% above a patient's baseline blood pressure using vasopressors (e.g., phenylephrine and dopamine) to reach a central venous pressure of 8–12 cm H_2O using intravenous fluids, and to allow hematocrit to remain in the low 30s. It is imperative to monitor and manage the potential risks of the above-mentioned hemodynamic therapy, including cardiac failure, electrolyte abnormality, cerebral edema, and bleeding diathesis resulting from dilution of clotting factors.

At some centers, endovascular treatment of vasospasm using balloon angioplasty and/or super selective injection of intra-arterial vasodilators is becoming common. The anesthesiologists should be prepared to manage possible systemic hypotension resulting from intra-arterial injection of vasodilators.

Seizures

Seizures occur in 10–20% of SAH patients, and these patients require anticonvulsant therapy. American Stroke Association recommends consideration of prophylactic anticonvulsant treatment in the immediate posthemorrhagic period; however, this is based on very little data and remains controversial. The routine long-term use of anticonvulsants for SAH patients is not recommended, but may be considered for patients with risk factors including prior seizures, parenchymal hematoma and/or infarction, or middle cerebral artery aneurysms.

Hyponatremia

Hyponatremia occurs in about 10–30% patients after SAH and can develop in the first 2 weeks after SAH. The majority of the cases occur as a result of cerebral salt-wasting syndrome (CSWS), although a smaller portion of patients may develop a syndrome of inappropriate anti-diuretic hormone (SIADH) after SAH. It is important to distinguish these two underlying causes of hyponatremia since intravascular volume is usually contracted in the former, but normal or elevated in the latter. For most SAH patients, therefore, hyponatremia should not be routinely treated with the conventional free-water-restriction approach since it may increase the risk for ischemia-induced injuries from intravascular volume contraction. It is reasonable to monitor intravascular volume status, frequently check serum electrolytes, and treat the volume contraction with isotonic fluids. Medical therapies such as hypertonic saline and fludocortisone acetate may be useful to correct severe hyponatremia.

Summary

Proper perioperative monitoring and management of SAH-induced complications is critical to help improve patients' outcome. Although there are only a few areas in the management of SAH for which there is conclusive evidence from randomized, controlled clinical studies, this chapter summarized the principles currently used to manage patients with aneurysmal SAH in the perioperative period.

Key Points

- Securing the airway and proper ventilation control may be required prior to the treatment of the ruptured cerebral aneurysm in patients with severe decline of consciousness and/or seizures.
- Close monitoring and adequate control of intracranial pressure and blood pressure are critical in prevention of aneurysm rerupture pre- and intraoperatively.
- Intracranial hypertension should be diagnosed and treated promptly.
- Caution against vasospasm should remain high in patients after SAH. It can be treated using conventional triple "H" therapy and/or endovascular interventions. It is important to monitor and be ready to manage treatment-related complications.
- Hyponatremia most likely develops as a result of cerebral salt-wasting syndrome after SAH. Appropriate treatment is important to avoid the risk of worsening brain ischemia after SAH.

Suggested Reading

Benderson JB, Connolly ES, Batjer HH, et al. Guidelines for the management of aneurysmal subarachnoid hemorrhage: a statement for healthcare professionals from a special writing group of
   the Stroke Council, American Heart Association. Stroke. 2009;40:994–1025.

Bendo AA, Kass IS, Hartung J, Cottrell JE. Anesthesia for neurosurgery. In: Barash PG, Cullen
   BF, Stoelting RK, editors. Clinical anesthesia. 5th ed. Philadelphia, PA: Lippincott, Williams
   & Wilkins; 2006. Chapter 28.

Drummond JC, Patel PM. Neurosurgical anesthesia. In: Miller RD, editor. Miller's anesthesia,
   vol. II. 7th ed. New York: Churchill Livingstone; 2009. Sect. 4: Chap. 63.

Rabinstein AA. The AHA guidelines for the management of SAH: what we know and so much we
   need to learn. Neurocrit Care. 2009;10(3):414–7. Epub April 24, 2009.

Stevens RD, Nyquisr PA. The systemic implications of aneurysmal subarachnoid hemorrhage.
   J Neurol Sci. 2007;261(1–2):143–56.

Chapter 9
Traumatic Brain Injury: Risk Assessment and Perioperative Management

Lingzhong Meng

Overview

Traumatic injury is the third leading cause of death in the USA. For traumatic brain injury (TBI), approximately 1.4 million cases are reported in the USA each year, among which roughly 50,000 patients die and 235,000 are hospitalized. For spinal cord injury (SCI), the incidence has remained stable over the past 30 years in North America, ranging between 27 and 47 cases per million, 55% of which are cervical spine (C-spine) injuries – the most common anatomic region for SCI. In a polytrauma patient, TBI or SCI is often involved. Indeed, approximately one-third of the fatalities after multisystem traumatic injury (150,000 deaths) each year is due to fatal head injuries; C-spine injuries occur in 1.5 to 3% of all major trauma patients.

Implications for the Neurosurgical Patients

The early diagnosis and management of TBI or SCI is of paramount importance in terms of preventing further injury immediately after initial injury and preserving neurologic function. However, life-threatening situations, including airway, breathing, and circulation (ABC), must take priority. Needless to say, protecting the injured brain or spinal cord during the ABC action is important. For example, avoid nasal intubation in patients with basilar skull fracture and use in-line manual stabilization in patients with unstable C-spine.

L. Meng, MD (✉)
Department of Anesthesiology & Perioperative Care, University of California Irvine
Medical Center, Orange, CA, USA
e-mail: meng.lingzhong@gmail.com

A.M. Brambrink and J.R. Kirsch (eds.), *Essentials of Neurosurgical Anesthesia & Critical Care*, DOI 10.1007/978-0-387-09562-2_9,
© Springer Science+Business Media, LLC 2012

Concerns and Risks

The management of TBI and SCI, especially in a serious polytrauma situation is challenging. The most pertinent and urgent perioperative concerns and risks in managing neurotrauma patients are as follows:

- Jeopardized airway: This may be caused by impaired consciousness, direct injury to face and neck, and/or full stomach and aspiration. Airway is always the number one priority.
- Inadequate ventilation and oxygenation: This may be caused by obstructed airway, depressed central drive, neuromuscular weakness caused by high C-spine injury, or thoracic injuries such as pulmonary contusion, pneumothorax, hemothorax, or multiple rib fractures. Avoiding hypercapnia will facilitate intracranial pressure management; avoiding hypoxemia is crucial in preventing secondary injury to both brain and spinal cord.
- Hypovolemia and hypotension: This often occurs in a multisystem trauma patient. Rarely, isolated brain and/or spinal cord injury cause massive bleeding if the patient is not pharmacologically anticoagulated before the injury. Nonetheless, treating hypotension via fluid resuscitation is the standard of care in neurotrauma patients.
- Anemia and coagulopathy: Acute and massive hemorrhage can cause concerning low hematocrit (inadequate O_2 content and delivery and low blood viscosity; threshold value unclear and under debate) and coagulation abnormality (worsening bleeding) in neurotrauma patients if relevant blood products are inadequately administered. Severe hypothermia and acidosis can further aggravate massive transfusion-associated coagulopathy. Also, severe TBI-associated coagulopathy is a well-known phenomenon. Therefore, early and goal-directed blood product therapy is important for severely injured neurotrauma patients (endpoint targets are controversial).
- Elevated intracranial pressure (ICP): Intracranial hemorrhage and cerebral edema can cause intracranial hypertension. The impaired cerebral perfusion pressure (CPP = Mean arterial pressure – ICP) causes decreased cerebral blood flow (CBF), which is detrimental to the already injured brain. Before surgical intervention, measures, such as head of bed up 30°, hyperventilation, mannitol, loop diuretics, hypertonic saline, cerebrospinal fluid drainage, or thiopental, etc., need to be instituted as soon as possible based on the severity of intracranial hypertension.
- Unstable C-spine: The implication of unstable or uncleared C-spine is twofold. One, it challenges the airway management. Two, it mandates spinal cord protection when transporting and positioning patients to prevent further injury.

The multiple relevant issues are summarized in the following discussion.

Glasgow Coma Scale and TBI Severity

Glasgow Coma Scale (GCS), first proposed by Teasdale and Jennett in 1974, is currently the most widely used clinical measure for severity of TBI. The GCS must

Table 9.1 Glasgow coma scale

Eyes opening	Spontaneous	4
	Speech	3
	Pain	2
	None	1
Verbal response	Oriented	5
	Confused	4
	Inappropriate	3
	Incomprehensible	2
	None	1
Motor response	Obeys commands	6
	Localize pain	5
	Flexor withdrawal	4
	Flexor posturing (decorticate rigidity)	3
	Extensor posturing (decerebrate rigidity)	2
	None	1
Total		3–15

be obtained through interaction with the patient and should be measured after initial resuscitation has been performed and prior to the administration of sedative or paralytic agents. A score of 14–15 is defined as mild TBI, 9–13 as moderate, 5–8 as severe, and 3–4 as critical (Table 9.1).

Primary Survey in Polytrauma Patients with Coexisting TBI and SCI

The advanced trauma life support (ATLS) primary survey should be used as the guideline for managing a patient after traumatic injury, and consists of simultaneous diagnostic and therapeutic activities intended to identify and treat life- and limb-threatening injuries, beginning with the most immediate. The ABCDE acronym of primary survey is shown in Fig. 9.1.

Airway Management After Traumatic Injury

A successful early resuscitation and a promising long-term outcome depend on expert airway management. This is especially true when TBI is present in the context of SCI in a multisystem trauma patient. The airway management algorithm after traumatic injury is presented in Fig. 9.2; however, variation can exist from institution to institution and provider to provider as long as the fundamentals are followed. Note that this algorithm differs from ASA algorithm in that: (1) reawakening the patient is seldom an option in a truly emergent situation, (2) awake fiberoptic intubation is often counterproductive in an uncooperative trauma patient,

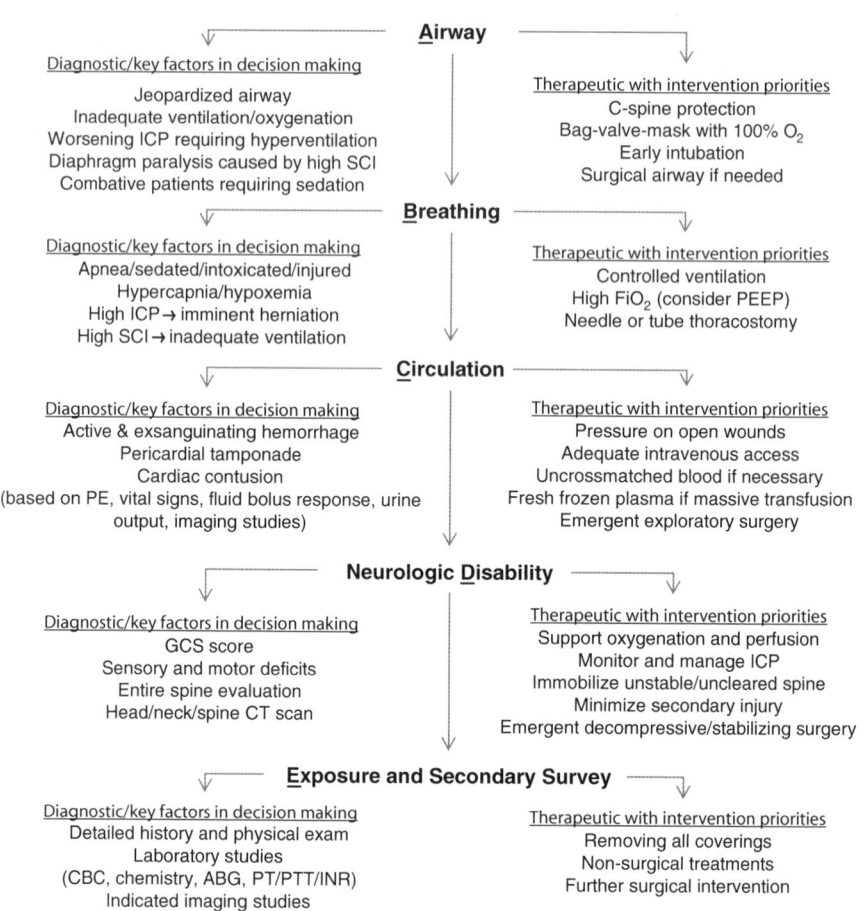

Fig. 9.1 Diagnostic and therapeutic principles of ATLS primary survey (ABCDE) in polytrauma patients with coexisting TBI and/or SCI. *ICP* intracranial pressure, *FiO₂* inspired oxygen fraction, *PEEP* positive end-expiratory pressure, *PE* physical exam, *GCS* glasgow coma scale, *CT* computed tomography, *CBC* complete blood count, *ABG* arterial blood gas, *PT* prothrombin time, *PTT* partial thromboplastin time, *INR* international normalized ratio, *FAST* focused assessment by sonography for trauma. (*Adapted from the Advanced Trauma Life Support curriculum of the American College of Surgeons.*)

and (3) glidescope is advantageous due to the fact that it requires less neck flexion/extension which is desirable in a patient with unstable or uncleared C-spine.

Resuscitation After Traumatic Injury with Coexisting TBI and SCI

Resuscitation, in a broad sense, refers to the restoration of normal physiology after injury. Resuscitation commences immediately after injury, beginning with the patient's own compensatory mechanisms, and continues for hours and even days

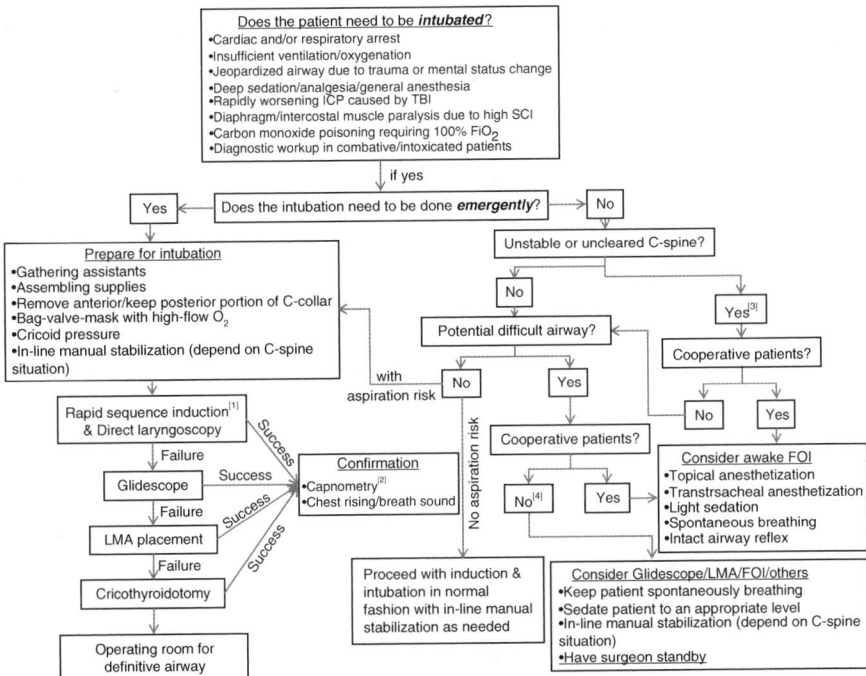

Fig. 9.2 Airway management algorithm in patients with traumatic injury [1]. The dose of anesthetic must be decreased in the face of hemorrhage, down to none at all in patients with severe hypovolemia; scopolamine or midazolam can be considered in order to inhibit memory formation in situations where none or very small dose of quick-offset anesthetics is being administered; etomidate is advocated due to its better cardiovascular stability profile; succinylcholine can be safely used in the first 24 h after traumatic injuries; ketamine is not advocated in patients with TBI who are not mechanically ventilated [2]. Capnometry may show low CO_2 level in low cardiac output situations [3]. In-line manual stabilization is the standard of care in the ATLS curriculum for unstable or uncleared C-spine [4]. If difficult airway is anticipated in an uncooperative patient, it is prudent to sedate the patient to an appropriate level while keeping him/her spontaneously breathing due to the dilemma that awake intubation is often counterproductive in a combative patient and making the patient apneic is risky; having alternative plans ready to be instituted is well-advised, which include glidescope, LMA, fiberoptic scope, and surgical airway by having a surgeon standby. *ICP* intracranial pressure, *FiO2* inspired oxygen fraction, *LMA* laryngeal mask airway, *FOI* fiberoptic intubation

thereafter. The cornerstone of clinical resuscitation after traumatic injury is fluid resuscitation to replete the depleted intravascular volume caused by acute hemorrhage. The early phase of resuscitation refers to the efforts of replacing intravascular volume and controlling active bleeding in a parallel or simultaneous manner, while the late phase of resuscitation deals with posthemorrhage fluid and/or blood product administration to optimize oxygen delivery and tissue perfusion.

The endpoint targets of early resuscitation are a matter of controversy due to the side effects caused by aggressive volume replacement, which include decreased blood viscosity, low hematocrit, and inadequate clotting factors, to name a few. Deliberate hypotension via restraining resuscitation volume is proposed in an effort to reduce the physiologic derangements caused by aggressive resuscitative approach;

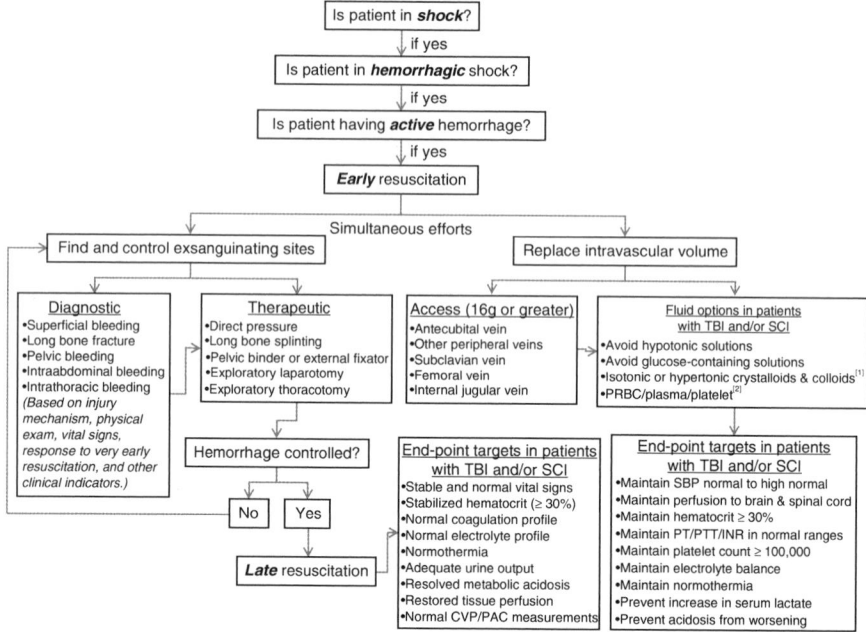

Fig. 9.3 Simplified resuscitation principles for a patient in acute hemorrhagic shock after polytrauma with coexisting TBI and/or SCI [1]. Both crystalloids and colloids are lacking oxygen-carrying capacity and coagulation capability. Colloids have a longer intravascular half-life and can restore intravascular volume more rapidly at a lower administered volume than crystalloids [2]. PRBC is the mainstay of treatment in hemorrhagic shock. Plasma is indicated for the treatment of coagulopathy that arises during resuscitation. One unit of plasma for each unit of PRBC is generally required in a massive transfusion situation (one blood volume or about 10 units of PRBCs); plasma is not usually necessary with the transfusion requirement of 1 to 4 units of PRBCs; the need for plasma is variable and better guided by coagulation studies when 5 to 9 units of PRBCs are given. Transfused platelets have a very short serum half-life and should generally be administered only to patients with visible coagulopathy or to TBI patients whose platelet counts are lower than 100,000. IV, intravenous; *PRBC* packed red blood cell, *SBP* systolic blood pressure, *CVP* central venous pressure, *PAC* pulmonary artery catheter, *PT* prothrombin time, *PTT* partial thromboplastin time, *INR* international normalized ratio

however, this approach is not encouraged in a polytrauma patient with coexisting TBI and/or SCI. Maintaining normal to high normal blood pressure, to maintain brain and/or spinal cord perfusion pressure, is the current standard of care in a patient with injured brain and/or spinal cord. Simplified resuscitation principles for a patient in acute hemorrhagic shock after polytrauma with coexisting TBI and/or SCI are presented in Fig. 9.3.

Development of Secondary Injury of Brain

Conventionally, primary injury refers to the brain damage incurred at the moment of impact and secondary injury to the damage that evolves over the ensuing minutes,

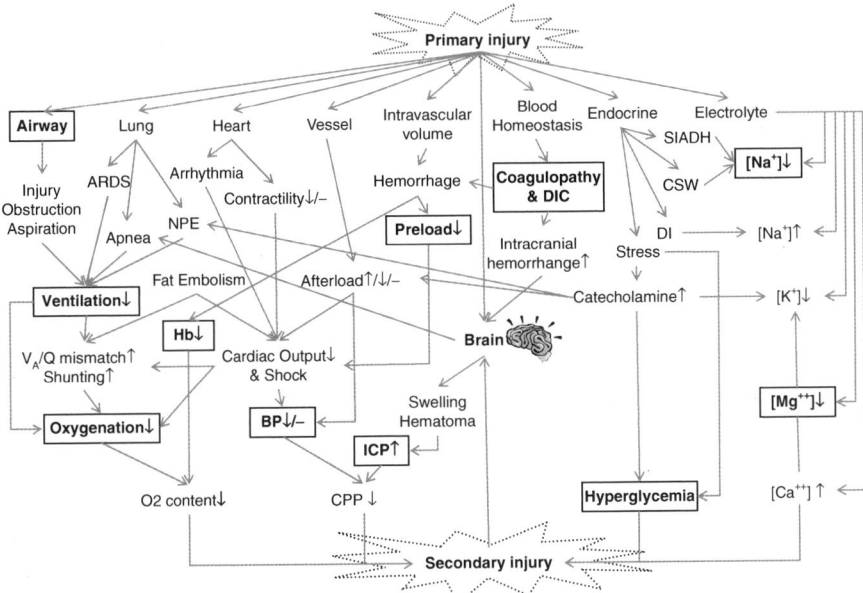

Fig. 9.4 Schematic illustration of the pathophysiologic processes after TBI with emphasis on the development of secondary injury. The open squares highlight the targets of clinical interventions. *ARDS* adult respiratory distress syndrome, *NPE* neurogenic pulmonary edema, *Hb* hemoglobin, V_A/Q ventilation over perfusion, *BP* blood pressure, *ICP* intracranial pressure, *CPP* cerebral perfusion pressure, *SIADH* syndrome of inappropriate antidiuretic hormone release, *CSW* cerebral salt wasting syndrome, *DI* diabetes insipidus, *DIC* disseminated intravascular coagulopathy, $[N_a^+]$ sodium, [K+] potassium, [Mg++] magnesium, $[C_a^{++}]$ calcium; ↑, increase; ↓, decrease; –, no change

hours, and days. The deleterious post-TBI multisystem sequelae, such as hypoxemia and hypotension, are the major contributing factors in secondary injury. The pathophysiologic mechanisms of secondary injury are illustrated in Fig. 9.4.

Multisystem Sequelae After TBI and Their Management

Once primary injury of brain incurred, management should focus on early diagnosis and treatment of deleterious multisystem sequelae in order to decrease the mortality, morbidity, and additional damage caused by secondary injury. A systemic approach is summarized in Table 9.2.

Nonsurgical Approaches of Spinal Cord Protection

Transfer of the patient with SCI to a level I trauma center as soon as possible is recommended. Considerable emphasis has been placed on the early immobilization of the entire spine of all patients with a potential SCI starting at the scene of injury.

Table 9.2 Multisystem sequelae and their managements after traumatic brain injury

Systems	Sequelae	Managements	Guideline recommendations for severe TBI[a]
Airway	Apnea Obstruction Injury Aspiration	Early endotracheal intubation	Level II: Pneumonia prophylaxis Level II: Early tracheostomy when feasible
Pulmonary	ARDS NPE Contusion Pneumothorax	Supportive Mechanical ventilation High FiO2 Consider PEEP Thoracostomy	Level II: Prophylactic hyperventilation not recommended Level III: Temporary hyperventilation for worsening ICP Level III: Avoid hypoxia (PaO_2 <60 mmHg or SaO_2 <90%) Level III: Avoid jugular venous saturation <50% or brain tissue oxygen tension <15 mmHg
Cardiovascular	Hypovolemia Arrhythmia Contusion Tamponade	Maintain normal to high normal BP Replace intravascular volume Avoid hypotonic solutions Avoid glucose-containing solutions Vasopressors Pericardial window	Level II: Avoid hypotension (systolic BP <90 mmHg) Level II: Avoid aggressively maintaining CPP >70 mmHg due to ARDS risk Level III: Avoid low CPP (<50 mmHg)
Brain	Primary injury Secondary injury ↑ICP ↓CPP	Monitor and control ICP Prevent secondary injury Decrease $CMRO_2$ Hypothermia[b] Hyperventilation	Monitor ICP via ventricular catheter connected to an external strain gauge Level II: Monitor ICP in all salvageable patients with a severe TBI (GCS score of 3–8 after resuscitation) and an abnormal CT scan Level II: Avoid ICP >20 mmHg Level II: Prophylactic barbiturates coma not recommended: barbiturate coma recommended for elevated ICP refractory to maximum standard medical and surgical treatment Level II: Prophylactic phenytoin or valproate not recommended for preventing late posttraumatic seizures (PTS)l: Anticonvulsants indicated to decrease the incidence of early PTS (within 7 days of injury)

Category	Subcategory	Treatment	Recommendation[a]
		Hyperosmolar therapy	Level III: Restrict mannitol use prior to ICP monitoring to patients with signs of transtentorial herniation or progressive neurological deterioration not attributable to extracranial causes
		CSF drainage	
		Surgical decompression	
		Barbiturate coma	
		IV anesthetic agents	
		Avoid inhalational agents	
Blood and Homeostasis	Acute hemorrhage	PRBC → keep Hct ≥30	Level III: Graduated compression stockings or intermittent pneumatic compression (IPC) stockings is recommended and should be combined with LMWH or low dose unfractionated heparin for DVT prophylaxis; however, there is an increased risk for expansion of intracranial hemorrhage
	Coagulopathy	FFP and Factor VIIa	
	DIC	DIC treatment	
	Thrombocytopenia	Platelet	
	DVT	Prophylaxis	
	Hyponatremia	NS or 3% NS slowly	
	Hypomagnesemia	Magnesium replacement	
Endocrine	Hyperglycemia	Insulin → keep BG <200 ml/dl	Level I: The use of steroids is not recommended for improving outcome or reducing ICP. In patients with moderate and severe TBI, high-dose methylprednisolone is associated with increased mortality and is contraindicated
	SIADH	Water restriction	
	CSW	Sodium replacement	
	DI	DDAVP	

ARDS adult respiratory distress syndrome, NPE neurogenic pulmonary edema, FiO_2 inspired oxygen fraction, PEEP positive end-expiratory pressure, ICP intracranial pressure, PaO_2 arterial oxygen partial pressure, SaO_2 arterial oxygen saturation, BP blood pressure, CPP cerebral perfusion pressure, $CMRO_2$ cerebral metabolic rate of oxygen, PRBC packed red blood cell, FFP fresh frozen plasma, DVT deep venous thrombosis, LMWH low molecular weight heparin; Hct hematocrit, BG blood glucose, SIADH syndrome of inappropriate antidiuretic hormone release, CSW cerebral salt wasting syndrome, DI diabetes insipidus, ↑ increase, ↓ decrease

[a] Based on "Guidelines for the Management of Severe Traumatic Brain Injury, 3rd Edition. Journal of Neurotrauma. 2007: 24 (Supplement 1)." Level I recommendations are based on the strongest evidence for effectiveness and represent principles of patient management that reflect a high degree of clinical certainty; level II recommendations reflect a moderate degree of clinical certainty; for level III recommendations, the degree of clinical certainty is not established.

[b] Temperature management is still a matter of controversy

The combination of a rigid cervical collar and supportive blocks on a backboard with straps or similar device to secure the entire spine is the current standard of care. An adequate number of personnel should be deployed to "log-roll" the patient with a potential unstable spine as a unit when repositioning, turning, or preparing for transfers.

Like TBI, SCI can cause multisystem sequelae (e.g., spinal shock with profound arterial hypotension), which are the major contributing factors in secondary injury of spinal cord. Early diagnosis and treatment of those deleterious consequences are the centerpieces in the post-SCI management. Airway management in a patient with potential SCI is confounded by multiple factors, including unstable or uncleared C-spine, combative/uncooperative patient, full stomach, and potential difficult airway. The airway management algorithm presented above is appropriate for SCI, as well as TBI.

There is no existing clinical evidence to definitively recommend the use of any neuroprotective pharmacologic agent, including steroids, in the treatment of acute SCI in order to improve functional recovery. However, the administration of glucocorticoid to a patient with a complete or partial neurologic deficit remains a relatively common practice. Nevertheless, methylprednisolone should be stopped as soon as possible, if it has been started, in neurologically normal patients and in those whose prior neurologic symptoms have resolved to reduce deleterious side effects.

Multisystem Sequelae After SCI and Their Management

The management of the deleterious post-SCI multisystem sequelae is summarized in Table 9.3.

Table 9.3 Multisystem sequelae and their managements after spinal cord injury

Systems	Sequelae	Managements[a]
Pulmonary	Weak or paralyzed respiratory muscles (depend on the level of injury); reduced lung volumes except for residual volume, atelectasis; high risks for infection and aspiration; pulmonary edema (cardiogenic, noncardiogenic); coexisting blunt chest trauma (pulmonary contusions, hemothorax, pneumothorax); respiratory failure (hypoxemia, hypercapnia)	Aggressive pulmonary hygiene; bronchodilator therapy; early use of fiberoptic bronchoscopy in cases of lobar atelectasis secondary to retained secretions; early endotracheal intubation or tracheostomy when feasible[b]; early institution of mechanical ventilation; admit patients with complete tetraplegia and injury level at C5 or rostral to ICU; ventilator-associated pneumonia prophylaxis

(continued)

Table 9.3 (continued)

Systems	Sequelae	Managements[a]
Cardiovascular	*Orthostatic hypotension* due to vasodilation caused by functional sympathectomy	Intravascular volume repletion (overzealous fluid administration can cause or worsen pulmonary edema.); vasopressor therapy; maintain BP with a balance of infusion and inotropes
	Spinal shock (characterized by hypotension, bradycardia, hypothermia, loss of somatic motor and sensory function, loss of voluntary rectal contraction, and a typical resolution over a period of days to a few weeks) caused by the imbalance of autonomic nervous system due to functional sympathectomy and unopposed parasympathetic activity	Exclude other injuries before assigning the cause of hypotension to neurogenic shock, determine the initial base deficit or lactate level to assess severity of shock and need for ongoing fluid resuscitation; invasive hemodynamic monitors; intravascular volume repletion and vasopressor therapy; treat persistent bradycardia
	Bradycardia due to loss of cardiac accelerator nerves (T1–T4) and unopposed parasympathetic nerves; profound bradycardia, even cardiac arrest, when stimulating the patient; supraventricular dysrhythmia; ventricular dysrhythmia	Anticipate bradycardia and hypotension during intubation of the tetraplegic patient; sedate the patient before stimulation such as tracheal suctioning; administer atropine; consider temporary pacemaker if atropine not working
Autonomic nervous system	Autonomic dysreflexia (or hyperreflexia) is a massive sympathetic response due to the loss of the modulation by the normal inhibitory impulses arising from brainstem and hypothalamus, characterized by vasoconstriction below the lesion and vasodilation above the lesion and often accompanied by bradycardia, ventricular dysrhythmias, and even heart block. It occurs in 85% of patients with spinal cord transactions above T5 and usually begins to appear about 2–3 weeks after injury	Change patient's position from supine to sitting; loosen any clothing or constrictive devices; quickly survey the individual for the instigating causes, place an indwelling urinary catheter if not in place or troubleshoot the catheter if in place, consider the possibility of fecal impaction and check the rectum for stool; consider antihypertensive treatment; consider deep general, epidural, or spinal anesthesia

(continued)

Table 9.3 (continued)

Systems	Sequelae	Managements[a]
Blood and homeostasis	DVT (40% of patients with complete SCI); PE (4–13% and primarily in the first month after SCI)	Prophylactic treatment for a minimum of 3 months; combination of mechanical compression devices and adjusted-dose of heparin, LMWH, or warfarin in all patients once primary hemostasis achieved[c]; consider placing an inferior vena cava filter[d]
Gastrointestinal	Ileus; gastroparesis; peptic ulcer disease; pancreatitis; acalculous cholecystitis; occult acute abdomen	Aspiration precaution; gastric decompression via nasogastric tube; antacids/H_2 blockers/sucralfate; provide appropriate nutrition
Genitourinary	Bladder flaccidity (early phase), bladder spasticity (late phase); recurrent UTI/urosepsis; nephrocalcinosis	Place an indwelling urinary catheter early and leave it in place at least until a stable hemodynamics achieved and strict attention to fluid status no longer needed
Muscle	Hyperkalemia from succinylcholine	Avoid the use of succinylcholine after the first 48 h post-SCI
Bone	Osteoporosis; hypercalcemia; heterotopic ossification and muscle calcification	Early physical therapy
Skin	Decubitus ulcers	Frequently assess areas at risk and provide meticulous care
Thermoregulation	Prone to hypothermia due to inability to conserve heat	Monitor and regulate temperature
Immunologic	Pneumonia; urosepsis; skin infection	Relevant prophylaxis and appropriate antibiotics

[a]Based on "Consortium for Spinal Cord Medicine: Early acute management in adults with spinal cord injury: a clinical practice guideline for health-care professionals. 2008"
[b]For those patients who are likely to remain ventilator dependent or to wean slowly from mechanical ventilation over an extended period of time
[c]Intracranial bleeding, perispinal hematoma, or hemothorax are potential contraindications to the administration of anticoagulants, but anticoagulants may be appropriate once bleeding has stabilized
[d]Only in those patients with active bleeding anticipated to persist for more than 72 h and begin anticoagulants as soon as possible, *DVT* deep venous thrombosis, *PE* pulmonary embolism, *LMWH* low molecular weight heparin, *UTI* urinary tract infection

Key Points

- Life-threatening situations, including airway, breathing, and circulation, are always the priorities in managing patients after traumatic injury.
- The early diagnosis and management of the coexisting TBI and/or SCI in a polytrauma patient is of paramount importance in terms of preventing further injury immediately after injury and preserving neurologic function.
- The early diagnosis and treatment of multisystem sequelae after traumatic injury, such as hypoxemia and hypotension, are crucial in preventing secondary injury after TBI or SCI, which should be the focus of attention after initial successful resuscitation.

Suggested Reading

Dutton RP, McCunn M, and Grissom TE. Anesthesia for trauma. In: Miller R, editor. Miller's anesthesia. 7th ed. Philadelphia: Elsevier Churchill Livingstone; 2010. p. 2277–2311.

Furlan JC, Fehlings MG. Cardiovascular complications after acute spinal cord injury: pathophysiology, diagnosis, and management. Neurosurg Focus. 2008;25:1–15.

Harris MB, Sethi RK. The initial assessment and management of the multiple-trauma patient with an associated spine injury. Spine. 2006;31:S9–15.

Lim HB, Smith M. Systemic complications after head injury: a clinical review. Anaesthesia. 2007;62:474–82.

Matjasko MJ, Stier GR, Schell RM, Cole DJ. Multisystem sequelae of severe head injury. Spinal cord injury. In: Cottrell JE, Smith DS, editors. Anesthesia and Neurosurgery. 4th ed. St. Louis, MO: Mosby; 2001. p. 693–747.

Moppett IK. Traumatic brain injury: assessment, resuscitation and early management. Br J Anaesth. 2007;99:18–31.

Chapter 10
Rare Neurologic Disorders and Neuromuscular Diseases: Risk Assessment and Perioperative Management

Nicholas Hirsch

Although many neurological conditions are rare even in neuroanesthetic practice, they have important implications for the conduct of anesthesia. This chapter concentrates on some of the more commonly encountered "rare" diseases (Table 10.1).

Neurodegenerative Diseases

Parkinson's Disease

Overview

- Parkinson's disease (PD) is characterized by triad of bradykinesia (difficulty initiating movement), increased muscle tone (cogwheel rigidity), and tremor (pill-rolling).
- Seen in 3% of population >65 years old, it is due to an imbalance of dopamine and acetylcholine (ACh) in the substantia nigra of the basal ganglia.
- Etiology usually unknown although may follow traumatic brain injury, cerebrovascular disease, carbon monoxide poisoning, and encephalitis. Drugs causing parkinsonism include phenothiazines, butyrophenones, and metoclopramide.
- Drug treatment of PD aims to increase levels of dopamine in basal ganglia and includes levodopa, dopamine agonists (e.g., bromocriptine, pergolide), and monoamine oxidase type B inhibitors (e.g., selegiline). Surgical treatment centers on deep brain stimulation (especially of subthalamic nucleus).

N. Hirsch, FRCA, FRCP, FFICM (✉)
Department of Neuroanesthesia, National Hospital for Neurology and Neurosurgery, London, UK
e-mail: nicholas.hirsch@uclh.nhs.uk

A.M. Brambrink and J.R. Kirsch (eds.), *Essentials of Neurosurgical Anesthesia & Critical Care*, DOI 10.1007/978-0-387-09562-2_10,
© Springer Science+Business Media, LLC 2012

Table 10.1 Rare neurologic diseases

Neurodegenerative diseases
- Parkinson's disease
- Amyotrophic lateral sclerosis

Demyelinating disease
- Multiple sclerosis

Neuromuscular diseases
- Guillain–Barré syndrome
- Myasthenia gravis
- Lambert Eaton myasthenic syndrome
- Critical illness neuropathy and myopathy

Muscle diseases
- Muscular dystrophies
- Myotonic dystrophy

Table 10.2 Physiological derangements seen in Parkinson's disease

System	Abnormalities
Respiratory	Upper airway/vocal cord dysfunction may result in postoperative laryngospasm
	Respiratory muscle impairment due to rigidity and bradykinesia
	Poor lung function due to repeated aspiration
Cardiovascular	Arrhythmias if on high doses of levodopa
	Orthostatic hypotension due to PD itself or chronic therapy with levodopa (causes reduction in blood volume and a decrease in norepinephrine production and stores)
	Autonomic instability especially if parkinsonism is associated with other neurodegenerative diseases (e.g., multisystem atrophy)
Gastrointestinal	Poor swallow in majority of patients with abnormal handling of saliva and increased risk of tracheal aspiration
	Increased incidence of reflux and constipation
	Poor nutritional status
Central nervous system	Bradykinesia, muscle rigidity, and tremor
	Depression
	Confusion, hallucinations

Implications for the Neurosurgical Patient

A number of physiological systems are affected in PD (Table 10.2).

Concerns and Risks

- Antiparkinsonian drug therapy must be continued throughout the perioperative period (via a nasogastric tube if necessary) as untreated severe PD can result in respiratory and bulbar failure.

- Drugs which worsen PD (e.g., metoclopramide, high-dose opioid agents) should be avoided.
- Thiopental, propofol, and suxamethonium are safe in PD patients.

Key Points

- Patients with Parkinson's disease require thorough preoperative assessment of their CNS and their respiratory and cardiovascular systems.
- Antiparkinsonian medication must be continued throughout the perioperative period.
- Drugs which exacerbate parkinsonism must be avoided.
- Careful cardiovascular monitoring is essential as autonomic nervous system involvement may be present.

Suggested Reading

Clarke CE. Parkinson's disease. Br Med J. 2007;335:441–5.
Nicholson G, Pereira AC, Hall GM. Parkinson's disease and anaesthesia. Br J Anaesth. 2002;89: 904–16.

Amyotrophic Lateral Sclerosis (Motor Neuron Disease)

Overview

- Amyotrophic lateral sclerosis (ALS) is characterized by degeneration of motor neurons throughout the central nervous system from motor cortex to anterior horn cell.
- Onset most common in late middle age and death usually occurs within 3 years.
- Patients may present with bulbar and pseudobulbar symptoms and signs (dysphagia, dysarthria, poor tongue movement, and emotional lability), with cervical symptoms (weakness and wasting of arm and hand muscles, fasciculation, and brisk reflexes) and lumbar symptoms (e.g., foot drop, difficulty climbing stairs).
- Death usually caused by pneumonia is secondary to respiratory muscle weakness and aspiration pneumonia. Riluzole, a glutamate antagonist, prolongs life expectancy by 3 months.

Implications for the Neurosurgical Patient

The anesthesiologist usually encounters the patient with ALS when anesthesia and surgery is required for an unrelated condition; the intensivist encounters the patient when the question of intensive care treatment of respiratory failure arises. This clearly brings profound ethical issues to the forefront.

Concerns and Risks

- Respiratory muscle weakness is invariable in the latter stages of ALS and many patients will be receiving intermittent mechanical ventilation either via a nasal mask or tracheostomy.
- Postoperative weaning from mechanical ventilation may prove to be impossible due to respiratory muscle weakness.
- Bulbar dysfunction predisposes to perioperative pulmonary aspiration and airway obstruction.
- Suxamethonium may result in severe hyperkalemia and must be avoided. Patients with ALS require reduced doses of nondepolarizing neuromuscular blocking agents.

Key Points

- Patients with ALS often have profound bulbar dysfunction increasing the perioperative risk of pulmonary aspiration.
- Respiratory muscle function is almost invariably affected and patients may be receiving respiratory support preoperatively. Postoperatively it may be impossible to wean the patient from mechanical ventilation and it is important that this possibility is discussed carefully with the patient and their relatives.
- Suxamethonium must be avoided as it may cause fatal hyperkalemia.

Suggested Reading

Bradley MD, Orrell RW, Clarke J, et al. Outcome of ventilatory support for acute respiratory failure in motor neurone disease. J Neurol Neurosurg Psychiatry. 2002;72:752–6.
Mitchell JD, Borasio GD. Amyotrophic lateral sclerosis. Lancet. 2007;369:2031–41.

Demyelinating Disease

Multiple Sclerosis

Overview

- Multiple sclerosis (MS) is the most common of the demyelinating diseases and is characterized by a wide spectrum of neurological symptoms and signs that are "disseminated in time and space."
- Symptoms and signs include visual disturbance (typically caused by optic neuritis; frequently first manifestation), sensory and motor disturbances (causing pain,

Table 10.3 Physiological derangements seen in multiple sclerosis

Abnormality	Comments
Disordered control of breathing, especially during sleep	Seen with brainstem involvement
Poor pharyngeal and laryngeal control predisposing to aspiration	Seen with lower cranial nerve involvement
Diaphragmatic weakness	Seen with cervical cord involvement
Generalized respiratory muscle weakness	May occur with baclofen treatment of spasticity
Postural hypotension	Seen with high thoracic cord lesions

numbness, weakness, spasticity, etc.), autonomic dysfunction, and behavioral changes.

- Most commonly affects women between ages of 20–40 years. 85% suffer from intermittent partial or complete relapses and remissions ("relapsing-remitting MS") while others exhibit a slowly progressive picture (primary progressive MS).
- Diagnosis is confirmed using magnetic resonance imaging and examination of cerebrospinal fluid.
- Acute relapses of MS are treated with high-dose corticosteroids and/or plasma exchange. Treatments shown to reduce recurrence rates of relapses include interferon beta-1a and -1b, azathioprine, and cyclophosphamide.

Implications for the Neurosurgical Patient

MS can affect all parts of the CNS resulting in respiratory and cardiovascular instability (Table 10.3).

Concerns and Risks

- Neurological deficits should be recorded carefully preoperatively.
- Bulbar and respiratory function must be assessed.
- Spinal anesthesia has resulted in worsening of neurological deficit although epidural anesthesia has been successfully used. Often avoided for medico-legal reasons.
- Suxamethonium may result in fatal hyperkalemia; nondepolarizing neuromuscular blocking agents have variable effects and require intraoperative monitoring.
- Increases in body temperature can result in exacerbation of MS and must be avoided.

Key Points

- MS may affect bulbar and respiratory function.
- Drug therapy of MS may influence anesthesia.
- Suxamethonium must be avoided and nondepolarizing neuromuscular blocking agents used with careful neuromuscular monitoring.
- Rises in body temperature should be avoided.

Suggested Reading

Dorotta IR, Schubert A. Multiple sclerosis and anesthetic implications. Current Opinions in Anaesthesiology. 2002;15:365–70.

Neuromuscular Diseases

Guillain–Barré Syndrome

Overview

- Guillain–Barré syndrome (GBS) is the most common cause of acute neuromuscular paralysis in the Western World and is usually the result of a postinfectious demyelinating polyneuropathy.
- In its classical form it is characterized by ascending limb weakness, areflexia and mild sensory symptoms (usually glove and stocking paresthesiae).
- 30% of GBS patients require tracheal intubation and mechanical ventilation because of respiratory and/or bulbar muscle paralysis.
- Diagnosis is based on history, examination, nerve conduction studies, and CSF examination.

Implications for the Neurocritical Care Patient

Patients often require prolonged periods of mechanical ventilation and tracheostomy is usually performed early. Suxamethonium may result in hyperkalemia and must be avoided. Autonomic involvement may result in labile blood pressure and tachy- and bradyarrhythmias. General management consists of meticulous nursing care, management of pain, early nutrition, and thromboembolic prophylaxis. Specific treatment consists of plasma exchange or intravenous immunoglobulin (IVIg) which are equally efficacious.

Key Points

- GBS is the most common cause of acute neuromuscular paralysis.
- 30% of patients will require mechanical ventilation, often for prolonged periods; tracheostomy should be performed early.
- Autonomic involvement may result in cardiovascular instability.
- Specific treatment involves plasma exchange or intravenous immunoglobulin which accelerate recovery.

Suggested Reading

Hughes RAC, Cornblath DR. Guillain-Barré syndrome. Lancet. 2005;366:1653–66.
Ng KKP, Howard RS, Fish DR, Hirsch NP, Wiles CM, Miller DH. Management and outcome of severe Guillain-Barré syndrome.Quarterly Journal of Medicine. 1995;88:243–50.

Myasthenia Gravis

Overview

- Myasthenia gravis (MG) is a disease of the neuromuscular junction (NMJ) in which IgG autoantibodies are directed toward the postsynaptic ACh receptor at the NMJ. The decreased ACh receptor density causes weakness and fatigability of skeletal muscle.
- 15% of patients with MG will require mechanical ventilation during the course of their disease; when this occurs it is called a *myasthenic crisis*. Deterioration may also be associated with overtreatment with anticholinesterase agents; this is referred to as *cholinergic crisis*. However, clinical presentation is often similar between crisis types.

Treatment of MG includes anticholinesterase drugs (e.g., neostigmine, pyridostigmine), immunosupression agents (e.g., prednisolone, azathioprine), and thymectomy. IVIg and plasma exchange are useful in the treatment of myasthenic crisis.

Implications for the Neurosurgical Patient

Patients with MG either present for thymectomy or for surgery unrelated to their condition; intensivists encounter MG patients when they present with myasthenic or cholinergic crises.

Concerns and Risks

- Patients with MG undergoing anesthesia require careful assessment of their respiratory reserve. A forced vital capacity of <2.9 L, bulbar dysfunction, and a long history of MG are associated with increased risk of needing postoperative mechanical ventilation.
- Drug treatment must be optimized preoperatively. Hydrocortisone should be given at induction if patients have been receiving corticosteroid therapy.
- Patients are relatively resistant to suxamethonium and are very sensitive to nondepolarizing neuromuscular blocking agents. Careful neuromuscular monitoring is mandatory.
- Patients in myasthenic crisis often require prolonged periods of mechanical ventilation while their MG is controlled with a combination of anticholinesterase and immunosuppressant drugs and intravenous immunoglobulin treatment.

Key Points

- Patients with MG often have poor respiratory reserve and require careful preoperative assessment and optimization of respiratory muscle function and drug treatment.
- Patients with MG are resistant to suxamethonium and sensitive to nondepolarizing neuromuscular blocking drugs. Their use should be titrated against effect using neuromuscular monitoring.

Suggested Reading

Meriggioli MN, Sanders DB. Autoimmune myasthenia gravis: emerging clinical and biological heterogeneity. Lancet Neurology. 2009;8:475–90.
O'Riordan JI, Miller DH, Mottershead JP, Hirsch NP, Howard RS. The management and outcome of patients treated acutely in a neurological intensive care unit. European Journal of Neurology. 1998;5:137–42.

Lambert Eaton Myasthenic Syndrome

Overview

- Lambert Eaton myasthenic syndrome (LEMS) is a disease of the NMJ in which IgG autoantibodies are directed toward the presynaptic voltage-gated calcium channel receptor. Blockage of these channels results in decreased release of ACh at the NMJ leading to muscle weakness.
- Ocular and proximal leg muscles are most commonly affected; respiratory muscle failure is rare.

- Autonomic involvement is common.
- 50–70% of patients have an underlying malignancy (most commonly small-cell carcinoma of the lung).

Implications for the Neurosurgical Patient

Patients most commonly present for resection of their bronchial tumor but may also be admitted for investigation of unexplained muscular weakness.

Concerns and Risks

- Patients often have symptoms and signs of underlying malignancy and smoking related illness.
- Patients with LEMS are extremely sensitive to both suxamethonium and the non-depolarizing neuromuscular blocking drugs and anticholinesterase agents may be ineffective at reversing the latter's actions.

Suggested Reading

Hirsch NP. Neuromuscular junction in health and disease. Br J Anaesth. 2007;99:132–8.

Critical Illness Polyneuropathy and Myopathy

Overview

- Critical illness polyneuropathy (CIP) is an acute axonal motor and sensory neuropathy that occurs in 50% of ITU patients; its incidence rises to almost 100% of patients with the severe sepsis.
- Clinical features of CIP include generalized muscle weakness and wasting with absent or reduced reflexes. Diagnosis requires exclusion of other causes of weakness and nerve conduction studies.
- Prevention of CIP includes rapid treatment of sepsis and possibly tight glycaemic control.
- Critical illness myopathy (CIM) is seen in a similar population to CIP.
- There may be an association between CIM and the use of corticosteroids and neuromuscular blocking drugs.
- Definitive diagnosis requires muscle biopsy.

Implications for the Neurointensive Care Patient

- CIP and CIM may coexist and are potent causes of failure to wean from mechanical ventilation.
- It may be difficult to differentiate between CIP and CIM and the term *polyneuromyopathy* has been suggested to encompass both entities.
- Treatment is largely supportive while awaiting recovery.

Suggested Reading

Zink W, Kollmar R, Schwab S. Critical illness polyneuropathy and myopathy in the intensive care unit. Nature Revies Neurology. 2009;5:372–9.

Muscle Diseases

Muscular Dystrophies

Overview

- The muscular dystrophies (MD) are a group of inherited muscle disorders characterized by progressive muscle weakness often ultimately resulting in respiratory failure.
- Duchenne muscular dystrophy (DMD) is the commonest (1 in 3,500 live male births) muscular dystrophy and is due to a deficiency of dystrophin, a protein necessary for sarcolemmal stability.
- Respiratory muscle failure and dilated cardiomyopathy in DMD often lead to death from cardiopulmonary causes. Associated scoliosis exacerbates respiratory dysfunction. Mean survival is 25 years.
- Patients are often receiving noninvasive nasal positive pressure ventilation (NPPV) especially during sleep.

Concerns and Risks

- Patients with DMD with impaired respiratory function are at high risk for death when exposed to sedation or general anesthesia.
- Patients with DMD have an *increased risk of a malignant hyperthermia* type reaction with associated rhabdomyolysis, hyperkalemia, and cardiac arrest when anesthetized with volatile anesthetic agents and suxamethonium.
- There is an increased need for cardiopulmonary support following surgery.
- Gastrointestinal pathology may lead to acute gastric dilatation.

Table 10.4 Systems affected by DM1

System	Abnormalities
Cardiac	Conduction defects which may result in sudden death. Cardiomyopathy, septal defects, and valvular disease
Respiratory	Respiratory muscle weakness with alveolar hypoventilation and poor cough. Reduced ventilatory to carbon dioxide. Central and obstructive sleep apnoea. Undue sensitivity to sedative and anesthetic agents
Gastrointestinal	Dysphagia, reduced rate of gastric emptying
Endocrine	Hypothyroidism, diabetes mellitus

Key Points

- Patients with DMD require thorough assessment of respiratory and cardiac function. An FVC < 30% of predicted is associated with an increased need for postoperative respiratory support.
- Total intravenous anesthetic techniques should be considered for induction and maintenance of anesthesia. *Volatile anesthetic agents and suxamethonium must be avoided.*
- Following extubation, a period of NPPV may be necessary.
- Postoperatively, patients must be cared for in a high-dependency setting. Supplemental oxygen therapy must be used with caution.
- A nasogastric tube should be in situ to treat gastric distension and immobility.

Suggested Reading

Birnkrant DJ, Panitch HB, Benditt JO, et al. American College of Chest Physicians consensus statement on the respiratory and related management of patients with Duchenne muscular dystrophy undergoing anesthesia or sedation. Chest. 2007;132:1977–86.

Myotonic Dystrophy

Overview

- Myotonic dystrophy (DM1) is an autosomal dominant disease of muscle characterized by myotonia (persistent contraction following exercise of a muscle). Prevalence is 1 in 20,000 of population.
- DM1 is a multisystem disease (Table 10.4).

Concerns and Risks

- Patients with DM1 are sensitive to the respiratory depressant effects of premedication, induction agents, and opioid drugs.

- Suxamethonium may result in an increased myotonia making laryngoscopy and ventilation impossible. Hyperkalemia following suxamethonium has been reported.
- If muscle wasting is present, nondepolarizing neuromuscular blocking drugs may have a prolonged action. Anticholinesterase drugs may precipitate increased myotonia.
- Surgical stimulation, cold, and shivering may increase myotonia.

Key Points

- Patients with DM1 require careful cardiorespiratory assessment.
- Reduced doses of sedative, induction, and analgesia agents are required.
- Suxamethonium should be avoided.
- Nondepolarizing neuromuscular agents should be carefully titrated using neuromuscular monitoring.
- Normothermia must be maintained perioperatively.

Suggested Reading

Russell SH, Hirsch NP. Anaesthesia and myotonia. Br J Anaesth. 1994;72:210–6.

Chapter 11
Perioperative Pharmacotherapy in Neurosurgery: Risk Assessment and Planning

Alejandro E. Delfino and Hernán R. Muñoz

There is a multiplicity of drugs that can be used during the perioperative period. Each has indications and adverse reactions that must be appreciated.

Inhaled Anesthetics

Overview

These drugs are widely used as fundamental components of general anesthesia.

Implications for the Neurosurgical Patient

In addition to their marked cerebrovascular effects, inhaled anesthetics produce important hemodynamic and respiratory changes in a dose-dependent manner that can have a significant impact on the neurologic patient.

Concerns and Risks

All inhalational anesthetics are potent cerebral vasodilators in a dose-dependent fashion; therefore, they have the potential to increase intracranial pressure (ICP).

A.E. Delfino, MD (✉) • H.R. Muñoz, MD, MSc
Department of Anesthesia, Escuela de Medicina, Pontificia Universidad Católica de Chile,
Santiago, Chile
e-mail: aedelfin@med.puc.cl

A.M. Brambrink and J.R. Kirsch (eds.), *Essentials of Neurosurgical Anesthesia & Critical Care*, DOI 10.1007/978-0-387-09562-2_11,
© Springer Science+Business Media, LLC 2012

Halothane is the most powerful cerebral vasodilator; however, currently it has limited use. It produces an increase in cerebral blood flow in association with a decrease in cerebrovascular resistance that can result in significant increases in ICP. Controlled hyperventilation can help to limit this effect.

Isoflurane, sevoflurane, and desflurane produce cerebral vasodilation and an increase in ICP, but the effects are clinically significant with doses higher than 1 MAC. Desflurane might produce more vasodilation than the others and has been proposed to be the inhaled agent of choice for brain protection in patients undergoing temporary cerebral artery occlusion during cerebrovascular surgery.

Nitrous oxide has a variable effect from zero to marked cerebral vasodilation and the potential to increase ICP depending on the initial $PaCO_2$ and the presence of adjuvant anesthetic drugs. Experimental evidence suggests that inhaled anesthetics cause neuro-apoptosis in the very young and the brain of the elderly. Nitrous oxide is the only inhaled agent that appears to worsen short-term outcome following transient focal cerebral ischemia.

Key Points

- Inhaled anesthetics as a group cause cerebral vascular dilation and increased ICP in high doses.
- Avoid halothane if possible.
- Use isoflurane, sevoflurane, or desflurane at a concentration ≤ 1 MAC.
- Use nitrous oxide cautiously.

Suggested Reading

Patel MP, Drummond JC. Cerebral physiology and the effects of anesthetic drugs. In: Miller RD, editor. Miller's anesthesia. 7th ed. Philadelphia: Elsevier Churchill Livingstone; 2010. p. 305–40.

Pasternak J, McGregor D, Lanier W, et al. Effect of nitrous oxide use on long-term neurologic and neuropsychological outcome in patients who received temporary proximal artery occlusion during cerebral aneurysm clipping surgery. Anesthesiology. 2009;110:563–73.

Intravenous Anesthetics

Overview

They are used virtually in every general anesthetic, either only at induction or also during maintenance. These drugs are responsible for the hypnosis, while opioids provide the analgesic component of general anesthesia (balanced anesthesia).

Implications for the Neurosurgical Patient

In general, intravenous anesthetics reduce the cerebral metabolic rate and oxygen consumption, and because they have no vasodilatory effects, both cerebral blood flow and ICP are proportionally reduced.

Concerns and Risks

The optimal anesthetic should maintain normal coupling between cerebral blood flow and metabolism, keep cerebrovascular autoregulation intact, and not increase cerebral blood volume and ICP, and, ideally, (potentially combined with other drugs) provide neuroprotective effects.

Barbiturates and propofol are used during temporary clipping of intracerebral arteries in cerebral vascular surgery (i.e., aneurysm and extra- to intracraneal by pass surgery) because of their allegedly neuroprotective effects in focal ischemia. When barbiturates are used as the primary anesthetic (usually by infusion), emergence may be delayed. In addition, propofol infusion (short- or long-term) infrequently can be associated with impaired free fatty acid utilization and mitochondria activity (propofol infusion syndrome) often presenting as acidosis, cardiac dysrhythmias, and myocardial dysfunction.

Alpha2-adrenoceptor agonists (e.g., dexmedetomidine) are now being used as a component of a balanced anesthesia and for sedation in the ICU. Although dexmedetomidine is associated with an easily managed level of sedation, rapid administration may be associated with hypertension and slow rate infusion with hypotension. In addition, there is the concern that dexmedetomidine might prevent normal cerebral vasodilation during hypoxemia.

Although etomidate is a reasonable choice for the induction of anesthesia in cardiovascularly compromised patients, it does not confer significant neuroprotection. A single dose of etomidate for the induction of anesthesia produces adrenal suppression that can be relevant in trauma and septic patients. As many neurologically impaired patients are receiving high-dose steroids as part of their underlying therapy, the adrenal suppression effects of etomidate might have less clinical significance in these patients. Etomidate during temporary clipping was associated with a reduction in brain oxygenation and should, therefore, be avoided in this context.

Opioids are necessary components for most surgical procedures, to afford the patient with appropriate intra- and postoperative analgesia. Although they inhibit the respiratory drive, the use of short-acting opioids (fentanyl, alfentanil, and remifentanil) is common in neurosurgical patients. Using the right dose and dosing frequency, even opioids with a long duration of action can be used safely (e.g., hydromorphone). The use of opioids and benzodiazepines requires caution, particularly toward the end of surgery, as they will impair respiratory drive leading to significant increments in $PaCO_2$ and ICP.

Table 11.1 shows the effect of different drugs on some important parameters.

Table 11.1 Effect of different intravenous anesthetics on some cerebral physiologic parameters and arterial pressure

	CBF	CMR	ICP	CO_2 reactivity	Arterial pressure
Barbiturate	⇓⇓	⇓⇓	⇓⇓	0	⇓
Propofol	⇓⇓⇓	⇓⇓	⇓	0	⇓⇓
Etomidate	⇓⇓	⇓⇓	⇓⇓	0	0
Benzodiazepines	⇓	⇓	⇓ or 0	⇓⇓	0
Ketamine	⇑	⇑ or 0	⇑	?	⇑
Opioids	0	0	0	⇓	⇓ or 0

CBF, cerebral blood flow; CRM, cerebral metabolic rate; ICP, intracranial pressure; ⇑/⇓, slight increase/reduction; ⇓⇓, significant reduction; ⇓⇓⇓, marked reduction; 0, without significant effect; ?, uncertain effect

Key Points

- Consider intracranial distensibility and hemodynamic parameters to choose the appropriate intravenous anesthetics.
- The use of benzodiazepines and opioids to sedate and treat pain in awake patients with closed head trauma must be done very carefully.

Suggested Reading

Jackson WL. Should we use etomidate as an induction agent for endotracheal intubation in patients with septic shock?: a critical appraisal. Chest. 2005;127(3):707–9.
Martyn JA. Neuromuscular physiology and pharmacology. In: Miller R, editor. Miller's anesthesia. 7th ed. Philadelphia: Elsevier Churchill Livingstone; 2010. p. 341–60.
Reves J, Glass P, et al. Intravenous anesthetics. In: Miller R, editor. Miller's anesthesia. 7th ed. Philadelphia: Elsevier Churchill Livingstone; 2010. p. 719–68.

Neuromuscular Blocking Drugs

Overview

Neuromuscular blocking drugs (NMBs) are used to facilitate tracheal intubation, to assure lack of movement during surgery and sometimes to facilitate mechanical ventilation in the ICU.

Implications for the Neurosurgical Patient

NMBs are used in virtually all the neurosurgical patients; however, they have several adverse effects that can be harmful for these patients.

Concerns and Risks

NMBs can be classified into two groups according to their mechanism of action.

(a) *Depolarizing NMBs*: succinylcholine is the only drug of this group in clinical use. Its rapid onset of action makes it particularly useful to obtain a rapid control of the airway. Some of its problems in neurologic patients include:

Transient increase in ICP that might be dangerous when it is already elevated. Adequate depth of anesthesia, normal arterial pressure, and controlled PaCO$_2$ are required to reduce this adverse effect.

Hyperkalemia: a single dose of succinylcholine (1–2 mg/kg) usually increases potassium plasma levels by approximately 0.5–1.0 mEq/L; however, in some patients with severe skeletal muscle trauma, denervation injury with skeletal muscle atrophy, upper motor neuron lesions, paraplegia, spinal cord injury or transection, stroke, and closed head trauma, severe hyperkalemia leading to cardiac arrest has been described. The mechanism for hyperkalemia appears to be linked to the stimulation of extra-junctional receptors which increase on the muscle surface secondary to the above-mentioned diseases.

(b) *Nondepolarizing NMBs*: include pancuronium, vecuronium, rocuronium, atracurium, and several others. With the advent of intraoperative electrophysiologic monitoring, use of nondepolarizing NMBs has become more limited. The use of these drugs is contraindicated during EMG monitoring (e.g., acoustic neuroma surgery and facial nerve monitoring) or motor evoked potentials (e.g., for spine surgery). Great caution must be used when administering nondepolarizing NMBs in patients who have previously experienced a cerebral vascular accident (i.e., ischemic stroke). In addition to the higher risk of hyperkalemia from depolarizing NMBs (see above), these patients are at high risk of being overmedicated with nondepolarizing NMBs, particularly if neuromuscular monitoring is done on the paretic extremity (because of the higher concentration of post-synaptic receptors in that extremity secondary to upregulation).

Residual paralysis secondary to their use is not a real adverse effect but undesired clinical practice and can lead to upper airway obstruction, hypoxemia, and hypercarbia within minutes. In addition, it has been associated with a higher rate of postoperative respiratory complications. To avoid this complication, the routine use of neuromuscular monitoring and careful clinical assessment before extubation is mandatory. Clinical manifestations include respiratory difficulty, problems swallowing secretions, and muscular weakness. Residual paralysis must be rapidly treated with anti-acetylcholinesterases.

Key Points

- Succinylcholine should be used with great caution and only if it cannot be substituted with a non-depolarizing neuromuscular blocking agent.
- Residual paralysis must be ruled out and properly treated before extubation to be sure that the patient is safe while spontaneously breathing.

Suggested Reading

Minton MD, Grosslight K, Stirt JA, et al. Increases in intracranial pressure from succinylcholine: prevention by prior nondepolarizing blockade. Anesthesiology. 1986;65(2):165–9.

Murphy GS, Szokol JW, Marymont JH, et al. Intraoperative acceleromyographic monitoring reduces the risk of residual neuromuscular blockade and adverse respiratory events in the post anesthesia care unit. Anesthesiology. 2008;109(3):389–98.

Inotropic and Vasoactive Drugs

Overview

The recognition that cerebral hypoperfusion is associated with adverse outcome in acute brain syndromes and during neurosurgery has led to an increase in the use of vasoactive drugs. Thus, some of the inotropes (adrenaline, dopamine, dobutamine, etc.) and vasoactive drugs (phenylephrine and noradrenaline) are extensively used in neurologic patients during surgery and ICU care. In some cases, vasodilators (sodium nitroprusside, nitroglycerin, calcium channel blockers, etc.) are also used.

Implications for the Neurosurgical Patient

Normally inotropic drugs have minimal or no direct effect on cerebral vessels; therefore, their effects on cerebral perfusion pressure (CPP), cerebral blood flow, intracranial volume, and ICP mostly depend on their effects on systemic hemodynamics. In patients with areas of brain with poor or lack of autoregulation (e.g., tumor, ischemia, or trauma), the maintenance of arterial pressure within a very tight range is critical. Sodium nitroprusside and nitroglycerin may worsen neurologic injury. While they do not have direct cerebrovascular vasodilatory effects, the reduction in arterial pressure may lead to vasodilation in areas of preserved autorregulation and, secondarily, to an increase in ICP: This will result in a reduction of CPP.

Concerns and Risks

Aggressive use of vasopressor drugs and fluids to raise arterial pressure can lead to systemic (pulmonary edema, cardiac failure, and myocardial ischemia) and neurologic (brain bleeding and edema) complications.

Intravenous, and to a lesser extent also by oral route, nimodipine as a prophylaxis of cerebral vasospasm after subarachnoid hemorrhage, can result in arterial hypotension. However, this does not contraindicate its use.

Key Points

- Treat and exclude reversible causes of hypotension before using vasopressor drugs to improve CPP.
- Limited experimental and clinical evidence suggests that norepinephrine might be the most appropriate catecholamine to augment cerebral perfusion in traumatic brain injury.
- Recommended therapy for severely elevated arterial pressure after acute stroke include labetalol, nicardipine, and nitroprusside (used with great caution in patients with elevated ICP). Hemodynamic goals are greatly different between hemorrhagic stroke (tight control to prevent rebleeding) and ischemic stroke (permissive hypertension to improve collateral flow).
- Any pharmacologic intervention to reduce elevated arterial pressure in neurologic patients has to be very slowly and should be intensively monitored. With continuous treatment regimes, careful and repeated reassessments are paramount with particular considerations of the treatment effects on CPP.

Suggested Reading

Pfister D, Strebel SP, Steiner LA. Effects of catecholamines on cerebral blood vessels in patients with traumatic brain injury. Eur J Anaesthesiol. 2008;42(Suppl):98–103.

Talbert RL. The challenge of blood pressure management in neurologic emergencies. Pharmacotherapy. 2006;26(8 Pt 2):123S–30S.

Diuretics and Hypertonic Saline

Overview

Diuretics, particularly mannitol and furosemide, and hypertonic saline are used in neurosurgical patients to reduce ICP and/or to obtain intraoperative brain relaxation.

Implications for the Neurosurgical Patient

Adverse effects are predictable and usually dose dependent. Therefore, these drugs can be applied safely to the neurosurgical patient if the clinician treats these known adverse effects in a preemptive fashion.

Concerns and Risks

Hypovolemia: secondary to diuretics can result in hypotension and reduced CPP.

Hypervolemia: secondary to the use of mannitol and/or hypertonic saline. Although this is rather a theoretical problem, it is transient and would only theoretically occur after rapid administration. The consequences of transient hypervolemia would be most significant in patients with a history of congestive heart failure.

Electrolyte disorders: secondary to a high urine output (hyponatremia and hypokalemia) or massive load of crystalloid solutions, particularly hypertonic saline. Mannitol causes sodium diuresis, which should be replaced to prevent hyponatremia. Loop diuretics (e.g., furosemide) cause hypokalemia, hypocalcemia, and hypomagnesaemia, which can cause cardiac arrhythmias and hypotension. When hypertonic saline is used for hyperosmolar treatment, it can produce hypernatremia and hyperchloremic metabolic acidosis. When using hypertonic saline (e.g., as a 3% solution) in the neurosurgical patient, many clinicians limit administration to a serum sodium not higher than 150 mEq/L. Hyperchloremic metabolic acidosis can be prevented by administering the 3% sodium as a 50% mix of chloride and 50% as acetate.

Key Point

- Monitor electrolyte status after a period of high urine output and/or hypertonic saline administration.

Suggested Reading

Rozet I, Tontisirin N, Saipin M, et al. Effect of equiosmolar solutions of mannitol versus hypertonic saline on intraoperative brain relaxation and electrolyte balance. Anesthesiology. 2007;107:697–704.

White H, Cook D, Venkatesh B. The role of hypertonic saline in neurotrauma. Eur J Anaesthesiol. 2008;42(Suppl):104–9.

Antiemetic Drugs

Overview

Post-craniotomy patients (this excludes transsphenoid hypophysectomy) are at high risk of postoperative nausea and vomiting (PONV). Despite the lack of a documented case of harm caused by retching or vomiting in these patients, an important number of patients undergoing general surgery fear the occurrence of PONV more than postoperative pain. However, the potential risk caused by vomiting, the associated arterial hypertension and high intra-abdominal/intra-thoracic pressure leading to high ICP suggests that avoiding/treating PONV in these patients is warranted.

Implications for the Neurosurgical Patient

Antiemetic drugs (AEDs) for PONV prophylaxis/treatment include several groups of drugs with an excellent safety profile in general surgery patients. However, some agents (e.g., droperidol and haloperidol) are associated with sedation. Droperidol is also an alpha-1 receptor agonist and may be associated with transient hypotension.

Concerns and Risks

Some adverse effects might be more relevant in neurosurgical patients.

Hyperglycemia: It is the most frequent known adverse effect after dexamethasone 8–10 mg IV. Steroid-induced hyperglycemia peaks between 8 and 10 h after IV administration and can exceed 200 mg/dL. Significant hyperglycemia has been demonstrated to impair neurologic outcomes and increases the risks for infection and impair wound healing. The use of dexamethasone for PONV in patients undergoing intracranial surgery should possibly not be considered the first-line therapy.

Sedation: A decrease in level of consciousness can occur secondary to droperidol and haloperidol and is more frequent within the first 6 h after its administration. It is dose-dependent and very uncommon after ≤1 mg IV of these AEDs. However, these drugs should be avoided in patients having craniotomy because the differential diagnosis of decreased level of consciousness may be unnecessarily complicated in the immediate post-craniotomy period.

Extrapyramidal side effects: They can be secondary to droperidol/haloperidol and metoclopramide, usually after higher than recommended doses. Rarely, administration of haloperidol, droperidol, promethazine, and metoclopramide may cause neuroleptic malignant syndrome. In the postoperative period of neurosurgical patient, this diagnosis must be considered in the presence of rigidity, autonomic dysfunction, hyperthermia, and mental status changes. If unrecognized and improperly treated the outcome could be fatal.

Headache: Occurs in 3–5% of patients given 5-HT(3) antagonists at the usual doses (such us ondansetron and granisetron) and must be taken into consideration for the differential diagnosis of headache in the neurological patient.

Key Points

- Monitor blood glucose levels after dexamethasone administration. Treat hyperglycemia in neurological patients to a goal of 130–180 mg/dL (current recommendations).
- Neurological and surgical causes of sedation, extrapyramidal signs, and headache must be ruled out before assuming that they are secondary to AEDs.

Suggested Reading

Lukins MB, Manninen PH. Hyperglycemia in patients administered dexamethasone for craniotomy. Anesth Analg. 2005;100:1129–33.
The NICE-SUGAR Study Investigators. Intensive versus conventional glucose control in critically ill patients. N Engl J Med. 2009;360(13):1283–9.

Anticonvulsants

Overview

A large number of patients undergoing a craniotomy are under or will be given anticonvulsants during the perioperative period. Possibly the most used are phenytoin, phenobarbital, and carbamazepine. However, benzodiazepines and thiopental can also be used, especially during active seizures.

Implications for the Neurosurgical Patient

Adverse effects are predictable and usually dose dependent. However, it must be remembered that, postoperatively, patients may have reduced protein binding (particularly affecting phenytoin) due to altered albumin and other drug-binding proteins making it imperative to monitor free drug concentrations in the perioperative period.

Concerns and Risks

Hypotension: secondary to almost all these drugs especially when administered quickly by the intravenous route. Hypotension is often accentuated when these drugs are administered during surgery, as they may act synergistically with anesthetic agents having the same cardiovascular effects.

Bradycardia/arrhythmia: phenytoin when injected fast can produce arrhythmia including asystole. This risk is accentuated when the drug is administered during the period of general anesthesia.

Sedation/respiratory depression: secondary to benzodiazepines and barbiturates. Respiratory depression can result in an increased arterial tension of CO_2 and hypoxemia in patients breathing spontaneously and thereby potentially in severe secondary brain injury.

Interaction with neuromuscular blockers (*NMBs*): chronic treatment with phenytoin and carbamazepine is associated with modest increase in acetylcholine receptor numbers, induced liver metabolism and increased release of acute phase reactant proteins that bind the NMDs, all causing reduced duration of neuromuscular blockade.

Key Points

- Administer slowly when active seizures are not currently present. Never inject phenytoin at a rate > 50 mg min^{-1}.
- When barbiturates and benzodiazepines are administered at a fast rate, check hemodynamic and respiratory status frequently until patients recovers; consider admission to the intensive care unit.
- Monitor intraoperative neuromuscular blockade more frequently in patients under treatment with phenytoin and carbamazepine.
- In the presence of severe cutaneous reactions in patients receiving anticonvulsants other than benzodiazepines, consider changing to a different family of drugs.

Suggested Reading

McNamara J. Drugs effective in the therapy of epilepsies. In: Hardman JG, Limbird LE, editors. Goodman and Gilman's the pharmacological basis of therapeutics. 10th ed. New York: McGraw-Hill; 2001.

Chapter 12
Specific Considerations Regarding Consent and Communication with Patients and Family Prior to Neurosurgery

Kenneth Abbey and Chloe Allen-Maycock

Overview

For any medical procedure, informed consent consists of four basic elements: (1) voluntariness, (2) competence, (3) informed, and (4) comprehended (capacity). For neuroanesthesia, satisfaction of the elements may be more difficult due to both the underlying pathology and the difficult choices facing patients undergoing neurosurgery. As a result of the unique nature of neurosurgical cases, anesthesiologists need to allow more time and need to take more care in obtaining consent for the anesthetics used in those cases.

A review of the elements for valid consent is useful for understanding the challenges faced in obtaining valid consent in neurosurgical cases. The classic criteria for voluntariness was set forth in the Nuremberg Code which stated that the patient should be "able to exercise free power of choice, without the intervention of any element of force, fraud, deceit, duress, overreaching, or other ulterior form of constraint or coercion." Several factors may impair the voluntary nature of informed consent. First, sedation is commonly encountered among preoperative patients and may constitute a form of constraint on a patient's ability to fully evaluate and participate in informed consent. Sedation may be obvious in the case of a sleepy patient who has received a large dose of anxiolytic, or may be more subtle, such as in a patient who has received a smaller dose of analgesic medication. The environment in which informed consent is obtained may also undermine voluntariness. Addressing informed consent in the operating room may make a patient more likely

K. Abbey, MD, JD
Department of Anesthesiology and Perioperative Medicine, Oregon Health &
Science University, Portland, OR, USA

C. Allen-Maycock, MD (✉)
Department of Anesthesiology, Legacy Salmon Creek Medical Center, PeaceHealth
Southwest Medical Center, Vancouver, WA, USA
e-mail: allenmaycock@comcast.net

A.M. Brambrink and J.R. Kirsch (eds.), *Essentials of Neurosurgical
Anesthesia & Critical Care*, DOI 10.1007/978-0-387-09562-2_12,
© Springer Science+Business Media, LLC 2012

to feel pressured to agree to a procedure. The anesthesia provider may also limit voluntariness by deliberately limiting anesthetic choices for the patient, based on the anesthesia provider's preference.

Patient competency is a legal term and designation. All adults are deemed competent unless designated otherwise by a court, and a declaration of incompetence is universally followed by appointment of a legal guardian. Patients that have been declared incompetent cannot consent, and consent must be obtained from their designated guardian.

Capacity is distinct from competency and is a determination made by the physician. The subject of informed consent should have "sufficient knowledge and comprehension of the elements of the subject matter involved as to enable him to make an understanding and enlightened decision." This requires that the patient have the capacity to provide informed consent and "implies that a patient has the ability to understand and weigh medical information and make decisions." The patient must be able to understand the medical problem and proposed treatment alternatives. For some procedures, this may be relatively simple. However, as the complexity of the medical problem and treatment increases, the patient's decision-making capacity may be exceeded. Likewise, as the complexity of the medical decision increases, so does the obligation of the physician to ensure that the patient has the capacity to understand the medical decisions and its implications.

Meeting the "informed" element of consent can be obtained by addressing the four key components of the PARQ discussion: (1) procedures, (2) alternatives, (3) risks, and (4) questions. The PARQ discussion can be utilized not only to provide information to the patient but also in determining the patient's ability to understand the concomitant risks and alternatives.

Implications for Neurosurgical Procedures

Obtaining informed consent from neurosurgical patients can be complex, due to the nature of the patient's diagnosis, the treatment options, and the increased likelihood for diminished decision-making capacity related to the neurosurgical procedure. First, voluntariness may be problematic for several reasons. Neurosurgical problems often present treatment choices without a "good" choice. For example, a patient with a brain mass must decide between surgery, which may leave the patient with a significant neurologic deficit or even death, or not having surgery and risk the tumor growing causing neurologic deficits and again possibly death. Family members may strongly support or oppose some options and may place pressure on the patient to choose a particular course.

Neurosurgical problems often compromise a patient's decision-making capacity, and any diagnosis or treatment that alters mentation may be associated with diminished capacity. Neurosurgical conditions most likely to decrease capacity include stroke and dementia. In cases of delirium, waxing and waning mental status creates a moving target for the assessment of medical decision-making capacity. Additionally, based on the degree of delirium, sedative medications may be required to maintain the patient's safety. The intensive care unit setting itself is associated with a high proportion of patients with diminished medical decision-making capacity. Conditions among patients in the ICU can range from postoperative sedation to ICU psychosis, which interfere to varying degrees with a patient's ability to evaluate medical decisions, but interfere nonetheless. Psychiatric diagnoses can also impair capacity. Unfortunately, many physicians caring for impaired patients may not appropriately identify them as such.

Much variability can exist within a given diagnosis or even between physicians evaluating whether a patient has capacity to provide informed consent. Other instruments that may be valuable in assessing capacity include the Mini-Mental State Examination (MMSE), which has been found to correlate with clinical judgments of incapacity. A score of <19 is associated with lack of capacity. The MacArthur Competence Assessment Tool for Treatment may also be utilized and specifically incorporates information related to a patient's decision-making situation. Unfortunately, these assessments can be time-consuming; the Mac-CAT takes about 20 min to perform.

Often, obtaining surgical consent implies consent for anesthesia, although the PARQ process for each should be distinct. It is possible, however, that a patient may be able to provide surgical consent without the capacity to consent to anesthesia. Again, it is incumbent on the anesthesia provider to weigh whether the patient has medical decision-making capacity, even if surgical consent has already been obtained from the patient.

Concerns and Risks

Neurosurgical patients comprise a group at risk for incomplete and/or inadequate informed consent. Taking the necessary time to assess a patient's ability to engage in and understand informed consent is fundamental to ensure the patient's ability to provide informed consent. Failure to obtain proper consent may subject the provider to a claim of battery (the tort of an inappropriate and unconsented touching).

Key Points
- Address each element of informed consent, including voluntariness, competence, informed and comprehended (capacity).
- It is incumbent upon physicians taking care of neurosurgical patients to ensure that informed consent is obtained.
- Neurosurgical patients comprise a high-risk group of patients who may have diminished medical decision-making capacity and may required additional time.
- Maintain a heightened awareness of factors potentially interfering with obtaining informed consent.

Suggested Reading

Appelbaum PS. Assessment of patients' competence to consent to treatment. N Engl J Med. 2007;357:1834–40.

Grisso T, Appelbaum PS. MacArthur competence assessment tool for treatment (MAC-CAT-T). Sarasota, FL: Professional Resource Press; 1998.

Kim SYH, Caine ED. Utility and limits of the mini mental state examination evaluating consent capacity in Alzheimer disease. Psychiatr Serv. 2002;53:1322–4.

Kim SYH, Karlawish JST, Caine ED. Current state of research on decision-making competence of cognitively impaired elderly persons. Am J Geriatr Psychiatry. 2002;10:151–65.

Raymont V, Bingley W, Buchanen A, et al. Prevalence of mental incapacity in medical inpatients and associated risk factors: cross-sectional study. Lancet. 2004;364:1421–7.

Terry PB. Informed consent in clinical medicine. Chest. 2007;131:563–8.

Trials of War Criminals before the Nuremberg Military Tribunals under Control Council Law No. 10. vol. 2. Washington, DC: U.S. Government Printing Office; 1949. p. 181–2.

Part III
Fundamentals of Adult Neurosurgery and Neuroanesthesia

Chapter 13
Preparing for Anesthesia in Neurosurgical Patients

Andrea M. Dower and Pirjo Manninen

Overview

Preparation for the treatment of patients with neurological disease involves multiple elements related to the patient, the procedure, the equipment required for both the surgical interventions and anesthesia, and the location where the procedure will be performed. The neurosurgical operating rooms and neuroradiological suites are highly complex and technical environments where healthcare professionals from various disciplines interact. Individuals from neurosurgery, anesthesia, nursing, neurophysiology, and radiology, each bring unique perspectives, demands, and contributions to the care of the patient. Effective communication among individuals and disciplines is essential to the safe and efficient function of the entire team. Communication failure can lead to catastrophic medical errors.

Patients with neurological disease often present with a wide range of pathological processes that may place additional demands on their management. Careful planning is required with respect to the anesthetic techniques, as well as the equipment requirements for anesthesia, surgery, and neurological monitoring. Infectious complications following neurosurgical procedures can significantly impact on patient outcome and require careful adherence to established protocols. In addition, neurosurgical and neuroradiological procedures may be carried out at sites remote from the operating room, necessitating thorough planning with respect to both the equipment and personnel required.

A.M. Dower, BSc, MD, FRCPC
Department of Anesthesia, McMaster University, Hamilton, ON, Canada

P. Manninen, MD, FRCPC (✉)
University of Toronto, Toronto Western Hospital University, Health Network,
Toronto, ON, Canada
e-mail: Pirjo.Manninen@uhn.ca

A.M. Brambrink and J.R. Kirsch (eds.), *Essentials of Neurosurgical Anesthesia & Critical Care*, DOI 10.1007/978-0-387-09562-2_13,
© Springer Science+Business Media, LLC 2012

Implications for the Neurosurgical Patient

Advanced planning is necessary to ensure that the layout of the room allows space for all necessary anesthetic, surgical, and radiological equipment including microscopes, imaging devices, and surgical instruments. There is a wide spectrum of neurosurgical procedures with positions ranging from prone to sitting. Each of these requires additional positioning tables and adjuncts to protect the patient and prevent possible injury. The final position of the patient for surgery as well as the locations of surgical access also need to be considered in deciding upon the placement of monitors, peripheral and central lines, and the endotracheal tube. Poor communication may result in delays and in possible harm to the patient.

Patient identification is essential. Lack of communication and lack of correct patient identification by all members of the intraoperative team can lead to catastrophic outcomes such as performing surgical procedures at the wrong surgical site or even on the wrong patient. Miscommunication has been identified as a major source of medical error leading to significant patient morbidity and mortality. Many hospitals have now introduced perioperative surgical safety checklists with a format similar to that used in the aviation industry. Importantly, this approach has been associated with a significant reduction in the incidence of wrong-site surgeries. All preoperative checks should include confirmation that informed consent has been obtained for the surgical procedure to be performed, as well as adjunctive investigations and treatments such as medical imaging, invasive monitoring, and possible blood transfusion.

Communication in the operating room can also be hampered by lack of team integration and collaboration. Prior to the commencement of anesthesia, communication between the anesthesiologist and surgeon must take place to ensure that each understands the medical concerns of the individual patient and the requirements from both for the specific operation. Communication between the neurophysiology team and anesthesiology team is also necessary to ensure that the form of anesthesia used allows for appropriate neuromonitoring. Simulators have also been used in an effort to improve teamwork in crisis situations such as major trauma. However, such endeavors are costly, time-consuming, and not readily available in all surgical centers.

The prevention of complications related to anesthesia begins with the preoperative assessment of the neurosurgical patient. Many neurosurgical procedures, such as treatment of a ruptured aneurysm, are performed on an urgent or emergent basis, thus limiting time for preoperative preparation. Every patient should have a complete assessment by an anesthesiologist to review all the concerns of neurological disease as well as other medical comorbidities. The continuation of routine medications and especially of neurological medications, such dexamethasone and antiepileptic agents, is essential to the prevention of perioperative complications. Psychological preparation of the patient is needed in all cases. A more detailed discussion is necessary in those cases requiring patient participation, such as an awake craniotomy, where lack of preparation may result in failure of the procedure or a bad outcome for the patient. Many procedures are complex and the patient and family need to be aware of the potential problems at the end of the procedure, such as postoperative pain, nausea, and vomiting, new neurological deficits, and even the possibility of prolonged intubation and ventilation.

A thorough preoperative assessment of the patient's airway is critical in preparation and in prevention of devastating complications in neurosurgical patients. Patients may present with acute or chronic cervical spine disease or trauma, placing them at increased risk of spinal cord injury with excessive neck motion. Controversy exists surrounding the optimal approach to airway management. No single technique has been shown to be superior in the setting of suspected cervical spine disease or injury, and the choice will be guided largely by the skill set of the anesthesia provider. The anesthesiologist should prepare various airway adjuncts and have skilled assistance readily available to aid in difficult airway management. Once intubation of the trachea has been confirmed, the endotracheal tube must be definitively secured to prevent the loss of the airway during positioning of the patient. A bite block should be used whenever there ia a risk of execussive tongue edema macroglossia and possible post-extubation airway obstruction such as in the prone position.

Neurosurgical anesthesia frequently entails caring for a patient with significant comorbidities during long, complex operative procedures. During this time, the responsibility of medication dosing, including antibiotics and anti-epileptic agents, falls to the anesthesiologist. Anesthetic medications should be prepared and labeled as per ASA guidelines with appropriately colored labels, generic drug names, and concentration. All medications must be positively identified by label checking prior to administration. Potent vasoactive agents must be correctly prepared, labeled, and infused through appropriate infusion pumps. Several medications, such as heparin and insulin, are commonly administered using the wrong concentration; therefore, some advocate that these drugs should only be administered after a double check of dose is conducted by another independent provider (e.g., nurse or surgeon). Fluid management is controversial and each patient must be assessed individually with respect to the amount and type of intravenous fluid administered. The potential for cerebral ischemia exists in most neurosurgical procedures.

The role of neurological protection by mechanisms such as hypothermia and selective use of anesthetic agents is controversial but should be considered in high-risk procedures. Most anesthetic agents, including barbiturates, propofol, sevoflurane, desflurane, and isoflurane, have been shown to offer some element of neuroprotection. The actual technique of the anesthetic inhalation versus total intravenous anesthesia and the actual anesthetic agents chosen are probably not of the greatest concern. The real aim is to prevent any complication as a result of deviation from the appropriate management for each case. Neuromonitoring may, however, influence the type of anesthetic planned. For instance, total intravenous anesthesia may be required in patients where motor evoked potential monitoring is used, while electromyography recordings preclude the ongoing use of muscle relaxants. This should be discussed with the surgeon and neurophysiologist prior to the commencement of anesthesia.

A comprehensive review of standard equipment should also be carried out prior to the commencement of anesthesia. A formed checklist is a useful tool to ensure a proper safety check of the anesthetic machine. Cardiac arrest carts equipped with defibrillators and drugs for emergency resuscitation must be located nearby and maintained regularly. A cross match of blood should be performed prior to commencement of surgery and the hospital blood bank should be notified in cases where massive transfusion is anticipated. Pressure bags or a rapid transfuser should be readily available. In multi-level spinal surgeries, a blood salvage system may be of assistance. The protocol for rapidly obtaining blood must be understood and implemented for each institution. Failure to follow correct protocol for blood transfusion may lead to catastrophic events. Failure to identify the patient at the time of blood collection and prior to the initiation of transfusion has been recognized as the most common cause of acute intravascular hemolytic transfusion reaction.

The patient's core temperature should be monitored to ensure normothermia. Hypothermia has been investigated as a means of neuroprotection but has only been shown to be effective in the setting of global cerebral ischemia. Hypothermia is associated with complications such as coagulopathy, myocardial ischemia, and wound infection, while hyperthermia may contribute to secondary cerebral injury. Appropriate warming devices such as heated air blankets and fluid warmers are often necessary. Many other additional monitoring devices are usually required to prevent complications related to prolonged procedures and complex surgery. Invasive monitoring such as intra-arterial lines and central venous catheters can assist hemodynamic monitoring and allow ease of intraoperative blood sampling. A precordial Doppler may be considered in those cases with a high risk of air embolism. Urinary catheters should also be placed in longer procedures for assessment of fluid balance and monitoring of disorders such as diabetes insipidus.

Surgical site infection is a catastrophic complication of neurosurgery. The North American Spine Society has established clinical guidelines with respect to antibiotic prophylaxis in spine surgery. These guidelines support the use of preoperative prophylactic antibiotics in both instrumented and uninstrumented spinal surgery. They do not advocate the choice of one antibiotic or dosing schedule over another. Broad-spectrum coverage is recommended in patients with risk factors for polymicrobial infection. A common regimen would involve administering cefazolin 1 g intravenously 30 min prior to incision. This may be increased to a dose of 2 g in patients weighing greater than 80 kg. Repeated doses of antibiotics must be administered in cases exceeding four hours in duration.

Numerous studies have examined the role of prophylactic antibiotics in patients undergoing craniotomy. While the majority of studies support this practice, there has been concern that those patients treated with prophylactic antibiotics are more likely to develop infections with resistant bacteria. Further controversy surrounds the efficacy of this practice in preventing meningitis. While the use of antibiotics has been demonstrated to reduce the rate of surgical incision infection, there have been differing results in studies examining the prevention of meningitis. It is generally accepted that antibiotic prophylaxis is indicated for the placement of ventricular shunts, though no specific guidelines have been formulated regarding choice of drug, drug dose, timing of administration, or duration of treatment. Both intraventricular and systemic antibiotics have demonstrated benefit.

Concerns and Risks

Errors in Patient Identification and Wrong-Site Surgery

In a recent national survey of practicing neurosurgeons, 25% admitted to having cut skin on the wrong side of the head at least once in their careers, and 32% admitted to having removed lumbar disk material at the wrong level. The Joint Commission on Accreditation of Healthcare Organizations (JCAHO) maintains a database of wrong site, wrong procedure, and wrong patient surgery. Of 150 cases reported as of 2001, 14% were neurosurgical. The JCAHO identified multiple risk factors for wrong-site operations including emergency cases, unusual physical characteristics, unusual time pressures, involvement of multiple surgeons, and multiple procedures. However, the majority of such cases were attributed to a "breakdown in communication."

Difficult Airway Management

In the 2005 ASA closed claims report on management of the difficult airway, 19% of claims were related to patients in the neurosurgical or spine surgical group. The majority of these events, however, occurred outside of the perioperative location. Patients who have undergone recent surgical procedures such as cervical fusion may present for urgent reintubation when the airway becomes compromised due to hematoma formation or edema. Any site of anesthesia delivery should always be equipped to allow safe and efficient management of the airway. In addition to standard airway equipment, a difficult airway cart should be readily available in close proximity. The ASA has established guidelines for difficult airway management that include suggestions for contents of a portable unit for difficult airway management. This should include a fiberoptic bronchoscope, local anesthetic for topicalization, and a surgical cricothyroidotomy kit. When failure to intubate is highly anticipated, a surgeon skilled in emergency tracheostomy should be standing by in the room where the procedure is scheduled to occur.

Infection

The estimated incidence of postoperative infection in neurosurgery varies, depending on the procedure performed. The National Nosocomial Infections Surveillance System maintains a national database of hospital-acquired infections and calculates infection rates associated with specific surgical interventions and patient risk factors. In a summary of data collected from 1992 to 2004, the rate of infection for craniotomy ranged from 0.91 to 2.4 per 100 cases depending on patient risk category. Infection rates following ventricular shunt insertion were much higher, ranging from 4.42 to 5.36 infections per 100 cases. Infection rates for spinal fusion varied widely from 1.04 to 6.35 infections per 100 cases, depending on individual patient risk. Identifiable risk factors for infection also vary, depending on the procedure performed. Risk factors for postoperative infection following spinal surgery include age greater than 60 years, smoking, diabetes, previous surgical infection, BMI greater than 25.5, and alcohol abuse. Risk factors for meningitis following craniotomy include leakage of cerebrospinal fluid, concomitant incision infection, male gender, and longer surgical duration. Clinical risk factors for surgical site infection include CSF leakage and external CSF drainage. Implications range from the need for prolonged antibiotic therapy to reoperation, sepsis, or death. Preventative measures include strict adherence to aseptic technique, maintenance of intraoperative normothermia, and perioperative antibiotic prophylaxis. However, the broad spectrum of procedures performed within the scope of neurosurgery does not allow for universal guidelines with respect to antibiotic use. Given the considerable morbidity and mortality associated with infectious complications, careful consideration must be given to the need for antibiotic treatment at the time of surgery.

Out-of-the OR Procedures

Increasing numbers of neurosurgical interventions are being carried out in radiology suites and other locations remote from the standard operating room. Preparation and the provision of essential equipment is critical. Other risks to patient and personnel exist here as well. Protection from radiation exposure is required. If anesthesia is in an MRI suite or if an intraoperative MRI is planned, the room must be prepared with all MRI safety recommendations. To prevent injury and even death to the patient or personnel, a thorough review of both the room and all people must be performed to ensure that all metal objects have been removed.

Patient Positioning

Neurosurgical cases are frequently of long duration, requiring heightened vigilance with respect to patient positioning. Peripheral nerve injuries are not uncommon complications. Care must be taken to appropriately cushion all pressure points, particularly in extreme positions such as park bench, prone, or sitting.

Key Points

- Effective communication between individuals and disciplines is essential to the safe and efficient function of the operating room team.
- Miscommunication in the operating room has been implicated in adverse patient events.
- Operative briefings guided by a surgical safety checklist can improve communication in the operating room and reduce errors in patient identification and wrong-site surgery.
- Patients must be appropriately prepared based on their neurological and medical concerns.
- Psychological preparation of the patients should include a discussion of the requirements of the intraoperative procedure, postoperative implications, and outcome.
- Adequate preparation of all aspects of the operating room is essential to their efficient and safe function.
- Appropriate resuscitative equipment should always be readily available prior to the commencement of anesthesia.
- Neurosurgical patients can present unique challenges to airway management.
- Potential challenges with airway management should be anticipated and airway adjuncts must be readily available.
- Positioning must be performed with care to prevent related complications.
- Neurosurgical procedures performed remote from the operating room require additional planning and safety precautions.
- Surgical site infection is a serious complication of neurosurgery. Risk factors for postoperative infection vary depending upon the specific neurosurgical procedure.
- The indication for preoperative prophylactic antibiotics should be judged on an individual basis with consideration to the procedure to be performed.

Suggested Reading

A follow-up review of wrong site surgery. http://www.jointcommission.org/SentinelEvents/SentinelEventAlert/sea_24.htm. Accessed 14 Jan 2009.

American Society of Anesthesiologists Task Force on Management of the Difficult Airway. Practice guidelines for management of the difficult airway; an updated report by the American Society of Anesthesiologists Task Force on Management of the Difficult Airway. Anesthesiology. 2003;98:1269–77.

Fang A, Hu SS, Endres N, et al. Risk factors for infection after spinal surgery. Spine. 2005;30:1460–5.

Jhawar BS, Mitsis D, Duggal N. Wrong-sided and wrong-level neurosurgery: a national survey. J Neurosurg Spine. 2007;7:467–72.

Korinek AM, Baugnon T, Golmard JL, et al. Risk factors for adult nosocomial meningitis after craniotomy: role of antibiotic prophylaxis. Neurosurgery. 2006;59:126–33.

Lietard C, Thebaud V, Besson G, et al. Risk factors for neurosurgical site infections: an 18-month prospective survey. J Neurosurg. 2008;109:729–34.

National Nosocomial Infections Surveillance System. National Nosocomial Infections Surveillance (NNIS) System Report, data summary from January 1992 through June 2004, issued October 2004. Am J Infect Control. 2004;32:470–85.

North American Spine Society evidence-based clinical guidelines for multidisciplinary spine care. http://www.spine.org/Documents/Antibiotic_Prophylaxis_Web.pdf. Accessed 10 Dec 2008.

Peterson GN, Domino KB, Caplin RA, et al. Management of the difficult airway: a closed claims analysis. Anesthesiology. 2005;103:33–9.

[ST-41] Statement on ensuring correct patient, correct site, and correct procedure surgery. http://www.facs.org/fellows_info/statements/st-41.html. Accessed 18 Aug 2008.

Additional Suggested Reading

Bratzler DW, Houck PM. Antimicrobial prophylaxis for surgery: an advisory statement from the National Surgical Infection Prevention Project. Clin Infect Dis. 2004;38:1706–15.

Crosby ET. Considerations for airway management for cervical spine surgery in adults. Anesthesiol Clin. 2007;25:511–33.

Patient and unit identification. http://www.transfusionmedicine.ca/. Accessed 29 Sept 2008.

Ratilal B, Costa J, Sampaio C. Antibiotic prophylaxis for surgical introduction of intracranial ventricular shunts: a systematic review. J Neurosurg Pediatr. 2008;1:48–56.

Valentini LG, Casali C, Chatenoud L, et al. Surgical site infections after elective neurosurgery: a survey of 1747 patients. Neurosurgery. 2008;62:88–96.

World Health Organization Surgical Safety Checklist. http://www.who.int/patientsafety/safesurgery/tools_resources/SSSL_Checklist_finalJun08.pdf. Accessed 27 Sept 2008.

Chapter 14
Basics of Neurosurgical Techniques and Procedures

Kenneth C. Liu, Murat Oztaskin, and Kim J. Burchiel

Overview

Neurosurgical procedures are a collaborative effort between surgical, anesthesiology, and nursing teams. Approaches to the cranial vault are generally designed to minimize retraction and manipulation of surrounding neural tissue and to provide the shortest distance possible from the surgeon's hands to the surgical target. Cranial procedures are unique in that the approach vector can take on any number of trajectories. The position of the patient's head is determined by the anatomic location of the lesion and the approach and exposure selected by the neurosurgeon. Similarly, approaches to the spine are dependent on the target of interest and are typically posterior, anterior, lateral, or some combination of the three.

Implications for the Neurosurgical Patient

Cranial Surgery

Cranial procedures are often performed with the patient's head in three-point fixation to minimize movement of the operative field during the procedure. Approaches are fashioned depending upon the goal of the operation and the anatomic area of interest. Lesions on the superficial aspect of the brain are most easily operated upon

K.C. Liu, MD (✉)
Departments of Neurological Surgery and Radiology, University of Virginia
Health System, Charlottesville, VA, USA
e-mail: KCL3J@hscmail.mcc.virginia.edu

M. Oztaskin, MD • K.J. Burchiel, MD
Dotter Interventional Institute, Oregon Health & Science University, Portland, OR, USA

A.M. Brambrink and J.R. Kirsch (eds.), *Essentials of Neurosurgical Anesthesia & Critical Care*, DOI 10.1007/978-0-387-09562-2_14, © Springer Science+Business Media, LLC 2012

by placing the lesion near the top of the operative field. If the lesion is frontal, the head is secured in the anatomic position. If the lesion is occipital, the head is secured in the prone position. If the lesion is lateral, the head is turned to provide easy access to the lesion. Surgery of deeper structures, such as the cranial nerves and the arteries at the base of the brain require retraction of neural structures to adequately visualize and manipulate the surgical target. Additionally, brain relaxation via CSF drainage catheters is often used to provide adequate operative corridors.

Cautery is primarily used to control bleeding in the surgical field by the induction of thermal damage to incompetent blood vessels. The majority of non-neurosurgical procedures rely on monopolar electrocautery, which creates a current between a handheld electrode and an electrode placed on the patient's skin. This typically creates an arc of electricity between the handheld electrode and the tissue in closest proximity. Because this runs a current through the patient's body, neurosurgeons are hesitant to use monopolar electrocautery in an electrically active organ such as the brain, for fear of inducing cortical arrhythmias and/or seizures. More commonly, bipolar cautery is used for hemostasis in cortical tissue where the current runs between two poles in the forceps-shaped handpiece, precluding the need to run electrical current through the entire body. While bipolar cautery is fairly well tolerated, the use of monopolar cautery should be used with caution in patients harboring an electrically active device such as a pacemaker or implanted automatic defibrillator. Other methods of hemostasis typically involve tamponading the bleeding area with a biologic agent (such as methoxycellulose) soaked in thrombin. These methods tend not to work as well when the patient is hypertensive.

In patients undergoing cerebrovascular procedures, intraoperative angiograms are occasionally performed to confirm obliteration of the vascular anomaly. These are typically accomplished using a transfemoral approach with a catheter coupled with a fluoroscope. Intracranial Doppler ultrasonography is also used to confirm patency of parent vessels especially after aneurysm surgery. Intraoperative optical angiography is another method, albeit fairly new, that is used to evaluate the circulation in the surgical field. Injection of a fluorescing agent systemically can be visualized through digital infrared processing via the surgical microscope.

Spinal Surgery

Spinal procedures are performed with the patient in the supine, prone, or lateral positions. Preoperative communication between the surgeon and the anesthesiologist is important to identify issues related to the perioperative management of the patient. For example, spinal procedures may be associated with significant blood loss. Anterior approaches to the thoracic and lumbar spine may involve a thoracotomy and benefit from the anesthesiologist utilizing a double-lumen endotracheal tube. Transoral approaches to the high cervical spine may require keeping the patient intubated postoperatively because of airway edema. Careful communication between all members of the surgical team is crucial to preventing perioperative and postoperative morbidity.

Stereotactic and Awake Cranial Procedures

Occasionally, patients are kept awake for a portion of or all of a neurosurgical procedure. Procedures such as deep brain stimulation involve the implantation of an electrode in thalamic or subthalamic structures for the treatment of movement disorders. These procedures are often done awake to facilitate the correct placement of these electrodes and to monitor patient progress during the procedure. For these cases, the patient's head is secured in a frame, and for someone to lie with their head secured for an hour or more, especially someone with a movement disorder, this can be difficult. Carefully titrated anesthesia is required to keep the patient comfortable but awake enough so that they can be adequately assessed neurologically. Careful hemodynamic monitoring and control at the time the electrode is placed is necessary as well.

More extensive awake procedures are performed when a lesion, such as a tumor, involves the eloquent cortex of the brain, usually the speech area or the motor cortex. Some centers utilize a fully awake approach for the entire procedure with a scalp block as the only form of anesthesia. Other centers use an anesthetized-awake-sedated technique. In this latter situation, the patient is usually ventilated via an LMA, which is removed after emergence from anesthesia once the brain is exposed (see Chap. 20). The patient then answers questions or performs physical tasks while the surgeons stimulate the cortex to delineate which areas can be safely removed without causing a neurologic deficit. Keeping a patient who is in pins calm and awake while their cerebral cortex is exposed can be a daunting task. Once the lesion is removed, the patient is sedated for the remainder of surgery.

Shunt and Generator Implantation

These cases are fairly noninvasive neurosurgically but can still be very stimulating for patients. Placement of CSF shunts from the cranium to the peritoneum involves prepping out the patient from head to abdomen. The large surface exposure is associated with significant convective heat loss for the patient and makes it difficult for the anesthesia team to maintain the patient's body temperature in a normal physiologic range. ECG leads and other monitoring devices must be kept out of the surgical field and are best placed on the back of the patient. Shunt tubing or lead wires are passed between stab incisions to keep the hardware subcutaneous. This portion of the procedure (tunneling in the subcutaneous tissue) can be very stimulating for the patient.

Electrophysiologic Monitoring

Monitoring of cranial nerves or the cortex is done in certain cases where the intended surgical approach puts certain nervous structures at risk. Cranial nerve monitoring often involves the use of electromyographic needles placed into the various targets of the nerves and requires a working neuromuscular junction. Neuromuscular blockade, therefore, is contraindicated in this regard. Cortical EEG monitoring electrodes are used in somatosensory evoked potentials (SSEPs) and motor evoked potentials (MEPs) monitoring. Various inhalational and intravenous agents such as propofol can drastically affect the EEG. Again, preoperative communication with the surgical and electrophysiologic monitoring team is important in identifying these pitfalls.

Concerns and Risks

Placing the patient in "pins" or three-point fixation is quite stimulating, and adequate analgesia should be in place before the patient's cranium is secure by the surgeon. Preemptive strategies that have been employed to prevent hypertension or patient movement during pin placement include intravenous administration of short-acting anesthetics (e.g., propofol bolus), short-acting narcotic (e.g., alfentanil), or local block (either scalp block or local application of anesthetic at pin sites). Occasionally, the pins can cause a skull fracture or rest on the patient's face. This should be avoided. Once the head is secured, the neck is often flexed or extended to provide optimum access to the surgical target. This can cause the endotracheal tube to move proximally or distally, and care should be taken to ensure that the patient remains adequately ventilated after the head is secured. Additionally, severe flexion can cause cerebral venous outflow obstruction, which can be problematic for both the surgeon and the anesthesiologist. Likewise, severe flexion or extension may rarely result in critical impairment of arterial blood flow to the brain or direct cervical neurologic injury with potentially devastating consequences for the patient. Adequate space between the patient's chin and chest should be ensured prior to proceeding with the operation. For prone cranial procedures, the patient's head is typically placed in fixation when they are supine prior to rolling them into the prone position. This roll provides an opportunity for disaster, as carefully placed tubes and lines can be inadvertently pulled during positioning. When the patient is placed in the prone position for cranial procedures, adequate padding of pressure points must also be performed to prevent the formation of pressure sores and nerve injury.

In order for the surgeon to expose a large enough working surgical corridor to lesions deep in the brain, brain relaxation is important. This can be achieved with intravascular osmolytes (e.g., mannitol and hypertonic saline) and temporary hyperventilation. The systemic side effects of these two methods must be kept in mind while trying to maintain adequate brain relaxation. CSF drainage catheters, placed either intracranially or intrathecally via a lumbar approach, are occasionally used to control intracranial pressures or assist in brain relaxation. Careful communication between anesthesiologist and surgeon regarding the level of placement of these drainage tubes (i.e., "pop-off" level) and how much fluid should be drained is of tantamount importance. Excessive drainage can cause subdural hematomas and in severe cases, herniation syndrome. When brain relaxation does not provide enough visualization, for instance during surgery of deeper structures at the base of the skull, metal retractors blades are used to gently retract neural tissue. Excessive retraction can cause occult bleeding beneath the retractor or bleed or place tension on cranial nerves that provide autonomic tone to the vascular tree. During intracranial surgery, changes in the patient's vital signs can be very abrupt and should be communicated to the surgeon.

Blood pressure management can be critical, especially during cerebrovascular procedures (aneurysms, carotids, and AVMs). During active bleeding, blood pressures should be kept low. When temporary occlusion of arteries is in place to control bleeding, it is helpful to keep blood pressure up to maintain adequate cerebral perfusion via collaterals to the areas of brain at risk for ischemia. Occasionally, during surgery of the brain stem or during surgery where there are rapid changes in intracranial pressure (decompression during trauma surgery or hydrocephalus surgery), changes in blood pressure and heart rate can be noted secondary to traction or disturbance of the baroreceptor areas in the brainstem. These are often transient in nature but can be severe enough to temporarily require vasoactive pharmacological support. Effective communication of the anesthesiologist with the surgeon can often facilitate surgical amelioration of the inciting factor (e.g., retraction, stimulation, and manipulation) that is causing the hemodynamic instability.

Spinal procedures often have the patient's arms in non-anatomic positions and care should be taken to ensure that there is not excessive traction on the brachial plexus. In situations where the patient is prone, care should be taken not to have the arms in an extended position. They should be flexed at the shoulder and elbow to prevent nerve and joint injury. Spinal procedures also often involve the use of a fluoroscopic unit (C-arm) to guide hardware placement. When the unit is moved in or out of the surgical field, the technician or surgeon can inadvertently place the unit on the patient's body. In addition, this movement may inadvertently result in premature removal of an intravascular catheter or disconnection of a physiologic monitoring. Vigilance is key to prevent complications from excessive pressure and traction from the fluoroscopy unit. Significant blood loss is associated with invasive spinal procedures and should be monitored carefully to optimize perioperative management. For posterior spinal operations, retraction of the paraspinal musculature is used to gain adequate exposure to the bony and neural elements of the spine. Prolonged retraction and prone positioning has been known to occasionally result in rhabdomyolysis or postoperative visual loss.

Key Points

- Positioning the patient for either a cranial or spinal operation requires careful communication with the surgical and nursing teams to minimize perioperative morbidity.
- Preoperative planning with the surgical team regarding the planned use of CSF drainage, the use of neuromuscular blockade, or if the patient will remain awake during the procedure is critical.
- Blood pressure management during cerebrovascular procedures is critical during periods of active hemorrhage and temporary ligation.
- Abrupt changes in vitals can occur with rapid changes in intracranial pressure or manipulation of the brain stem and lower cranial nerves.

Suggested Reading

Fletcher S, Lam A. Anesthesia: preoperative evaluation. In: Winn HR, editor. Youmans neurological surgery. 5th ed. Philadelphia: Elsevier; 2004.

Goodkin R, Mesiwala A. Surgical exposure and positioning. In: Winn HR, editor. Youmans neurological surgery. 5th ed. Philadelphia: Elsevier; 2004.

Jenkins III AL, Deutch H, Patel NP, Post KD. Complication avoidance in neurosurgery. In: Winn HR, editor. Youmans neurological surgery. 5th ed. Philadelphia: Elsevier; 2004.

Chapter 15
Positioning the Patient for Neurosurgical Operations

Alexander Zlotnik, Monica S. Vavilala, and Irene Rozet

Overview

Patient positioning for surgery should provide surgical comfort and optimization of surgical exposure, while minimizing positioning-related risks and complications. The most common complications of patient positioning include pressure sores and peripheral nerve damage (brachial, sacral, lumbar plexus, ulnar, radial, sciatic, and common peroneal nerves injuries). Besides length of surgery, preexisting pressure ulcers, extremes of age (neonates, elderly), major comorbidities, thin body habitus, morbid obesity, and/or smoking are risk factors for positioning related pressure ulcers. Most commonly, pressure ulcers occur at the ischium, trochanter, or heel. Other specific complications related to positioning for neurosurgical procedures include cerebral edema and bleeding, visual loss, quadriplegia, venous and paradoxical air embolism, pneumocephalus, and macroglossia.

A. Zlotnik, MD
Department of Anesthesiology and Critical Care, Soroka University Medical Center,
Ben Gurion-University of the Negev, Beer-Sheva, Israel

M.S. Vavilala, MD
Departments of Anesthesiology and Pain Medicine and Neurological Surgery, Radiology,
University of Washington and Harborview Injury Prevention and Research Center,
Harborview Medical Center, Seattle, WA, USA

I. Rozet, MD (✉)
Department of Anesthesiology, and Pain Medicine, University of Washington and
VA Paget Sound Health Care System, Seattle, WA, USA
e-mail: irozet@u.washington.edu

A.M. Brambrink and J.R. Kirsch (eds.), *Essentials of Neurosurgical Anesthesia & Critical Care*, DOI 10.1007/978-0-387-09562-2_15,
© Springer Science+Business Media, LLC 2012

Implications for the Neurosurgical Patients

Neurosurgical procedures are often lengthy. Therefore, attention must be paid to patient positioning. Proper positioning requires an adequate anesthetic depth (or adequate comfort for the patient having an awake procedure), maintenance of ventilation and hemodynamic stability within the desired physiologic range. The most commonly utilized positions in neurosurgery, their risks and preventive measures for positioning related complications for neurosurgical procedures are described in Tables 15.1 and 15.2.

Table 15.1 Summary of benefits with positioning for neurosurgical procedures

Supine position
1. Optimal approach to frontal lobe and anterior spine
2. The safest position; does not require disconnection of the endotracheal tube and invasive monitors during repositioning, good approach to the patient's airway
3. Minimal risk for genital and breast injuries
4. Minimal risk for VAE, pneumocephalus, and visual loss
5. Less risk for postoperative upper airway edema compared with sitting and prone

Lateral position
1. Optimal approach to the temporal lobe
2. Good approach to the patient's airway
3. Minimal risk for head position-related injury
4. Minimal risk for genital and breast injuries
5. Minimal risk for VAE and pneumocephalus
6. No risk of visual loss
7. Less risk for postoperative upper airway edema compared with sitting and prone

Prone position
1. Optimal posterior approach to spine and posterior fossa
2. Less risk for VAE compared with sitting (12% of the cases)
3. Less risk for pneumocephalus and quadriplegia compared with sitting
4. Less risk for brain ischemia, if invasive blood pressure transducer is not in an appropriate level. Blood pressure transducer shall be positioned and zeroed at the level of ear canal (the scull base) rather at the level of atrium to reflect and maintain adequate cerebral perfusion

Sitting position
1. Optimal approach to posterior fossa and posterior cervical spine
2. The best surgical exposure and anatomic orientation, low ICP, good CSF and venous outflow, minimal bleeding, reduced risk for cranial nerve damage, less need for diuretic therapy, and blood transfusions
3. Easy access to airway
4. No risk for visual loss
5. Excellent respiratory/ventilatory conditions

Three-quarters position
1. The position is used for posterior fossa and parieto-occipital surgery and resembles lateral position
2. The risk of VAE is lower compared with sitting position
3. Acceptable access to airway

ICP intracranial pressure, *VAE* venous air embolism, *CSF* cerebrospinal fluid

Table 15.2 Summary of specific risks with positioning for neurosurgical procedures and their preventions

Risks of positioning	Preventive measures
Supine position	
1. Impaired venous return from the head leading to brain edema and macroglossia, and nerve damage due to head positioning (rotation, or flexion, or extension)	1. Avoid head rotation more than 45° in relation to body axis. Elevate head by 15–30°. Zero invasive blood pressure transducer at the level of the Circle of Willis
2. Upper airway edema after spinal surgery (anterior approach, longer than 5 h)	2. Avoid an excessive surgical retraction. Monitor high-risk patients within 36 h after the surgery
3. Brachial plexus injury	3. Avoid an excessive traction down of the shoulders. Place the roll under the dependent shoulder
Lateral position	
1. Brachial plexus injury and compression of dependent axillary artery	1. Place axillary roll under the upper chest and away from axilla. Avoid an excessive traction of shoulders
2. Common peroneal and saphenous nerve injuries	2. Place pillows between knees and ankles. No tubing or catheters should be allowed under or between the legs
Prone position	
1. Difficult positioning necessitating the patient disconnection from monitoring and ventilation	1. Pulse oximeter and arterial line should be left in place whenever possible. Preoxygenate the patient before positioning to increase safe time
2. Access to the airway is poor. Copious secretions may weaken fixation of ETT	2. Verify position and safely secure ETT and check connections of respiratory circle. Consider using at additional adhesives with tape, and combination of tie and tape fixation of the ETT. Periodically check that tie is not interfering with surgical field and not compromising venous outflow, suction oral secretions. Provide a free access to tubing and connections
3. High intraabdominal pressure may impair ventilation and hemodynamic stability	3. Frames supporting the chest and leaving abdominal wall free should be used (Jackson table and frame are the best choice, also Wilson, Relton-Hall, and Andrews frame may be used)
4. Postoperative visual loss	4. Protect eyes. Avoid any external pressure on eyes, recheck it every 30 min. For high-risk patients avoid low arterial blood pressure (probably less than 85 mmHg systolic for normotensive patients or within 25% of the patient's baseline level), anemia (no lower threshold for blood transfusion is recommended to date), and prolonged head down position leading to venous congestion
5. Brachial plexus injury	5. Avoid excessive traction and hyperextension of shoulders and arms
6. Risk of VAE	6. Avoid steep head up position
7. Risk of upper airway and tongue edema; cranial nerves damage	7. Avoid excessive head flexion. Maintain at least 2–3 finger-breadths of thyromental distance. Avoid foreign bodies in the pharynx (TEE probe, oral airway). Properly-sized oro/nasogastric tube is usually safe

(continued)

Table 15.2 (continued)

Risks of positioning	Preventive measures
Sitting position	
1. Risk of VAE and paradoxical air embolism	1. Use prehydration with crystalloids and colloids before the induction and positioning to maintain adequate circulating blood volume, pneumatic anti-shock trousers, PEEP, precordial Doppler for the monitoring, and right atrial catheter for air aspiration. Sitting position is dangerous with open foramen ovale
2. Hemodynamic instability due to decreased venous return	2. Use prehydration, wrap the legs with elastic bandages, and slow, incremental adjustment of table position
3. Edema of upper airway and tongue (macroglossia); cranial nerves damage	3. Avoid excessive head flexion. Maintain at least 2–3 finger-breadths thyromental distance. Avoid foreign bodies in the pharynx (TEE probe, oral airway). Properly-sized oro/nasogastric tube is not a concern
4. Common peroneal and sciatic nerve damage	4. Knees should be partially flexed. The buttock gel pad prevents an excessive pressure on the sciatic nerve
5. Impairment of brain perfusion	5. Invasive blood pressure transducer should be zeroed at the level of the Circle of Willis. Blood pressure transducer shall be positioned and zeroed at the level of ear canal (the scull base) rather at the level of atrium to reflect and maintain adequate cerebral perfusion. Maintain CPP at 60–80 mmHg
6. Pneumocephalus and tension pneumocephalus	6. Discontinue nitrous oxide before the dural closure
Three-quarters position	
1. Brachial plexus injury due to both compression of brachial plexus on the dependent side and stretching of non-dependent shoulder toward the legs for better surgical exposure	1. Place axillary roll under the upper chest and away from axilla. Avoid an excessive traction of non-dependent shoulder
2. Other risks are similar to *lateral* position	

ETT endotracheal tube, *TEE* transesophageal echocardiography, *VAE* venous air embolism, *PEEP* positive end-expiratory pressure, *CPP* cerebral perfusion pressure

Head Positioning

Patient positioning for craniotomies and the majority of spine procedures begins with positioning of the head. Special attention is paid to the skeletal fixation of the head with the pins fixation device, providing both immobility of the head and surgical comfort. Application of a skeletal fixation device has a profound stimulating effect, leading to tachycardia and hypertension. Therefore, deepening the plane of general anesthesia and/or infiltration of local anesthetic of the skin at the anticipated pin sites in conjunction with a scalp block with local anesthetic is required before pinning. To maintain hemodynamic stability preventing both hypertensive and tachycardic responses as well as hypotension which potentially may compromise cerebral perfusion pressure (CPP), the anesthetic given should be carefully titrated using standard or invasive blood pressure monitoring. Risks of using the head holder with pins include bleeding, air embolism (especially in sitting position), scalp and eye laceration, and cervical spine injury during inadvertent patient movement. Patients should be adequately anesthetized until the head holder is removed. If the surgical procedure is planned to be done with the patient awake and in a pinned head holder, adequate local anesthetic at the pin sites (skin and periostium) and placement of a scalp blocks allows for adequate patient comfort. Risks of *head* malpositioning include decrease in blood flow in vertebral and carotid arteries, potentially causing brain stem and cervical spine ischemia, quadriparesis, and quadriplegia. Hyperflexion may reduce anterior–posterior size of the hypopharynx, causing ischemia of the base of the tongue, leading to pharyngeal and tongue edema. This complication is more common when foreign bodies [transesophageal echocardiography (TEE) probe, oral airway] are used. Maintaining 2–3 finger-breadths thyromental distance is recommended during neck flexion. The head can be safely rotated between 0 and 45° lateral to the left and right from the body's sagittal axis. If more rotation is needed, a supportive chest roll should be placed under the opposite shoulder. Impairment of cerebral venous outflow may occur as a result of improper head positioning due to an external pressure on the neck [like with the neck collar, or endotracheal tube (ETT) fixation device], or "head down" position, and can potentially cause intraoperative brain swelling resulting in poor surgical conditions, increase in intracranial pressure (ICP) in enclosed brain areas (distant to surgical site), enhanced surgical bleeding, and even cerebral hemorrhage or ischemia. Fifteen degrees head up position is generally optimal during neurosurgery to allow adequate venous drainage. Neck vein distention, elevated ICP, and jugular bulb pressure are signs of inadequate head and neck positioning.

Body Positioning

There are five basic body positions utilized in neurological surgery: "supine," "lateral," "prone," "sitting," and "three-quarters." Each position has special considerations with respect to desired effects (Table 15.1) and risks (Table 15.2), such as compromise in ventilation and hemodynamic stability.

Concerns and Risks

The risks, complications, and ways to prevent them during patient positioning for the neurosurgical procedure are summarized in Table 15.2.

Although the incidence of perioperative visual loss (POVL) has not been reported higher than 0.2%, POVL represents one of the most devastating complications of modern spine surgery in prone position. The predisposing factors include prolonged duration of surgery, significant blood loss, and intraoperative hypotension. The preventive measures of intraoperative management are listed in Table 15.2. To avoid an excessive blood loss and hemodynamic instability, high-risk patients should be identified, and staging of the surgery should be considered early, allowing the patient to recover during 4–7 days between surgeries (sometimes to complete an extensive

Key Points

- Deepen anesthesia and use local anesthetic before application of the device for skeletal fixation of the head is recommended to prevent hyper-dynamic cardiovascular response.
- Avoid hyperflexion of the head to prevent quadriplegia and airway edema, maintain minimum 2–3 finger-breadths of thyromental distance. Avoid the head rotation more then 45°.
- Head up position of 15° is optimal for neurosurgical procedures. Neck vein distention, elevation of ICP, and bulking brain are signs of inappropriate head and neck positioning and an obstruction of the venous outflow from the brain.
- Properly secure the tracheal tube and respiratory circuit in place before positioning, since access to patient's airway is difficult in prone position.
- Postoperative visual loss is a devastating complication of prone positioning. Eyes should be properly protected and checked every 30 min to avoid an external pressure over the eyeballs. Severe anemia and low blood pressure should be avoided.
- Avoid hypotension in sitting position by preventing and rapidly correcting hypovolemia, wrapping of the legs with elastic bandages, and slow, incremental adjustment of table position.
- In sitting position, transduce mean arterial pressure (MAP) corrected to the Circle of Willis (interauricular plane) to provide a CPP above 60 mmHg.
- Prevent tension pneumocephalus in sitting position by discontinuing nitrous oxide before dural closure. Clinical signs of postoperative tension pneumocephalus include delayed awakening, new neurological deficit, headache, and signs of increased ICP. Consider immediate head CT for differential diagnosis. Twist drill hole and dural puncture for decompression may be considered for treatment, if needed.
- Use protective padding whenever possible, particularly for upper extremities. Use chest rolls in lateral position.
- If feasible, monitor somatosensory evoked potentials (SSEPs) for early detection of ischemia due to peripheral nerve damage, and reposition, if needed.
- Assess and document patient's neurological condition pre- and postoperatively.

spine surgery with instrumentation may require four separate procedures). Postoperatively, the vision should be assessed when the patient is awake. In case of any concern regarding potential POVL, an urgent ophthalmologic consultation should be obtained.

Suggested Reading

American Society of Anesthesiologists Task Force on the Prevention of Perioperative Peripheral Neuropathies. American Society of Anesthesiologists Task Force on the prevention of perioperative peripheral neuropathies: practice advisory for the prevention of perioperative peripheral neuropathies. Anesthesiology. 2000;92:1168–82.

Black S, Ockert DB, Oliver WC, et al. Outcome following posterior fossa craniectomy in patients in the sitting or horizontal positions. Anesthesiology. 1988;69:49–56.

Miller RD, editor. Miller's anesthesia. 6th ed. Philadelphia: Churchill Livingston; 2006. p. 2134–42. Chapter 53.

Orliaguet GA, Hanafi M, Meyer PG, et al. Is the sitting or the prone position best for surgery for posterior fossa tumours in children? Paediatr Anaesth. 2001;11:541–7.

St-Arnaud D, Paquin MJ. Safe positioning for neurosurgical patients. AORN J. 2008;87:1156–68. quiz 69–72.

Chapter 16
The Intraoperative Team: Getting the Most Out of Collaborative Care in the Operating Room

Debra A. Reeves

Overview

As surgery continues to become increasingly complex both technologically and procedurally, effective collaboration among intraoperative team members remains an important way to decrease errors and increase patient care safety. Multiple studies in recent years have shown that communication failure is the central issue in many critical incidents where patients experienced complications that could have been prevented.

Identifying and overcoming the barriers to effective collaboration that are inherent in the Operating Room system, as well as having a basic understanding of the perioperative nurse's role in caring for the surgical patient, are important in preventing and managing complications in the neurological surgery patient.

Effective collaboration in the operating room can be defined as optimization of the care of the patient through mutual understanding and respect of the individualized but interdependent roles of each intraoperative team member, as they work together toward a common goal of accomplishing a safe and successful surgical procedure.

There are many barriers to effective collaboration in the operating room. It is a dynamic environment which is frequently noisy and sometimes chaotic. Multiple team members are simultaneously carrying out tasks that relate to their own agenda within the overall care of the surgical patient. Through the course of the workday, intraoperative team members change during breaks or at shift ends forcing the team to form and reform multiple times. New team members may or may not have similar levels of knowledge and experience but are expected to maintain the highest level of functioning while caring for the patient. Each transfer of care between team members carries with it a risk of communication breakdown.

D.A. Reeves, RN, BS, BSN (✉)
Division of Perioperative Services, Oregon Health & Science University, Portland, OR, USA
e-mail: reevesd@ohsu.edu

A.M. Brambrink and J.R. Kirsch (eds.), *Essentials of Neurosurgical Anesthesia & Critical Care*, DOI 10.1007/978-0-387-09562-2_16,
© Springer Science+Business Media, LLC 2012

In addition to a difficult physical environment, a surgical schedule runs with an underlying time pressure. The need for decreased costs, increased efficiency, and rapid turnovers for timely accomplishment of procedures creates a hurried atmosphere. Team functioning suffers when team members feel rushed with a resultant increase in risk of error.

Both the scrub person and circulating nurse have well-defined roles during a surgical procedure. The scrub person, who could be either a Surgical Technologist or a Registered Nurse (RN), focuses primarily on the surgical field. The Scrub Tech or Nurse is responsible for managing the surgical instruments and implants, handing them to the surgeon as they are needed, and assisting with the surgery when necessary, while maintaining the integrity of the sterile field.

The circulating nurse is an RN who has received an average of 6 months of additional training in surgical nursing. During training, the nurse learns basic information about the procedures most common to each surgical specialty, the risks inherent in all procedures such as infection, blood loss, and inability to maintain normothermia, as well as the additional risks caused by the administration of anesthesia, the effects of prolonged immobility on blood flow and skin integrity, and the risks of nerve damage due to positioning of the patient to optimize surgical exposure. The surgical nurse is trained with the holistic view that they function as the patient's primary advocate during a time when they are unable to speak for themselves. The circulating nurse is also responsible for managing the equipment used within the surgical suite and must know how to operate and where to place items such as pneumatic drills, electrocautery units, lasers, microscopes, and positioning devices for example. Nurses who specialize in neurological surgery have received additional training specific to neurological surgery procedures and additional considerations for the patient undergoing neurological surgery.

This chapter, written from the perspective of a neurological surgery circulating nurse, outlines the data that is gathered and analyzed by the nurse to determine the needs of the patient and plan for their care during the procedure. Risks common to various types of neurological surgery procedures and interventions to prevent or manage possible complications will be included. A list of suggestions for overcoming the barriers to effective collaboration will follow in the "Risks and Concerns" section.

Implications for the Neurological Surgery Patient

Earlier chapters have discussed preparation for surgery, the basics of surgical techniques and patient positioning. The following section provides information detailing how the circulating nurse prepares and executes a plan of care for a neurological surgery patient in a sequential format.

- Review the planned procedure:

  - Check scheduling form information, clarify with surgeon if inconsistencies are found.

- Determine equipment, instruments, implants, and supplies that will be required.
- Determine the availability, including ETA if not currently available.
- Configure the equipment and positioning devices in the room as necessary for operative exposure.
- Determine the normal risks for the patient due to the type of procedure:

  (a) Hypothermia, DVT, infection; all surgeries.
  (b) Skin breakdown; procedure scheduled longer than 4 h.
  (c) Massive blood loss; aneurysm/AVM, intracranial bleed, tumor in cavernous sinus.
  (d) Air embolus; sitting craniotomy.

- Determine additional risks for the individual patient:

  - Review the patient's H&P, current labs, and allergies.
  - Interview the patient and conduct preoperative assessment including:

    (a) Confirmation that the patient understands what procedure is planned.
    (b) Confirmation of allergies and previous surgeries, e.g., joint replacements.
    (c) Discussion of other pertinent history, current pain level, and any emotional or spiritual needs.

  - Assess for increased risk of skin breakdown using sensory perception, moisture, activity/mobility, nutrition, and friction and shear as well as age criteria (e.g., Braden Scale score).
  - Assess for increased risk of infection: history of MRSA, VRE, trauma, and current infection.
  - Assess for increased risk of DVT: positive history, suspended anti-coagulant therapy.
  - Assess for increased risk of blood loss; highly vascular tumor, suboptimal lab values.

- Review patient and procedural data with the anesthesia provider:

  - Need for awake or fiber-optic intubation; unstable C-spine, limited neck mobility.
  - Need for additional invasive lines; arterial line, central line, large bore IV.
  - Discuss any need for deviation from standard preoperative antibiotic.
  - Discuss probability of need for blood products and confirm availability if necessary.
  - Discuss level of readiness and ongoing communication during the procedure.
  - Plan for any known high risks.

- Initiate plan of care from time into the OR through procedure end

  - Accompany the patient to the operating room or receive the patient in the room.
  - Provide warm blanket, apply DVT prevention, offer emotional support.

- Assist Anesthesia Provider during intubation.
- Place foley catheter (if indicated), perform initial count with scrub person.
- Assist with positioning of the patient for the procedure:

  (a) Cushion pressure points, bony prominences, and vulnerable nerves with gel devices. Place support devices such as chest rolls, Mayfield headrest, pillows, overhead arm support boards, etc. Place additional devices as needed for patient safety or operative exposure such as warming blanket, safety belt, tape, traction devices, etc.

- Assist with surgical skin prep and draping of patient for the procedure.
- Participate in surgeon lead pause (or time-out) and document according to policy.
- Connect electrical devices and move equipment into final position at commencement of procedure.
- Assess room for safe and functional placement of electrical cords, equipment, etc. and adjust as needed.
- Pre-check blood products with Anesthesia Provider if there is high probability of need.
- Call OR charge nurse for assistance if patient experiences airway emergency, code, massive blood loss, or other serious unexpected event.
- Communicate all necessary information to team members at every patient hand-off during the procedure and when calling report to PACU using a consistent format.

Risks and Concerns

In the absence of effective collaboration, the risk of error during surgery increases as well as the possibility that the patient will experience a preventable complication. Historically, the operating room has been a hierarchical and sometimes personality driven environment. Although current surgical culture has shifted away from old attitudes and beliefs, being able to create high functioning intraoperative teams on a daily basis will probably always be somewhat of a challenge.

Improving the communication among team members is the key to implementing the solutions listed below. Ideally, all intraoperative team members would contribute equally to the effort, but any team member can make a difference. Here are some characteristics of good communication: it should be professional, respectful, accurate, comprehensive, timely, and specific without personal emotional content, and always with the goal of exchanging the information needed to provide safe care for the patient.

Following is a list of some common barriers to collaboration and suggestions for overcoming them:

- The perioperative environment

  - *Noise*: Reduce distracting environmental sounds at key times and ask for quiet when crucial information is being exchanged.
  - *Chaos*: Coordinate activities with other team members to help avoid distraction when critical tasks are performed.
  - *Time pressure*: Organize tasks, delegate appropriately, and communicate changes in patient condition or procedure plan as they occur.

- The intraoperative team

  - *Team work*: Understand individual roles of surgical team members, resolve interpersonal issues as they arise, encourage team members to voice questions, and concerns.
  - *Team member changes*: Communicate to assess knowledge/experience levels, share relevant information, and encourage questions, comments, concerns.

Key Points

Intraoperative Team Collaboration:

- *Anticipate*: Review the procedure, possible complications specific to the procedure and to the patient.
- *Communicate*: Exchange information with all team members. Confirm any procedural or patient variables.
- *Plan*: Determine the needs for care of the patient, e.g., lines, equipment, instruments, implants, and availability of each. Plan coordination of activities, discuss concerns.
- *Respond*: Take action early when potential problems are identified, utilize resources to avoid complications.
- *Collaborate effectively*: Encourage clear, thorough, respectful, and frequent communication throughout the procedure. Ask for debriefing after adverse outcomes or near-misses.

Suggested Reading

Amato-Vealey E, Barba M, et al. Hand-off communication: A requisite for perioperative patient safety. AORN J. 2008;88(5):763–70.

Helmreich R, Schaefer HG. Team performance in the operating room in Bogner, MS. Human error in medicine. Hillsdale, NJ: Lawrence Erlbaum; 1994. p. 225–53.

Lefevre F, Woolger J. Surgery in the patient with neurologic disease. Med Clin North Am. 2003;87:257–71.

Lingard L, Espin S, et al. Communication failures in the operating room: an observational classification of recurrent types and effects. Qual Saf Health Care. 2004;13:330–4.

Powel SM, Hill RK. My co-pilot is a nurse-using crew resource management in the OR. AORN J. 2006;83(1):178–202.

Part IV
Critical Situations During Anesthesia for Brain Surgery in Adults

Chapter 17
The "Tight Brain": Cerebral Herniation Syndrome

Leslie C. Jameson, Paul D. Mongan, Daniel J. Janik, and Tod B. Sloan

Overview

"Tight brain" is a euphemistic reference to elevation in intracranial pressure (ICP) caused by expansion in the intracranial volume beyond its ability to compensate. This can be seen in patients with mass lesions or acute trauma during a craniotomy when acute changes in neurophysiology cause increased brain swelling and in the intensive care unit. Treatment rests on understanding the physiology of the intracranial compartments.

ICP is the sum of the partial pressures of the intracranial (IC) contents: brain tissue (approximately 80% of normal total volume), cerebrospinal fluid (CSF) (8–12%), and venous and arterial blood volume (6–8% and 2–4% respectively). Normal ICP is between 5 and 10 mmHg with intracranial hypertension (ICH) defined as pressures above 20 mmHg. ICH is usually categorized as mild (20–29 mmHg), moderate (30–40 mmHg), or severe (>40 mmHg). As in all closed containers, pressure increases as volume expands beyond the ability of other components to contract. Normal physiologic events increase ICP briefly with little consequence; however, pathologic

L.C. Jameson, MD (✉)
Department of Anesthesiology, University of Colorado at Denver School of Medicine,
Aurora, CO, USA
e-mail: leslie.jameson@ucdenver.edu

P.D. Mongan, MD
Department of Anesthesiology, University of Colorado at Denver, School of Medicinal,
Aurora, CO, USA

D.J. Janik, MD
Department of Anesthesiology, University of Colorado at Denver School of Medicine,
Aurora, CO, USA

T.B. Sloan, MD, MBA, PhD
Department of Anesthesiology, The University of Colorado Denver School of Medicine,
Aurora, CO, USA

A.M. Brambrink and J.R. Kirsch (eds.), *Essentials of Neurosurgical Anesthesia & Critical Care*, DOI 10.1007/978-0-387-09562-2_17,
© Springer Science+Business Media, LLC 2012

Table 17.1 Causes of intracranial pressure increase

| Physiologic causes | Pathologic causes | |
	Acute	Chronic
• Increased abdominal/ thoracic pressure (valsalva, cough) • Relative hypoventilation (sleep, sedation) • Drug effect (general anesthetics, limited antibiotics) • Increased metabolic demands (seizures, fever) • Hypervolemia (fluid overload, head down position) • Hypoperfusion vasodilation (anemia, ischemia)	• Intraparenchymal hemorrhage (hemorrhagic stroke, aneurysm rupture, postoperative intracranial hemorrhage) • Traumatic hemorrhage (epidural hematoma, acute subdural hematoma) • Acute cerebral edema (acute hyponatremia, hepatic coma, Reye's syndrome, cerebral contusion from traumatic brain injury (TBI), severe hypertension)	• Slow growing lesion (brain tumor-primary, metastatic, abscess) • Disturbance in CSF absorption, production or flow (hydrocephalus, idiopathic intracranial hypertension) • Chronic subdural hematoma • Congenital anomalies (Arnold Chiari malformation, stenosis of aqueduct of Sylvii)

increases in ICP can produce brain injury. Whereas slow increases in ICP can be caused by gradual volume increases (e.g., tumor and hydrocephalus) and often require little therapeutic action, rapid increases (e.g., intracranial hemorrhage, cerebral edema, and some metabolic derangements (e.g., hepatic coma, hyponatremia, and severe hyperglycemia)) (Table 17.1) require urgent therapy in a critical care unit or surgical suite. During craniotomy, treatment will be required to reduce brain swelling to facilitate surgery and occasionally allow for dural closure at the end of surgery.

Prevention

ICP management for anesthesiologists and critical care physicians is mitigation of the progression of an existing process and requires aggressive physiological and pharmacologic therapy until, in many cases, surgical intervention (e.g., tumor excision, shunt placement, and decompressive craniectomy) can occur.

Crisis Management

Pathophysiology and Clinical Presentation

The most common cause of increased ICP is expansion of the extracellular and intracellular components of the brain parenchyma. These volumes are maintained by an effective blood–brain barrier (BBB); blood vessels allow only small molecules (e.g., Na^+, K^+, and glucose) to be exchanged between the extracellular fluid and the intravascular space (Chap. 3). Extracellular edema, usually in the white

Table 17.2 Signs and symptoms of increased ICP

Mild elevation (20–29 mmHg)	Moderate elevation (30–40 mmHg)	Severe elevation (>40 mmHg)
• Unrelenting positional headache • Nausea and vomiting • Papilledema • Blurred vision • Loss of retinal venous pulsations	• Confusion and agitation • Drowsiness progressing to lethargy • Decreased papillary response (constriction, dilation), Sluggish • Seizures • Spontaneous hyperventilation • Focal motor weakness	• Progressive decreased consciousness • Anisocoria (asymmetric pupils) • Tonic eye deviation • Seizures • Decerebrate posturing • Cushing's reflex • Abnormal respiratory pattern • Hypotension • Death

matter, occurs when there is fluid transfer across the BBB due to increased permeability. Edema can be caused by increased active fluid leakage (vasogenic edema, angiogenesis factors from brain tumors), passive fluid transfer from reduced osmotic pressure (osmotic edema), elevated venous pressure (compressive edema), and elevated CSF pressure (hydrocephalic edema). Therapeutic actions that reduce fluid transfer include increased serum osmotic pressure, decreased venous pressure, and reduced CSF pressure. Intracellular edema (particularly in neurons) is usually due to cellular injury or ischemia leading to the loss of membrane integrity then swelling and eventually cell death (cytotoxic edema; Chaps. 9 and 18).

The CSF volume is regulated by the balance of production, passive filtration, and active transport of the noncellular components of blood at the choroid plexus and absorption by the arachnoid villa in dural sinusoids. Obstruction of CSF flow through drainage channels and increases in cerebral venous pressure (CVP) expand the CSF volume (Chap. 1).

Expansion of intracranial blood volume also increases ICP. Any situation that increased CVP such as, obstruction of jugular veins (excessive neck rotation), increased intrathoracic pressure, valsalva and a head down position will increase intracranial venous blood volume and ICP. Arterial volume contributes to elevated ICP when physiologic or drug-induced perturbations cause vasodilation. Physiologic demands that increase cerebral metabolic rate (CMR) increase ICP; likewise, direct vasodilators such as nitroprusside increase ICP. Pharmacological and physiological changes that reduce arterial volume lower ICP. These actions are most effective in normal brain since autoregulation in damaged brain is often lost.

The clinical presentation of the "tight brain" depends to some degree on the speed of ICP increase. When expansion is slow, a volume reduction of 80 cc in intracranial volume can occur before elevation in ICP begins, but, with rapid expansion, the ability of the brain to accommodate is reduced. Symptoms begin when intracranial volume expansion leads to an ICP increase. The relationship between the volume increase and the consequent ICP increase is termed elastance (change in pressure per unit change in volume).

Symptoms of mild ICH are intractable headache that worsens with lying flat, breath holding or valsalva (Table 17.2). With moderate ICH, symptoms progress to

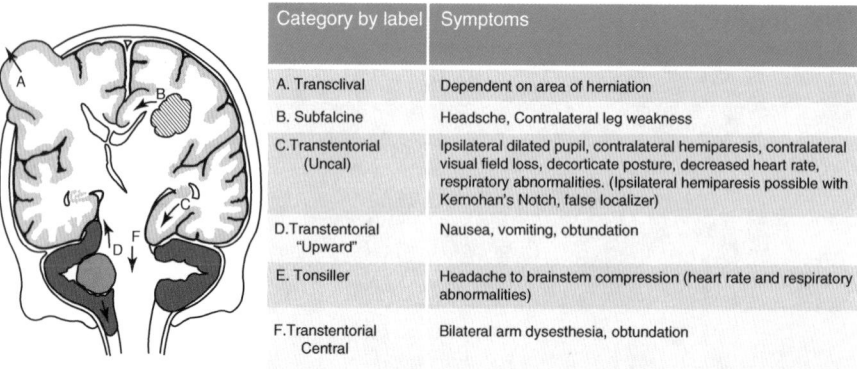

Category by label	Symptoms
A. Transclival	Dependent on area of herniation
B. Subfalcine	Headsche, Contralateral leg weakness
C.Transtentorial (Uncal)	Ipsilateral dilated pupil, contralateral hemiparesis, contralateral visual field loss, decorticate posture, decreased heart rate, respiratory abnormalities. (Ipsilateral hemiparesis possible with Kernohan's Notch, false localizer)
D.Transtentorial "Upward"	Nausea, vomiting, obtundation
E. Tonsiller	Headache to brainstem compression (heart rate and respiratory abnormalities)
F.Transtentorial Central	Bilateral arm dysesthesia, obtundation

Fig. 17.1 Brain herniation syndromes. With brain swelling, brain tissue is pushed across immobile structures resulting in several clinical symptoms. Many, if not most, brain herniation symptoms occur in combination (adapted from http://rad.usuhs.mil/rad/herniation/herniation.html)

nausea, vomiting, dizziness, blurred vision, difficulty concentrating, memory lapses, and occasionally abnormal respiratory patterns. The patient may have an abnormal fundoscopic exam or systemic hypertension due to the autoregulatory attempt to maintain cerebral perfusion pressure (CPP) (CPP = mean arterial blood pressure–ICP). Papilledema is a nonspecific sign since only 3.5% of traumatic brain injury (TBI) patients with elevated ICP have papilledema. With only moderate elevations in ICP, localizing signs on a neurologic exam usually depend on the primary etiology (e.g., left subdural hematoma results in right motor weakness).

When the volume expansion exceeds the brain's ability to compensate, shifting of intracranial tissues into other compartments or herniation will occur (Fig. 17.1). This may force tissue across tentorial structures (falx cerebri, tentorium cerebelli, and foramen magnum) and often results in permanent neurologic disability or death. Symptoms of herniation include obtundation, posturing, third and sixth cranial nerve palsy (third CN: pupil dilation, impaired light reflex; both: disconjugate gaze), Cushing's reflex (severe hypertension, bradycardia, increased ICP), spontaneous hyperventilation, abnormal respiratory pattern (irregular or apnea), and ultimately hypotension and death (Table 17.2). Decerebrate posture (rigid extension of arms, legs, arching of the back and downward pointing toes) can occur with any brainstem injury but is often seen with central transtentorial herniation.

Patient Assessment

While signs and symptoms can be suggestive of increased ICP, a more definitive diagnosis requires imaging and possibly ICP monitoring. Computed tomography (CT) is the standard imaging technique due to advances in technology, speed, resolution and point of care availability for diagnosis and monitoring with head trauma, basilar skull fracture, epidural or subdural hematoma, intraparenchymal and subarachnoid hemorrhage, cerebral edema, and cerebral contusion. Magnetic resonance

Table 17.3 Indications for ICP monitoring

- GCS < 8 after resuscitation
- Abnormal head CT with the evidence of brain edema/mass lesion effect
- Rapid neurologic deterioration plus clinical signs of increased ICP
- GCS > 8 but unable to follow serial neurologic examination due to
  - Drugs, anesthesia, prolonged nonneurologic surgery
  - Prolonged ventilation or use of PEEP (e.g., ARDS)
- Post-neurosurgery for the removal of intracranial hematoma
- Normal CT scan plus 2 of the following
  - Age older than 40 years
  - Decerebrate or decorticate posturing
  - Systolic blood pressure less than 90 mmHg

imaging (MRI) may be useful in some selected pathologies, especially for the initial evaluation or presurgical imaging for tumors. Characteristic findings for elevated ICP on brain images are loss of ventricles, decreased CSF around cerebrum (basal cisterns), midline shift, herniation, increased perilesion edema, and loss of definition of gyri or other brain structures.

ICP monitoring confirms the diagnosis of ICH. Algorithms (Table 17.3) that combine Glasgow coma scale (GCS) (Chap. 9), a directed neurologic exam, patient characteristics, and CT findings identify patients where the benefits of ICP monitoring outweigh the significant risks. CT findings alone cannot predict who is at risk for developing ICH. About 60% of TBI patients who have an abnormal CT will have ICH. Only 4% of patients with a normal CT scan and no additional risk factors will develop increased ICP; however, 60% of patients with a normal CT *and* two risk factors will develop ICH. Patients who require prolonged general anesthetics or other therapies that prevent adequate neurologic assessments require an ICP monitor. During preoperative assessment, patients who meet the criteria for ICP monitoring should be assumed to have ICH.

ICP monitoring can be performed using an intraventricular, intraparenchymal, or subdural/epidural device. The preferred method is an intraventricular catheter placed in the lateral ventricle since it provides the best quality pressure tracing and can demonstrate the IC elastance by reflecting ICP changes with vascular pulsations. An intraventricular catheter can drain CSF in the ICU or OR to permit the reduction of ICP. When the lateral ventricle is compressed, CSF drainage becomes difficult and accurate pressure measurement lost. Changes in the waveform pattern allow recognition of impending critical ICP elevations. Plateau waves, sudden and rapid ICP elevation to >40 mmHg that for 5–20 min followed by an abrupt ICP decrease, are caused by the loss of the brain's ability to appropriately autoregulate. The cascade of events is active vasodilation → increased CBV → ICH → decreased CPP. Finally, active vasoconstriction reverses these events. Plateau waves portend severe refractory ICH. Appearance of B waves, spontaneous slow waves (0.5–2 Hz) with an amplitude of about 20 mmHg, act as a warning sign of decreased intracranial elastance.

The subdural/epidural "bolt" monitor is a saline filled hollow screw placed through the skull into the subdural/epidural space. It has less risk of brain injury with placement than the intraventricular catheter but is considered less reliable.

It becomes ineffective when occluded by brain or other material and will not allow CSF removal. When surgery is performed, an intraparenchymal fiberoptic catheter can be placed to monitor ICP when ventriculostomy catheters cannot be inserted. These also cannot be used to drain CSF, and calibration may drift over time.

Intervention/Treatment

Prevention or treatment of existing ICH or herniation depends on directed management to reduce intracranial volumes. During craniotomy, the management goal is apparent with bulging brain or difficulty accessing the surgical lesion. In the ICU, therapy goals are to maintain ICP < 20–25 mmHg while maintaining CPP > 60 mmHg. Table 17.4 shows management techniques to reduce specific intracranial component volumes. A chronic mild elevation may require little change in medical management or anesthetic technique should surgery be performed. Acute management of a patient with clinical signs of severe ICH usually involves the administration of hyperosmotic solution (mannitol or hypertonic [e.g., 3%] saline), furosemide, intubation, a brief period of hyperventilation, head elevated position (if blood pressure allows) and sedation if agitated.

Normal responses to physiologic change should be assumed only in normal brain (Chap. 1). Mean arterial blood pressure (BP) should be maintained between 60 and 90 mmHg (or higher if needed to maintain CPP; measured at the acoustic meatus). Hyperventilation, the most rapid method available to reduce intracranial blood volume, acts via vasoconstriction due to the production of a respiratory alkalosis, however, renal compensation and adaptation of the CSF pH correct the alkalosis and eliminates the effectiveness over an 8 h period making it an effective temporary measure until other methods to correct the ICP are effective. Adequate oxygenation should be assured. A CT to guide therapy, which can be surgical intervention, placement of an intraventricular catheter, excision of a hemorrhagic lesion or continued medical management, is needed. Patients with known space occupying lesions, hemorrhagic lesions and aneurysm or arterial venous malformation bleeding often proceed immediately to the operating room once a diagnosis is made (Chaps. 8, 19, 23, and 26).

If the patient is to undergo surgery, anesthetic management of the tight brain (Table 17.4) requires meticulous continuation of previous medical interventions including (1) patient positioning: maintain head elevation, prevent increases in central venous pressure or jugular venous obstruction; (2) ventilation: use of minimum peak airway pressure, avoidance of positive end-expiratory pressure, maintenance of previous $PaCO_2$, avoidance of hypoxemia; and (3) fluids: use of modest fluid administration of normotonic saline, hyperosmotic solutions. All of these strategies are important in minimizing further injury. Close attention to ICP or brain swelling can guide therapy. Choosing anesthetic drugs that are unlikely to increase in ICP is crucial. Generally it is acceptable to administer volatile anesthetics below 0.75 MAC. Volatile anesthetics increase CBF and ICP. Opioids produce minimal change as long as blood pressure and ventilation are maintained. Intravenous anesthetic

Table 17.4 The effect of common medical and surgical actions on ICP

Action	Effect on brain	ICP response
Physiologic		
↓ PaCO$_2$ 25–30 mmHg (<8 h)	Arterial vasoconstriction	↓
↓ PaCO$_2$ 25–30 mmHg (>8 h)	None	↔↑
↓ PaO$_2$ (<50 mmHg)	↑ CBF/volume	↑
↑ BP	Arterial vasoconstriction	↔↓
↓ BP	Arterial vasodilatation	↑
↑ CVP	Venodilatation	↑
Jugular venous obstruction	↑ Venous volume	↑
Head elevation	↓ Venous volume	↓
Agitation/seizures	↑ CMR/arterial volume	↑
Drugs to reduce parenchyma volume		
Mannitol	↓ Interstitial fluid	↓
Hypertonic saline (3%)	↓ Interstitial fluid	↓
Furesomide	↓ CSF production, cellular edema	↓
Dexamethasone – TBI	No effect – TBI	↔
– Tumor intraoperative	↓ interstitial fluid	↓
Drugs used for anesthesia or sedation effects		
Volatile anesthetics (>0.75 MAC)	↑ Arterial/venous volume	↑
Nitrous oxide	↑↔ CMR	↔↑
Intravenous anesthetics		
Propofol	↓ CBF/CMR	↓
Barbiturate	↓ CBF/CMR	↓
Dexmedetomidine	↓ CBF	↓
Ketamine	↑ CBF, ↑ CMR	↑↔
Narcotics	↓ CBF/CMR	↔
Benzodiazepines	↓ CBF	↓↔
Muscle relaxants		
Nondepolarizing	None	↔
Succinylcholine	↑ CVP	↑ (Brief)
Cardiovascular drugs		
Vasodilators	↑ Vascular volume	↑
Vasoconstrictors	↔↓ Vascular volume	↔↓
Surgical interventions		
Intraventricular catheter	Removal of CSF	↓
Remove space occupying lesion (tumor, hematoma)	Removal parenchymal tissue	↓
Decompressive craniectomy	Removal parenchymal tissue	↓

CBF cerebral blood flow, *CMR* cerebral metabolic rate, *BP* mean blood pressure, *CVP* central venous pressure

sedative agents, with the exception of ketamine, reduce CMR and arterial volume reducing ICP. A propofol-based total intravenous anesthetic (TIVA) is often advocated when moderate to severe ICH is present, when herniation is eminent, or where treatment of an intraoperative tight brain is required (especially when a decompressive craniectomy is required (removal of cranium with possible brain resection to decompress brain volume)). Avoiding hypotension and maintenance of BP to support an adequate CPP reduces the risk of hypoperfusion injury to marginally perfused cells.

Key Points

- Normal intracranial components are CSF (10–12%), blood (8–10%), and parenchyma (80%).
- "Tight brain" is an excess intracranial volume causing an increase in ICP.
- The clinical presentation ICH depends on the speed of ICP increase.
- Brain herniation is the shifting of brain tissue across tentorial structures (falx cerebri, tentorium cerebelli, and foramen magnum).
- Increases in cerebral venous and mean intrathoracic pressure increase ICP.
- CT is recommended methodology to assess pathology causing elevated ICP.
- An ICP monitor should be placed in patients with an abnormal CT scan or a normal CT scan and two additional risk factors (over 40 years, posturing, hypotension or unable to follow a neurologic exam).
- Acute management of ICH includes mannitol/hypertonic saline (3%), furosemide, brief hyperventilation, head elevation, and neutral head position.
- Therapies that increase CMR, jugular venous pressure, vasodilation, and increased airway pressures should be avoided.
- Use of anesthetic drugs which reduce CMR and vasoconstriction are desirable.

Suggested Reading

Balestreri M, Czosnyka M, et al. Association between outcome, cerebral pressure reactivity and slow ICP waves following head injury. Acta Neurochir Suppl. 2005;95:25–8.

Brain Trauma Foundation; American Association of Neurological Surgeons et al. Guidelines for the management of severe traumatic brain injury. J Neurotrauma. 2007;24 Suppl 1:S1–106.

Cole CD, Gottfried ON, et al. Total intravenous anesthesia: advantages for intracranial surgery. Neurosurgery. 2007;61(5 Suppl 2):369–77. discussion 377–8.

Jantzen JP. Prevention and treatment of intracranial hypertension. Best Pract Res Clin Anaesthesiol. 2007;21(4):517–38.

Loh M, Patel M. Brain herniation. 2009. http://emedicine.medscape.com/article/337936. Retrieved 24 Jan 2009.

Milhorat T, Pan J. The blood brain barrier and cerebral edema. In: Cottrell J, Smith D, editors. Anesthesia and neurosurgery. Philadelphia: Mosby; 2001. p. 115–27.

Petermann G, Smirniotopoulos J, et al. Brain herniation. 2009. http://rad.usuhs.mil/herniation/herniation.html. Retrieved 24 Jan 2009.

Randell T, Niskanen M, et al. Management of physiological variables in neuroanaesthesia: maintaining homeostasis during intracranial surgery. Curr Opin Anaesthesiol. 2006;19(5):492–7.

Chapter 18
Cerebral Ischemia: Options for Perioperative Neuroprotection

Martin Soehle

Brain or cerebral ischemia is defined as any critical reduction in cerebral blood flow (CBF) that affects the entire brain (global cerebral ischemia) or parts of it (regional or focal cerebral ischemia). As a consequence, the supply of oxygen (and nutriments) to the brain decreases since the arterial supply of oxygen (D_aO_2) is directly related to CBF:

$$D_aO_2[mlO_2 \, / \, min] = C_aO_2[mlO_2 \, / \, ml] \times CBF[ml \, / \, min]$$

where C_aO_2 refers to the content of oxygen in the arterial blood ($C_aO_2 \approx 0.2$ ml O_2/ml blood).

Under resting conditions in an unanesthetized patient, global CBF is approximately 750 ml/min (50 ml/100 g/min) and is unevenly distributed between grey matter (CBF $\approx$ 90 ml/100 g/min) and white matter (CBF $\approx$ 20 ml/100 g/min). The supply of oxygen to the brain ($D_aO_2 \approx 150$ ml O_2/min $\approx$ 10 ml O_2/100 g/min) exceeds its demand (cerebral metabolic rate of oxygen CMRO$_2 \approx$ 50 ml O_2/min $\approx$ 3.3 ml O_2/100 g/min) by a factor of three, under normal conditions. However, during brain ischemia, CBF is critically reduced (CBF < 250 ml/min $\approx$ 18 ml/100 g/min) which means that the deterioration of oxygen and glucose supply does not meet the brain's demand anymore. As a consequence, the neuron's (and glial cell's) function ceases, as indicated by an isoelectric electroencephalogram (EEG) (CBF ~ 16 ml/100 g/min) or lapsed evoked potentials (CBF ~ 12 ml/100 g/min). A further reduction in CBF (<90 ml/min $\approx$ 6 ml/100 g/min) will finally cause irreversible damage to the cell's themselves resulting in cell necrosis and brain infarction.

Common causes for cerebral ischemia in the context of craniotomy are related to arterial hypotension, occlusion of cerebral vessels – as intended (e.g., during

M. Soehle, MD, PhD, DESA (✉)
Department of Anaesthesiology and Intensive Care Medicine,
University of Bonn, Bonn, Germany
e-mail: martin.soehle@ukb.uni-bonn.de

A.M. Brambrink and J.R. Kirsch (eds.), *Essentials of Neurosurgical Anesthesia & Critical Care*, DOI 10.1007/978-0-387-09562-2_18,
© Springer Science+Business Media, LLC 2012

temporary clipping) or not (to control intraoperative bleeding) – or excessive retraction of the brain. Some of those may be affected by the anesthesiologist, whereas others are not. The following text is focused on the former.

Brain Ischemia due to Arterial Hypotension

Overview

The incidence of intraoperative cerebral ischemic events which are caused by arterial hypotension is unknown. Although short episodes of arterial hypotension occur frequently, it is hypothesized that they seldom lead to cerebral ischemia as long as those events are short and treated immediately.

In the healthy adult brain with its preserved cerebral autoregulation, CBF will not be affected by changes in arterial blood pressure (ABP), at least in the ABP range between 50 and 150 mmHg. However, every drop in ABP below the lower autoregulation threshold (mean ABP~50 mmHg) may result in a deterioration of CBF with the risk of cerebral ischemia. It must be noted that the lower threshold is shifted toward higher values in patients with a history of arterial hypertension.

In the diseased brain, cerebral autoregulation is frequently impaired to an extent which is usually unknown in a given patient unless it has been tested by means of transcranial Doppler (TCD) or intracranial pressure-related reactivity (PRx) studies. Moreover, many anesthetics – especially volatile anesthetics – impair autoregulation in a dose-dependent manner.

In clinical practice one should anticipate that every episode of arterial hypotension poses the risk of brain ischemia. Hence, any drop in mean ABP below 60 mmHg (or ~70 mmHg in suspected intracranial hypertension) should be recognized and treated immediately. The two main reasons for arterial hypotension are an excessive depth of anesthesia and hypovolemia due to intraoperative blood loss.

Prevention

- Place an arterial catheter into the radial artery (preferred location; alternatives: brachial, dorsalis pedis, or femoral artery) for continuous ABP monitoring to enable an immediate diagnosis of arterial hypotension.
- Chose anesthetics that allow the anesthesia provider to rapidly adapt the depth of anesthesia to the changing intensity of surgical stimuli; for instance, prefer drugs with short elimination half times. Be prepared for a substantial blood loss by having adequate venous access and readily available fluid and blood for replacement.
- Preserve cerebral autoregulation by avoiding high doses of volatile anesthetics (keep dose<1 MAC).

Crisis Management

Whereas the diagnosis of arterial hypotension is easily obtained based on the actual ABP readings, there is no common agreement below which ABP threshold it is to be treated. With respect to the lower limit of cerebral autoregulation (MABP ~ 50 mmHg) and some safety margin, an ABP-threshold for treatment of 60 mmHg seems reasonable. A higher threshold (70–80 mmHg) should be considered in patients with suspected intracranial hypertension or a history of arterial hypertension. Arterial hypotension is treated by removing its cause.

Treatment of Excessive Anesthetic Depth

Depth of anesthesia is usually increased prior to painful stimuli such as endotracheal intubation, placement of the Mayfield head-holder, skin incision, and craniotomy. Arterial hypotension typically occurs thereafter as soon as the stimulus decreases. It is treated by reducing the depth of anesthesia which may take some time depending on the pharmacokinetic and pharmacodynamic properties of the anesthetics used. During this period of adjusting anesthetic depth, it is justified to use vasopressors; for example, phenylephrine boli of 50–100 μg. However, the use of vasopressor must not replace the adaptation of the anesthetic depth.

Treatment of Hypovolemia

An average craniotomy is associated with a blood loss of approximately 300–500 ml since skin and subgaleal tissues are well perfused. In adults, this is usually not associated with hypovolemic shock and the blood loss can easily be replaced by fluid therapy. As in other fields of anesthesia, there is no consensus (and no clear evidence) with respect to the type of fluids (crystalloids vs. colloids) recommended which is best for volume resuscitation. Profound bleeding may occur without prior warning at any time during craniotomy. In particular, craniotomy in the vicinity of the dural sinus and preparation of cerebral vessels (for instance, during surgery for aneurysms or arteriovenous malformations but as well for tumor resection) are associated with a high risk of sudden and profound bleeding causing arterial hypotension and cerebral ischemia. Ongoing or significant sudden blood loss should not be treated solely by vasopressors or catecholamines which could disguise the extent of hypovolemia and cause lactic acidosis because of diminished splanchnic perfusion. Instead, hypovolemia is treated by volume replacement. It seems reasonable – though not proven by evidence – that small amounts of blood loss (<500 ml) are treated by crystalloids; whereas, larger amounts (>500 ml) are substituted by colloids (solely or in combination with crystalloids). A fast and consistent volume therapy is presumably more important than the type of fluid used for correction of the volume deficit. Eventually, transfusion of packed red blood cells may be indicated to maintain a sufficient oxygen content in the arterial blood in order to assure tissue oxygenation.

Depending on patient age and comorbidity, transfusion of packed red blood cells is indicated at hemoglobin concentrations ranging between 6 g/dl (young patient without comorbidity) and 10 g/dl (elder patient with coronary heart disease), although there is no agreement within neuroanesthesiologists with respect to transfusion triggers. Fresh frozen plasma or thrombocyte concentrates should be given whenever coagulation factor activity drops below 50%, or thrombocyte count below 80,000/μl, respectively.

Key Points (See Table 18.1)

Table 18.1 Overview of brain ischemia, its etiology, prevention, and management

Extent of cerebral ischemia	Etiology of cerebral ischemia	Prevention of cerebral ischemia	Management of cerebral ischemia
Global	Arterial hypotension due to	• Place arterial line for continuous ABP recording	• Maintain cerebral autoregulation: Avoid more than 1 MAC of volatile anesthetics
	• Inadequate anesthetic depth	• Use short-acting anesthetics	• Decrease anesthetic depth • Give phenylephrine (50–100 μg boli) meanwhile
	• Hypovolemia caused by intraoperative bleeding	• Expect sudden and profound blood loss at any time	• Apply neither vasopressors nor catecholamines • Replace volume with crystalloids and/or colloids • Transfuse packed red blood cells if hemoglobin conc. drops below 6–10 g/dl

Focal/ regional	Vessel occlusion	• Record EEG to monitor burst suppression or isoelectric EEG	• Reduce brain metabolism:
			  – Increase anesthetic depth (use propofol, thiopental, or volatile anesthetics)
			  – Induce hypothermia (not recommended)
			• Maintain homeostasis (target):
			  – Avoid hypoxia ($paO_2 > 70$ mmHg)
			  – Avoid arterial hypotension (MABP > 60 mmHg)
			  – Avoid hyperglycemia (glucose < 150 mg/dl)
			  – Maintain normocapnia ($35 < p_aCO_2 < 40$ mmHg)

- Appreciate that every drop in ABP might be associated with cerebral ischemia. Therefore, treat arterial hypotension immediately and consistently.
- In adult patients maintain mean ABP of at least 60 mmHg during craniotomy. Higher values (MABP > 70 mmHg) should be achieved in patients with intracranial hypertension or a history of arterial hypertension.
- Treat arterial hypotension causally: Decrease depth of anesthesia in case of a diminishing surgical stimulus and replace volume in case of intraoperative bleeding.
- Vasopressors or catecholamines may be used during the short period of time until depth of anesthesia has been adapted to the actual surgical stimulus or while the initial period of volume resuscitation. However, do not use vasopressors and catecholamines as the sole treatment in case of blood loss since this would disguise the extent of hypovolemia.
- Expect profound bleeding at any time during surgery, but especially during craniotomy, preparation of cerebral vessels, and tumor resection.

Brain Ischemia due to Cerebral Vessel Occlusion

Overview

During surgery, cerebral vessels might be occluded intentionally (e.g., during temporary clipping in aneurysm surgery) or to control intraoperative bleeding. Even in the process of otherwise uneventful cerebrovascular reconstruction – such as clipping, coiling, or glueing – perforant arteries or parent vessels might be occluded unintentionally. As a consequence, immediate (focal or regional) ischemia occurs in the brain tissue supplied by the occluded vessel. Since the cause of ischemia (that is the vessel occlusion) can neither be affected nor reversed by the anesthesiologist, the therapy aims at making the brain less vulnerable to ischemia and to prevent further (secondary) ischemic events.

Cerebral ischemia leads to an under-supply of the brain with respect to oxygen and nutriments. Theoretically, this would be attenuated if the brain's demand could be lowered by means of reducing its metabolism. Mechanisms to diminish brain metabolism include general anesthesia and hypothermia. An alternate experimental approach strives for reducing the brain's susceptibility to ischemia by a mechanism termed "ischemic pre-/postconditioning." This is explained in more detail in a section below.

As already mentioned, a reduction of CBF below the ischemic threshold of 250 ml/min ($\approx$18 ml/100 g/min) does not result in an immediate neuronal and glial death. Rather, their function is shut down as can be seen by an isoelectric EEG and lapsed evoked potentials; whereas, their structural integrity remains intact. Only if CBF drops further (below 90 ml/min ≈ 6 ml/100 g/min), neurons and glial cells will become necrotic inevitably and brain infarction will occur.

Prevention

• Apply intraoperative neuromonitoring such as somatosensory evoked potential monitoring, EEG, jugular bulb oxygen saturation monitoring, or cerebral microdialysis for early detection and monitoring of cerebral ischemia.

Crisis Management

Cerebral ischemia happens unrecognized unless it is detected by neuromonitoring. However, it is frequently suspected by the neurosurgeon when occluding a cerebral vessel. Nevertheless ischemia is often not detected until postoperative neurologic examination or imaging reveal signs of cerebral infarction.

The anesthesiologist should consider to reduce brain metabolism in case of suspected or confirmed focal cerebral ischemia, as presented below.

Hypothermia reduces brain metabolism such that every degree Celsius by which body temperature is decreased, results in a metabolism reduction of approximately 7%. Hence, hypothermia of 33°C – as used in the majority of studies – would diminish brain metabolism by roughly one quarter. However, this effect is much less pronounced (possibly even halved) in both the diseased and the anesthetized brain. Nevertheless, mild hypothermia (33°C) improves favorable neurologic outcome after cardiac arrest (*global cerebral ischemia*) with a number needed to treat of 4–13. In contrast, prophylactic intraoperative mild hypothermia (33°C) during aneurysm clipping (*focal cerebral ischemia*) following subarachnoid hemorrhage failed to improve neurologic outcome but was associated with an increased rate of infections according to the IHAST-study. Therefore, mild hypothermia is not indicated as a prophylactic measure during aneurysm surgery but may be considered in selected cases as an *ultima ratio*-therapy following vessel occlusion. Moderate (30°C) or deep hypothermia cannot be recommended due to its high complication rate in terms of cardiac arrhythmias, cardiovascular instability, coagulation impairment, and severe infections.

The majority of anesthetics (among others, propofol, etomidate, barbiturates, benzodiazepines, and volatile anesthetics) reduce brain metabolism in a dose-dependent manner and to a similar extent as hypothermia: For instance, 1 MAC of isoflurane halves the brain metabolism which is equivalent to a hypothermia of 30°C.

Historically, barbiturates were first observed to suppress the brain's activity as indicated by burst suppression or even an isoelectric EEG. They are without effect in global ischemia; however, they reduce the neurologic injury in animal models of focal ischemia. Barbiturates were once considered as a gold standard of neuroprotection; however, the optimal dosing has never been determined and, hence, no uniform recommendation exists. A dose of 5 mg thiopental/kg body weight seems to be effective to elicit a burst suppression EEG and to decrease CBF by approximately 45% for a period of approximately 10 min. However, thiopental is associated with cardiovascular depression, profound immunosuppression, and prolonged awakening, especially when given repeatedly in high doses. Hence, the neuroprotective effect of thiopental due to the reduction in metabolism may be neutralized by the adverse effect of arterial hypotension. Nowadays, the neuroprotective effect of barbiturates is considered as modest and as overestimated in the past. It is not recommended as a routine measure but may be considered as an *ultima ratio* option in selected cases.

The ability of propofol to reduce ischemic injury in animal models has been found similar to that achieved with barbiturates but is associated with less cardiovascular depression. An interindividual variable dosage of approximately 15–18 mg/kg body weight/h of propofol is required to achieve an isoelectric EEG. Etomidate reduces cerebral metabolism as well but has been shown to increase infarct volume and to cause adrenal insufficiency. Therefore, etomidate is not recommended to reduce brain injury.

Volatile anesthetics contain neuroprotective properties which seem to be irrespective of the agent used. However, the high concentrations of volatile anesthetics required for an isoelectric EEG will reduce ABP and impede both cerebral autoregulation and metabolic coupling. In contrast, the intravenous anesthetic propofol maintains autoregulation and coupling even at higher doses, which makes it the preferred drug to maximally reduce brain metabolism.

Intraoperative monitoring of EEG is a valuable technique to confirm that the actual chosen dosage of anesthetic is sufficient to suppress the brain's function. Here, therapy should aim for an isoelectric EEG, which is associated with more cerebral protection than burst suppression. For convenience, a bifrontal EEG montage should be used, which might be difficult in some cases of frontal craniotomies. As induction of an isoelectric EEG by anesthetics is associated with more or less pronounced arterial hypotension (depending on the kind of anesthetic chosen), application of vasopressors such as phenylephrine or norepinephrine is usually required to maintain a sufficient cerebral perfusion. To avoid overdosage, the anesthetic dose should be titrated just enough to elicit an isoelectric EEG.

So far, the neuroprotective effect of anesthetics seems to be effective in short and mild to moderate cases of brain ischemia. However, anesthetics seem to be ineffective in severe and prolonged ischemia, independent if global or focal in extent. Moreover, their neuroprotective effect seems to be transient and disappears when investigating the long-term outcome. In general, most evidence regarding the neuroprotective effects of anesthetics has been obtained from experimental animal studies; whereas, little is known about their neuroprotective effects in humans.

Hence, clinical anesthesia should focus on maintaining homeostasis especially with respect to normoxia ($p_aO_2 > 70$ mmHg), mean ABP (>60 mmHg), serum *glucose* levels (<150 mg/dl) and normocapnia ($35 < p_aCO_2 < 40$ mmHg) since hypoxia, hypotension, hyperglycemia and hypo- as well as hypercapnia have been shown to aggravate cerebral ischemia.

Hypocapnia ($p_aCO_2 < 30$ mmHg) as induced by hyperventilation causes vasoconstriction and may reduce CBF below the ischemic threshold. Here, the decrease in CBF is proportionally to that in p_aCO_2, hence hyperventilation from a p_aCO_2 of 40 to 30 mmHg, lowers CBF by one quarter. On the other hand, hypercapnia ($p_aCO_2 > 40$ mmHg) produces cerebral hyperemia due to vasodilatation, which increases intracranial pressure which in turn reduces CBF.

Induced or permissive arterial hypertension may theoretically increase collateral CBF during temporary vessel occlusion, at least in case of an impaired cerebral autoregulation. However, according to the 2009 AHA guidelines for the management of SAH, there are insufficient data on induced hypertension during vessel occlusion to make specific recommendations.

Key Points (See Table 18.1)

- Therapy of focal ischemia caused by vessel occlusion aims at reducing the brain's metabolism and thus making the brain less susceptible to ischemia. This may be achieved by hypothermia and anesthetics.
- Routine application of mild intraoperative hypothermia (~33°C) does not improve outcome in aneurysm surgery following subarachnoid hemorrhage.
- Induced arterial hypertension may be considered reasonable to augment collateral CBF during temporary vessel occlusion, but there are insufficient data to make specific recommendations.
- The neuroprotective effects of barbiturates have been overestimated in the past. Propofol and volatile anesthetics cause a similar reduction in brain metabolism.
- Anesthetics provide a sustained neuroprotection only under circumstances of mild or modest ischemia, however not in severe ischemia.
- Homeostasis should be maintained during the entire course of anesthesia. Especially hypoxia, arterial hypotension, hyperglycemia, hypo- and hypercapnia have been shown to aggravate cerebral ischemia.

Neuroprotection by Means of Pre- and Postconditioning

A modern, yet experimental approach aims at reducing the brain's susceptibility to ischemia by a mechanism termed "cerebral preconditioning." This is based on the observation that a short period of (sublethal) cerebral ischemia results in a decreased vulnerability of the brain to subsequent prolonged (and potentially lethal) ischemia. Moreover, not only previous ischemia but certain drugs seem to elicit this preconditioning effect. Among these are quite different pharmacological substances such as volatile anesthetics (isoflurane and sevoflurane), antibiotics (erythromycin), hematological factors (erythropoietin) and succinic dehydrogenase inhibitors (3-nitropropionic acid). However, the preconditioning potency, the optimal dosage and time point of application remains to be determined for these drugs.

After temporary ischemia, cerebral reperfusion takes place which is often characterized by an initial period of hyperemia. Just recently, it has been reported that repetitive interruptions of this reperfusion by short periods of (sublethal) ischemia reduces the injury as caused by the initial prolonged and potentially lethal ischemia. This mechanism has been termed ischemic postconditioning analogous to the previous mentioned preconditioning. Again, postconditioning might be elicited not only by ischemia itself but by pharmacological substances (such as isoflurane) as well. Both pre- and postconditioning offer fascinating perspectives for neuroprotection; however, it is unknown so far whether its effects are of clinical relevance and whether they will find their way into clinical medicine.

Suggested Reading

Brain Metabolism

Fitch W. Brain metabolism. In: Cottrell JE, Smith DS, editors. Anesthesia and neurosurgery. 4th ed. St. Louis: Mosby; 2000. p. 1–16.

Hypothermia

Holzer M, Bernard SA, Hachimi-Idrissi S, Roine RO, Sterz F, Müllner M. Hypothermia for neuroprotection after cardiac arrest: Systemic review and individual patient data meta-analysis. Crit Care Med. 2005;33:414–8.
Todd MM, Hindman BJ, Clarke WR, Torner JC. Mild intraoperative hypothermia during surgery for intracranial aneurysm. N Engl J Med. 2005;352:135–45.

Neuroprotection by Anesthetics

Head BP, Patel P. Anesthetics and brain protection. Curr Opin Anaesthesiol. 2007;20:395–9.
Koerner IP, Brambrink AM. Brain protection by anesthetic agents. Curr Opin Anaesthesiol. 2006;19:481–6.

Pre-/Postconditioning

Kitano H, Kirsch JR, Hurn PD, Murphy SJ. Inhalational anesthetics as neuroprotectants or chemical preconditioning agents in ischemic brain. J Cereb Blood Flow Metab. 2007;27:1108–28.

Pignataro G, Meller R, Inoue K, Ordonez AN, Ashley MD, Xiong Z, et al. In vivo and in vitro characterization of a novel neuroprotective strategy for stroke: ischemic postconditioning. J Cereb Blood Flow Metab. 2008;28:232–41.

Chapter 19
Massive Hemorrhage During Craniotomy: Emergency Management

Lawrence Lai and Audrée A. Bendo

Overview

The brain is a highly vascular organ, receiving approximately 20% of cardiac output at rest. Thus, rapid exsanguination can result from uncontrolled hemorrhage during a craniotomy. The reported morbidity and mortality from hemorrhage is very high, varying between 5–27% and 0–4%, respectively, in one series and between 8% and 1%, respectively, in another. Therefore, the anesthesiologist must anticipate and prepare for potential massive intraoperative hemorrhage during craniotomy. Intraoperative hemorrhage is more likely to occur during surgical procedures that involve the intracranial vasculature, such as clipping of aneurysms and resection of arteriovenous malformations (AVMs).

Aneurysms

The incidence of aneurysm rupture varies with the size and the anatomic location of the aneurysm. In one series, approximately 8% of aneurysm ruptures resulted in frank hemorrhagic shock. In another study, 7% of the ruptures occurred before dissection of the aneurysm, 48% during dissection, and 45% during clip application. Intraoperative rupture is associated with increased perioperative morbidity and mortality.

L. Lai, MD (✉) • A.A. Bendo, MD
Department of Anesthesiology, The State University of New York Downstate Medical Center,
Brooklyn, NY, USA
e-mail: Lawrence.Lai@downstate.edu

A.M. Brambrink and J.R. Kirsch (eds.), *Essentials of Neurosurgical Anesthesia & Critical Care*, DOI 10.1007/978-0-387-09562-2_19,
© Springer Science+Business Media, LLC 2012

Arteriovenous Malformations

AVMs present clinically one-tenth as frequently as aneurysms. Cerebral edema or hemorrhage may occur either during endovascular embolization or surgical resection of AVMs. "Normal perfusion pressure breakthrough" (NPPB) is a theory explaining why intraoperative or postoperative cerebral edema/hemorrhage occurs in AVM's. With the abrupt removal of the shunt (i.e., AVM) from the circulation either by embolization or by surgery, the increase in CBF into previously hypoperfused areas can lead to cerebral edema and hemorrhage at normal perfusion pressure.

Preparation for/Prevention of Intraoperative Hemorrhage

The anesthesiologist must be prepared to manipulate the blood pressure and transfuse blood products emergently during a craniotomy. In patients at high risk for intraoperative hemorrhage, *patient preparation* should include the following:

Insertion of:

• Intra-arterial cannula
• Two large bore (16- or 14-gauge) peripheral IVs
• Central venous catheter
• A type and cross (4 units packed red blood cells [PRBC])

To accurately reflect the cerebral perfusion pressure (CPP = mean arterial pressure (MAP) – intracranial pressure (ICP)), the arterial pressure transducer is placed at mid-head level (usually the level of the external auditory meatus) to approximate the MAP at the level of the circle of Willis.

Intraoperative Management

Several studies suggest that perioperative hypertension (HTN) and coagulopathy (to be discussed under Clinical Presentation/Patient Assessment) are factors that predispose craniotomy patients to intracranial bleeding. Intraoperatively, acute hypertensive episodes may occur during

• Induction
• Epinephrine-containing local anesthetic administration
• Head-pin application
• Periosteal dissection
• Brain manipulation and
• Emergence

Therefore, it is important to recognize and vigilantly *prevent* abrupt and major increases in MAP that may cause rupture of a vascular lesion, cerebral vessel or aneurysm and subsequent hemorrhage. (The incidence of aneurysm rupture during induction of anesthesia is reported to be 1–2%). As a general rule, the patient's blood pressure should be maintained within 15–20% of the baseline value, and prophylaxis for the normal hypertensive response to intubation or application of the pin head-holder should be instituted before starting either of these procedures.

During the *induction sequence,* minimize the hypertensive response to laryngoscopy and intubation with administration of

- Intravenous lidocaine (1.5 mg/kg, 90 s prior to suppress laryngeal reflexes)
- A β-adrenergic antagonist (esmolol or labetalol)

Prior to *pin head-holder application,* prevent a hypertensive response by administering

- Thiopental (3–5 mg/kg) or propofol (2–3 mg/kg) or
- Alfentanil (500–1,000 mcg) or
- Scalp block

To minimize straining or bucking on the endotracheal tube, particularly during movement of the head when the surgical dressing is applied,

- Intravenous lidocaine, 1.5 mg/kg, is effective, but its duration of action is only about 3–5 min; it can be safely repeated if necessary.

Induced hypotension during *emergence* is recommended to prevent emergence HTN and elevated ICP. The following intravenous agents are recommended:

- Labetalol, given in 5–10 mg increments
- Esmolol, given in 0.1–0.5 mg/kg increments, until blood pressure is controlled
- Hydralazine and nicardipine may also be administered, but can cause cerebral vasodilation and increased ICP

Crisis Management

Pathophysiology and Clinical Presentation

Hemorrhage may be multifactorial, and the most common etiologies are

1. Tissue damage from trauma or aneurysm rupture
2. Dilution of coagulation factors/platelets resulting from massive blood and fluid resuscitation
3. Hypothermia
4. Metabolic acidosis
5. Anticoagulation medications
6. Effects of comorbid illness and preexisting hemostatic defects

Tissue Thromboplastin

The injured brain can liberate sufficient thromboplastin, or tissue factor, into the circulation to result in consumptive coagulopathy. Thromboplastin complexes with factor VII to initiate thrombin formation, which ultimately leads to the coagulation of blood.

Hypothermia

Since the coagulation cascade enzymes are temperature dependent, hypothermia may "slow" enzyme reactions, thus producing coagulopathy. Aside from causing fibrinolysis, hypothermia also adversely affects platelet function by inducing a change in platelet shape and inhibition of aggregation.

Comorbid Illness and Preexisting Haemostatic Defects

Patients with severe liver disease demonstrate multiple coagulation defects since the liver is the sole source of synthesis of all the coagulation factors (except factor VIII and von Willebrand factor). Factor VII levels are most severely affected and this is manifested as an abnormally high International Normalized Ratio (INR). Treatment includes

- Maintenance of platelet count above 50,000
- Administration of antifibrinolytics, such as aminocaproic acid and tranexamic acid, if fibrinolysis is suspected
- Replacement of fibrinogen and clotting factors with either cryoprecipitate, fresh frozen plasma (FFP), or the off-label use of recombinant activated Factor VII (rFVIIa) in select patients

rFVIIa is an effective pro-hemostatic agent for use in patients with congenital or acquired hemophilia. Its efficacy has led to the off-label use of rFVIIa in patients with massive hemorrhage, liver disease, DIC, and patients on anticoagulants. Two studies have shown that rFVIIa has reduced PRBC transfusion and improved early survival in trauma patients with massive hemorrhage.

Patient Assessment

Diagnostic tests to monitor during hemorrhage include

- Hemoglobin and hematocrit (changes delayed; normal values during acute hemorrhage can be misleading)
- Platelet count
- Prothrombin time (PT), INR, activated partial thromboplastin time (aPTT)

- Fibrinogen level
- Ionized calcium levels (to monitor for citrate intoxication)
- Serum osmolality (to monitor effects of mannitol treatment and massive fluid resuscitation)
- Thromboelastogram (TEG), which measures whole blood thrombus formation and lysis, will provide valuable information on platelet function and the presence of fibrinolysis

Intervention/Treatment

Successful anesthetic management requires effective communication with the surgeon and other members of the perioperative care team. The patient's vital signs, laboratory values (CBC, electrolytes, and coagulation) and operative conditions must be closely monitored. When frank hemorrhage occurs, aggressive fluid resuscitation and blood transfusion must begin immediately. At the same time, the anesthesiologist must be aware of any preexisting condition that may predispose the patient to coagulopathy and uncontrolled bleeding.

Fluid Management

Circulating blood volume should be restored with isotonic crystalloids solutions. The main concern is the development of cerebral edema 24–48 h after resuscitation.

Current intraoperative fluid management recommendations include

- Maintaining normal serum osmolality
- Avoiding profound reduction in colloid osmotic pressure
- Restoring circulating blood volume with glucose-free crystalloid solutions
- Maintaining normovolemia to preserve CPP

Crystalloids

Isotonic

Blood loss is replaced initially with 3 mL of isotonic crystalloid (e.g., normal saline) for each milliliter of blood loss. Fluids administered to replace blood loss should be near iso-osmolar with respect to plasma (295 mOsm/L). Normal saline (NS) (308 mOsm/L) and lactated Ringer's solution (LR) (273 mOsm/L) are often used. However, lactated Ringer's is slightly hypotonic and contains a small amount of Ca^{2+}, which can counteract the citrate anticoagulant in PRBCs. Normal saline in large volumes can cause hyperchloremic metabolic acidosis, which can cause coagulopathy. In the setting of large-volume fluid administration, isotonic solutions of balanced electrolytes, such as Plasmalyte-A and Normosol-R, have the advantage of a pH of 7.4, no Ca^{2+}, and normal osmolarity (295 mOsm/L).

Crystalloid replacement:

- Advantages: inexpensive, readily available, nonallergenic, noninfectious
- Disadvantages: lacks oxygen-carrying capacity, lacks coagulation capability, limited intravascular half-life

Hypertonic

Hypertonic saline solutions are used by some clinicians for rapid volume resuscitation of hypovolemic trauma victims with brain injury and intracranial HTN. Hypertonic saline will draw fluid into the vascular space from the interstitium. However, be aware that sustained hyperosmolarity (e.g., >320 mOsm/L) caused by any fluid has the potential to result in rebound swelling of the brain if allowed to rapidly auto-correct. Another risk is the induction of pontine demyelination (Na increase max. 0.5–1 mmol/L/h). Frequently, hypertonic sodium chloride: acetate solutions are chosen in order to reduce the chloride load and thereby the incidence of hyperchloremic metabolic acidosis.

Colloids

There are few clear indications for the administration of albumin or synthetic colloids. However, colloid infusion is often recommended in neurosurgical patients based on the assumption that increasing colloid osmotic pressure will decrease cerebral edema. If the blood–brain barrier is intact, colloid osmotic pressure exerts little effect. Compared to sodium ions, colloids contribute minimally to osmolality and osmotic pressure. There is new evidence that hypertonic salt solutions combined with colloids may more effectively reduce ICP and restore intravascular volume in neurosurgical patients.

- Dextran and various starch-containing solutions should be avoided because they interfere directly with both platelets and the factor VIII complex, and have a small risk of causing an anaphylactoid reaction.
- Several reported instances of bleeding have been attributed to hetastarch administration. However, all of them have involved circumstances in which the manufacturer's recommended limit was exceeded. Therefore, the manufacturer's recommended limit (20 mL/kg/24 h) should be observed, when administered.

To replace fluids, use:

- Isotonic crystalloid solutions (NS, LR, Plasmalyte-A, or Normosol-R)
- Combination of crystalloids and/or colloids

Avoid using:

- Dextran and various starch-containing solutions
- Dextrose-containing solutions, unless specific indication for its use, e.g., hypoglycemia; can exacerbate ischemic damage and cerebral edema
- Hypotonic solutions (i.e., 0.45% saline) can result in brain edema

Blood Products

The major risk of aggressive fluid administration is dilution of circulating blood volume, and this has led to the increased use of blood products.

Whole Blood

The American Association of Blood Banks (AABB) states that the primary indication for whole blood is for patients who are actively bleeding and have sustained a loss of greater than 25% of their total blood volume. Less severe degrees of hemorrhage may be effectively treated with PRBCs. Many blood banks follow the AABB guidelines, and whole blood cannot be obtained in the operating rooms except by special request.

Packed Red Blood Cells

ASA Practice Guidelines for Blood Component Therapy conclude that

- Transfusion is rarely indicated when the hemoglobin concentration is greater than 10 g/dL
- Transfusion is almost always indicated when the hemoglobin concentration is less than 6 g/dL
- Determination of whether intermediate hemoglobin concentrations (6–10 g/dL) justify or require RBC transfusion should be based on the patient's risk for complications of inadequate oxygenation

PRBCs are the mainstay of treatment of hemorrhagic shock. However, one concern has been that if large volumes of PRBCs reconstituted with a crystalloid are given, serum albumin deficiencies may result. However, administration of saline-reconstituted PRBCs for losses of blood less than 2,500 mL/70 kg usually does not induce low levels of albumin, although fibrinogen concentration can be decreased in the recipient.

Advantages:

- With an average hematocrit of 60–70%, a unit of PRBCs will restore oxygen-carrying capacity
- Effectively expands intravascular volume

Disadvantages:

- Risk of transfusion reactions; thus, cross-matching is desirable when time allows (typically about 1 h)
- Type O blood (the "universal donor") can be given to patients of any blood type with little risk of a major reaction. O-negative blood will not sensitize women of childbearing age to the rhesus antigen (if O-positive blood is given in this situation, prophylactic administration of anti-Rh_0 antibody is indicated)

- Risk of transmission of infectious agents
- Risk of hypothermia – PRBCs are stored at 4°C and will lower the patient's temperature rapidly (0.25°C per unit transfused) if not infused through a warming device or mixed with warmed isotonic crystalloid at the time of administration
- Impair immune function of the recipient.

The following is recommended for administration of PRBCs:

- Premixing with crystalloid will reduce the viscosity of PRBCs and allow more rapid administration.
- Reconstitute PRBCs with a warmed crystalloid or via a warming device.

    - Do not use solutions that contain calcium, as clotting can occur.
    - Lactated Ringer's solution is not recommended for use as a diluent.
    - Do not use a diluent that is hypotonic with respect to plasma (if so, the RBCs will swell and eventually lyse).
    - Solutions recommended for dilution of PRBCs are 0.9% saline, Normosol-R with a pH of 7.4, or Plasmalyte-A.

- For PRBC infusions, roughly 1 mL PRBC is used for each 2 mL of blood lost, plus crystalloid. The following equation is used to calculate the necessary volume of PRBCs to be infused:

$$PRBC_{infused} = \frac{[(Hct_{desired} \times 55 \times weight(kg)) - (Hct_{observed} \times 55 \times weight(kg))]}{0.60}.$$

Plasma

Fresh frozen plasma contains all the plasma proteins, particularly factors V and VIII, and is an excellent volume expander. The practice of administering PRBCs and FFP to the same patient should be discouraged, because this adds to the cost and doubles the infection exposure. When conditions are appropriate, whole blood (if available) should be given. Some indications for FFP administration (ASA Task Force 2 guidelines):

1. Replacement of isolated factor deficiencies
2. Reversal of warfarin effect
3. Coagulopathy that arises during massive blood transfusion
4. Correction of bleeding in the presence of increased (>1.5 times normal) PT or PTT

Plasma is usually not necessary after 1–4 units of transfused PRBCs because most patients have sufficient coagulation factor reserves to compensate for this amount of blood loss. Patients who lose one blood volume, or about 10 units of PRBCs, will require 1 unit of plasma for each unit of PRBCs. It is at the clinician's discretion whether plasma is needed when 5–9 units of PRBCs are transfused.

FFP should be administered to correct any deviation from normal laboratory values in an actively hemorrhaging patient, because hemorrhage exacerbates coagulopathy, thereby causing further hemorrhage.

The following is recommended for administration of FFP:

- 10–15 mL/kg of FFP is administered to achieve a minimum of 30% of plasma factor concentration, except for urgent reversal of warfarin anticoagulation, for which 5–8 mL/kg of FFP usually suffices.
- FFP must be warmed during administration.
- Coagulation parameters (PT, INR, PTT, fibrinogen) should be measured frequently during resuscitation.
- Plasma and PRBCs should be administered prophylactically in a 1:1 ratio to any patient with obvious massive hemorrhage, even before confirmatory laboratory studies are available.
- Plasma requires blood typing but not cross-matching; delay in the availability of plasma is caused by the need to thaw frozen units before they can be administered. Prethawed plasma (thawed fresh plasma as opposed to fresh frozen plasma) can be issued quickly in response to an emergency need.

Platelets

Platelets should be transfused in clinically coagulopathic patients (platelet level <50,000 cells/mm^3).

- Massively hemorrhaging patients may suffer from consumption of coagulation factors.
- Transfused platelets have a short serum half-life (3–4 days).
- Each single unit of platelets may only be expected to increase the count by 10,000–20,000 cells/mm^3.
- Platelets should not be administered through filters, warmers, or rapid infusion devices, since this will cause platelets to adhere to the devices and reduce the number of platelets reaching the patient.

Citrate Intoxication

Citrate is a common anticoagulant added to banked blood to bind free calcium, (an essential element in the clotting cascade) in order to prevent clotting. Transfusion of multiple units of banked blood causes a marked reduction in circulating serum calcium, and this can cause "citrate intoxication." Besides a further impairment on the coagulation potential, hypocalcemia in citrate intoxication can have a negative inotropic effect on the heart, causing hypotension despite adequate resuscitation. Thus, ionized calcium should be measured regularly, and calcium should be given in a separate intravenous line from the transfusion line, as needed.

Hemostatic resuscitation does not end when active hemorrhage is controlled. It is important to look beyond normal vital signs as endpoints of resuscitation to more accurate indicators of tissue perfusion, such as arterial pH, base deficit, and lactate level. Massively transfused patients that achieve a normal lactate rapidly after resuscitation have substantially better outcomes.

Key Points

- Rapid exsanguination can result from uncontrolled hemorrhage during a craniotomy.
- The anesthesiologist must be prepared to manipulate the blood pressure and transfuse blood products emergently during a craniotomy.
- It is important to vigilantly prevent abrupt and major increases in MAP that may cause rupture of a vascular lesion and subsequent hemorrhage, especially during induction and emergence.
- Hemorrhage may be multifactorial, and it is important to keep in mind the effect of dilution of coagulation factors/platelets resulting from massive blood and fluid resuscitation.
- The anesthesiologist should use diagnostic tests to monitor the patient during hemorrhage.
- Fluids administered to replace blood loss should be near iso-osmolar with respect to plasma (295 mOsm/L).
- To replace fluids, use isotonic crystalloid solutions (NS, LR, Plasmalyte-A, or Normosol-R), or a combination of crystalloids and/or colloids.
- Avoid using dextran and various starch-containing solutions, dextrose-containing solutions, and hypotonic solutions (i.e., 0.45% saline).
- Transfusion is rarely indicated when the hemoglobin concentration is greater than 10 g/dL and is almost always indicated when it is less than 6 g/dL.
- FFPs should be used to reverse warfarin or correct a coagulopathy that arises during massive blood transfusion.
- Platelet transfusion should be reserved for clinically coagulopathic patients with a documented low platelet level (<50,000 cells/mm^3).
- Rapid transfusion of banked blood carries the risk of inducing "citrate intoxication" in the recipient.
- Hemostatic resuscitation does not end when active hemorrhage is controlled.

Suggested Reading

American Society of Anesthesiologists Task Force on Perioperative Blood Transfusion and Adjuvant Therapies. Practice guidelines for perioperative blood transfusion and adjuvant therapies: an updated report by the American Society of Anesthesiologists Task Force on Perioperative Blood Transfusion and Adjuvant Therapies. Anesthesiology. 2006;105:198.

Basali A, Mascha EJ, Kalfas I, Schubert A. Relation between perioperative hypertension and intracranial hemmorrhage after craniotomy. Anesthesiology. 2000;93:48–54.

DeLoughery DG. Coagulation defects in trauma patients: etiology, recognition and therapy. Crit Care Clin. 2004;20:13–24.

Dutton RP, McCunn M. Anesthesia for trauma. In: Miller RD, editor. Miller's anesthesia. 6th ed. Philadelphia, PA: Elsevier; 2005. p. 2463–6.

Ferrara A, MacArthur J, Wright H, et al. Hypothermia and acidosis worsen coagulopathy in the patient requiring massive transfusion. Am J Surg. 1990;160:515–8.

Miller RD. Transfusion therapy. In: Miller RD, editor. Miller's anesthesia. 6th ed. Philadelphia, PA: Elsevier; 2005. p. 1799–827.

Rusa R, Zornow MH. Fluid management during craniotomy. In: Cottrell JE, Young W, editors. Cottrell's neuroanesthesia. 5th ed. Philadelphia, PA: Elsevier; 2009.

Chapter 20
Challenges During Anaesthesia for Awake Craniotomy

Judith Dinsmore

Overview

Awake craniotomy enables the intra-operative assessment of a patient's neurological status. This allows the safe mapping of resection margins in epilepsy surgery, the accurate localisation of electrodes for deep brain stimulation and the excision of space occupying lesions in eloquent cortex. Awake craniotomy is becoming more popular as it is associated with a lower requirement for high dependency care, shorter hospital stay and reduced costs. In tumour surgery, awake testing allows maximum resection with minimal post-operative neurological deficit. The anaesthetic techniques for awake craniotomy have evolved along with the surgical indications but significant challenges remain. The anaesthetic goals are the provision of adequate analgesia and sedation, with a safe airway, haemodynamic stability, optimal operating conditions and an alert, cooperative patient for intra-operative neurological assessment. Various techniques have been described but they fall into three main categories:

- Local anaesthesia
- Conscious sedation
- Asleep–awake–asleep (AAA) technique airway instrumentation.

Overall, awake craniotomy is safe and well tolerated, but many complications have been described which are summarised in Table 20.1. Several studies have looked at complication rates, but, due to differing case mixes and the variety of anaesthetic techniques used, the incidences vary widely. Fortunately, catastrophic complications are very rare.

J. Dinsmore, MBBS, FRCA (✉)
Department of Anaesthesia and Intensive Care Medicine, St. George's University of London, London, UK
e-mail: judith.dinsmore@btinternet.com

A.M. Brambrink and J.R. Kirsch (eds.), *Essentials of Neurosurgical Anesthesia & Critical Care*, DOI 10.1007/978-0-387-09562-2_20,
© Springer Science+Business Media, LLC 2012

Table 20.1 Complications of awake craniotomy

Complications
- Respiratory
  - Airway obstruction
  - Respiratory depression
- Cardiovascular
  - Hypotension
  - Hypertension
- Neurological
  - Seizures
  - Neurological deficit
  - Brain swelling
- Other
  - Pain
  - Nausea and vomiting
  - Local anaesthetic toxicity
  - Excessive sedation/unco-operative patient
  - Air embolism

Prevention

The key to success is careful patient selection, an anaesthetic plan tailored to the individual case and meticulous attention to detail. Both the neurosurgeon and the anaesthetist should be experienced in awake craniotomy and familiar with the technique chosen. To minimise complications, the following points should be considered:

Communication

- Operative aims should be discussed beforehand and likely problems anticipated. What is the expected duration of the entire procedure, of awake testing and what is the modality to be tested intra-operatively? Is there raised intracranial pressure (ICP), what is the anticipated blood loss, etc?

Patient Selection and Preparation

- Patients must have had a full explanation of what is involved, understand exactly what is expected of them and be able to tolerate lying still for the procedure.
- An uncooperative patient is the only absolute contraindication to this technique.

- Relative contraindications include morbid obesity, gastro-oesophageal reflux, a difficult airway or highly vascular tumours. However, the risk of complications will be increased so the decision to go ahead should be carefully considered.
- Coexisting medical problems should be optimised and routine medication continued, including on the day of surgery. Anticonvulsant prophylaxis, dexamethasone, and either ranitidine or omeprazole should be prescribed.

Anaesthetic Technique

The technique chosen must be the one considered most appropriate for that particular procedure, the patient's age and any associated co-morbidity. Routine monitoring for craniotomy should be used. Drapes are taped out of the way to allow access to the patient's face and for testing. A warming blanket helps to prevent shivering; padding of pressure areas and a calm relaxed atmosphere in theatre minimise patient discomfort and anxiety. Urinary catheterisation is required, if mannitol is to be given or the duration of surgery prolonged. Antiemetic prophylaxis must be given to all patients, and a loading dose of paracetamol provides useful additional analgesia.

Local Anaesthetic

Whatever technique is chosen, effective local anaesthesia is essential. This can be achieved by field infiltration of the incision area and pins sites or by individual nerve blockade with long-acting agents such as bupivacaine or ropivacaine (lidocaine for speed of onset and with epinephrine 1:200,000). Local anaesthesia alone removes the risk of excessive sedation or airway compromise. The elderly are often very sensitive to the sedative and respiratory depressant effects of sedative agents. Burr hole procedures or a small craniotomy are often well tolerated under local anaesthetic. However;

- Many patients will not tolerate a long, uncomfortable procedure without sedation.
- Scalp infiltration with large volumes of local anaesthetic or scalp blocks carry the potential risk of local anaesthetic toxicity in patients already seizure prone.
- Ropivacaine is less cardiotoxic and is advocated by some as agent of choice.

Sedation

Historically, midazolam, fentanyl and droperidol were most commonly used for sedation. Today, propofol is the most popular agent providing controllable sedation, a rapid smooth recovery and, when stopped, minimal interference with electrocorticographic recordings. It is often used as a target-controlled infusion (TCI) in combination with remifentanil. The very short context sensitive half-life of remifentanil ensures reliable elimination whatever the duration of infusion. Dexmedetomidine, an α_2-adrenergic receptor agonist, is increasingly used. It has rapidly titratable sedative, analgesic and sympatholytic effects without respiratory depression. It can be used as a sole agent (0.3–0.6 g/kg/h), an adjunct (0.01–1.0 g/kg/h) or a rescue agent. However,

- Sedation can be notoriously difficult to accurately control.
- Airway compromise is more common in patients who are obese.
- Neurolept analgesia has a higher incidence of seizures, nausea and vomiting but a lower incidence of respiratory depression when compared with propofol sedation.
- There is a learning curve associated with the use of remifentanil in spontaneously breathing patients. Propofol and remifentanil used for sedation are associated with frequent respiratory complications, but these decrease with experience.
- Sedative synergism has been reported between dexmedetomidine and midazolam.

Asleep–Awake–Asleep

The AAA technique with or without airway intervention is becoming more popular. Typically, propofol and remifentanil TCI are titrated against patient response, haemodynamic parameters and possibly BIS monitoring. The remifentanil is reduced to 0.005–0.01 g/kg/min (1–2 ng/ml) for awake testing. The patient need only be awake for intra-operative testing, minimising discomfort. In addition, haemodynamic and respiratory parameters are easier to monitor and control providing optimal operative conditions. However,

- The AAA technique without airway instrumentation is associated with more respiratory complications: apnoeas, arterial desaturation and a higher $PaCO_2$.
- Time to wake up may be prolonged. However, remifentanil significantly reduces propofol requirements, allowing a median wake up time of 9 min.

Airway Management

There is the risk of hypoventilation or airway obstruction with any sedation technique. Patient positioning may limit access and further contribute to airway compromise.

- There must always be a plan for securing the airway, if necessary.
- Airway adjuncts range from a nasopharyngeal airway to an endotracheal tube.
- The laryngeal mask airway is popular for AAA techniques. It is easy to insert and remove, well tolerated at lighter planes of anaesthesia, and it allows ventilation to be controlled, providing optimal operative conditions.

- The cuffed oropharyngeal airway (e.g. "King Airway") seems to be most useful in the lateral position.
- Non-invasive positive pressure ventilation (biphasic positive airway pressure and proportional assist ventilation) has been used successfully for awake craniotomy as has pressure support ventilation for patients with obstructive sleep apnoea.

Crisis Management

The Acutely Restless Patient

The restless patient poses a risk to themselves (especially with head fixation) and theatre staff. An uncooperative patient may also result in failure of intra-operative testing. Table 20.2 summarises the possible causes, patient assessment and management.

Nausea and Vomiting

Nausea and vomiting are relatively common but are usually preventable. Table 20.3 summarises the possible causes, patient assessment and management.

Table 20.2 The restless or uncooperative patient

Causes
- Anxiety
- Excessive sedation
- Pain
- Urinary retention
- Hypoxia or hypercapnia
- Seizures
- Neurological deterioration

Assessment
- Is the patient safe?
- Is sedation level (BIS?) and analgesia adequate for the stage of procedure?
- Check airway
- Exclude hypoxia or hypercapnia
- Check pulse and BP
- Is there seizure activity or evidence of a new neurological deficit?

Treatment/intervention
- Reassure
- Give oxygen and make patient safe
- Treat remediable causes – pain, urinary retention
- Decrease or increase sedation (at what stage is the surgery?)
- Dexmedetomidine and remifentanil are useful rescue agents

Table 20.3 Nausea and vomiting

Causes
- Past history
- Deep-seated lesions
- Surgical manipulation
- Pain
- Hypotension
- Anaesthetic technique (neurolept is associated with more nausea than propofol)
- Raised ICP

Assessment
- Check airway
- Check pulse and BP
- Look for surgical cause such as dural traction
- Are there signs of raised ICP?
- Has prophylactic anti-emetic been given?

Treatment/intervention
- Reassure patient
- Correct hypotension, e.g. IV fluids or vasopressors
- Give adequate analgesia
- A combination of anti-emetics may be needed
- Change anaesthetic?

Hypoxia/Airway Obstruction

Hypoxia presents with cyanosis or decreased SaO_2 and may result in bradycardia, hypertension or drowsiness. Both hypoxia and airway obstruction will increase ICP. Table 20.4 summarises the possible causes, patient assessment and management.

Seizures

Seizures may present with a sudden loss of consciousness, generalised seizures or development of new neurological deficit. The anaesthetised patient may have unexplained tachycardia, hypertension or a sudden rise in $EtCO_2$. Development of a new neurological deficit may be post-ictal and should be observed before surgery continues. Table 20.5 summarises the possible causes, patient assessment and management.

Hypertension

Table 20.6 summarises the possible causes, patient assessment and management.

Table 20.4 Hypoxia/airway obstruction

Causes
- Reduced oxygen delivery
- Respiratory depression (two sedation or opioids)
- Airway obstruction
- Aspiration
- Laryngospasm
- Bronchospasm
- Risk factors include: obesity, gastro-oesophageal reflux or pre-existing lung disease

Assessment
- Check airway, respiratory rate, tidal volume, $EtCO_2$ and FiO_2
- Is the patient cyanosed?
- Exclude measurement error (oximeter position?)
- Look for disconnection of oxygen delivery or breathing system
- Listen for air entry, wheeze or crepitations
- Check sedation level
- Measure ABGs looking for $PaCO_2$ or PaO_2

Treatment/intervention
- Give 100%
- Relieve airway obstruction (airway, LMA or ET tube as appropriate)
- If respiratory depression – reduce/stop sedation or opiates
- If laryngospasm – increase the depth of sedation, CPAP, succinylcholine?
- Treat aspiration or bronchospasm as appropriate

Table 20.5 Seizures

Causes
- Cortical stimulation
- Sub-therapeutic anticonvulsant levels
- Local anaesthetic toxicity
- Neurolept sedation is associated with a greater rate of seizures compared with propofol

Assessment
- Check airway, breathing and circulation
- If the patient's head is immobilised in pins ensure safety
- Check if the patient has had anticonvulsant prophylaxis

Treatment/intervention
- Secure airway and give O_2
- Stop cortical stimulation (cold saline to cortex?)
- If seizures continue treat – propofol 0.75–1.25 mg/kg, thiopentone 1–1.5 mg/kg or low-dose benzodiazepine
- For prolonged seizures phenytoin 10–15 mg/kg or phenobarbitone 200 mg (and repeated to max of 15 mg/kg)

Table 20.6 Hypertension

Causes
• Pain
• Inadequate sedation
• Hypoxaemia
• Hypercapnia
• Raised ICP
• Pre-existing hypertension
Assessment
• Establish cause and exclude artefact
• Is it associated with painful stimulus?
• Is there adequate sedation and analgesia?
• What is the pulse and BP?
• Is there hypoxia, what is the SaO_2 or $EtCO_2$?
• Is there evidence of raised ICP?
Treatment/intervention
• Treat underlying cause
• Give analgesia
• Increase sedation
• Optimise ventilation
• Antihypertensives, e.g. labetolol 5–10 mg boluses should then be used as necessary

The Acutely Swollen Brain

Bulging dura on lifting the craniotomy flap is often due to peritumour oedema. Table 20.7 summarises the possible causes, patient assessment and management.

Venous Air Embolism

There are several reports of venous air embolism (VAE) during awake craniotomy. Patients present with tachypnea, refractory coughing or chest pain, or in the anaesthetised patient, a sudden reduction in $EtCO_2$. Table 20.8 summarises the possible causes, patient assessment and management.

Table 20.7 The acutely swollen brain

Causes
- Inadequate corticosteroids
- Airway obstruction
- Hypercapnia
- Hypoxia
- Hypertension
- Raised venous pressure

Assessment
- Check airway
- What is the SaO_2 and $EtCO_2$ (check ABGs)
- Assess level of sedation
- Is the patient coughing or straining?
- Check pulse and BP
- Has patient had corticosteroids?
- Venous outflow obstruction

Treatment/intervention
- Establish patent airway
- Increase FiO_2 and reduce $PaCO_2$ by increasing ventilation
- Control BP (see above)
- Try head up tilt 30; consider in-line position; consider removal of jugular venous catheter
- Dexamethasone 8–12 mg
- Give mannitol 0.25–0.5 g/kg or furosemide 0.25–0.5 mg/kg

Table 20.8 Venous air embolism

Causes
- Head up position
- Spontaneous ventilation
- Airway obstruction

Assessment
- Have a high index of suspicion
- $EtCO_2$
- Hypoxia
- Hypotension
- Arrhythmias
- Precordial Doppler

Treatment/intervention
- Inform surgeon
- Flood operative field
- Stop N_2O
- Lower operative site below level of the heart
- Protect airway and FiO_2
- Maintain BP with fluids or vasopressors
- Other supportive treatment as needed

Key Points

- Awake craniotomy is safe and well tolerated but careful patient selection is vital.
- Prepare carefully and do not rush.
- Assess the patient yourself, check history, allergies and airway.
- The prevention of complications is easier than their treatment.
- Meticulous attention to detail and good communication are the keys to success.
- Always have a back-up plan.
- Know your limits and do not be afraid to ask for help.

Suggested Reading

Dinsmore J. Anaesthesia for elective neurosurgery. Br J Anaesth. 2007;99:68–74.

Frost EA, Booij LH. Anesthesia in the patient for awake craniotomy. Curr Opin Anaesthesiol. 2007;20:331–5.

Keifer JC et al. A retrospective analysis of a remifentanil/propofol general anesthetic for craniotomy before awake functional brain mapping. Anesth Analg. 2005;101:502–8.

Serletis D, Bernstein M. Prospective study of awake craniotomy used routinely and nonselectively for supratentorial tumors. J Neurosurg. 2007;107:1–6.

Skucas AP, Artru AA. Anesthetic complications of awake craniotomies for epilepsy surgery. Anesth Analg. 2006;102:882–7.

Chapter 21
Perioperative Challenges During Stereotactic Neurosurgery and Deep Brain Stimulator Placement

Mitchell Y. Lee and Marc J. Bloom

Overview

Stereotactic surgery is based on three-dimensional coordinates, which accurately localize the area of interest. With the advancement of radiology, essentially any specific region within an organ can be localized with stereotactic equipment. In neurosurgery, stereotactic technique is especially beneficial since the localization allows for conduct of minimally invasive surgery, thereby preserving other important structures in brain.

Stereotactic surgery can be performed with or without a head frame. Frameless systems such as Brain Lab or Cygnus PFS are often used as a navigation aid during a standard craniotomy for the neurosurgeons. A frame-based system allows the neurosurgeon not only to establish the frame of the reference but also to mount a guiding device to minimize the margin of error when approaching a deep target within the brain. The use of the frameless system affects anesthesiologists minimally; therefore, the discussion will focus on *frame-based systems*.

The head frame presents several issues that need to be considered by the anesthesiologist preoperatively. During the patient interview, the anesthesiologist should evaluate whether the patient can tolerate local anesthesia and the prolonged time in the head frame. Once the head frame is applied, the patient is transferred to and from the radiology suite for the imaging studies, which may take several hours. Patients often complain of pain at the pin sites, neck stiffness, claustrophobia, and headache. Since the patient may be transferred from one area to another

M.Y. Lee, MD
Department of Anesthesiology, New York University School of Medicine, New York, NY, USA

M.J. Bloom, MD, PhD (✉)
Department of Anesthesiology, New York University School of Medicine, Langone
Medical Center, New York, NY, USA
e-mail: Marc.Bloom@nyumc.org

A.M. Brambrink and J.R. Kirsch (eds.), *Essentials of Neurosurgical Anesthesia & Critical Care*, DOI 10.1007/978-0-387-09562-2_21, © Springer Science+Business Media, LLC 2012

area by a nonclinical transport aid, it is critical that the patient has completely emerged from any sedation or analgesic medications that were administered during the imaging period.

Patients with airway difficulty or history of obstructive sleep apnea should be accompanied by an individual with appropriate clinical training (e.g., nurse or physician). The airway must be considered not only during the time of the head frame placement but also when the patient presents for the actual stereotactic procedure. In the worst case scenario, the difficult airway patient should be considered for general anesthesia for the entire event from the placement of the head frame to imaging and surgery. Every part involved should be organized so that the patient is exposed to the minimal amount of anesthetic medications.

Deep brain stimulation (DBS) is performed for the patients with movement disorders such as Parkinson's disease or essential tremor. Although stereotactic coordinates allow the neurosurgeon to reach the exact target with great accuracy, the chosen target may or may not be the optimal location for stimulation to alleviate clinical symptoms. Therefore, once the target is reached, trial stimulation allows the surgeon to confirm appropriate probe location. To assess the optimal area for the placement of the stimulating probe, the patient is instructed to withhold any medication that controls the symptoms. The importance of not taking the medication (e.g., anti-Parkinson medication) must be emphasized during the preoperative visit. Since the anesthesiologist instructs the patient which medications to take for the day of the surgery, the half-life and the timing of the individual medication also must be considered since some Parkinson's medications may take more than 24 h to clear. Careful history taking will also allow the anesthesiologist to understand the timing of symptom deterioration with dose-holding based on the patient's past experience with forgetting to take their therapeutic medication(s). The symptomatic patients are often anxious and uncomfortable; tremors may not only cause discomfort but also may be severe enough to disturb the operation. These patients require extensive reassurance and presurgical preparation.

Prevention

Airway

If general anesthesia is to be induced, the head frame is a major obstacle for airway management. Once the head frame is placed, even mask ventilation becomes difficult. Most of the head frames have a removable front section. However, the opening is not often large enough to accommodate an adult-sized mask. The space between the front of the face and the head frame can be adjusted at the time of the placement. If the space is too narrow, the mask may not fit underneath the frame and a smaller mask or deflated mask can be used. A quick reminder by any member of the operative team at the time of the frame placement (preprocedural pause) will save a lot of trouble later. Allen wrench or other equipment for the removal of the frame must be available at all times.

Proper positioning with a shoulder roll, a wedge, and a head support will result in the patient being fixed in a sniffing position but may not give an adequate space to manipulate a standard laryngoscope during the time of anesthetic induction and tracheal intubation. Fiberoptic bronchoscope, glide scope, video laryngoscope, and intubating laryngeal mask airway (LMA) (or standard LMA and hollow stylette, e.g., Aintree) have all been used to intubate the trachea in patients fixed in a stereotactic head holding device. The fiberoptic bronchoscope is one of the most effective tools in advanced airway management. However, effective use of this tool requires advanced technical ability, which may take years to achieve an appropriate level of competence for effective airway management in patients who have their head fixed in a stereotactic holding device. In addition, the fiberoptic bronchoscope is expensive to purchase and has a high cost for maintenance, which often limits its usage. The Glidescope is a lighted fiberoptic camera on a strongly curved laryngoscope blade that projects an image to attached video screen. Visualization of the vocal cords is simple, but inexperienced users often find it very difficult to place the endotracheal tube through the cords because of limited mouth opening and the acute turn that the tube must take between the lips and vocal cords. The intubating LMA has a large enough lumen to accept a standard wire-reinforced endotracheal tube and a preformed curve that directs the tube through the vocal cords. Unfortunately, it is difficult to establish reproducible competency with the intubating LMA and has a higher failure rate than a fiberoptic bronchoscope. It is also possible to intubate the trachea through a classic LMA, using a hollow stylette (e.g., Aintree) loaded on to a fiberoptic bronchoscope. Once the stylette is positioned in the trachea, the bronchoscope and LMA are removed, and an endotracheal tube (e.g., Parker endotracheal tube) is advanced into the trachea over the stylette, which is then also removed.

Once the head frame is attached to the OR table, it becomes impossible to manipulate the head. Do not transfer the patient to the operating table until airway management is complete. As for prone or lateral position, the endotracheal tube must be taped securely. A circumferential taping, however, should be avoided to ensure adequate venous drainage from the head and face, as facial swelling could prevent an ability to safely extubate the trachea at the end of surgery. Other airway complications include apnea, airway obstruction, endotracheal tube malposition and obstruction, and accidental extubation.

Positioning

For both stereotactic surgery and deep brain surgery, sitting position or reverse-Trendelenberg position with the neck flexion is often required. Although the procedure requires a smaller craniotomy or a Burr hole, venous air embolism is a known risk. Early detection and prevention of further venous air embolism is the best course of action. Precordial Doppler may be used for the stereotactic surgery, but for the DBS procedure, the Doppler may interfere with the neurophysiology monitoring. If this is the case, precordial Doppler use can be limited to the initial opening and the exposure of the brain. For an awake or sedated patient, air embolism may present as coughing, chest discomfort, or sudden sense of anxiety. For such minimally invasive surgery, central venous catheter is not usually indicated. If venous air embolism was to occur, the treatment options are Trendelenberg position, flooding of the surgical field, and packing the area with Gelfoam or bone wax.

For DBS placement procedures, the patients are often kept awake or minimally sedated. Sedated patient should be positioned so that there is an adequate space for breathing and ventilation. The positioning should allow the patients to be as comfortable as possible, and lumbar support, arm rests, leg support, and possible Foley catheter should be considered. At some institutions, the services of a professional massage therapist have been utilized during the procedure to alleviate the discomfort for staying in one posture for a prolonged time.

Crisis Management

Seizures

Stereotactic surgery: If seizure activity is suspected, intubated patients should be treated with induction agents such as propofol or barbiturates (e.g., thiopental). Other treatments include benzodiazepine or cool saline irrigation to brain.

DBS in awake patients: If a seizure occurs in the awake or sedated patient, clinical judgment will be required to determine whether the seizure will be of short duration and simply observed or prolonged and require administration of a short-acting benzodiazepine and potentially airway management.

The alpha-2 receptor agonist, dexmedetomidine may be proconvulsant, especially if given as an intravenous bolus and inhalational gas is used. However, dexmedetomidine has been used for patients with a seizure history without problems at the normal clinical dosage. No real evidence exists to establish if intravenous dexmedetomidine is protective for seizures.

Hemorrhage

Due to the small size of the opening, any bleeding can be dangerous. Bleeding may result in hematoma formation deep at the target site, anywhere along the path of the probe transit through brain parenchyma or at the brain surface (e.g., subdural near the site of the craniectomy). Most often hematoma is diagnosed from postprocedure neuro-radiology studies and has no clinical importance. Rarely, the patient may present with acute neurologic deterioration from procedure-related cerebral hemorrhage. In these cases, immediate support with airway management, blood pressure control, and position change must be achieved. If significant subarachnoid blood accumulates, (rare) postoperative vasospasm should be considered and treated as indicated.

Nausea and Vomiting

Prevention of nausea and vomiting is key. Nausea and vomiting during the procedure may make it impossible for the neurosurgeon to appropriately position the brain probe and is very unpleasant for the patient. In addition, with the patient's head fixed in the stereotactic holder, it may be impossible to prevent aspiration of regurgitated material. It is, therefore, critical that strict NPO guidelines be followed for these patients. In choosing pharmacologic agents to prevent nausea and vomiting during the procedure, care must be taken to avoid administration of medication that interacts negatively with anti-Parkinson therapy. For example, metoclopramide (Reglan) may exacerbate Parkinson symptoms due to its effect on central dopaminergic receptors. Other medications such as phenothiazines (e.g., Compazine [prochlorperazine]), butyrophenones (Droperidol) also are included in this group. Ondansetron (Zofran) and dexamethasone combination can be very effective with minimal risk of complication. Newer agents such as Aprepitant, an NK1 antagonist, may be prescribed prior to surgery as a preventative measure.

Cardiovascular

The Parkinson patients who take bromocriptine or pergolide may experience severe and precipitous hypotension during the induction of general anesthesia (central dopamine receptor stimulation and peripheral vasodilatation), particularly in the presence of other antihypertensives, as, for instance angiotensine converting enzyme (ACE) inhibitors. Careful review of the medication is a must where this group of patients is concerned. Severe bradycardia and cardiac arrhythmia have been reported during DBS surgery. Therefore, adequate venous access must be assured to allow rapid intravenous administration of cholinergic antagonists (e.g., atropine) and vasoactive drugs (e.g., epinephrine and ephedrine). Intraoperative arterial line placement may not be necessary for many of the procedures, but access to emergent arterial line should be ensured.

Other Complications

Stereotactic surgery is based on establishing the frame of reference. If any objects or maneuvers interfere with the reference points, stereotactic surgery will fail. Operating room tables or the frame bracket cannot be moved or disturbed. The "Cygnus" system depends on X-ray detectable fiducial markers and they may not be moved. Since the fiducials are placed on the skin, any changes to the surface anatomy may affect the reference point. The "Brain Lab" system incorporates facial features as well as fiducial markers. Tape on the eyes, local anesthetic for scalp block or processed EEG monitor sensors such as BIS strip may interfere with the setup of the reference point. Effective communication between anesthesiologist and surgeons as well as OR technicians is a must to prevent inadvertent disruption of stereotactic reference points.

During the DBS procedure, even the slightest electrical noise may interfere with the neurophysiology monitor. Common sources of electrical noise in the operating room that interfere with neurophysiologic monitoring include cellular phone use, florescent lighting, or any instrument or device (e.g., convective warmers) connected to an electrical outlet. Battery operated monitors and infusion pumps should be considered for use during cases requiring neurophysiologic monitoring to minimize the risk of noise from AC power sources affecting the monitoring.

Key Points

- Minimally invasive procedures such as stereotactic surgery and DBS procedures can present significant challenges to the anesthesiologists.
- Understanding the patient population, different types of surgical procedures, the preoperative preparation, and the complications is essential.
- Airway management can be difficult in patients with head frames and requires careful planning and expertise.
- Functional brain surgery frequently requires an awake procedure, which requires close cooperation between patient, anesthesiologist, and surgeon and poses significant risks.
- Complications include seizures, cerebral hemorrhage, intraoperative nausea, and vomiting followed by tracheal aspiration, and sudden cardiovascular deterioration.

Suggested Reading

Dinsmore J. Anaesthesia for elective neurosurgery. Br J Anaesth. 2007;99(1):68–74.

Fabregas N, Craen RA. Anaesthesia for minimally invasive neurosurgery. Best Pract Res Clin Anaesthesiol. 2002;16(1):81–93.

Nichoson G, Pereira AC, Hall GM. Parkinson's disease and anaesthesia. Br J Anaesth. 2002;89:904–16.

Oda YMP et al. The effect of dexmedetomidine on electrocorticography in patients with temporal lobe epilepsy under sevoflurane anesthesia. Anesth Analg. 2007;105:1272–7.

Spiekermann BF et al. Airway management in neuroanaesthesia. Can J Anaesth. 1996;43(8): 820–34.

Venkatraghavan L et al. Anesthesia for functional neurosurgery. J Neurosurg Anesthesiol. 2006;18:64–7.

Chapter 22
Perioperative Challenges During Posterior Fossa Surgery

Martin Schott, Dieter Suhr, and Jan-Peter A. H. Jantzen

Overview

The posterior fossa contains vital brainstem centers for respiration, the cardiovascular system and consciousness as well the cranial nerves and their nuclei. This high concentration of delicate structures, added to the poor accessibility, makes posterior cranial fossa surgery a major challenge for the neurosurgeon. When such surgery is performed in the sitting position, additional neuroanesthesiological risks ensue, notably midcervical myelopathy and venous air embolism (VAE). This chapter is based on the authors' personal experience with more than 2,500 posterior fossa procedures performed in the sitting or semi-sitting position.

A wide spectrum of lesions may require surgical exploration of the posterior cranial fossa (e.g., tumors like acoustic neurinomas, meningeomas or metastases, traumatic contusiones or hemorrhages, aneurysms or AV-malformations), as well as development anomalies (e.g., Chiari malformation I and II).

Posterior fossa surgery can be performed in different positions, such as the sitting position to facilitate access to the cerebellum, cerebellopontine angle or brainstem. Alternative positions include the prone (midline suboccipital) or modified lateral position (park bench). There are no valid outcome data and prospective studies to support superiority of one position technique over another. The choice depends on the clinical experience and preference of the local practitioners.

Martin Schott, MD (✉) • J.A.H. Jantzen, MD, PhD, DEAA
Department of Anesthesiology, Intensive Care and Pain Management,
Academic Teaching Hospital Hannover Nordstadt, Hannover, Germany
e-mail: martin.schott@germanynet.de

D. Suhr, MD
Department of Anesthesiology, International Neuroscience Institute (INI),
Hannover, Germany

A.M. Brambrink and J.R. Kirsch (eds.), *Essentials of Neurosurgical Anesthesia & Critical Care*, DOI 10.1007/978-0-387-09562-2_22,
© Springer Science+Business Media, LLC 2012

Clinical Characteristics of Mass Lesions and Neurosurgical Procedures in the Posterior Fossa

- Small amount of mass (e.g., hematoma/edema) can be rapidly fatal due to the paucity of space and the immediate compression of the brainstem leading to catastrophic neurological compromise.
- Immediate proximity of brainstem and cranial nerves can cause intraoperative hemodynamic instability (hyper-/hypotension, arrhythmia, etc.), sensations (coughing, deep inspiration, etc.) and postoperative cranial nerve dysfunction (dysphagia, etc.).
- Positioning (e.g., sitting position, semiprone, or park bench position) can lead to special complications, most notably air embolism, hypotension, or obstruction of jugular venous outflow. Craniotomy in the posterior fossa, especially in the sitting position, causes a set of unique and potential hazardous problems.

Preoperative

- Deterioration of the neurological status and/or cranial nerve dysfunction
- Obstructive hydrocephalus

Intraoperative

- VAE and paradoxic air embolism (PAE)
- Complications due to positioning

  - Peripheral nerve injuries
  - Hemodynamic alteration and instability
  - Jugular venous outflow obstruction
  - Midcervical quadriplegia

- Brainstem injury
- Impairment of ventilation and airway

Postoperative

- Compression or herniation of the brainstem or midbrain structures
- Cranial nerve injury
- Brainstem injury
- Pneumocephalus and tension pneumocephalus
- Swelling of the upper airway (e.g., tongue, due to venous obstruction)

Table 22.1 Incidence of clinically significant complications in the sitting position vs. horizontal position

• Venous air embolism[a]	30–76% vs. 12%
• Paradoxic air embolism[a]	Rare[b]
• Arterial hypotension	19–36% vs. 24–38%
• Pneumocephalus	100% vs. 57%
• Tension pneumocephalus	3%
• Midcervical quadriplegia	Rare[b]

[a] The incidence varies according to the method of detection
[b] The exact incidence is unknown

The incidence of complications in relation of the position in posterior fossa surgery is shown in Table 22.1.

Prevention

The first step to prevent complications in the management of posterior fossa surgery is adherence to the standards: careful and accurate preoperative evaluation, meticulous maintenance of perioperative homoeostasis, and improvement of surgical conditions.

Secondly, perioperative management aims at *prevention* of specific crises as outlined in Table 22.2).

Crisis Management

Pathophysiology and Clinical Presentation

Anesthesia and critical care for posterior fossa surgery requires a detailed understanding of anatomy and pathophysiology.

Preoperative Crisis

• Deterioration of the neurological status preoperatively and/or cranial nerve dysfunction:

Pathophysiology: patients with posterior fossa lesions are more sensitive to sedatives and analgetics in particular with increasing mass effect of the lesion.
Symptoms: altered state of consciousness and difficulties to maintain a patent airway.

Table 22.2 Guide of perioperative management

crisis	Methods to prevent the crisis
Preoperatively	
Deterioration of the neurological status/ cranial nerve dysfunction (A.1)	• Examination of the cranial nerves IX, X, and XII • Avoid sedatives and opioid analgetics in the presence of raised ICP • Use these agents with caution in patients with any posterior fossa lesion
Obstructive hydrocephalus (A.2)	• Perform ventriculostomy or external ventrical drainage prior to induction of general anesthesia
Intraoperatively	
Venous air embolism (VAE) (B.1)	• Use sensitive monitors to detect air entrainment (<0.25 ml): Precordial Doppler and/or transoesophageal echocardiography (TEE) • Central venous line placed in the right atrium at its junction with the superior vena cava (correct catheter position confirmed by intravascular ECG or TEE) • Surgeon should tolerate a gradient as small as possible between the heart and site of surgery • Use a careful surgical technique (e.g., apply bone wax) • Identify venous structures by temporary compression of the jugular veins • Avoid nitrous oxide • Avoid hypovolemia • Avoid hyperventilation
Paradoxical air embolism (PAE) (B.1)	• Exclude a patent foramen ovale by TEE or transcranial Doppler (TCD) • Avoid sitting position in patients with known patent foramen ovale or pulmonary AV-fistula • Avoid high PEEP (>10 cm H_2O) • Avoid hypervolemia
Damage due to positioning General aspects (B.2)	• Meticulous attention to positioning and the use of neurophysi-ological monitoring (SSEP, MSEP, BAEP, EEG, etc.) helps to avoid injuries • Avoid excessive neck rotation and flexion (minimum 1–2 in.-space between chin and sternum) • Exclude severe degenerative diseases of the cervical spine (X-Ray, CT, functional test)
Peripheral nerve injuries (B.2)	• Care must be taken to pad all pressure points (elbow, fibula, heels, etc.) and to avoid stretching or compression of the plexus and peripheral nerves
Midcervical quadriplegia (B.2)	• Avoid excessive neck rotation and flexion (see general aspects above)
Jugular venous outflow obstruction and swelling of the upper airway (B.2)	• Avoid excessive flexion of the neck and allow venous drainage (see general aspects above)

(continued)

Table 22.2 (continued)

crisis	Methods to prevent the crisis
Hemodynamic alteration and instability (B.2)	• Maintain normovolaemia by i.v.-fluids and use vasopressors to avoid hypotension caused by positioning and ensure cerebral perfusion • Ensure abdominal and femoral venous return • Transducer level should be skull base to estimate CPP
Brainstem/cranial nerve injury (B.3)	• Use sensory-evoked potentials (SEP) (cortical integrity), brainstem auditory-evoked potentials (BAEP) (N. VIII) or/and electromyography (EMG) (N. VII; in incomplete neuromuscular blockade) • Alert the surgeon immediately when autonomic disturbances occur
Impairment of ventilation (B.4)	• Secure airway (e.g., proper fixation of the armored endotracheal tube) and ensure free access to the airway • Allow adequate diaphragma excursion
Postoperatively	
Deterioration of the neurological status (C.1, C.2, C.3)	• Monitor all patients in an intensive care setting • Beware that a small degree of edema or bleeding in the posterior fossa can lead to catastrophic neurological compromise • Leave the patient intubated if postoperative deterioration or damage to cranial nerves (IX, X, XII) is anticipated
Pneumocephalus (C.4)	• Avoid using nitrous oxide • Beware, especially in the sitting position
Swelling of the upper airway (e.g., tongue) (C.5)	• Avoid excessive flexion of the neck and allow venous drainage • Consider tongue edema before extubation, delay extubation to allow the edema to resolve

• Obstructive hydrocephalus:

Pathophysiology: infratentorial mass can obstruct the outflow of CSF and markedly increase the ICP.
Symptoms: continued impairment of neurological function.

Intraoperative Crisis

• Venous air embolism:

Pathophysiology: There is subatmospheric pressure in a noncollapsible vein (e.g., dural sinus or diploic vein) when the head is elevated above the heart; the pathophysiological consequences depend on the volume, rate of air entry and pulmonary clearance, as well as on the cardiac function; cardiac output decreases in response to the increased right ventricular afterload, resulting in *acute right heart failure* and/or reduced left ventricular filling.
Symptoms: bubbles in the transoesophageal echocardiography (TEE), roaring sounds of the Doppler signal, decrease of end-tidal CO_2 and increase of $paCO_2$

reflecting increased dead space, decrease of arterial oxygen saturation, arterial
hypotension, low output, cardiac arrest.

- Paradoxical air embolism:

  Pathophysiology: see VAE, presence of a patent foramen ovale or pulmonary
      shunts/AV-fistula, air can traverse to the arterial circulation.
  Symptoms: stroke and/or coronary occlusion (may be apparent postoperatively).

- Hemodynamic alteration and instability:

  Pathophysiology: venous pooling (by hydrostatic and position effect) influenced
      by patient factors (intravascular volume status, BMI, depressant effects of
      anesthetic agents, etc.).
  Symptoms: arterial hypotension.

- Midcervical quadriplegia:

  Pathophysiology: myelopathy presumably due to flexion with compression of
      the anterior spinal artery; preexisting degenerative disease of the cervical
      spine probably disposes patients.
  Symptoms: quadriplegia.

- Brainstem injury:

  Pathophysiology: direct surgical manipulation, traction, or ischemia of the brain-
      stem centers, as well as cranial nerves or their nuclei; damage to respiratory
      centers is almost always associated with hemodynamic instability.
  Symptoms: hyper-/hypotension, arrhythmia (tachy-/bradycardia); sudden shifts
      of autonomic discharge (unpredictable alternation between bradycardia/
      asystole and tachycardia/hypertension).

Postoperative Crisis

- Compression of the brainstem by edema or hematoma formation:

  Pathophysiology: a small amount of mass (e.g., hematoma/edema) can be rapidly
      fatal due to the paucity of space and the immediate compression of the brain-
      stem or herniation (downward through the foramen magnum or upward
      through the tentorium).
  Symptoms: delayed awakening and continued impairment of neurological func-
      tion, respiratory and cardiovascular derangement (including apnoea or abnor-
      mal breathing pattern, persistent hypertension, etc.).

- Cranial nerve dysfunction:

  Pathophysiology: direct surgical trauma, traction, manipulation or ischemia cause
      temporary or permanent dysfunction (particularly cranial nerves IX, X, XII).
  Symptoms: difficulties to swallow or to maintain a patent and protected airway
      (dysphagia, aspiration, stridor, respiratory distress).

- Brainstem injury:

  Pathophysiology: see above (intraoperative crisis).
  Symptoms: abnormal breathing pattern or inabilitiy to maintain a patent airway after extubation.

- Pneumocephalus/tension pneumocephalus

  Pathophysiology: air is retained in the cranial cavity after all craniotomies, located over the cerebral convexities, in the ventricles and/or posterior fossa; air is usually resorbed with symptomatic improvement within 1–3 days (*pneumocephalus*). Intracranial gas expansion may result in elevated intracranial pressure and mass effect (*tension pneumocephalus*; mechanisms include presence of N_2O which diffuses into preexisting air-filled spaces ["valve effect"] and rewarming of the patient.
  Symptoms: delayed awakening and continued impairment of neurological function (confusion, lethargy, reduced consciousness/coma, nausea and vomiting, seizures).

- Upper airway edema

  Pathophysiology: edema of the mucosa due to venous and lymphatic obstruction.
  Symptoms: tongue and soft tissue edema with inability to maintain a sufficient airway (cardinal symptom: inspiratory stridor).

Patient Assessment

Preoperative Assessment

Obstructive hydrocephalus is evident in preoperative CT or MRT scan and should be treated pre- or intraoperatively. Any preoperative premedication in patients with posterior fossa lesions must be individualized, taking into account physical status and ICP.

Intraoperative Assessment

Routine monitoring includes electrocardiography, pulse oximetry, capnography, temperature, urinary catheter and relaxometry. Strictly recommended in posterior fossa surgery are an intra-arterial line (beat-by-beat measurement of systemic blood pressure to estimate cerebral perfusion pressure and assessment of $paCO_2$) and a central venous line (e.g., application of catecholamines, aspiration of air). Supplementary monitoring is directed toward the detection and treatment of VAE when the risk of VAE is high: Precordial Doppler, TEE, and the use of central venous line as a right atrial catheter.

Postoperative Assessment

Three typical scenarios occur in the management of patients undergoing posterior fossa surgery: (1) early awakening and extubation, (2) postoperative neurologic status is worse than preoperative, and (3) anticipation of cranial nerve dysfunction.

Scenario 1: Early Awakening and Extubation

The aim of emergence is early awakening to allow assessment of the neurological status. Important criteria for extubation are normal vital signs including normothermia, a level of consciousness that allows management of secretions, absent airway edema, and intact protective airway reflexes.

Scenario 2: Postoperative Neurologic Status Is Worse than Preoperative

When the postoperative neurologic status is worse than preoperative, emergency evaluation and treatment is indicated. Time to diagnosis is a critical determinant of outcome.

Approach to the scenario:

- Maintenance of adequate ventilation and oxygenation (reintubate if necessary)
- Consider measures to lower ICP
- *Quickly obtain a computed tomography* (CT) to rule out structural causes of intracranial hypertension, including hematoma, edema, tension pneumocephalus, and hydrocephalus
- *Important differential diagnosis* to be ruled out:

    - Metabolic derangement (e.g., hypoglycemia, hyponatremia)
    - Pharmacologic/persistent anesthetic effect (caused by anesthetic agents, muscle relaxants; central anticholinergic syndrome)
    - Seizure (e.g., nonconvulsive)
    - Paradoxical air embolism (consider MRI)

Scenario 3: Anticipation of Caudal Cranial Nerve Dysfunction

Certain scenarios (e.g., prolonged surgery, surgery near the brainstem) carry a high likelihood of postoperative worsening of the neurological status secondary to cerebral edema or pneumocephalus. In these cases prolonged intubation may be necessary until neurologic function will allow extubation.

Approach to the scenario:

- Return of protective airway reflexes (including swallowing, sticking out the tongue) is essential
- Extubation under fiberoptic control, withdrawal of the endotracheal tube to hypopharynx
- Fiberoptic examination to assess laryngeal function and ability to swallow

Intervention/Treatment

Treatment in crisis of posterior fossa surgery is mostly supportive.

Treatment for Air Embolism

- Inform the neurosurgeon immediately about the air embolism
- Surgical field can be flooded with saline or packed; bone wax may be applied to the skull edges
- Request assistance
- Temporary bilateral jugular vein compression (in communication with the neurosurgeon, to identify the source of air embolus)
- Ventilate the patient with 100% oxygen, discontinue N_2O
- Aspirate air from the right atrium-central-venous line

If the Above Procedures Fail

- Lower patient's head if at all possible
- Regularly reevaluate the patient status (hemodynamic, blood gas analysis)
- Management of acute right heart failure and/or reduced left ventricular filling

    - Treat hypotension with vasopressors to secure sufficient coronary perfusion
    - Apply PEEP cautiously (>8–10 cm H_2O); excessively high PEEP levels may promote paradoxical air embolism
    - Be cautious with intravascular volume (only in hypovolemia)

- Persistent circulatory instability should provoke surgeon to terminate surgery rapidly
- Circulatory arrest requires return to the supine position to apply ACLS algorithms
- Continue postoperative ventilation, check for signs of pulmonary edema

Treatment of Sudden Hemodynamic Instability (Surgical Intervention Near Brainstem)

- Alert the surgeon to interrupt manipulation, which will alleviate the disturbance/ problem immediately in most cases
- When the hemodynamic situation has stabilized, prophylactic measures should be considered (e.g., glycopyrrolate, ephedrine or atropine in bradycardia or β-adrenic blockade, if sympathic reflexes are involved)

Treatment of Tension Pneumocephalus

- Ventilation with 100% O_2
- Burr hole to release trapped air under local or general anesthesia
- Rapid improvement occurs with the release of gas under pressure

Key Points

- Even a small amount of mass (e.g., hematoma/edema) can cause severe neurologic compromise due to the paucity of space and the immediate compression of the brainstem. Patient positions that permit surgical access to the posterior fossa are associated with unique difficulties, notably due to the risk of VAE, jugular venous outflow obstruction, and pneumocephalus.
- Intracranial hypertension may develop secondary to increased abdominal pressure, venous congestion, or outflow obstruction (hyperflexion/-rotation of the neck) and arterial hypotension; precautionary measures need to be applied to minimize these effects.

Suggested Reading

Black S, Ockert DB, Oliver Jr WC, Cucchiara RF. Outcome following posterior fossa craniectomy in patients in the sitting or horizontal positions. Anesthesiology. 1988;69:49–56.

Patel SJ, Wen DY, Haines SJ. Posterior fossa: surgical considerations. In: Cottrell J, Smith D, editors. Anesthesia and neurosurgery. 4th ed. St. Louis: Mosby; 2001. p. 335–52.

Porter JM, Pidgeon C, Cunningham AJ. The sitting position in neurosurgery: a critical appraisal. Br J Anaesth. 1999;82:117–28.

Smith DS, Osborne I. Posterior fossa: anesthetic considerations. In: Cottrell J, Smith D, editors. Anesthesia and neurosurgery. 4th ed. St. Louis: Mosby; 2001. p. 319–33.

von Gösseln HH, Samii M, Suhr D, Bini W. The lounging position for posterior fossa surgery: anesthesiological considerations regarding air embolism. Childs Nerv Syst. 1991;7:368–74.

Chapter 23
Perioperative Challenges During Release of Subdural and Epidural Hemorrhage

Walter van den Bergh and Olaf L. Cremer

Overview

Following head injury, blood may accumulate between the inner surface of the skull and the dura (epidural hematoma, EDH – Fig. 23.1), between the dura and the arachnoid membrane (subdural hematoma, SDH – Fig. 23.2), in the subarachnoidal space or within the brain parenchyma itself. Although the findings in individual patients will vary significantly, some characteristics that are considered "typical" for the presentation of patients with acute EDH, acute SDH, and chronic SDH are summarized in Table 23.1. Specifics of intraparenchymal or subarachnoidal hemorrhage are covered elsewhere in this book.

While many intracranial hematomas, depending on their size and rate of growth, can be managed by careful monitoring, expanding mass lesions that cause shift and clinical deterioration typically require urgent surgical decompression. The prognosis in such patients critically depends on the extent of primary intracranial damage, as well as the timing of surgery, the occurrence of secondary physiological insults during the ensuing hours and days, and the presence of injuries to other organs.

Risks

The injured brain is extremely vulnerable to the occurrence of systemic factors that contribute to secondary injury, such as arterial hypotension, hypoxemia, hypercapnia and hypocapnia, hyperglycemia, coagulopathy, and pyrexia. Perioperative

W. van den Bergh, MD, PhD (✉)
Department of Intensive Care, Academic Medical Center, Amsterdam, The Netherlands
e-mail: w.m.vandenbergh@amc.nl

O.L. Cremer, MD, PhD
Department of Intensive Care Medicine, University Medical Center Utrecht,
Utrecht, The Netherlands

A.M. Brambrink and J.R. Kirsch (eds.), *Essentials of Neurosurgical
Anesthesia & Critical Care*, DOI 10.1007/978-0-387-09562-2_23,
© Springer Science+Business Media, LLC 2012

Fig. 23.1 Epidermal hematoma

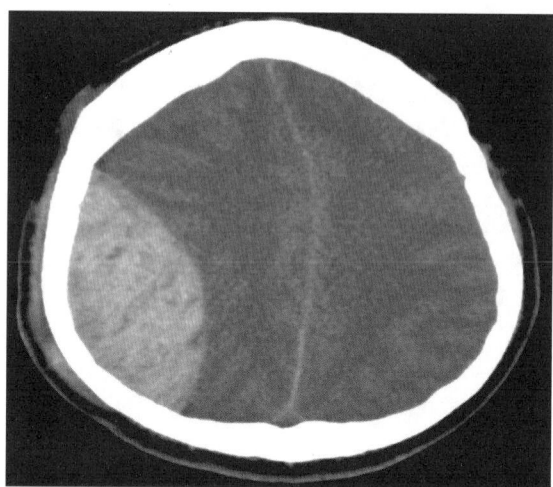

Fig. 23.2 Subdural hematoma

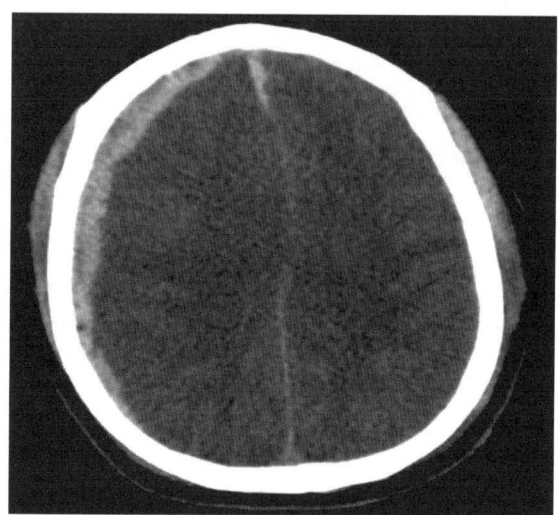

management should, therefore, be primarily directed toward avoiding or reversing the derangements that are associated with poor neurological outcome. This chapter addresses several common problems that may occur prior to or during release of acute SDH and EDH, more specifically:

- Raised intracranial pressure and brain swelling
- New or recurrent bleeding
- Neurogenic pulmonary edema (NPE)

Table 23.1 Etiology, typical findings, and mortality of epidural and subdural hematomas

Type	Etiology	Associations	Presentation	Neurologic findings	Mortality
Epidural, acute	• Middle meningeal artery rupture • Venous bleeding from fractured cranial bone	• Young age • High-velocity trauma • 85%: cranial bone fracture	• 18%: brief loss of consciousness with lucid interval followed by sudden deterioration (minutes to hours) • 35%: immediate loss of consciousness with rapid, progressive deterioration	• 84%: lethargy, headaches, nausea • 50%: ipsilateral mydriasis • 62%: contralateral hemiparesis • Coma	20–60%
Subdural, acute	• Shearing of bridging veins	• All ages • High speed rotational or linear acceleration–deceleration injury • Underlying brain contusion and/or brain stem injury	• Immediate loss of consciousness • Subacute loss of consciousness (within minutes to hours) • Cerebral contusion produces focal symptoms • Brainstem damage (60%) resulting in respiratory disorders and pulse and systemic blood pressure fluctuations • Acute psychotic manifestations and disorientation for varying periods of time • Convulsive seizures (25%) (late complications)	• Focal deficits (associated with brain contusions) • Cardiorespiratory instability (associated with brain stem lesions) • Acute psychosis or disorientation • Seizures • Coma	50%
Subdural, chronic	• 50%: spontaneous or only minimal trauma	• Elderly and alcoholics with brain atrophy • Anticoagulant use	• Insidious onset of symptoms (days to weeks)	• Altered mental status • Headache • Focal deficits • Reduced level of consciousness	<20%

- Perioperative seizure
- Sudden arterial hypotension upon opening of the dura.

The perioperative management of a *chronic* SDH is less complicated, and satisfactory outcomes are usually easier to achieve than with acute intracranial bleeding. This topic will not be further discussed in this chapter.

Raised Intracranial Pressure and Brain Swelling

Prevention

Early assessment, intubation, and resuscitation of patients with severe traumatic brain injury should be performed according to generally accepted trauma life support principles. If clinical signs of intracranial hypertension are present or if the head CT scan shows evidence of mass lesions with midline shift or obliteration of the basal cisterns, urgent craniotomy may be indicated. While waiting to bring the patient to the OR, the anesthesiologist or intensivist must aim to minimize ischemic-hypoxic brain injury primarily by preventing any further increase in ICP:

- Treat stress and pain (give sedatives, anesthetics, and/or opioids)
- Maintain head-up position (30°)
- Prevent venous outflow obstruction (neutral head position, avoid compression on jugular region)
- Maintain systolic blood pressure > 90 mmHg or cerebral perfusion pressure (CPP) between 50 and 70 mmHg
- Maintain normothermia (treat pyrexia)
- Maintain normoventilation (hyperventilation is not recommended)
- Maintain $PaO_2 > 60$ mmHg or O_2 saturation > 90%
- Prevent hyponatremia/low-serum osmolality; use normal or hypertonic saline and/or colloids for IV fluid resuscitation
- Avoid unnecessary endotracheal suctioning.

When indicated, induction of anesthesia and securing of the airway must be done in a controlled manner to avoid inadvertent deterioration of ICP. The following considerations apply:

- Etomidate 1–2 mg/kg causes less cardiovascular depression and may be preferable to propofol or thiopental in hemodynamically unstable patients.
- All volatile anesthetics may cause vasodilation and hypotension.
- Nitrous oxide should probably not be used.
- Use muscle relaxants prior to intubation; succinylcholine (1.5 mg/kg) has traditionally been the drug of choice for rapid sequence induction but is associated with brief increases in ICP and serum potassium; high-dose rocuronium (1.0–1.2 mg/kg) may be a more suitable alternative.

Table 23.2 Management of raised intracranial pressure and brain swelling

Clinical findings	Patient assessment	Intervention/treatment

• Decreased level of consciousness
• Pupillary asymmetry
• Focal or lateralizing neurological signs
• Hemodynamic instability
  – Hypertension-bradycardia
	• Standard hemody-namic and respiratory monitoring
	• Intraarterial pressure monitoring
	• Consider need for central venous access and CVP monitoring
	• Order laboratory studies
	  – Arterial blood gas analysis
	  – Sodium or osmolality
	  – Coagulation studies
	• If available use ICP monitoring with intraparenchymous probe or ventriculos-tomy to allow venting of CSF
		• Increase level of anesthesia (consider bolus infusion of propofol or barbiturate)
		• Pressors and fluid loading to maintain adequate CPP
		• Hypertonic solutions
		  – Saline 3–7.5% as a 150–300 cc bolus
		  – Mannitol 20% 0.25–1 g/kg bolus infusion
		  – Maintain serum osmolality < 320 mOsm/L
		• Hyperventilation
		  – Target pCO_2 25–27 mmHg
		  – Hyperventilation is only temporarily effective and may worsen cerebral ischemia
		  – If jugular venous oximetry is available maintain SjvO2 > 55%
		• Consider moderate hypothermia
		  – Target temperature 32°C

- Avoid bucking/coughing (maintain sufficient level of anesthesia, consider muscle relaxants, spray lidocaine on vocal cords or give iv 60–90 s prior to airway instrumentation).
- Avoid shivering (maintain sufficient level of anesthesia, give opioids, consider muscle relaxants).

Crisis Management

Cerebral swelling and edema following brain injury may result from intracellular fluid accumulation (cytotoxic edema), fluid extravasation (vasogenic edema), hyperemia/vascular engorgement (vasodilatation), or, rarely in the context of EDH and SDH, an obstruction of cerebrospinal fluid outflow. Thus, the underlying causes leading to swelling of brain tissues are cellular energy failure, inflammation, and blood–brain barrier disruption. In the perioperative setting, specifically during evacuation of an SDH, profound edema of the ipsilateral hemisphere may occur because of a sudden reduction in ICP with its associated abrupt increase in the capillary transmural pressure, which promotes the development of hydrostatic edema. Although drugs may cloud recovery and impair reflexes, it is crucial that perioperative ophthalmoplegia should never be attributed to drugs alone but should always instigate further examination.

Table 23.2 lists various recommendations for crisis management of intracranial hypertension. It is important to consider that hyperventilation should only be used as a temporary measure in the case of impending herniation, because hypocapnia/alkalosis-induced vasoconstriction may worsen ischemia in vulnerable parts of the brain. Furthermore, ICP-lowering effects during sustained hypocapnia are only transient (4–12 h), because compensatory reductions in cerebral extracellular bicarbonate levels restore pH over time. The success of hyperosmolar therapy (e.g., mannitol) depends on preserved blood–brain barrier function. If its semipermeable properties are seriously compromised (e.g., in areas of contusion or hemorrhage), the osmotic agents may pass from the blood into the interstitial space, where they might produce reverse osmotic shifts and cause "rebound" intracranial hypertension. Mannitol has traditionally been administered as a repeated 0.25–1 g/kg bolus infusion. In critical cases, it can be combined with a loop diuretic, but care must be taken to maintain normovolemia. Hypertonic saline is an alternative osmotic agent that may be effective particularly for early fluid resuscitation in hypovolemic trauma patients and in the cases of refractory intracranial hypertension. It is important to stress that steroids are not recommended for the treatment of posttraumatic cerebral edema and may in fact be associated with increased mortality.

Uncontrolled or Recurrent Bleeding

A postoperative hematoma is present in approximately 50% of patients who show clinical deterioration *within 6 h* of craniotomy. About 20% of postoperative hematomas develop more than 1 day after the procedure, especially in the cases of emergency surgery.

Risk factors for recurrent bleeding include:

- Intraoperative or immediate postoperative hypertension (within 12 h)
- Intraoperative blood loss > 500 mL
- Age > 70 years
- Hypoxia and hypercapnia
- Coughing
- Increased prothrombin time, low-fibrinogen level, low-platelet count

Prevention

One of the most effective ways to reduce the risk of perioperative bleeding complications is by strict blood pressure management. Patients with recurrent bleeding are 3.6 times more likely to be hypertensive than matched controls. Moreover, the risk of postoperative intracranial hemorrhage is strongly associated with patients being normotensive intraoperatively but hypertensive postoperatively. In the postoperative period, systolic blood pressure is, therefore, commonly managed in the range of 120–150 mmHg. Short-acting intravenous antihypertensive drugs are

Table 23.3 Management of uncontrolled or recurrent bleeding

Clinical findings	Patient assessment	Intervention/treatment
– 60%: decreased level of consciousness – 90%: elevated ICP (when monitored) – focal findings	Order coagulation studies: – Prothrombin time – Platelets – Hb – Fibrinogen – Ca^{2+}	– Treat arterial hypertension – Maintain temp > 35°C – Give packed red cells – Give fresh-frozen plasma – Give platelets – Maintain ionized calcium > 1.0 mmol/L – Consider prothrombin complex concentrate (PPSB) – Consider desmopressin (DDAVP) 0.3 µg/kg – Consider recombinant activated Factor VII (eptacog alfa) – Consider use of controlled hypotension

generally preferable (e.g., labetalol). Other measures to reduce the risk of bleeding include:

• Avoid jugular venous obstruction
• Maintain head-up position (e.g., 30°)
• Prevent hypothermia (keep temp > 35°C)
• Order coagulation studies and maintain:

– Hb > 6 mmol/L
– (Activated) prothrombin time < 1.5 × reference
– Platelets > 50 × 10⁹/L
– Fibrinogen > 0.8 g/L
– Ionized Ca⁺⁺ > 1.0 mmol/L

• Antagonize anticoagulants as appropriate
• Minimize stress during recovery from anesthesia:

– Maintain body temperature > 36.5°C to prevent shivering
– Prevent pain.

Crisis Management

Treat hypertension aggressively in all cases of intraoperative or immediate postoperative bleeding, but do not over-treat: maintain a minimally acceptable CPP of 50–70 mmHg in the face of elevated ICP (arterial BP measurements suggested). Adrenergic antagonists, such as labetolol, are the agents of choice (Table 23.3).

Neurogenic Pulmonary Edema

Prevention

In patients with acute traumatic brain injury, impaired pulmonary function is a common but poorly understood complication. Over one half of patients will develop NPE to various extents. The mechanisms leading to NPE are probably related to a massive sympathetic adrenergic discharge at the time of injury, which results in increased pulmonary microvascular hydrostatic pressures and capillary permeability. Alpha-adrenergic blockade (e.g., with phentolamine) prevents the formation of NPE in an experimental setting, but no specific measures are known to be beneficial in the clinical situation.

Crisis Management

Treatment must be focused on the underlying disorder. As NPE resolves within 48–72 h in the majority of affected patients, management can be done in a supportive and conservative fashion. Mechanical ventilation is likely necessary in the majority of patients to assure adequate oxygenation and ventilation and to prevent iatrogenic lung injury. To avoid excessively high-inflation pressures, tidal volumes between 5 and 8 mL/kg are used (lung protective ventilation strategy). With the use of low-inflation volumes, positive end-expiratory pressure (PEEP) is added to prevent atelectasis. High levels of PEEP may be required to treat severe hypoxemia. Caution is advised; however, since high levels of PEEP can compromise cerebral venous return and increase intracranial hypertension. For the same reasons, the peak inspiratory (plateau) pressure should be kept below 30–35 cm water, and normocapnia should be maintained to avoid further increases in intracranial pressure. Several pharmacological agents such as alpha-adrenergic antagonists, beta-adrenergic blockers, dobutamine, and chlorpromazine are advocated by some authors, but assessment of their effectiveness is difficult because NPE is usually a self-limited condition that ameliorates spontaneously (Table 23.4).

Seizures

Prevention

The rationale for routine seizure prophylaxis is that there is a relatively high incidence of posttraumatic seizures in traumatic brain injury patients. The incidence of early posttraumatic seizures varies between 4 and 25% in untreated patients. Both acute epidural and SDHs are risk factors for developing posttraumatic seizures.

Table 23.4 Management of neurogenic pulmonary edema

Clinical findings	Patient assessment	Intervention/treatment
– Onset within minutes to hours following trauma – Sudden onset of dyspnea – Mild hemoptysis – Protein-rich pulmonary edema	– Order laboratory studies (including arterial blood gas analysis) – Order chest X-ray – Assess need for mechanical ventilation	– Maintain adequate level of sedation – Treat intracranial hypertension – Start mechanical ventilation using adequate PEEP to keep the lung open – Consider ventilation with TV less than 6 mL/kg of predicted body weight might – Consider head of bed elevation – Consider use of diuretics (treat hypervolemia) – Consider use of intravenous alpha-/beta-adrenergic receptor antagonists (phentolamine, labetolol, esmolol)

Anticonvulsants are indicated to decrease the incidence of posttraumatic seizures (within 7 days of injury). However, early posttraumatic seizures are not associated with worse outcomes and anticonvulsants have been associated with adverse side effects. Most clinicians consider a loading dose of phenytoin 20 mg/kg IV followed by a daily maintenance dose if seizures have been witnessed or suspected to have occurred after injury. If no further seizures occur, taper and discontinue the phenytoin after 1 week.

Crisis Management

Airway management is critical to avoid exacerbating status epilepticus through hypoxia. If endotracheal intubation under neuromuscular blockade is necessary, use a short-acting non-depolarizing agent such as rocuronium (1.0–1.2 mg/kg for rapid sequence induction). Give lorazepam 0.2 mg/kg and repeat every 5 min. Consider a loading dose of phenytoin 20 mg/kg at the same time. If a status epilepticus persists, give midazolam with a loading dose of 0.2 mg/kg followed by an infusion of 0.2–2.0 mg/kg/h or administer propofol 3–5 mg/kg as a bolus, then 1–15 mg/kg/h to achieve seizure control. Should the patient not be controlled with propofol, administer pentobarbital 20 mg/kg at 0.2–0.4 mg/kg/min as tolerated, followed by an infusion of 0.25–2.0 mg/kg/h as determined by EEG monitoring. The administration of volatile anesthetics can be considered as a last resort to control intractable seizure activity in emergency situations (Table 23.5).

Table 23.5 Management of seizures

Clinical findings	Patient assessment	Intervention/treatment
• Tonic–clonic convulsions • Loss of consciousness (no convulsions may be apparent)	• Check airway, breathing, and circulation • If the patient's head is immobilized in pins, ensure safety	• Secure airway (if applicable) • Increase FiO_2 • Give lorazepam 0.2 mg/kg IV, (repeat as necessary) • Give phenytoin 20 mg/kg loading dose IV • Consider additional agents as required (propofol, barbiturates)

Table 23.6 Management of arterial hypotension during opening of the dura

Clinical findings	Patient assessment	Intervention/treatment
Sudden arterial hypotension Sudden tachycardia Decrease of end-tidal CO_2	Order laboratory studies • Hb/Ht • Sodium or osmolality	Give fluids Consider vasopressors Decrease depth of anesthesia

Sudden Arterial Hypotension upon Opening of the Dura

Prevention

To ensure intraoperative hemodynamic stability, it is essential to maintain good communication between anesthesiologist and surgeon throughout all stages of the procedure, as hypovolemic hypotension may be unmasked as the stimulus for hypertension if suddenly released during opening of the skull. The following considerations apply:

• Ensure adequate venous access
• Frequently check the operative status; communicate with the surgeons
• Give fluid loading before decompression occurs
• Have catecholamines (pressors) on standby.

Crisis Management

Fluid administration that reduces osmolality should be avoided. Small volumes (1–3 L) of lactated Ringer's may be used. When larger volumes are needed, a combination of isotonic crystalloids (e.g., normal saline) and colloids is preferred. Hypertonic saline is useful when there is hypotension and increased ICP. Circulation support to influence CBF is achieved best by increasing blood pressure, as cardiac output appears not to be varying with CBF. The drug of choice to increase blood pressure is phenylephrine (provided that the fluid status is adequate or is corrected in parallel). Patients with low-myocardial reserve may require an inotrope, such as dopamine or (nor)epinephrine (Table 23.6).

Key Points

- The prevention of complications is easier than their treatment
- Maintain good communication between all team members
- Maintain blood pressure, temperature, coagulation studies, electrolytes, and blood gases within their normal ranges
- Maintain CPP between 50 and 70 mmHg (if ICP monitoring is available).

Suggested Reading

Brain Trauma Foundation; American Association of Neurological Surgeons; Congress of Neurological Surgeons. Guidelines for the management of severe traumatic brain injury. J Neurotrauma. 2007;24 Suppl 1:S1–106.

Maas AI, Stocchetti N, Bullock R. Moderate and severe traumatic brain injury in adults. Lancet Neurol. 2008;7(8):728–41.

Perry JJ, Lee JS, Sillberg VAH, Wells GA. Rocuronium versus succinylcholine for rapid sequence induction intubation. Cochrane Database Syst Rev 2008;(2):CD002788. doi:10.1002/14651858. CD002788.pub2.

Chapter 24
Perioperative Challenges During Cerebrovascular Surgery

Jeremy D. Fields, Kenneth C. Liu, and Ansgar M. Brambrink

Overview

Cerebrovascular surgery accounts for a significant proportion of neurosurgical interventions. This chapter focuses on the most common and challenging: aneurysm repair, arterio-venous malformation (AVM) resection, and cerebrovascular bypass surgery.

- Aneurysm repair:

    - Surgical procedure: clip placed across neck of aneurysm to exclude aneurysm from blood flow, thereby preventing rupture
    - Indications:

        (a) Any ruptured aneurysm
        (b) Symptoms from mass effect
        (c) Elective surgery for unruptured aneurysms:

            * Incidental aneurysms >6 mm in the anterior circulation (except posterior communicating artery: PCOM)

J.D. Fields, MD (✉)
Departments of Neurology and Dotter Interventional Institute, Oregon Health &
Science University, Portland, OR, USA
e-mail: fieldsje@ohsu.edu

K.C. Liu, MD
Departments of Neurological Surgery and Radiology, University of Virginia Health System,
Charlottesville, VA, USA

A.M. Brambrink, MD, PhD
Departments of Anesthesiology and Perioperative Medicine, Neurology and Neurologic Surgery,
Oregon Health & Science University, Portland, OR, USA

A.M. Brambrink and J.R. Kirsch (eds.), *Essentials of Neurosurgical Anesthesia & Critical Care*, DOI 10.1007/978-0-387-09562-2_24,
© Springer Science+Business Media, LLC 2012

* Any size aneurysm of the PCOM or posterior circulation
* Any aneurysm in a patient with a history of ruptured aneurysm or a strong family history of subarachnoid hemorrhage (SAH)

- AVM resection:

  - Surgical procedure: clips placed across feeding vessels and AVM nidus excised
  - Indications:

    (a) AVMs are generally resected if risk of surgery is acceptable, based on the quality of the individual surgeon, location of the AVM, and the pattern of arterial feeders and venous drainage
    (b) Prior symptomatic bleeding in past (annual risk of bleeding is substantially increased)

- Cerebral bypass surgery:

  - Extracranial–intracranial bypass surgery:

    (a) Surgical procedures:

        * Donor vessels: superficial temporal (STA), occipital (OA), or proximal external carotid (ECA)
        * Recipient vessels: middle cerebral artery (MCA), anterior cerebral artery (ACA), posterior cerebral artery (PCA), superior cerebellar (SCA), posterior inferior cerebellar (PICA)
        * Anastomosis:

            (1) Direct: donor ECA vessel sewn directly to branch intracranial vessel
            (2) Indirect:

                ○ Donor ECA vessel sewn to pial surface
                ○ Over time, collateral circulation forms, connecting ECA vessel to intracranial circulation

    (b) Indications:

        * High-grade stenosis or occlusion of the internal carotid artery (ICA), MCA, PCA, or basilar artery in patients with demonstrated inadequate cerebral reserve (hemodynamic stroke, diamox CT or MR perfusion studies, PET)
        * Moyamoya disease

  - Adjunct to aneurysm repair or skull base tumor resection:

    (a) Surgical procedures:

        * EC–IC bypasses, as above
        * Direct bypass from one major intracranial vessel to another; choice of graft depends on flow characteristics

        (1) Low flow: generally use STA, OA, or ECA (used for M3-branches of MCA)

        (2) Intermediate flow: radial artery or saphenous (used for P2 or M2-branches of MCA)

        (3) High flow: large caliber saphenous vein graft (used for M1/M2 branches of MCA or for ICA bypass)

  (b) Indications:

      * Preservation of blood flow via the bypass when aneurysm clipping requires sacrifice of a critical portion of a cerebral blood vessel

      * Tumors encasing or invading major arteries at the skull base; bypass allows adequate distal cerebral blood flow

– Transposition of vertebral artery: used for patients with symptomatic vertebral artery stenosis at origin

Prevention

The most feared perioperative complications are as follows:

- Intracranial hemorrhage from an unsecured vascular malformation (cerebral aneurysm or AVM) prior to definitive surgical treatment.
- Ischemic stroke from inappropriate cerebral perfusion during surgery, a complication that cannot be reliably detected because the patient is under anesthesia and the neurologic exam is unavailable.
- Complications from increased or rapidly decreased ICP.
- Retraction injury (particularly in skull base surgeries), which may result in cerebral edema, ischemia, or hemorrhage; this type of injury may be mitigated by interventions to "relax" the brain tissue, by reducing total brain tissue or CSF volume.

Based on the above analysis, the basic goals for the prevention of perioperative complications during cerebrovascular surgery are as follows:

- Prevent aneurysm/AVM rupture
- Maintain cerebral perfusion pressure (CPP) and cerebral blood flow (CBF)
- Control ICP and decrease brain tissue volume ("brain relaxation") to improve surgical approach/visualization

General considerations for prevention include the following:

- Controlled induction and maintenance of anesthesia

  – Adequate doses of opioids to prevent hemodynamic response to laryngoscopy and endotracheal tube placement (e.g., 3–7 mcg/kg of fentanyl); lidocaine IV can also be used as an adjunct

  – Use esmolol during induction to prevent blood pressure spikes

- Additional doses of opioids or hypnotic drugs to deepen anesthesia during placement of head pins
- When practical, avoid succinylcholine in patients with high ICP

- Choice of anesthetic agents:

  - Volatile anesthetics cause cerebral vasodilation and increase ICP to varying degrees; sevoflurane may have the least effect on CBF and ICP of all volatile anesthetics; many anesthesiologists currently advocate for a combination of IV hypnotics and volatile anesthetics in order to control unwanted side effects, and benefit from certain pharmacodynamic characteristics (see below); others advocate for total IV anesthesia using propofol based on their observation of reduced ICP and improved cerebral perfusion pressure; nitrous oxide should be avoided during cerebrovascular surgery due to its negative effects on CBF and ICP and its physical characteristics
  - In patients with known or suspected elevated ICP, volatile anesthetics should be limited or avoided entirely in favor of short-acting intravenous medications, typically propofol in combination with short-acting opioids or with sub-MAC doses of desflurane, a combination which was shown to improve brain tissue oxygenation. Etomidate is associated with less favorable effects on cerebral blood flow and brain tissue oxygenation and should not be used as a component for maintenance in an intravenous anesthesia regime for these patients. Propofol is associated with the most pronounced reduction in CBF of all IV agents
  - Newer agents such as dexmedetomidine and ketamine are being explored as alternatives to more traditional ones
  - Agents with rapid emergence are preferred in order to allow neurological examination immediately after surgery (examples are propofol/remifentanil, volatile anesthetic/fentanyl, thiopental/fentanyl)
  - High doses of sevoflurane or isoflurane will lower the seizure threshold

- Ventilation:

  - EtCO2 monitoring should always be performed and used to manage the pCO2 levels throughout surgery
  - Check ABG regularly during surgery to correlate EtCO2 to pCO2
  - Mild hyperventilation (pCO2 30–35) is indicated (1) in patients with suspected or known increased ICP (2) for "brain relaxation" (3) to counteract cerebrovascular vasodilation caused by volatile anesthetics

- Enhanced surgical access:

  - Mannitol 50–75 g (0.5–1 g/kg) or 3% hypertonic saline 250 ml given prior to surgical incision for "brain relaxation"; particularly during opening of the dura, careful titration of osmotherapy and its effects on blood pressure (mannitol may decrease blood pressure; hypertonic saline may increase it) is necessary in patients with unsecured cerebral malformations in order to maintain a stable aneurysmal transmural pressure gradient and prevent rupture (see below for details)

- Use of CSF diversion via ventriculostomy, lumbar drain, or direct CSF drainage via craniotomy

- Positioning:

  - If possible, keep head at least 20 cm above heart to prevent decreased venous outflow from the brain and elevated ICP

- Bleeding:

  - Although rare, massive and rapid blood loss can occur during surgical manipulation of cerebral blood vessels
  - It is, therefore, essential to have adequate vascular access and blood products available

- Monitoring:

  - Cerebrovascular surgeries should be monitored using ASA standard monitoring plus invasive arterial blood pressure (placed prior to induction, if not too stimulating for the patient) and urine output measurement
  - Central venous access should be considered, for cerebral venous pressure (CVP) monitoring, for hemodynamic management, and for fluid resuscitation; particularly in patients who are at high risk of vasospasm requiring subsequent hypertensive therapy. Although subclavian access is associated with higher frequency of pneumothorax, it may be preferable in patients with high intracranial pressure to maintain optimal cerebral venous return and maybe associated with lower frequency of catheter associated bloodstream infections
  - In patients with ruptured aneurysms or AVM, ICP monitoring with an external ventricular drain allows for both ICP measurement and CSF removal. It is very important to ensure that ICP monitors are closed prior to position changes and subsequently leveled with respect to the patient's tragus in order to prevent over- or underdrainage of CSF
  - Electrophysiological intraoperative monitoring:

    (a) Somatosensory evoked potentials (SSEPs), brainstem auditory evoked potentials (BAEP), and electroencephalography (EEG) are most commonly used modalities
    (b) May allow for early detection of ischemia

- Fluid management:

  - Isotonic or hypertonic fluids as needed; consider high fluid and electrolyte loss secondary to osmotherapy
  - Dextrose-containing fluids are contraindicated for fluid management as hyperglycemia may accentuate brain injury in the setting of ischemia

- Hemodynamic management:

    - The goal is arterial normotension (ensuring CPP > 60 mm Hg) prior to securing the aneurysm or AVM
    - After the aneurysm or AVM is secured the blood pressure goals are specific for each scenario and described below

- Temperature management:

    - Some centers still provide mild hypothermia (33–35°C) during craniotomy for aneurysm or AVM repair despite lack of confirmation of neuroprotective benefit in a randomized trial
    - Prior to awakening, patients should be normothermic to avoid postanesthesia shivering

- Controlled emergence:

    - Blood pressure often increases during emergence and should be controlled to baseline values
    - Rapid emergence allows immediate neurological examination

In addition, specific considerations relate to particular surgical procedures:

- During repair of cerebral aneurysms:

    - Maintenance of stable transmural pressure gradient (TMPG):

        (a) TMPG = pressure within blood vessels − pressure outside = MAP-ICP
        (b) Higher TMPG increases risk of rupture
        (c) Therefore, marked decreases in ICP, particularly in the context of elevated arterial blood pressure, may increase the risk of rebleeding

    - Interventions during "temporary clipping":

        (a) Vascular clips are applied temporarily to parent artery in order to improve surgical visualization for application of permanent clip to aneurysm
        (b) No intervention necessary if temporary clip is applied for less than 2 min
        (c) If > 2 min:

            * Increase FiO2 to 100%
            * Increase inspired concentration of desflurane (consider phenylephrine to maintain blood pressure at or above baseline level). Others suggest an immediate bolus dose of barbiturates or propofol, although convincing support from clinical studies is lacking and in particular propofol appears not to be an effective neuroprotectant

        (d) If >10–15 min:

            * Consider slightly augmenting blood pressure to preserve perfusion via collaterals

* Discuss with surgical team the necessity for administration of anesthetic agents (e.g., desflurane) to induce burst suppression on EEG. In this situation, many anesthesiologists provided IV barbiturates, e.g., thiopental, or IV propofol, but the evidence from clinical studies is highly controversial regarding this practice. Recent clinical studies suggest that the combination of desflurane and propofol results in better brain tissue oxygenation than propofol alone
* Ischemic stunning may result in need for postoperative management in the ICU, including continued mechanical ventilation and adequate sedation

– Fluid management:

(a) Only isotonic or hypertonic fluids should be administered
(b) Prior to clipping, replace overnight fluid losses and maintain rate to account for hourly losses and diuresis from mannitol
(c) After clipping, replace intraoperative fluid loss and bolus additional fluids for goal euvolemic to mildly hypervolemic state in order to improve cerebral perfusion distal to aneurysm clipping

– Blood pressure management:

(a) Prior to aneurysm clipping, maintain blood pressure in a low normal range unless significant vasospasm is present, in which case higher blood pressure goals are desirable
(b) After clipping, target blood pressure may be liberalized to a level slightly above baseline (improved collateral perfusion)

– Criteria for extubation in OR:

(a) Good preoperative level of consciousness (without sedation)
(b) Mild brain swelling during surgery
(c) Short period of temporary clipping
(d) Adequate strength, demonstrated by sustained head lift, strong hand grasp or leg lift
(e) Awake and able to accurately follow commands
(f) Evidence of leak at 20 cm of water pressure (or less), with the endotracheal tube cuff deflated

• During AVM resection:

– Postoperative blood pressure management

(a) Elevations in blood pressure postoperatively are associated with increased bleeding from the AVM resection cavity, and may exacerbate normal perfusion pressure breakthrough (edema or hemorrhage resulting from increased perfusion following removal of the AVM; discussed further below)

(b) Aggressive postoperative blood pressure control has been shown to substantially decrease postoperative hematoma formation as well as the risk for brain edema formation

(c) The most vulnerable period for hematoma formation is probably during emergence from anesthesia; the risk for brain edema formation remains elevated for at least 48 h after surgery

- Cerebral bypass procedures:

  - Blood pressure management

    (a) Most likely periods of hypotension (relative or absolute) will occur during induction of anesthesia and during temporary clipping of recipient vessel

    (b) During these time periods, arterial hypotension – even over short periods – is likely to result in watershed ischemia and subsequent cerebral infarction

    (c) During temporary clipping, either maintain or slightly augment blood pressure (up to about 20% of baseline)

    (d) During ischemic time (while the artery to be bypassed is clamped and graft not yet completed), blood pressure may be augmented to 20% above baseline and burst suppression EEG may be considered

    (e) After graft placement, blood pressure targets in the first 2–3 days should be low to normal. This will prevent graft leakage and excessive cerebral perfusion but preserve graft patency; reasonable goals are systolic blood pressure (SBP) 100–120 in normotensive individuals; SBP 120–140 with a history of hypertension)

  - Antiplatelet agents, and intraoperative heparin are often used to preserve graft patency

    (a) For elective procedures a common regimen is aspirin 325 mg po per day

    (b) For emergency procedures, aspirin may be loaded as either 325 mg po (or via NGT) or 650 mg rectally

Crisis Management

During cerebrovascular surgery, certain complications may rapidly result in a life-threatening crisis which require immediate intervention. The most critical are (1) acute raise in ICP and impending brain herniation, (2) CSF overdrainage, (3) seizures; (4) intracranial homorrhage; and (5) stroke

- Elevated ICP, very tight brain, or herniation out durotomy

  - Check for venous outflow obstruction at the internal jugular vein (e.g., tape around neck for securing an endotracheal tube, head turning)

- Administer osmolar therapy (mannitol 0.5–2 g/kg, or hypertonic saline 3% 250 ml; some authors have advocated the administration of 30 ml of hypertonic saline 23.4%)
- Switch from volatile agents to total intravenous anesthesia (e.g., propofol + fentanyl) at high doses
- Drain additional CSF if drain in place
- Mild hyperventilation (arterial pCO2 30–35)
- Consider thiopental bolus 1 g ± infusion 4–5 mg/kg/h (or adequate doses of propofol) to reach burst suppression EEG
- Consider hypothermia 33–35°C

- CSF overdrainage in patients with external ventricular drain (EVD) or lumbar drain

  - Overdrainage of CSF can lead to downward herniation
  - If suspected, immediately clamp EVD or lumbar drain
  - Consult with neurosurgeon regarding need for intrathecal instillation of saline

- Seizure

  - Perioperative seizure may occur with any type of intracranial surgery
  - If prolonged seizures are suspected at any time during the perioperative period, treat with lorazepam 0.05–0.1 mg/kg, and load with a longer-acting medication (fosphenytoin (20 PE/kg), levetiracetam (1,000–1,500 mg), or valproate 20 mg/kg)
  - If seizures continue despite the above measures, patient should be immediately intubated and begun on high-dose propofol or midazolam infusion; seizures during surgery are extremely rare and require deepening of anesthesia. In the anesthetized and paralyzed patient, seizures should be considered if the patient demonstrates significant hypertension that cannot be attributed to surgical stimulation
  - Subclinical seizures are an important differential diagnosis when the patient fails to wake up after brain surgery

Some high-risk complications are specific for particular types of cerebrovascular surgeries and require specific interventions.

In patients undergoing aneurysm repair:

- Intraoperative aneurysm rupture:

  (a) Risk:

  * About half of the aneurysms tear or rupture while the clip is placed; this usually does not result in substantial blood loss
  * The risk of perioperative rupture without immediate access to the aneurysm by the surgeon (i.e., during induction or during preparation) is about

11% in patients with previously ruptured aneurysms (i.e., status post SAH) and 1% in elective cases (previously unruptured aneurysm)

* In 8% of cases in which intraoperative rupture occurs without immediate access to the source of bleeding, hemorrhagic shock results (<1% of total surgeries)

(b) Intervention: aggressive transfusion of blood products
(c) Blood pressure goals during intraoperative rupture are controversial and communication with surgeons is essential:

* If control of bleeding cannot be immediately accomplished, permissive arterial hypotension (MAP 40–60) may facilitate hemostasis (frequently clipping of aneurysm or temporary clipping of the parent artery is delayed in this situation secondary to poor visualization)
* Even if arterial hypotension is the goal, fluid resuscitation should target euvolemia
* Once temporary or definitive clips are applied:

    (1) Consider thiopental and hypothermia to decrease metabolic demand
    (2) Consider blood pressure augmentation MAP 70–90 for increased collateral circulation

* In patients with significant vasospasm or elevations in intracranial pressure, blood pressure should be preserved at preoperative baseline

– Neurogenic pulmonary edema

(a) Occurs in about 5% of patients with SAH, generally in the first 48 h
(b) Treat with supportive care, modified lung-protective ventilation (low MDAL volume, high PEEP with attention to possible effects on ICP, avoid hypercapnia to allow adequate ICP control)

– Cardiac dysfunction

(a) Cardiac arrhythmias are extremely common in SAH, and include signs of myocardial ischemia (ranging from nonspecific T-wave abnormalities to diffuse ST segment elevations or depressions) as well as brady- or tachyarrhythmias
(b) Neurocardiogenic stress cardiomyopathy occurs in up to 30% of patients; in most cases pressors with inotropic effects are preferred, e.g., norepinephrine
(c) Pharmacologically induced arterial hypotension: Nimodipine is a peripheral calcium channel blocker that is administered for 21 days. This oral agent may decrease the risk of vasospasm after SAH and may have neuroprotective attributes
(d) During surgery, if nimodipine results in a significant decrease in blood pressure, it should be held temporarily

In patients undergoing AVM repair:

– Intraoperative rupture:

    (a) Massive hemorrhage is possible; respond with aggressive transfusion of blood products to maintain a hemoglobin level of 8–10 g/dl

– Postoperative hemorrhage:

    (a) Goal low normal blood pressures
    (b) If significant mass effect, consider osmotherapy (hypertonic saline or mannitol), hyperventilation (pCO_2 30–35), and emergent return to the operating room

– Perioperative brain ischemia:

    (a) Cerebral steal: cerebral ischemia resulting from shunting of blood through AVM and away from adjacent normal tissue may cause symptomatic ischemia. If some arterial feeders are occluded and others are not, this will change blood flow characteristics through AVM, and increase perfusion in adjacent areas of brain which have been chronically adapted to lower perfusion pressures, resulting in postoperative "Normal perfusion pressure breakthrough":

        * Postoperative cerebral edema (or, in severe cases, intraparenchymal hemorrhage) attributed to cerebral hyperemia from exposure of areas of the cerebral vasculature with relative hypotension preoperatively (due to shunting from AVM) to increased perfusion pressures postoperatively (once the shunt is eliminated)
        * Occurs in <5% of cases

Cerebral bypass:

– Intraoperative graft thrombosis:

    (a) Rare; detected by surgeon under direct visualization
    (b) Check activated clotting time (ACT) if available, heparanize patient, and check coagulation parameters afterward
    (c) Surgeon will place temporary clips and reexplore grafts

– Postoperative graft thrombosis:

    (a) More common than intraoperative thrombosis
    (b) May be treated with blood pressure augmentation, or rarey, with endovascular thrombectomy/thrombolysis

Key Points

- Intracranial hemorrhage is the most feared complication
  - Prepare for hemodynamic compromise with adequate monitoring and availability of blood products
  - Postoperative hemorrhage generally requires immediate reoperation
- Tight control of intra- and perioperative blood pressure is essential
  - Lower blood pressures and avoidance of blood pressure spikes are usually desirable when bleeding complications are a concern
  - Higher blood pressures and avoidance of hypotension are critical when cerebral ischemia is a concern
  - Anticipate, to prevent blood pressure spike during endotracheal intubation, placement of head pins, and surgical incision
  - Anticipate hypotension after induction of anesthesia and sudden absence of surgical stimulation
- Consider anesthetic strategies with limited use of highly soluble volatile anesthetics rapid emergence
- Establish continuous communication with surgical team, particularly during acute crisis

Suggested Reading

Bendo AA. Intracranial vascular surgery. Anesthesiol Clin North America. 2002;20:377–88.

Hashimoto T, Young WL. Anesthesia-related considerations for cerebral arteriovenous malformations. Neurosurg Focus. 2001;11:e5.

Hindman BJ, Bayman EO, Pfisterer WK, Torner JC, Todd MM, IHAST Investigators. No association between intraoperative hypothermia or supplemental protective drug and neurologic outcomes in patients undergoing temporary clipping during cerebral aneurysm surgery: findings from the Intraoperative Hypothermia for Aneurysm Surgery Trial. Anesthesiology. 2010;112(1):86–101.

Jellish WS. Anesthetic issues and perioperative blood pressure management in patients who have cerebrovascular diseases undergoing surgical procedures. Neurol Clin. 2006;24:647–59, viii.

Randell T, Niskanen M. Management of physiological variables in neuroanaesthesia: Maintaining homeostasis during intracranial surgery. Curr Opin Anaesthesiol. 2006;19:492–7.

Randell T, Niemela M, Kytta J, Tanskanen P, Maattanen M, Karatas A, et al. Principles of neuroanesthesia in aneurysmal subarachnoid hemorrhage: The Helsinki experience. Surg Neurol. 2006;66:382–8. Discussion 388.

Sekhar LN, Natarajan SK, Ellenbogen RG, Ghodke B. Cerebral revascularization for ischemia, aneurysms, and cranial base tumors. Neurosurgery. 2008;62:1373–408. Discussion 1408–10.

Chapter 25
Perioperative Challenges During Pituitary Surgery

Shuji Dohi

Overview

Surgery on the pituitary gland may cause problems related to surgical intervention per se, as well as changes in endocrine function during and after surgery. The pituitary gland (hypophysis) is located in the sella turcica at the base of the brain in close proximity to the sphenoid sinus, hypothalamus, optic chiasm, and vessels (internal carotid artery, cavernous sinus).

The two components of the pituitary gland are the anterior pituitary (adenohypophysis) and posterior pituitary (neurohypophysis). The hypothalamus controls the function of the pituitary gland by virtue of vascular connections between the hypothalamus and anterior pituitary and nerve fibers between the hypothalamus and posterior pituitary.

Risk and Incidence

Pituitary tumors account for approximately 18% of all primary brain tumors. Of these, approximately two-thirds of pituitary tumors have a final diagnosis of adenoma. The three most common disorders of pituitary hyperfunction are those related to excesses of prolactin (amenorrhea, galactorrhea, and infertility), adrenocorticotropic hormone (ACTH) (Cushing's disease), or growth hormone (GH) (acromegaly) (Table 25.1).

S. Dohi, MD, PhD (✉)
Department of Anesthesiology and Pain Medicine, Gifu University Graduate
School of Medicine, Gifu, Japan
e-mail: shu-dohi@kujiran.jp

A.M. Brambrink and J.R. Kirsch (eds.), *Essentials of Neurosurgical
Anesthesia & Critical Care*, DOI 10.1007/978-0-387-09562-2_25,
© Springer Science+Business Media, LLC 2012

Table 25.1 Incidence of tumors in the pituitary region

Type of tumor	Incidence/percent
Pituitary tumors	10% of all autopsies
	10–15% of all brain tumors
	Majority of supra-sellar tumors
• Nonfunctional pituitary tumor	~30%
• Functional pituitary tumor	~70%
– Prolactin-producing tumor	43%
– Growth Hormone-producing tumor	17%
– ACTH-producing tumor	7%
– Thyroid producing tumor	3%
– LH-, FSH-producing tumor	Rare
Craniopharyngeomas	0.5–1:100,000/year
	1–3% of all brain tumors
	13% of all supra-sellar tumors

Table 25.2 Complications associated with pituitary surgery

Surgical approach	Complications
Trans-cranial	DI, CSF leakage, ischemia in forebrain, air embolism
Trans-sphenoidal	DI, numbness of upper lip and teeth, visual loss, nasal CSF leakage
Trans-nasal (endoscopic; "minimally invasive")	DI, skin lesion due to endoscopy, venous air embolism

DI diabetes insipidus

Risk for anesthesia and surgery is related to surgical approach, as well as to individual manifestation of patients' disorder as shown in Table 25.2. Trans-cranial approach with supra-sellar invasion may cause cerebral-spinal fluid (CSF) leakage and visual loss. Trans-sphenoidal and trans-nasal approach may cause numbness of upper lip and teeth, nasal CSF leakage, and venous air embolism. Neurogenic diabetes insipidus (DI) could occur with any approach.

In acromegalic patients, difficulty of airway management occurs approximately three times more often than the other pituitary disorders (9.1% vs. 2.6%). Patients with Cushing's disease and those with a prolactinoma are no more difficult to intubate than patients with nonfunctioning tumors.

Neurogenic DI occurs in approximately 20% of patients undergoing transsphenoidal resection of a pituitary adenoma in the immediate postoperative period. In addition, surgery in the sella turcica may also cause hypofunction of the hypothalamic-pituitary axis, vision disturbance, bleeding and local edema. Though rare, air embolism could occur during surgery in patients in semi-Fowler (being head with 20–30 cm higher than the lower part of the body) or lounging position (position in a chair with head bend back on a sofa).

Pathophysiology and Anticipated Problems

Anticipated problems following pituitary surgery are dependent upon pathophysiological changes associated with tumor-induced altered endocrine function in combination with endocrine changes associated with general surgical stress. Hypothalamic stress results in two categories of responses: rapid effects mediated through the sympathetic nervous system and adrenal medulla, and neuroendocrine responses mediated through the pituitary gland and adrenal cortex.

Although neither nonfunctional nor functional adenomas usually cause ICP to increase, the tumor growth in the restricted space of the sella turcica may represent clinical signs such as visual disturbance, as it impinges on the optic chiasm.

Acromegaly is a rare chronic disease of mid-life caused by excess secretion of adeno-hypophyseal GH, causing enlargement of bone, connective tissue, and viscera. Physical signs are most remarkable in the hands, feet, face, mandible, and head. Increase in subcutaneous connective tissue thickens the lips, skin folds, and tongue, and often causes glossoptosis. As a result, the large tongue and hypertrophied tissues in and around the upper airway reduce the airway space and predispose patients to airway obstruction. Thus, tracheal intubation is three times more common in patients with acromegaly.

The most common cause of Cushing's disease before age 40 is a pituitary tumor (in patients older than 60 years, the most likely cause is adrenal carcinoma). Associated problems include mild diabetes, hypertension, degenerative vascular disease, and heart disease, particularly in patients with hyperadrenocorticism. In Cushing's disease, hypokalemia, hypernatremia, increased intravascular fluid volume, and skeletal muscle weakness are commonly manifested. Prevention of long-term consequences involves early diagnosis, removal of the tumor, while treating secondary events (e.g., hypertension).

During Anesthesia and Surgery

In patients with acromegaly, the anesthesiologist must anticipate difficulty with airway management due to a large tongue, abundant soft tissue folds, and enlarged facial structures. As induction of general anesthesia in these patients carries a higher risk (cannot ventilate/cannot intubate scenario after induction), it is most conservative to intubate the trachea with the patient awake and breathing spontaneously; most commonly with a fiberoptic approach and local anesthesia.

Once the trachea is intubated, it is safest to maintain general anesthesia including muscle paralysis. This helps to prevent injury from patient movement while in head-pins (e.g., Mayfield head-holder), and during surgery through the rigid Hardy nasal scope. It is important to remember to consider reducing the initial dose of muscle relaxant and compulsively dose these drugs based on train-of-four testing, in view of skeletal muscle weakness in Cushing patients.

Emergence from Anesthesia and Postoperative Period

Tissue edema caused by surgical trauma may further decrease the oropharyngeal space and contribute to the upper airway obstruction after airway extubation. Prior to extubation, the clinician should at minimum confirm that there is a leak around the endotracheal tube, at a pressure below 20 cm H_2O, after the cuff is deflated. Some experts also advocate that an extubation catheter should be placed in the trachea prior to extubation in order to facilitate rapid reintubation in the event that extubation results in acute airway obstruction. Similarly, other experts advocate that extubation should be done in these high-risk patients over an intubating broncho-scope. Last, it is always prudent to make sure that extubation of high-risk patients is done at a time when an experienced surgeon would be available to establish a surgical airway of extubation and initial noninvasive techniques for reintubation fail. Thus, it is important to at least communicate plans for extubation of high-risk patients with the neurosurgeon. It is optimal to have that surgeon at the patient's bedside during the extubation.

Neurogenic diabetes insipidus (DI) could occur in patients undergoing trans-sphenoidal resection of pituitary adenomas in the immediate postoperative period. This could occur due to surgical trauma on posterior pituitary where antidiuretic hormone (ADH) is secreted. Treatment is complicated because the natural course of DI occurs in two phases in the first 24–48 h postoperatively: high urine output followed by reduced urine output, and then the chronic degree of DI is established, without apparent correlation to the initial degree of increased or reduced urine output.

Prevention

The basic principles of pituitary surgery remain unchanged with the other neuro-surgical patients. They include the provision of optimal operative conditions, maintenance of cerebral perfusion pressure and cerebral oxygenation during anesthesia, and speedy recovery from anesthesia. Anesthesiologists must maintain optimal physiologic condition of each patient-airway, respiratory and cardiovascular condition, fluid and plasma electrolytes, and metabolic condition.

As mentioned above, airway management may be challenging in patients with acromegaly, and fiberoptic intubation of the awake and spontaneously breathing patient is likely the safest approach. In all cases, the patients should be monitored with ECG, noninvasive BP, pulse oximetry, and ETCO2. More invasive monitoring (e.g., invasive arterial pressure monitoring) should be considered in patients with significant comorbidities (e.g., ischemic heart disease).

Crisis Management (Clinical Presentation)

Complications with Airway Management and Ventilation

Patients who, by physical examination or history, appear to be difficult to intubate or mask ventilate should always be managed conservatively for airway management in the awake state. In others, prior to inducing anesthesia, it is important to have the patient in an ideal sniffing position. It is also critical to have easy access to airway adjuncts in the event of an emergency situation, including oral and nasal airways, an LMA (or other supraglottic device), Glidescope (or equivalent), flexible fiberoptic endoscopy equipment and supplies necessary for establishing an emergency surgical airway. Failure of mask ventilation and tracheal intubation in the anesthetized state should invoke use of the ASA difficult airway algorithm.

If the clinician decides that it is safe to intubate the airway after induction of anesthesia, it is advisable to induce anesthesia with agents that have a short half-life or are easily reversed in the event difficulties with intubation arise by surprise. Mask ventilation may be facilitated with the use of an oral airway. Whenever possible, neuromuscular blocking agents should be withheld until the clinician confirms their ability to mask-ventilate the patient. Some centers recommend the placement of a sponge in the pharynx during surgery to prevent blood from entering the airway during trans-nasal or trans-sphenoidal approach.

Despite attempts to suction the airway and pharynx prior to extubation, there is often blood draining from the surgical site into the mouth. Emergence and extubation are facilitated with the patient in a head-up position and awake. It is critical to assure that the patient will be awake and strong enough after extubation to manage secretions and blood from the surgical site. The increased volume of secretions in the airway of these patients may predispose them to laryngospasm.

Cardiovascular Complications

Hypertension is anticipated during placement of the patient in the Mayfield head-holder (particularly when the peri-osteal pins are placed) and when the surgeon is administering the topical/local anesthetic in the nostrils. Typically, surgeons use epinephrine (1:200,000) with cocaine on cotton to cause local anesthesia and vasoconstriction. The degree of hypertension can be minimized by closely monitoring patients so that treatment can be provided in a timely fashion. Invasive arterial pressure monitoring is indicated in patients with cardiovascular co-morbidities in whom transient significant hypertension is likely to cause significant myocardial ischemia. Next, it is important to preemptively deep the level of anesthesia with a short-acting agent (e.g., alfentanil, propofol) or using direct acting agents (e.g., esmolol, nitroglycerin, nitroprusside) to mitigate the degree of hypertension.

Table 25.3 Diagnosis of diabetes insipidus

Urine	
Specific gravity	<1.005
Output	>250 mL
Osmolarity	<200 mOsm/kg
Serum	
Osmolarity	>300 mOsm/kg
Sodium concentration	>150 mg/L

Severe hypotension may rarely occur during surgical intervention due to accidental surgical injury of the cavernous sinus and carotid artery, both of which are immediately lateral to the area of surgery. Invasion of either of these structures by the surgeon may require institution of a massive transfusion protocol in order to save the patient's life. In addition, severe hypotension may occur secondary to venous air embolus. Whereas surgical invasion of the cavernous sinus or carotid artery are associated with significant hemorrhage in the surgical field, venous air embolus is associated with a dry surgical field. If a venous air embolus is suspected, the anesthesiologist must communicate their concern with the surgeon, ask the surgeon to flood the surgical field, and support the blood pressure pharmacologically.

Endocrine Failure

Pituitary surgery may result in significant hormonal deficiency requiring acute and/ or chronic therapy.

Deficiency in production of ACTH will result in reduced production of cortisol from the adrenal glands. Cortisol is necessary for maintaining vascular tone and affects bone density, growth, kidney function, the immune system, and behavior and cognition. Secondary adrenal insufficiency from inadequate ACTH production can be life threatening if untreated because of significant electrolyte (particularly sodium and potassium) abnormalities and hypotension. The treatment of choice is hydrocortisone; first, intravenously and then by oral administration. In the acute postoperative period, the patient should receive at least 100 mg/day in order to help address the stress of surgery. Ultimately, most adults take a dose of hydrocortisone of 20–25 mg/day, with most given in the morning to mimic the normal physiology of cortisol release.

Diabetes insipidus (DI) is characterized by decreased release of ADH (ADH, vasopressin) from the posterior pituitary gland, which results in reduced water retention by the kidneys and in urine output that is in excess of the fluid needs of the patient. ADH deficiency leads to DI which is characterized by excessive urination and thirst. DI is occasionally caused by the mass effect of adenomas but is more frequently associated with more invasive tumors that damage the hypothalamus or from pituitary surgery itself. Diagnostic components of DI are provided in Table 25.3.

Patients often present with three phases of DI in the immediately postoperative period. Initially urine output is very high, and treatment includes fluid and electrolyte replacement (carefully following serum electrolyte concentrations) and intravenous infusion of ADH. This is often followed by a period of marked reduction in urine output, and ADH infusion should be stopped. Ultimately, the patient will reach their state of chronic ADH reduction. In this final phase, the patient should be treated with once or twice a day dosing of ddAVP, which can be administered orally or via nasal spray preparation. Dose of ddAVP should be determined after careful assessment of the patient's fluid status and serum electrolyte (particularly sodium) concentration measurements

After the acute postoperative period, clinicians must also carefully assess the need for replacement of other pituitary hormones including thyroid-stimulating hormone (TSH), GH, follicle-stimulating hormone (FSH), luteneizing hormone (LH), prolactin, and oxytocin. It is rare to need to replace any of these hormones in the acute postoperative period. However, left untreated, chronic reduction in TSH may result in significantly reduced metabolism and cause hypothermia, coma, and death.

Complications Secondary to Structural Disruption

In the immediate postoperative period (until the time of hospital discharge), it is important to monitor for the effects of surgery on anatomic structures in the area of surgery. Disruption to the optic chiasm may be diagnosed by loss of peripheral visual fields immediately after emergence from anesthesia. In this situation, radiologic evaluation is necessary to determine if this deficit is due to formation of a hematoma that may require immediate surgical evacuation. More delayed loss of visual fields may occur as a result of edema and require only supportive care.

It is also important to carefully inspect the nasal cavity and lips for evidence of excessive surgical injury. Injury from the exposure may rarely require plastic surgery intervention.

CSF Leak

Although the pituitary gland is outside of the CSF space, it is in close proximity, and surgical intervention may result in dural leak. If a dural injury is observed at the time of surgery (up to 30% of patients), it is common for the surgeon to place a fat graft in the surgical site to promote healing of the disruption. Postoperative CSF leak is diagnosed in up to 6% of patients after evaluation for postoperative rhinorrhea. Since CSF contains glucose but mucus does not, nasal or ear leakage should be tested for glucose. A laboratory glucose value >30 mg/mL identifies CSF. Risk of persistent CSF leak includes meningitis and secondary neurologic injury. Treatment includes reoperation to try to seal the leak or placement of a lumbar subarachnoid drain to reduce the pressure on the surgical tear, to allow for normal healing/scarring.

Key Points

- Airway management is likely to be difficult in patients with excess production of GH. A conservative, awake approach to airway management in these patients is recommended.
- Significant hypertension is anticipated during placement of the Mayfield head-holder and during topicalization of the nasal mucosa with epinephrine and cocaine, which should be treated expectantly.
- Intraoperative treatment with hydrocortisone will prevent the post-operative physiologic consequences of low ACTH levels in the immediate postoperative period. Before extubation, confirm no material or blood clots on the base of the patient's pharynx, in addition to confirm no airway obstruction due to additional edema.
- Treatment of DI in the postoperative period must take into consideration the three phases of this disease in patients immediately following pituitary surgery.
- Postoperative diagnosis of either visual field abnormality or CSF leak requires immediate evaluation and treatment.

Suggested Reading

Ali Z, Prabhakar H, Bithal PK, Dash HH. Bispectral index-guided administration of anesthesia for transsphenoidal resection of pituitary tumors: a comparison of 3 anesthetic techniques. J Neurosurg Anesthesiol. 2009;21:10–5.

Atkinson JL, Young Jr WF, Meyer FB, Davis DH, Nippoldt TB, Erickson D, et al. Sublabial trans-septal vs transnasal combined endoscopic microsurgery in patients with Cushing disease and MRI-depicted microadenomas. Mayo Clin Proc. 2008;83:550–3.

Dinsmore J. Anaesthesia for elective neurosurgery. Br J Anaesth. 2007;99:68–74.

Nemergut EC, Zuo Z. Airway management in patients with pituitary disease: a review of 746 patients. J Neurosurg Anesthesiol. 2006;18:73–7.

Ovassapian A, Doka JC, Romsa DE. Acromegaly-uses of fiberoptic laryngoscopy to avoid tracheostomy. Anesthesiology. 1981;54:429–30.

Schmitt H, Buchfelder M, Radespiel-Tröger M, Fahlbusch R. Difficult intubation in acromegalic patients: incidence and predictability. Anesthesiology. 2000;93:110–4.

The Committee of Brain Tumor Registry of Japan: Report of brain tumor registry of Japan (1969–1993) 10th edition. Neurol Med Chir. 2000;40:1–102.

Chapter 26
Perioperative Challenges During Craniotomy for Space-Occupying Brain Lesions

Chanannait Paisansathan and Verna L. Baughman

Overview

In 2007, primary malignant and benign brain tumors were newly diagnosed in about 51,410 Americans and resulted in 12,740 deaths. The majority of brain tumors are located within the supratentorial compartment. The most commonly reported histology is meningioma, followed by glioblastoma and astrocytoma. Nonprimary brain masses include metastasis lesions from other malignancy origin and brain abscess. Surgery remains the mainstay of treatment. Patients present to the operating room for surgical diagnosis (biopsy) and for curative resection or debunking. Chemotherapy and radiation are used as adjunct therapies, depending on the type of the tumor and location. This chapter focuses on the complications associated with craniotomy for space-occupying lesions during preoperative, intra-operative, and postoperative periods.

Preoperative Complications

Space-occupying lesions (brain tumors and abscess) can cause symptoms related to mass effect, parenchymal infiltration, and tissue destruction. Headache is the most common presenting symptom. When the illness is severe nausea, vomiting or focal neurological deficit, and global suppression of mental status will occur. Seizures happen in 15–95% of patients depending on the type of brain tumor. Commonly, these lesions are accompanied with disruption of blood–brain barrier and edema.

C. Paisansathan, MD
Department of Anesthesiology, University of Illinois at Chicago, Chicago, IL, USA

V.L. Baughman, MD (✉)
Departments of Anesthesiology and Neurosurgery, University of Illinois Medical Center, Chicago, IL, USA
e-mail: VBaughma@uic.edu

A.M. Brambrink and J.R. Kirsch (eds.), *Essentials of Neurosurgical Anesthesia & Critical Care*, DOI 10.1007/978-0-387-09562-2_26, © Springer Science+Business Media, LLC 2012

Cerebral autoregulation is usually impaired in the tumor bed. Hypertension can lead to worsening of brain edema and can cause bleeding. A rapid rise in intracranial pressure (ICP) can exceed brain compensatory mechanism and produce fatal brain herniation.

Premedication

Patients with no evidence of significant increase in ICP will benefit from anxiolytic and/or small dose of narcotics prior to surgery to treat anxiety. Stress can aggravate vasogenic edema and ICP due to an increase in cerebral metabolism and blood flow. However, careful titration is required to avoid hypoventilation, which is associated with hypercapnia and hypoxia. To facilitate anxiolysis, it is best to use drugs that are known to have specific antagonists (e.g., benzodiazepines and opiates), as patients with brain tumors may have an exaggerated sedative effect from even small doses of these agents.

Intraoperative Complications

Induction and Maintenance of Anesthesia

The anesthetic management goals are to avoid a secondary brain insult during surgery, to optimize operating conditions, to permit brain function monitoring and to promote rapid emergence from anesthesia for neurological assessment.

The independent risk factors for brain swelling during craniotomy are $ICP > 13$ mmHg, the degree of midline shift, and tumor histology. The drugs used for induction and maintenance of anesthesia have not been identified as independent risk factors, although there is some suggestion that propofol produces more favorable characteristics in cerebral hemodynamics [ICP, cerebral perfusion pressure (CPP) and arteriovenous oxygen difference ($AVDO_2$)] compared with inhalational anesthesia during nornocapnia to mild hypocapnia ($PaCO_2$ 30–40 mmHg).

Brief hyperventilation ($PaCO_2$ 25–30) is useful to improve surgical working condition by decreasing brain bulk; however, this may be accompanied by a risk of hypoperfusion of injured brain. Mannitol and hypertonic saline in equiosmolar concentration can achieve similar brain relaxation. Serum osmolality should not exceed 320 mOsm/l. However, they produce the opposite electrolyte imbalance. Mannitol (0.25–1 g/kg) causes acute hyponatremia and increases serum potassium due to an intracellular to extracellular shift. Conversely, hypertonic saline causes an increase in blood sodium with acute but transient hypokalemia. Theoretically, both agents can initially increase intravascular volume and cause heart failure or pulmonary edema in patients with poor cardiovascular reserve. The need for osmotic diuresis should be discussed with neurosurgeon when the lesion is small and/or a neuro-navigating system is used.

Location of the lesion is the primary determinant for the use of neurophysiologic monitoring. The common techniques employed with supratentorial lesions are electro-encephalogram (EEG), somatosensory-evoked potentials (SSEPs), electromyography (EMG), and motor-evoked potentials (MEPs). Communication between anesthesiologist, neurophysiologist, and neurosurgeon is essential for successful monitoring to prevent neurological injury from resection. The anesthetic technique and use of muscle paralysis must be planned with these monitoring techniques in mind.

Fast recovery from anesthesia is desirable in neurosurgical patients to diagnose surgical complications such as bleeding, brain swelling, and cerebral ischemia. Ideally, patients should be extubated within 15 min after surgery. There is no clear advantage of IV agents (propofol/narcotics) over inhalation agents (isoflurane, sevoflurane, desflurane). Systemic hypertension often occurs during emergence and may predispose to cerebral edema and/or intracranial bleeding. Coughing and straining on the endotracheal tube must be minimized. Intravenous lidocaine and nonanesthetic agents [e.g., β blockers, α–β blockers and calcium channel blockers] are used successfully to blunt the hemodynamic response during emergence and endotracheal extubation.

Postoperative Complications

The most worrisome complication at the end of surgery is delayed emergence. Patients should be able to perform simple neurological functions such as motor movement, eye opening, and recovery of airway reflex within 10–15 min after termination of the anesthesia. If not, patients should remain intubated and search for nonanesthetic causes such as brain edema, intracerebral hematoma, deep vein occlusion, cerebral ischemia, tension pneumocephalus, seizure and metabolic or electrolyte disturbances. In patients who do not emerge from anesthesia as expected, obtaining an urgent CT scan is helpful for diagnosing intracranial events.

Other complications which can occur in the postoperative period include inadequate pain control, nausea/vomiting, seizure, postoperative wound infection, and pseudoankylosis of the mandible after supratentorial craniotomy.

Prevention

Preoperative Complications Prevention

Patients with evidence of vasogenic edema associated with tumors should receive steroid treatment which reduces peritumor edema and symptoms. Anticonvulsant level should be determined before the craniotomy, if possible, so that an additional dose can be administered if the level is subtherapeutic (phenytoin level goal: total = 10–20 mcg/ml, free = 1–2 mcg/ml). There is conflicting evidence regarding

Table 26.1 Preoperative prevention

Preoperative complication	Prevention
Brain edema	Dexamethasone 4 mg q 6 h
Seizure prophylaxis	Phenytoin
	– Loading dose 15–20 mg/kg
	– Maintenance 300 mg daily
Increase ICP	Avoid hypoventilation
	Avoid large-dose narcotics or benzodiazepines
Gastrointestinal effects	H_2 blocker

the benefit of adding short duration phenytoin treatment to other anti-seizure medication for the prevention of post craniotomy seizures. Patient complaints of headache should be treated with caution. Large dose of narcotics or benzodiazepines might lead to respiratory depression, hypercarbia, and increase ICP. Consider the initiation of H_2 blocker and/or metroclopramide treatment in the preoperative period because increase ICP can decrease gastric emptying and steroid treatment increases gastric acid secretion (Table 26.1).

Intraoperative Complications Prevention

Massive intraoperative blood loss from tumor removal along with the combination of osmotic diuresis can result in hypovolemia and hypotension. Adequate IV access is essential. Consider CVP placement for tumor resection which are located near the venous sinuses due to a risk of venous air embolus, procedures scheduled for longer than 6 h and for vasoactive drug infusion. Invasive arterial blood pressure monitoring is suggested for CPP monitoring and analysis of blood gases, electrolytes, and glucose. Arterial transducer height should be at the level of the Circle of Willis. CPP should be kept >60 mmHg to prevent cerebral ischemia from brain retraction during surgery.

Brain edema and swelling is not desirable. Impeding of cerebral venous drainage can occur after positioning for craniotomy. Inadequate ventilation might lead to hypoxia, hypercarbia, and increased cerebral blood flow. Any factors which contribute to increased cerebral metabolism such as seizure and pain will couple with cerebral blood flow and result in a "tight" brain.

Electrolyte imbalance and hyperglycemia from steroid administration and stress related to craniotomy can occur. Hyperglycemia has been reported to increase morbidity and mortality in critically ill patients and worsen neurological outcome. A single dose of 10 mg dexamethasone given intraoperatively can significantly increase blood glucose in diabetic and nondiabetic patients alike. However, the concept of tight glucose control (80–120 mg/dl) in the neurosurgical patient populations remains controversial (Table 26.2).

Table 26.2 Intraoperative prevention

Complication	Prevention
Intraoperative hemorrhage	• Adequate IV access: 2 large-bore
	• CVP is optional
	• Arterial line
Intraoperative hypotension	• Check volume status
	– Blood loss
	– Overdiuresis
	• Monitor for air embolus
	– Precordial Doppler
	– Transesophageal echocardiogram (TEE)
	– Et CO_2
	• Check for cardiovascular compromise
	– Severe bradycardia or arrhythmia
	– Myocardial ischemia
Increase brain edema and swelling (tight brain)	• Check patient position
	• Seizure
	• Deepen anesthesia
	• Hypoxia
	• Hypercarbia
Electrolyte imbalance (Na^+, K^+ and glucose)	• Monitor electrolytes every 1–2 h
	• Monitor glucose hourly if on insulin infusion
	• Check serum osmolality if using large dose of mannitol/ hypertonic saline or diabetes insipidus suspected

Postoperative Complication Prevention

Brain edema after craniotomy can result in herniation and death. Contributing factors include excessive brain retraction and subtotal resection of malignant tumors, especially glioblastoma. Proper surgical technique to identify venous and arterial structures will minimize complications associate with major vein thrombosis and arterial injury. Smooth emergence from anesthetic is crucial to prevent the disruption of hemostasis at the tumor bed. Postoperative pain should be treated with caution and postoperative nausea and vomiting prophylaxis is recommended for neurosurgical patients (Table 26.3).

Crisis Management

Preoperative Crisis Management

Brain Herniation (Transfalx, Transtentorium, Transmagnum)

Supratentorial brain tumors are often slow growing with the increase in volume compensated by a parallel volume reduction in the blood and CSF compartments (because brain is incompressible). A change in any one of the intracranial compartments, such

Table 26.3 Postoperative prevention

Complication	Prevention
Brain edema	– Avoid excessive brain retraction
	– Avoid excessive IV fluid
Postoperative hematoma	– Smooth emergence (avoid hypertension, coughing, straining)
	– Avoid excessive brain shift
Major vein thrombosis and arterial injury	– Proper surgical technique
Inadequate pain control	– Local anesthetic scalp infiltration
Nausea and vomiting	– PONV prophylaxis
	– Consider adding propofol infusion as part of anesthetic regimen
Postoperative wound infection	– Prophylaxis antibiotic
Ankylosis of the mandible	– Limited jaw opening posttemporal craniotomy, resolves after 3–4 weeks

Table 26.4 Preoperative crisis management

Acute brain herniation treatment in the preoperative period	
Airway	Intubate
	Hyperventilate (acute effect last 6–12 h)
	Keep $PaCO_2 \sim 28$–32 mmHg
	$PaO_2 > 100$ mmHg
	Avoid PEEP
Position	Neutral head position
	Elevate head 15–30°
Hemodynamics	Optimize cerebral perfusion pressure (CPP = MAP-ICP)
	↑MAP ~ 90–100 mmHg if no cerebral hemorrhage
Brain extracellular volume reduction	Diuretics
	• Mannitol
	• Hypertonic saline
	• Furosemide
	Steroids for tumor
	Extraventricular drain (EVD) placement

as hemorrhage into the tumor or an increase in cerebral blood flow (from hypoxia, hypercarbia or seizure), will lead to an exhaustion of compensatory mechanism and an acute rise in ICP with potential for brain herniation. Patients can present with signs and symptoms such as mental status depression, decrease in Glasgow coma score, Cushing triad (hypertension, reflex bradycardia, and abnormal respiratory pattern), new focal neurological deficit, and/or fix/dilated pupils, all of which need immediate intervention to prevent further brain injury or fatal brain herniation (Table 26.4).

Table 26.5 Intraoperative crisis management

Complication	Crisis management
Intraoperative hemorrhage	Blood products available, consider giving clotting factors early if disseminated intravascular coagulopathy is suspected
Intraoperative hypotension	– Blood replacement – Fluid bolus (250–500 cc) – Vasoactive drugs – Keep CPP > 60 mmHg – Watch for over hydration due to risk of cerebral edema
Venous air embolus	– Notify surgeon/flood surgical field – Aspirate air from CVP – Hemodynamic support, vasoactive drugs (phenylephrine, dopamine, epinephrine) – Cardiac resuscitation
Cardiovascular compromise (severe bradycardia, arrythmia)	– Alert surgeon – Treat bradycardia with atropine or epinephrine – Treat ↑ICP if cause cardiovascular compromise
Increase brain edema and swelling(tight brain)	– Elevate head 15–30° – Anticonvulsant therapy – Bolus thiopental or propofol – Consider switching to intravenous anesthesia – ↑FiO_2, avoid PEEP, hyperventilate – Mannitol, furosemide, hypertonic saline
Electrolyte imbalance (Na^+, K^+ and glucose)	– Consider DDAVP if DI is suspected – Replace K^+ if < 3.0 mEq/l – Treat glucose with insulin if > 160 mg/dl

Intraoperative Crisis Management

Blood and volume resuscitation should be readily available in the event of bleeding and hypotension. Monitor for signs of venous air embolus. Hyperventilate, elevate the head, and administer diuretic, narcotic and a bolus of thiopental or propofol if the brain is swelling. Closely monitor electrolytes and glucose intraoperatively (Table 26.5).

Postoperative Crisis Management

Postoperative hematoma after supratentorial craniotomy can occur at the operative site due to incomplete tumor bed hemostasis or with remaining vascular tumor. Remote bleeding such as subdural and/or epidural hematoma and cerebellar hemorrhage has been reported. Major venous thrombosis can produce a delayed hemorrhagic stroke. Arterial injury, on the contrary, produces an immediate neurological deficit. Pneumocephalus is common but tension pneumocephalus is rare in nonsitting craniotomy. Significant intracranial air postcraniotomy can be present even 7 days after surgery. Thus, administering nitrous oxide to a patient with a recent craniotomy (within 3 weeks) is not recommended (Table 26.6).

Table 26.6 Postoperative crisis management

Complication	Crisis management
Brain edema	• Proper head position • Hyperventilation • Steroid, diuretics

Postoperative hematoma	• Treat hypertension [β blocker, vasodilator)
	• Prevent coughing, straining (lidocaine 1.5 mg/kg)
	• Administer neuromuscular reversal agent after removal of head pins
	• Avoid excessive brain shift
	  – Gradually normalize $PaCO_2$
	  – Gently rehydrate to facilitate brain expansion

Major vein thrombosis and arterial injury	• Mannitol (10–20 cc/h of 20% solution) and rehydration may improve the rheologic profile sufficiently to prevent complete venous occlusion
Inadequate pain control	• Titration of long-acting opiates in conjunction with acetaminophen
Nausea and vomiting	• Dexamethasone 4 mg • 5 HT3 antagonist, NK1
Postoperative wound infection	• Antibiotic should be administered within 1 h prior to skin incision (2 h for vancomycin)
Ankylosis of the mandible	• Anticipate subsequent difficult airway • Consider fiberoptic intubation

---

Key Points

- Thorough evaluation for severity of increased ICP, neurologic function, location of a space-occupying lesion, along with patient's medical condition is essential for minimizing neurological injury during surgery.
- The anesthetic goals for craniotomy in patients with space-occupying lesions are for smooth induction, maintenance of adequate CPP, maximization of surgical exposure, maintenance of normal neurophysiological functions and homeostasis (water, electrolyte and glucose) followed by rapid emergence with controlled hemodynamic and minimized coughing and straining during tracheal extubation.

Suggested Reading

Berger MS, Hadjipanayis CG. Surgery of intrinsic cerebral tumors. Neurosurgery. 2007;61(SHC Suppl 1):SHC 279–305.

Bruder NJ, Ravussin PA. Anesthesia for supratentorial tumors. In: Newfield P, Cottrell JE, editors. Handbook of neuroanesthesia. 4th ed. Philadelphia, PA: Lippincott Williams& Wilkins; 2007. p. 111–32.

Burnstein R, Banerjee A. Anesthesia for supratentorial surgery. In: Gupta AK, Gelb AW, editors. Essentials of neuroanesthesia and neurointnsive care. Philadelphia, PA: Saunders Elsevier; 2008. p. 106–10.

CBTRUS. Statistical report: primary brain tumors in the United States, 2000-2004. Hindsdale, IL: Central Brain Tumor Registry of the United States; 2008.

Pasternak JJ, Lanier WL. Neuroanesthesiology review-2007. J Neurosurg Anesthesiol. 2008;20(2):78–104.

Part V
Critical Situations During Anesthesia for Spinal Surgery in Adults

Chapter 27
Perioperative Challenges in Patients with Unstable Spine

Carl Helge Nielsen

Overview

Blunt trauma from high speed motor vehicle accidents, falls from excessive heights, dives into shallow water, and penetrating trauma from gunshot wounds cause the majority of spine lesions; most of these do not involve permanent injury. Spinal cord injury occurs in 12,000–15,000 people per year in the USA; about 10% of these injuries cause permanent damage. Most spinal cord injuries occur in young men between the age of 15 and 25 years. About 5% occur in children.

Nearly 10% of patients with spinal cord injury have a second nonadjacent fracture elsewhere in the spine. Approximately 55% of spine injuries occur in the cervical spine; the remaining 45% are evenly distributed between the thoracic, thoracolumbar, and the lumbosacral regions. Instability of the spine is defined as the loss of the ability of the spine to tolerate physiologic loading without incurring neurologic deficit, pain, or progressive structural deficit. Patients with a suspected spine injury need to be immobilized, and their injuries, including life-threatening lesions, are attended to while movement of the spinal column is kept at a minimum. The immobilization is maintained until a spine injury is excluded.

Prevention

Plans to reduce both the number and the severity of unstable spine injuries are of paramount importance, albeit outside the scope of this text. The primary goal of resuscitation is to protect the spinal cord by reducing additional and secondary injuries.

C.H. Nielsen, MD (✉)
Department of Anesthesiology, Washington University School of Medicine,
St. Louis, MO, USA
e-mail: nielsenc@wustl.edu

A.M. Brambrink and J.R. Kirsch (eds.), *Essentials of Neurosurgical Anesthesia & Critical Care*, DOI 10.1007/978-0-387-09562-2_27,
© Springer Science+Business Media, LLC 2012

267

Thus, basic resuscitation and spine stabilization at all times are crucial. This requires that the anesthesiologist have intimate knowledge about the pathophysiology and the risks and benefits of multiple alternative approaches to both acute trauma care and anesthesia techniques. Spinal immobilization is a priority in multiple trauma; "spinal clearance" is not.

Specific pharmacologic management of patients with acute spinal cord injury in the USA focuses on the benefits of initiation of very high dose steroid therapy within 8 h after the injury. Improved degree and rate of neurologic recovery has been shown by using 30 mg/kg bolus of methylprednisolone over 15 min followed by an infusion of 5.4 mg/kg/h for 23 h. The National Acute Spinal Cord Injury Study (NASCIS) in 1990 showed that high-dose methylprednisolone (30 mg/kg) given within 8 h of ASCI improved neurological function. However, some patients showed no improvement and no patient recovered neurological function completely. This study has resulted in the widespread clinical use of high-dose steroids in ASCI, although controversy persists.

Crisis Management

Pathophysiology and Clinical Presentation

Symptoms from an unstable spine are in a wide range from mild local site pain to quadriplegia and death. They depend both on the severity of the injury and the level of involvement. Instability above the first thoracic spinal segment may show features of upper limb involvement. Above the fourth cervical vertebra, instability may lead to respiratory compromise. Involvement of the conus presents predominantly with bowel and bladder involvement. Patients may additionally present with varying degrees of autonomic dysfunction.

Both experimental and clinical observations of spinal cord injuries have demonstrated a spectrum of pathology that evolves over the days following the injury; this has led to the concept that the injury process is a result of both primary and secondary insults.

Primary mechanism of cord injury can be due to four kinds of mechanical forces:

- Impact with persisting compression; e.g., fractures, dislocations, and disc herniations.
- Impact with no persisting compression; e.g., hyperextension injuries.
- Distraction; e.g., hyperflexion injuries.
- Laceration/transection: Penetrating injuries, fracture dislocation.

Secondary injury mechanisms that may be involved are

- Systemic shock: Profound hypotension and bradycardia (often lasting for days) follows cord injury and may further compromise an already damaged cord.

- Local microcirculatory damage may occur due to mechanical disruption of capillaries, hemorrhage, thrombosis, and loss of autoregulation.
- Biochemical damage may occur due to excitotoxin release (glutamate), free radical production, arachidonic acid release, lipid peroxidation, eicosanoid production, cytokines, and electrolyte shifts.

All these factors (along with edema) lead to loss of energy-producing ability with consequent loss of impulse transmission, cell swelling, membrane lysis, and cell death.

Patient Assessment

Instability must be assumed (and the spine stabilized) in any patient with

- Complaints of a sense of instability (patient holds his head in the hands).
- Vertebral column pain.
- Tenderness over the midline or the spinous processes.
- Neurologic deficit.
- Altered mental status.
- Any suspected spine injury notwithstanding lack of proof.

The initial assessment of patients presenting with trauma is called the primary survey. During this assessment, life-threatening injuries are identified, and, simultaneously, resuscitation is begun. A simple mnemonic, "ABCDE," is used as a memory aid as to the order in which problems should be addressed.

1. Airway maintenance with cervical spine protection
2. Breathing and ventilation
3. Circulation with hemorrhage control
4. Disability (neurologic evaluation)
5. Exposure and environment

When the primary survey is completed, resuscitation efforts are well established, and the vital signs are normalizing, the secondary survey can begin.

The secondary survey is a head-to-toe evaluation of the trauma patient, including a complete history and physical examination, including the reassessment of all vital signs. Each region of the body must be fully examined. X-rays indicated by examination are obtained.

If at any time during the secondary survey the patient deteriorates, another primary survey is carried out, as a potential life threat may be present.

Spinal shock is the term for all the phenomena surrounding physiologic or anatomic transection of the spinal cord that results in temporary loss or depression of all or most spinal reflex activity below the level of the injury. Ditunno et al. proposed a four-phase model for spinal shock (Table 27.1).

Two additional considerations are particularly important to the anesthesiologist in the chronic phase: supersensitivity of cholinergic receptors and autonomic hyperreflexia.

Table 27.1 Phases of spinal shock

Phase	Time	Physical exam finding	Underlying physiological event
1	0–1 Day	Areflexia/hyporeflexia	Loss of descending facilitation
2	1–3 Days	Initial reflex return	Denervation supersensitivity
3	1–4 Weeks	Hyperreflexia (initial)	Axon-supported synapse growth
4	1–12 Months	Hyperreflexia, spasticity	Soma-supported synapse growth

In response to denervation, cholinergic receptors proliferate beyond the end plates of voluntary muscle fibers, eventually to invest the entire cell membrane. The muscle becomes "supersensitive" and contracts maximally in response to a concentration of acetylcholine of only 25% that is needed to initiate contraction in normal muscle. Potassium ion is released suddenly along the entire length of the fiber rather than gradually as the action potential propagates. This produces a rapid rise in serum potassium levels. Succinylcholine induces an identical response and may be associated with a serum potassium increase of 4–10 meq/L. Although succinylcholine is safe during the first day of paraplegia, it should be avoided completely after the third day.

The chronic phase in which spinal reflexes reappear is characterized by autonomic hyperreflexia in a high proportion of patients. Cutaneous, proprioceptive, and visceral stimuli, such as urinary bladder distention, may cause violent muscle spasm and autonomic disturbances. The symptoms of autonomic hyperreflexia are facial tingling, nasal obstruction, and severe headache, shortness of breath, nausea, and blurred vision. The signs are hypertension, bradycardia, dysrhythmias, sweating, cutaneous vasodilatation above and pallor below the level of the spinal injury, and occasionally loss of consciousness and seizures. The precipitous blood pressure increase may lead to retinal, cerebral, or subarachnoid hemorrhage, increased myocardial work and pulmonary edema. Patients with chronic spinal cord lesions above T-6 are particularly at risk for this response: 85% will display autonomic hyperreflexia at some time during the course of daily living. Of course, surgery is a potent stimulus to autonomic response even in patients who give no history of the problem.

Intervention Treatment

The recommendations from Advanced Trauma Life Support are used: Aggressive resuscitation and management of life-threatening injuries, as they are identified, is essential to maximize patient survival.

Assume a cervical spine injury in any patient with multisystem trauma, especially when there is associated altered level of consciousness or a blunt injury above the clavicle. Measures to establish and/or maintain a patent airway must be instituted with cervical spine protection. New neurologic deficits occur 7.5 times more frequently with an unrecognized injury, and up to 10% of patients with a cervical spine injury will suffer a new neurologic deficit if not immobilized.

Pre-hospital care personnel usually have immobilized the patient before transport to the hospital. The patient with an injured spine must be fitted with a semi-rigid cervical collar, placed on a spine board, foam bolsters positioned at each side of the head, and straps used to maintain the neutral position.

Supplemental oxygen is provided. Airway patency may be achieved with simple maneuvers; basic chin lift and jaw thrust maneuvers are applied while force is limited to prevent movement of the immobilized cervical spine. Airway compromise or altered mental status with a Glasgow Coma Scale score 8 or less require endotracheal intubation. There are no clear guidelines for the optimal method to secure the airway in patients with cervical spine injuries, with the exception that that the head and neck must be kept in neutral position throughout the intubation procedure. Numerous approaches and devices to secure an airway in patients with an unstable spine have been suggested and were often presented in small series with high success rates. That said, it is essential that an anesthesiologist master a couple of these alternative approaches in addition to the standard intubation techniques with direct laryngoscopy, fiber optic intubation, and blind nasal intubation. The goal is to facilitate endotracheal intubation without causing further injury to the unstable spine. Intubation while the patient wears the semi-rigid collar and the head is strapped down between the foam blocks is often impossible. The anterior part of the collar and the straps and blocks may be removed as long as head movement is avoided. This is accomplished with manual in-line axial stabilization (MIAS); note that the recommendation has changed *so traction (MIAT) is not recommended*. MIAS is applied by holding the sides of the neck and mastoid processes and exerting a gentle downward (posterior) pressure. During the intubation process the person who provides MIAS must counteract the forces applied by the person who performs the intubation. Rapid sequence induction/intubation with cricoid pressure application should be used whenever indicated. Patients with cervical cord injury should be treated with glycopyrrolate prior to intubation to prevent the bradycardia that often occurs from unopposed parasympathetic stimulation during airway manipulation in these patients. The risk of failed intubation with inability to ventilate the patient must always be considered; it usually necessitates a surgical airway.

The patients with an unstable spine but otherwise stable vital signs who present for urgent or semi-elective procedures are commonly intubated with the use of fiberoptic techniques. Fiberoptic intubation of an awake, minimally sedated patient can often be achieved after adequate topical anesthesia of the airway. This method is preferred because the patient can immediately afterwards follow commands and demonstrate that postintubation movement of the extremities is unchanged from before.

For very anxious patients and for those where movement to command is desired after final positioning on the operation table, fiberoptic facilitated intubation may be preferable while they are under anesthesia. An ultra short anesthetic provides analgesia and will keep the patient appropriately controlled while the intubation and positioning is accomplished, yet it wears off rapidly and the patient can demonstrate movement to command. The extremely unstable patients additionally may have somatosensory evoked potentials monitored both before and after intubation and positioning to document that neither procedure caused noticeable compromise. Team work, cooperation, and collaboration between the anesthesia, monitoring, and surgical teams are essential.

Rapid and accurate assessment of the patient's hemodynamic status is critical. Immediate replenishment of intravascular volume is followed with continued maintenance of an adequate intravascular volume and appropriate blood pressure to assure spinal cord perfusion. Anemia must be avoided. The bladder must be kept decompressed and an NG tube is used to decompress the stomach.

Key Points

- Primary survey with ABCDE while the spine is stabilized
- General management considerations
  - Neurogenic shock
    - (a) Traumatically induced sympathectomy with spinal cord injury
    - (b) Symptoms include bradycardia and hypotension
    - (c) Treatment: Volume resuscitation to maintain systolic BP>90 mmHg (euvolemia)
    - (d) May need phenylephrine (50–300 μg/min) or norepinephrine maintain BP
  - Gastrointestinal tract
    - (a) Ileus is common and requires use of a nasogastric tube
    - (b) Stress ulcer prevention using medical prophylaxis
    - (c) Bowel training includes a schedule of suppositories and maybe initiated within 1 week of injury
  - Deep vein thrombosis
    - (a) Start mechanical prophylaxis immediately
    - (b) Initiate chemical prophylaxis after acute bleeding has stopped
  - Bladder dysfunction
    - (a) Failure to decompress the bladder may lead to autonomic dysreflexia and a hypertensive crisis
    - (b) The bladder is emptied by intermittent or indwelling catheterization
    - (c) Antibiotic prophylaxis for the urinary tract is not advised
  - Decubitus ulcers
    - (a) Skin breakdown begins within 30 min in the immobilized hypotensive patient
    - (b) For prolonged transport, the injured patient must be removed from the hard spine board and placed on a padded litter
    - (c) Frequent turning and padding of prominences and diligence on the part of caretakers are essential to protect the insensate limbs
    - (d) All bony prominences are inspected daily
    - (e) Physical therapy is started early to maintain range of motion in all joints to make seating and perineal care easier

Suggested Reading

American College of Surgeons, editor. Advanced trauma life support student manual. Chicago: American College of Surgeons; 1997.

Deogaonkar M. Spinal cord injuries concepts of surgical management and rehabilitation. http://www.rehabindia.com/spinal-cord-injuries.htm. Accessed January 2009.

Desjardins G. Injuries to the cervical spine. http://www.trauma.org/archive/anaesthesia/cspinean-aes.html. Accessed January 2009.

Grande CM, editor. Textbook of trauma anesthesia and critical care. St. Louis: Mosby; 1993.

Smith C. Cervical spine injury and tracheal intubation: a never ending conflict. Trauma Care. 2000;10:20–6.

Wounds and Injuries of the Spinal Column and Cord. http://www.usaisr.amedd.army.mil/ewsh/Chp20SpinalWounds&Injuries.pdf. Accessed January 2009.

Chapter 28
Airway Crisis Associated with Cervical Spine Surgery

Edward Crosby

Overview

Airway problems encountered in anesthesia for cervical spinal surgery typically cluster into two major categories: the underlying spinal pathology increases the likelihood of *difficult airway* or surgery and prone positioning result in soft tissue swelling and acute *airway compromise postoperatively*. Less commonly, *intra-operative difficulties* arise, typically related to endotracheal tube migration or kinking resulting from surgical positioning.

Surgeries on the cervical spine can be divided into two broad categories, decompressive and stabilizing interventions. Simple decompression of a nerve foramen or discectomy is typically done via an antero-lateral approach with the patient in the supine position. Decompression of the canal itself is more commonly done via a posterior approach with the patient in a prone position, although anterior approaches are used. Stabilization procedures (with instrumentation) may be carried out after decompression to stabilize a spine compromised by the surgical intervention or done primarily to treat a spine rendered unstable by disease or injury. They may involve an anterior or posterior approach (or rarely both); the posterior approach is again carried out with the patient in the prone position.

Preoperative Airway Complications

Patients presenting for cervical surgery have a higher incidence of difficult laryngoscopy and intubation than in a normal population; the likelihood of difficulties increases as movement become more restricted and patients with occipito-atlanto-axial

E. Crosby, MD, FRCPC (✉)
Department of Anaesthesia, University of Ottawa, Ottawa, ON, Canada
e-mail: ecrosby@sympatico.ca

A.M. Brambrink and J.R. Kirsch (eds.), *Essentials of Neurosurgical Anesthesia & Critical Care*, DOI 10.1007/978-0-387-09562-2_28, © Springer Science+Business Media, LLC 2012

Table 28.1 Variables associated with airway complications after spinal surgery

- Rheumatoid arthritis
- Difficult intubation
- Surgical exposure involving > 3 levels
- Surgical exposure involving C2, C3, C4
- Occipito-cervical fusions
- Combined anterior posterior approach
- Blood loss > 300 ml
- Operative time > 5 h

complex disease have the highest prevalence of difficulty. In patients <60 years, limitations in cervical spine movement are associated with an increased likelihood of difficult mask ventilation.

Intraoperative Airway Complications

Intraoperative airway complications are typically related to either migration or kinking of the tube. The head is often flexed on the neck to improve surgical access for posterior operations in the prone position. This shortens the trachea and may result in migration of the tube into a mainstem bronchus. Flexing the head may also force the jaw closed; if the patient has full dentition, this may result in the tube being kinked or crushed by the teeth and an obstructed airway. Compromise of the tube lumen may not be immediately evident and may manifest intraoperatively with increasing airway pressures and difficulty with ventilation.

Postoperative Airway Complications

Airway complications are common after anterior cervical spine surgery and range from acute airway obstruction to chronic vocal cord dysfunction. Variables associated with an increased likelihood of postoperative airway complications are included in Table 28.1. Unilateral vocal cord paralysis resulting from recurrent laryngeal nerve palsy is the most common airway complication after anterior cervical spine surgery; it should rarely result in any important degree of airway compromise.

Airway complications also occur after spine surgery performed in the prone position; these result primarily from supraglottic and laryngeal edema and to a lesser degree from macroglossia. Decreased venous and lymphatic drainage of the head and upper airway is implicated as an etiological factor; prolonged operations and extreme flexed positioning may increase the risk. Patients with rheumatoid arthritis seem particularly susceptible to postoperative edema. A hematoma in the soft tissues of the neck is common after cervical spine surgery but rarely results in clinically important airway compromise. Larger hematoma may result in laryngeal and supraglottic edema, necessitating reintubation of the trachea on an urgent basis.

Prevention

Preoperative Airway Complications

A careful preoperative review will allow for the identification of many patients at risk for difficult intubation. Particularly relevant in the history is the presence of rheumatoid arthritis or ankylosing spondylitis, especially with disease which is longstanding and severe. Previous difficulties with laryngoscopy and intubation are also common in this population and likely predictive of repeat difficulties if the same strategy for airway management is chosen. The airway examination should emphasize evaluation of the usual features, but the Mallampati classification is a particularly useful predictor of difficult laryngoscopy in patients with cervical spine disease; a high score provides evidence of poor cranio-cervical extension and predicts difficulty. Although sophisticated imaging techniques can provide detailed information about the airway, even simple radiographs may be useful. Reduced separation of the posterior elements of the first and second cervical vertebrae on lateral radiographs is associated with difficult laryngoscopy. Once the evaluation is complete, a decision should be made as to whether the evaluation is reassuring regarding the ease of laryngoscopy. In the event that the evaluation is not reassuring, a plan for both intubation and extubation should be formulated which address the non-reassuring elements of the evaluation.

Intraoperative Airway Complications

Endotracheal tubes should be well secured and protected after correct placement has been confirmed. The use of a bite block or oral airway will provide protection to the tube intraoperatively and protect it from being crushed between the teeth; the use of an armored tube alone will not prevent this from occurring. The circuit should be supported so as to reduce the dependent weight acting on the endotracheal tube; this may be done by securing the circuit to the operating table or the apparatus supporting the head.

Postoperative Airway Complications

Extubation is as risky a proposition as intubation in these patients; the airway will be no less difficult to manage than at intubation and will possibly be more so. Consideration should be given to a period of postoperative ventilation to allow the

Table 28.2 An approach to postoperative airway care after cervical spine surgery

- Anticipate postoperative complications in at-risk patients
- Consider postoperative ventilation in high-risk surgical scenarios
- Employ tube exchangers for higher risk extubations
- Observe patients in high-surveillance units postoperatively
- Aggressively evaluate complaints of respiratory distress
- Administer drying agents if respiratory symptoms are present
- Ensure the immediate availability of difficult intubation cart
- Perform or arrange for endoscopic evaluation of the airway if airway symptoms persist
- Maintain a low threshold for airway intervention if symptoms seem progressive
- Arrange for timely notification of surgeon if airway interventions anticipated

swelling to subside, if high-risk characteristics are evident (Table 28.2). If a decision has been made to extubate the trachea of a high-risk patient immediately postoperatively, placement of an airway exchange catheter and a period of observation in a high surveillance unit is the most prudent management strategy. Signs and symptoms of respiratory distress often herald the development of airway edema and should prompt immediate evaluation of the airway. The development of a quiet or muffled voice is an ominous sign and should be dealt with as an airway emergency.

Management of a symptomatic hematoma is controversial. Airway compromise is often a result of supraglottic edema and, although frequently recommended, releasing the staple or suture line to evacuate the hematoma often has little apparent effect on the degree of compromise and the symptoms of distress. Consideration should be given to urgent tracheal intubation to stent the airway open, and, once the airway is secured and protected, a decision may be made regarding subsequent wound management.

Crisis Management

Pathophysiology and Clinical Presentation of Airway Complications

Preoperative Airway Complications

Difficulties with airway management at induction typically result from disease-related anatomical derangements and limitations in safe cervical spinal movement. It may not be possible to safely and optimally position a patient for direct laryngoscopy and an alternate strategy for tracheal intubation is advisable. Intraoperative complications more commonly are technical in nature and related to displacement of the tracheal tube or compromise of its lumen. Ensuring that it is appropriately placed, well secured and protected from kinking will reduce the potential for technical difficulties. A circuit leak should prompt immediate evaluation of tube integrity and placement; a fiberoptic bronchoscope (FOB) is indispensable in this regard. Increasing airway pressures and a concomitant reduction in the ventilation volumes should also trigger evaluation of the tracheal tube in addition to the usual review of the patient and apparatus.

Postoperative Airway Complications

Operative procedures performed upon patients in the prone position predispose to the development of airway edema. Venous drainage of the tongue, face, and airway is via veins which enter the internal jugular vein (IJV); the IJV is liable to kinking when the neck is maximally flexed. This may lead to partial or complete obstruction of the vessel and edema in the tissues drained by this system. Anatomical abnormalities of the skull base may predispose patients to venous obstruction at lesser degrees of flexion; the extreme positioning required to obtain surgical access to the skull base may increase the risk of this complication. Postoperative edema and hematoma formation may be associated with airway compromise through similar mechanisms.

Patient Assessment

Preoperative Airway Complications

Preoperative airway assessment should consist of both a history and physical examination. The occurrence of prior airway difficulties is predictive of recurrent difficulties during the new intervention being planned. Physical examination should review the usual features but a detailed assessment of neck mobility is advised. The Mallampati evaluation may be particularly useful in this population as an assessment of neck movement and predictor of difficult laryngoscopy. Detailed imaging is often available for these patients and should be reviewed. Loss of the gaps between the occiput and posterior arch of C1 and the posterior arches of C1 and C2 are associated with difficult direct laryngoscopy.

Postoperative Airway Complications

Postoperative airway compromise as a result of edema is often subtle in its initial presentation. As well, patient symptoms may be present in the absence of clear signs of hematoma or airway compromise. Complaints of dyspnea and insistence on either semi-recumbent or sitting positions are concerning; these should result in the continued observation of the patient in a high surveillance unit and evaluation of the state of the airway; a FOB facilitates this evaluation. This evaluation may be done with the patient in the sitting position; a nasal approach is useful and well tolerated.

A change in the quality of the voice should prompt immediate airway evaluation and consideration of tracheal intubation. Early administration of drying agents (e.g., glycopyrolate 0.4–0.6 mg IV) may facilitate subsequent airway evaluations and interventions.

Intervention and Treatment

Preoperative Airway Complications

Airway management is not predicted to be difficult in patients presenting for cervical spinal surgery who have reassuring airway assessments and well-preserved spinal mobility. However, patients for whom the assessments are not reassuring require management plans for both intubation and extubation which account for the anticipated difficulties. Awake intubation is more commonly chosen for patients with severe limitations in movement, myelopathy, unstable or fractured spines, and spinal stenosis. The FOB is prominently featured in the management of these patients and may be used in both awake and asleep patients. However, a multitude of devices have been demonstrated to provide safe and effective airway care in these patients, including lighted stylets, rigid fiberoptic endoscopes (e.g., Bullard), the intubating laryngeal mask airway, and fiberoptic stylets and experience rather than dogma should dictate choice.

Postoperative Airway Complications

Patients who present with airway compromise postoperatively require assessment on an urgent basis. Symptoms of airway distress may be out of proportion to observed signs of swelling and edema and should prompt early airway evaluation. If supraglottic or laryngeal edema is present on examination, continued observation in a high surveillance unit is mandatory and consideration should be given to tracheal intubation to protect the airway. Patients may progress to severe degrees of edema and airway compromise before the condition is recognized; it is likely that they will insist on sitting, and both position and agitation may complicate airway interventions. Awake intubation with an FOB may be attempted but will likely be complicated by the degree of airway distortion. If the patient has already suffered a respiratory arrest at the time of intervention, the degree of distortion is likely to be extreme. Surgical establishment of an infraglottic airway may be lifesaving for a patient in extremis. The surgical approach will likely be compromised by swelling in the neck and distortion of the anatomy. An urgent call for both a surgeon and the surgical kit should be made in a timely fashion. If respiratory arrest is imminent or apparent, airway interventions should not be delayed awaiting the arrival of a surgeon. Emergency intervention with the use of a direct laryngoscope and a gum elastic bougie to probe for the tracheal lumen may allow for successful tracheal intubation despite the lack of recognizable anatomy.

Key Points

- Patients presenting for cervical spine surgery have an increased incidence of difficult airway.
- Significant limitations in cervical spine movement are predictive of difficult airway.
- Prolonged or extensive cervical spine surgery and the use of the prone position are associated with postoperative airway compromise.
- Extubation should be considered a high-risk intervention in these patients and planned accordingly.
- The use of an airway exchange catheter should be considered in high-risk extubations.
- At risk patients should be monitored in high surveillance nursing units postoperatively.
- Symptoms of respiratory distress may be out of proportion to observed signs of airway compromise.
- Airway distortion may be severe by the time assessment of symptoms occurs.
- The use of a gum elastic bougie during direct laryngoscopy may be useful in a severely distorted airway.

Suggested Reading

Preoperative Assessment and Management of the Airway

Calder I, Calder J, Crockard HA. Difficult direct laryngoscopy in patients with cervical spine disease. Anaesthesia. 1995;50:756–63.

Manninen PH, Jose GB, Lukitto K, Venkatraghavan L, El Beheiry H. Management of the airway in patients undergoing cervical spine injury. J Neurosurg Anesthesiol. 2007;19:190–4.

Mashour GA, Stallmer ML, Kheterpal S, Shanks A. Predictors of difficult intubation in patients with cervical spine limitations. J Neurosurg Anesthesiol. 2008;20:110–5.

Postoperative Respiratory Complications

Sagi HC, Beutler W, Carroll E, Connolly PJ. Airway complications associated with surgery on the anterior cervical spine. Spine. 2002;27:949–53.

Terao Y, Matsumoto S, Yamashita K, Takada M, Inadomi C, Fukusaki M, et al. Increased incidence of emergency airway management after combined anterior-posterior cervical spine surgery. J Neurosurg Anesthesiol. 2004;16:282–6.

Management of Postoperative Respiratory Complications

Combes X, Dumerat M, Dhonneur G. Emergency gum elastic bougie-assisted tracheal intubation
    in four patients with upper airway distortion. Can J Anesth. 2004;51:1022–4.
Mort TC. Continuous airway access for the difficult extubation: the efficacy of the airway exchange
    catheter. Anesth Analg. 2007;105:1357–62.

Chapter 29
Spinal Cord Injury During Spinal Surgery

Masahiko Kawaguchi

Overview

Perioperative spinal cord injury (SCI) is a devastating complication, and its reported incidence can vary from 0 to 3%, depending on the pathological profiles and surgical approach. Its incidence seems to be especially high after spinal surgery, such as spinal stabilization following trauma or neoplastic disease, or correction of scoliosis. The neuronal/axonal injury can result in motor, sensory, and/or autonomic impairment. In addition to a direct insult to the spinal cord by surgical procedure, anesthesia-related factors can also deteriorate SCI, which is pre- and intraoperatively developed. In order to improve neurological outcome after spinal and spine surgery, prevention, identification, and treatment of SCI is critical. Maintenance of mean arterial pressure (MAP), application of methylpredonisolone, and neuromonitoring, including somatosensory-evoked potential (SEP) and motor-evoked potential (MEP), would be important strategies. However, anesthetic and neuromuscular blocking agents and physiological alterations can affect the results of neuromonitoring, which may interfere with an early detection of pending SCI and consequently delay its treatment. Therefore, proper understanding of its influences on each neuromonitor can be a key for anesthetic managements to reduce the incidence and severity of SCI after spinal surgery.

M. Kawaguchi (✉)
Department of Anesthesiology, Nara Medical University, Kashihara, Nara, Japan
e-mail: drjkawa@naramed-u.ac.jp

A.M. Brambrink and J.R. Kirsch (eds.), *Essentials of Neurosurgical Anesthesia & Critical Care*, DOI 10.1007/978-0-387-09562-2_29,
© Springer Science+Business Media, LLC 2012

Prevention

In the setting of underlying pathological entity of spinal cord at a risk for injury and ischemia (in the setting of underlying pathology of risk of SCI and ischemia), careful anesthetic management is required. Hyperextension of the neck during intubation in patients with severely tight spinal canals and potentially unstable cervical spines should be avoided. Transfer and positioning of the patients should be performed with a careful control of spine. Hypotension should be avoided because it can lead to a decrease of spinal cord perfusion. Vasopressors should be used to maintain the MAP>80 mmHg, although no ideal MAP has been determined. The maintenance of hematocrit may also be required. Although it is still controversial, several authors recommend the use of methylpredonisolone when the spinal cord is at high risk for injury or when surgical insult within the spinal cord is going to be done.

Successful neuromonitoring is one of the most important strategies to prevent permanent SCI. Early recognition of impending SCI can help to identify and promptly reverse the precipitating cause. Types of intraoperative neuromonitor to be used and its technique may vary depending on the pathological profiles, surgical procedures and availability of electrophysiological monitoring staffs and equipments. However, current evidence indicated that MEP is the most valuable tool to monitor functional integrity of descending motor pathways, although it may be combined with SEP and wake-up test. A schema on MEP is described in Fig. 29.1. Spinal MEP can be recorded through epidural electrodes and D-wave is used for

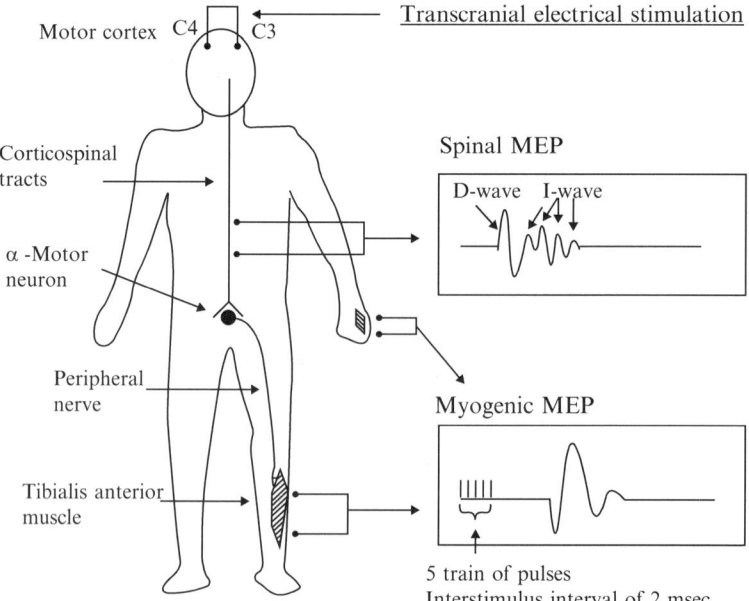

Fig. 29.1 Schema of spinal and myogenic MEPs

monitoring because it is not affected by the anesthetic agents and neuromuscular blocking agents. Myogenic MEP can be recorded from the muscles as compound muscle action potentials (CMAPs). Since the myogenic MEP is very sensitive to suppression by most anesthetic agents, a choice of anesthetic agents should be carefully performed. Intravenous anesthesia using propofol and fentanyl/remifentanil seems to be a good choice to obtain reliable myogenic MEPs. In contrast, inhalational anesthetics suppress MEP amplitude in a dose-dependent manner. Neuromuscular blocking agents should be avoided except for intubation or tightly controlled at a level of 25–50% of twitch height (T1) by a continuous infusion. In patients with preoperative motor deficits, the use of ketamine with minimum influences on myogenic MEP may be considered when a proper control MEP is difficult to obtain under propofol-based anesthesia.

Crisis Management

Pathophysiology and Clinical Presentation

Perioperative SCI involves a direct and indirect physiological insult to the spinal cord. A direct insult may include compression, impaction, laceration, distraction, and ischemia, which can develop during the induction of anesthesia, positioning of patients, and postoperative course, as well as during the surgical procedure. An indirect insult may result from reduction of spinal cord blood flow and oxygen delivery, edema, and inflammation, and may be secondary to a cascade of biochemical and cellular processes initiated by a direct insult. Postoperative causes of SCI include an epidural hematoma and infection, which can initially present with symptoms such as back pain, radicular pain, sensory disturbances, weakness, and paralysis.

Patient Assessment

To recognize the intraoperative development of SCI under general anesthesia, the use of neuromonitoring is critical. Although still debated in detail, examples of the criteria for significant MEP and SEP changes, which signal impending or manifest SCI, are shown in Table 29.1.

Usually myogenic MEP can be reduced or abolished in an early phase of SCI. In such situations, it is important to check whether changes in myogenic MEPs can truly be attributed to ongoing SCI or whether anesthesia-related factors are impairing the signal quality. Before initiating SCI-targeted treatment, other factors that may attenuate myogenic MEPs should be checked. Confounding variables that may affect the recording of myogenic MEPs and their appropriate managements are shown in Table 29.2.

Table 29.1 Criteria for significant MEP and SEP changes

Neuromonitor	Significant changes as an alarm
Myogenic MEP (CMAPs)	A reduction in amplitude to less than 25% of control or the complete lost
Spinal MEP (D-wave)	A reduction in amplitude to less than 50% of control
SEP	A reduction of amplitude to less than 50% of control
	An increase in latency by 10% of control
Wake-up test	Motor weakness or paralysis

Table 29.2 Variables affecting myogenic MEPs

Factors affecting myogenic MEPs	Management
Electrodes failure	Check electrodes
Stimulus parameters	Check stimulus parameters
Anesthetics	Check the depth of anesthesia
	Keep the level of anesthesia constant
	Avoid inhalational anesthetics
	Avoid nitrous oxide >50%
Neuromuscular blockade	Check the level of neuromuscular blockade
	Keep the level of neuromuscular blockade constant
	Avoid the use of neuromuscular blocking agents
Hypothermia	Maintain normothermia
MAP reduction	Maintain MAP >80 mmHg
Reduction of hematocrit (anemia)	Maintain hematocrit >30%

Intervention/Treatment

Once the development of SCI has been recognized by neuromonitoring, prompt and aggressive intervention is warranted. First, the concerns regarding impending or manifest SCI, based on the results of electrophysiological monitoring, should be immediately communicated to the surgeons. If surgical interventions such as particular instruments, screws, or deformity correction can be identified, these causes must be reversed immediately. If MAP is less than 80 mmHg or significantly below the preoperative value, the MAP should be corrected to levels at least above 80 mmHg using vasopressors. If profound perioperative blood loss has resulted in anemia and hypovolemia, means to correct the hematocrit and achieve normovolemia must be initiated. Although still controversial in the context of surgery, methylprednisolone can be considered as soon as possible after the recognition of SCI. The National Acute Spinal Cord Injury Study (NASCIS) trials indicated that high-dose methylprednisolone given within 8 h of SCI was safe and modestly effective in improving motor recovery after the insult.

Key Points

- Hyperextension of the neck during intubation, transfer and positioning of the patients, hypotension, and anemia can be causes of SCI, so that careful anesthetic management is required.
- Electrophysiological monitoring such as MEP and SEP is critical in the detection of SCI during spinal surgery.
- Understanding of the effects of anesthetic agents and physiologic alterations on electrophysiological monitoring is imperative for successful neuromonitoring.
- Maintenance of the MAP >80 mmHg and of the hematocrit > 30% appears important for minimizing the risk of SCI.
- Methylprednisolone can be applied as the prevention in patients with high risk for SCI and once acute SCI has been recognized by neuromonitoring or clinical evaluation.

Suggested Reading

Ahn H, Fehlings MG. Prevention, identification, and treatment of perioperative spinal cord injury. Neurosurg Focus. 2008;25(5):E15.

Bracken MB. Methylprednisolone and acute spinal cord injury: an update of the randomized evidence. Spine. 2001;26(24 Suppl):S47–54.

Deletis V, Sala F. Intraoperative neurophysiological monitoring of the spinal cord during spinal cord and spine surgery: A review focus on the corticospinal tracts. Clin Neurophysiol. 2008;119:248–64.

Langeloo DD, Journee HL, de Kleuver M, Grotenhuis JA. Criteria for transcranial electrical motor evoked potential monitoring during spinal deformity surgery. A review and discussion of the literature. Clin Neurophysiol. 2007;37:431–9.

Chapter 30
Blood Loss During Spinal Surgery

Matthew T.V. Chan and Patricia K.Y. Kan

Overview

Blood loss during surgery of the spine varies enormously. Although the experience of surgeons is often considered as a major determining factor, there are other risk factors that may predict excessive blood loss during surgery (Table 30.1). Intuitively, substantial blood loss is expected in a prolonged multilevel procedure that requires extensive decortication of the vertebrae and stripping of paravertebral muscles for surgical exposure and instrumentation. However, bleeding could be significant even in a single-level laminectomy during revision surgery, surgery for tumor excision, traumatic injury or infective diseases. Bleeding is also more likely in elderly because the vascular channels are wide open due to osteoporosis and the epidural venous plexus are more fragile.

Clearly, the consequences are related to the extent of blood loss and the underlying physiologic condition of the patient. In general, the mechanisms of adverse effects are due to

- Hemodynamic changes associated with fluid shift
- Anemia
- Depletion of platelets and clotting factors resulting in consumptive coagulopathy
- Adverse reactions related to the treatment administered, especially associated with transfusion of blood or blood products (Table 30.2)

In addition, bleeding will obscure operative field, and may have negative impact on surgical outcome. The associated coagulopathy and hyperfibrinolysis may lead

M.T.V. Chan, MBBS, FANZCA, FHKCA, FHKAM (✉)
• P.K.Y. Kan, MBBS, FANZCA, FHKCA, FHKAM
Department of Anaesthesia and Intensive Care, The Prince of Wales Hospital,
The Chinese University of Hong Kong, Shatin, NT, Hong Kong SAR
e-mail: mtvchan@cuhk.edu.hk

A.M. Brambrink and J.R. Kirsch (eds.), *Essentials of Neurosurgical
Anesthesia & Critical Care*, DOI 10.1007/978-0-387-09562-2_30,
© Springer Science+Business Media, LLC 2012

Table 30.1 Risk factors for substantial blood loss after spine surgery

Procedure characteristics	• Surgery for tumor excision
	• Surgery for trauma of the spine
	• Surgery for infection (such as tuberculosis, osteomyelitis)
	• Revision surgery
	• ≥3 vertebral segments fusion
	• Instrumentation
Patient characteristics	• Age > 70 years
	• Obese patients
	• Patients with known clotting defects
	• Children with neuromuscular scoliosis

Table 30.2 Complications associated with transfusion of allogenic blood products

Mechanism	Adverse effects	Incidence per unit blood transfused
Immunologic	*Acute reaction*	
	Urticaria	1:50–100
	Febrile, nonhemolytic transfusion reaction	1:300
	Anaphylaxis	1:150,000
	Acute hemolysis	1:25,000
	Transfusion-related acute lung injury	1:5,000
	Delayed reaction	
	Red cell alloimmunization	1:100
	Immune modulation/suppression	Unknown (extremely rare)
	Delayed hemolysis	Unknown (extremely rare)
	Graft-versus-host disease	Unknown (extremely rare)
Nonimmunologic	*Acute reaction*	
	Hypothermia	1:100
	Hypervolemia	1:200
	Coagulopathy	1:200
	Delayed reaction	
	HIV	1:1,000,000–2,000,000
	HTLV I and II	1:625,000
	Bacterial contamination	1:5,000,000
	Hepatitis C, hepatitis B	1:100,000–2,000,000

to postoperative hematoma, thus, predisposing patients to infection and potentially compressive neurologic injury (e.g., epidural hematoma). Although the causative relationship has not been established, severe blood loss is commonly considered as risk factor for postoperative visual loss following major spine surgery.

Perioperative management should therefore aim to control the source of bleeding and restore hemodynamics to pre-surgical values to ensure tissue perfusion with sufficient delivery of oxygen and nutrients and to enhance hemostasis. However, at the same time, it is important to minimize exposure to allogenic blood and blood products.

Prevention

Minimizing Blood Loss

Preventing hemorrhage during surgery requires communication and close collaboration between the spine surgeons and anesthesiologists throughout the perioperative period. The following strategies may be adopted:

- A detailed preoperative evaluation to identify patients with potential bleeding diathesis. This is particularly important to patients receiving nonsteroidal anti-inflammatory drugs. These agents are known to impair platelet function and are best avoided or switched to selective COX-II blockers during the week prior to surgery. Patients with coronary artery disease and stroke are often taking potent antiplatelet agents, such as aspirin and clopidogrel, either alone or in combination. Although it is clear that these agents prevent major cardiac events in the nonoperative setting, there is uncertainty whether the risk of perioperative bleeding will outweigh the benefits. Similarly, preoperative use of low-molecular-weight heparin and coumadin for the prevention of deep venous thrombosis has to be seriously questioned in patients undergoing surgery at risk of substantial bleeding. The other drugs that should receive equal attention are those "over-the-counter" herbal products and traditional Chinese medicine. Many of them, such as ginkgo and ginseng, are known to affect coagulation and should be discontinued long before (e.g., 2 weeks) surgery. It is also important to ensure patients with known clotting defects actually received the appropriate treatment before surgery (e.g., desmopressin for von Willebrand disease).
- In patients with vascular tumors, one should consider prophylactic embolization prior to invasive surgery.
- Where feasible, minimally invasive spine surgery should be considered. Compared with conventional open procedure, minimally invasive surgery avoids disruption of surrounding tissue and therefore minimizes approach-related bleeding.
- In the operating room, patient must be carefully positioned to avoid impediment of venous drainage and subsequent engorgement of epidural veins.
- Acute normovolemic hemodilution (ANH) may decrease total loss of hemoglobin during surgery. In this technique, blood is removed (down to a hematocrit value of 20–30%) using appropriate blood collection bags, and circulating volume is restored with crystalloids or colloids at the beginning of surgery (prior to an anticipated episode of bleeding). The blood is then appropriately stored during surgery. The blood collected is returned to the patient as physiologically needed during surgery or after hemostasis is achieved. Therefore, only diluted blood with lower hematocrit is being lost during surgery. Additional advantages of ANH are that it uses patient's own blood and that the clotting factors and platelets (often absent from autologous blood) in it will improve hemostasis.
- Controlled hypotension, aiming to reduce systolic arterial pressure between 60 and 80 mmHg, has been advocated to decrease intraoperative blood loss.

However, both controlled hypotension and ANH are contraindicated in patients with significant cardiac morbidity. Unfortunately, activity of spine patients is often limited because of pain and deformity. It is therefore difficult to predict the individual who may not be able to tolerate these maneuvers. Given the prevalence of coronary artery and cerebrovascular disease in the general population and the emerging cases of postoperative visual loss after spine surgery (see Chap. 32), the risk of controlled hypotension and ANH should not be overlooked.

- Meticulous hemostasis is always required to decrease blood loss. Locally applied vasoconstrictors, bone wax, fibrin sealants, and hemostatic collagen and cellulose are commonly used for control of bleeding. Hemostasis may also be enhanced with administration of hemostatic drugs. Table 30.3 summarizes the clinical uses, mechanisms of action and potential side effects of these agents. In the literature, prophylactic use of tranexamic acid, aprotinin or recombinant activated factor VII (rFVIIa) significantly decreases blood loss and the need for allogenic blood transfusion. However, they also increase the risk of thromboembolism, especially in patients with proven history or at risk of atherosclerosis or thrombosis. Aprotinin also increases the risk of other serious side effects, such as heart failure, renal failure, acute coronary syndrome, and stroke. Because of these adverse reactions, aprotinin is currently withdrawn from the market, and is only restricted to investigational use under a limited user agreement. The efficacy data on epsilon-aminocaproic acid (EACA) and desmopressin are, however, less consistent, owing to the small number of patients in the trials. Desmopressin is a specific treatment for von Willebrand disease and mild hemophilia A. Other than this, there is no evidence that desmopressin will decrease blood loss or rate of transfusion after spinal surgery. Currently, tranexamic acid and rFVIIa should only be given to patients when massive hemorrhage is anticipated.

Minimizing Allogenic Blood Transfusion

Despite the best attempt to reduce intraoperative blood loss, a substantial proportion of patients undergoing complex spine surgery will require blood transfusion. The following techniques have been advocated to minimize the potential risk of allogenic transfusion (Table 30.2).

- There is ample evidence to suggest that preoperative anemia predicts perioperative blood transfusion. It is important to identify and correct nutrient deficiency with supplemental iron, vitamin B, and folate therapy. Preoperative recombinant human erythropoietin (rHuEPO) administration (weekly subcutaneous injection 40,000 IU for 3 weeks) elevates hemoglobin and, thus, reduces allogenic transfusion. Thromboembolism and red cell aplasia (due to the development of autoantibodies) are the potential adverse effects of rHuEPO. Fortunately, these events are uncommon.
- Liberal transfusion should be avoided. Current evidence suggested that a hemoglobin concentration above 8 g/dl has little effect on perioperative morbidity.

Table 30.3 Clinical uses and mechanisms of action of hemostatic agents

Drug	Dosage	Mechanism of action	Side effects	Results of clinical investigations
Tranexamic acid	Loading dose 10 mg/kg during induction of anesthesia Maintenance dose 1–2 mg/kg/h	Lysine analogue that inhibits the binding of plasmin to fibrin	Thromboembolism Seizure at high doses (e.g. >100 mg/kg)	Study results support its prophylactic use
Epsilon-aminocaproic acid (EACA)	Loading dose 150 mg/kg during induction of anesthesia Maintenance dose 10–15 mg/kg/h	As above	Thromboembolism	Mixed results, most studies do not support its use
Aprotinin	Loading dose 1–2 × 10⁶ KIU during induction of anesthesia Maintenance dose 0.25–0.5 × 10⁶ KIU/h	Direct inhibition of plasmin, kallikrein, trypsin, and factor XIIa	Renal failure, coronary ischemia, cerebrovascular thromboembolism	Aprotinin has been withdrawn recently due to an increase in adverse events
Desmopressin (deamino-8-D-arginine-vasopressin, DDAVP)	Slow infusion 0.3 µg/kg over 30 min	Release of von Willebrand factor	Possible increase in myocardial infarction	Useful in specific disease (Type 1 von Willebrand disease and mild hemophilia A), may be effective in chronic renal failure
Recombinant activated factor VII (rFVIIa)	30–120 µg/kg every 2 h for three doses	Binds with subendothelial tissue factor that in the exposed vessel wall. The binding complexes subsequently generate thrombin that in turn facilitate conversion of fibrinogen to fibrin	Thromboembolism	Approved for the treatment of bleeding in patients with hemophilia. Limited data on its use for prophylaxis and treatment of bleeding during surgery

However, the actual decision of transfusion should also consider cardiac and cerebrovascular status of the patient and the rate of active bleeding.

- In preoperative autologous donation programs, patients donate several units of blood before surgery. During and after surgery, patients received their own stored blood when clinically indicated. The major drawback of this technique is that it only applies to elective surgery when procedures are planned weeks ahead. It should also be clear that the risk of clerical error, bacterial contamination and complications associated with stored blood are not modified as compared with autologous blood transfusion.
- Perioperative red cell salvage involves collection of blood shed during surgery and reinfused to the patients following appropriate filtering and treatment. The technique could be applied to emergency surgery and has been shown to reduce allogenic transfusion, but the effect is small. Although somewhat controversial, most authors warn against using perioperative red cell salvage in surgery for infective or malignant disease because of concern that this would result in systemic dissemination of the infection or cancer.
- Hemoglobin-based oxygen carrier solution (e.g., hemopure) is an attractive option to minimize allogenic transfusion. Currently these products are developed from stabilized human or animal hemoglobin. Although most clinical studies have demonstrated the efficacy of the blood substitute, recent reports on the increased incidences of deaths and myocardial infarction casts doubt on the future development of these agents.

Crisis Management

The cardinal signs for acute hemorrhage during spine surgery are hypotension, tachycardia, and oliguria (Table 30.4). Given its nonspecific nature, a number of events may mimic acute hemorrhage. Table 30.5 summarizes the potential differential diagnoses, patient assessment, and management of major blood loss during spine surgery. While it is easy to identify sudden massive hemorrhage, insidious concealed bleeding may be difficult to recognize. The treatment priority is to control the source of bleeding and then to replace blood volume, hemoglobin, and clotting factors.

Hypothermia, electrolyte abnormalities (particularly calcium), acidosis and coagulation factor deficiency must be seriously considered and treated when large amount of blood has been transfused (e.g., greater than 5 units of red cells). Table 30.6 shows the causes, assessment, and treatment for the adverse events associated with massive transfusion.

In the most uncommon event when hemolytic reaction is suspect during blood transfusion, an outline of treatment is listed in Table 30.7.

Table 30.4 Classes of the American College of Surgeons for acute hemorrhage

	Class I	Class II	Class III	Class IV
Blood loss				
Volume	≤750	750–1,500	1,500–2,000	≥2,000
Percent of total blood volume	≤15%	15–30%	31–40%	≥40%
Arterial pressure[a]	Normal	Normal	Decreased	Decreased
Pulse pressure	Normal/increased	Decreased	Decreased	Decreased
Pulse rate (beats/min)	>100	>100	>120	≥140
Urine output (ml/h)	>30	20–30	5–10	Negligible

[a]Pulse pressure = systolic–diastolic arterial pressure

Table 30.5 Patients with acute intraoperative bleeding

Differential diagnoses	Assessment	Treatment/intervention
• Inadvertent overdose of anesthetic and/or vasodilator therapy • Pulmonary embolism • Other forms of obstructive shock (e.g., pneumothorax, cardiac temponade) • Anaphylaxis (including transfusion reaction) • Always consider bleeding from other sites, especially in patients with multiple trauma (e.g., ruptured spleen)	• Confirm the vital signs • Exclude other causes of hemodynamic disturbances • Estimate blood loss (blood in suction bottle, surgical sponges, under the drape and on the floor, see Table 30.4) • Check hemoglobin concentration • Check coagulation status (both clinical – oozing from the wound and laboratory parameters – platelet count, activated partial thromboplastin time, prothrombin time, fibrinogen and thromboelastography) • Check responses to therapy (including plasma electrolytes and arterial blood gas)	• Communicate with the surgeons of the problem, and severity of blood loss • Ensure adequate vascular access if not already secured • Communicate with blood bank for adequate supply of blood and component therapy • Avoid hypertension to facilitate surgical control of bleeding (consider wound packing while preparing for transfusion or establishing equipments for cell salvage) • Restore blood volume and maintain perfusion pressure with vasopressors as soon as hemostasis is achieved • Reverse prior anticoagulation therapy (e.g., protamine for prophylactic heparin administration) • Start transfusion when hemoglobin concentration <8 g/dl and there is evidence of ongoing bleeding • Prevent and promptly treat the complications associated with massive transfusion (acidosis, hypothermia, and coagulopathy)

Table 30.6 Complications associated with massive transfusion

Complications	Causes/consequences/assessment	Treatment/intervention
• Hypothermia	• Heat loss due to exposure to refrigerated blood and cold operating room environment • Decrease clotting factor activity by 10%/°C decrease in core temperature • Depressed myocardial contractility when core temperature is <32°C	• Use only warmed fluids, blood, and blood products • Apply forced air warming devices, heated blankets
Electrolyte disorders		
• Hyperkalemia	• Infusion of aged stored blood in large amount • Tissue hypoperfusion • Tall peaked T wave when plasma potassium concentration>6 mmol/l	• Stop potassium containing solution • Administer dextrose 50%, 100 ml with actrapid 10 units *ivi* • Calcium gluconate 10%, 10 ml *ivi*
• Hypocalcemia	• Consequence of citrate toxicity when large amount of blood is infused (>1 unit every 10 min) • Prolonged QT interval	• Calcium gluconate 10%, 10 ml *ivi*

• Metabolic acidosis	• Tissue hypoperfusion
	• Hyperchloremic acidosis as a result of excessive saline infusion
		• Fluid resuscitation and vasopressor therapy is required to improve tissue perfusion
		• Temporary measures included:
		  – Hyperventilation to maintain arterial carbon dioxide tension between 28 and 30 mmHg
		  – Sodium bicarbonate 8.4%, 50–100 ml infusion *ivi* to maintain pH>7.2

• Coagulopathy	• Dilutional coagulopathy and hyperfibrinolysis	• Administer fresh frozen plasma 10 ml/kg, platelet concentrates 10 ml/kg, cryoprecipitate 10 units when PT>1.5, platelet count <50×10⁹/l and fibrinogen concentration <1 g/l, respectively • Consider other hemostatic agents (see Table 30.3; e.g., Tranexamic acid 10 mg/kg; rFVIIa 90 μg/kg)

Table 30.7 Treatment for acute hemolytic reaction after blood transfusion

Causes	Assessments	Treatment/intervention

• Infected blood transfusion
• Transfusion-related acute lung injury
• Mismatched (incompatible) blood transfusion
	• Many of the signs are concealed during general anesthesia, but the following should raise the possibility of hemolytic reactions:
	  – Hypotension, tachycardia
	  – Bronchospasm, urticaria
	  – Bleeding diathesis
	  – Hemoglobinuria due to an elevated plasma-free hemoglobin
		• Stop transfusion
		• Maintain arterial pressure and intravascular volume with fluid and vasopressor
		• Treat bronchospasm with bronchodilator
		• Maintain urine output with mannitol 20%, 0.5 g/kg over 10–30 min, furosemide 10–20 mg *iv* if urine output remains unsatisfactory.
		• Force alkaline diuresis with sodium bicarbonate 8.4%, 50–100 ml infusion
		• Avoid further transfusion, if feasible
		• Check hemoglobin concentration and coagulation status, correct clotting defects promptly
		• Return unused blood and send blood samples from the patients to the laboratory for further investigations

Key Points

- Detailed preoperative preparation to identify patients at risk of massive hemorrhage during spine surgery; correct anemia and stop medications and supplements that may impair coagulation.
- In patients at high risk of massive bleeding during surgery, preoperative autologous donation should be considered.
- During surgery, hypertension should be avoided. ANH is safe down to a hematocrit value of 30%. Lower hematocrit or controlled hypotension is considered risky in patients with known or at risk of coronary artery disease.
- Tranexamic acid may be used prophylactically to decrease blood loss. When bleeding becomes massive, consider giving rFVIIa.
- During an episode of massive bleeding, the treatment priority is to control the source of bleeding. When bleeding slows down, blood volume and hemodynamic stability should be restored
- During massive transfusion, hypothermia, acidosis and coagulopathy must be treated promptly.

Suggested Reading

Bormanis J. Development of a massive transfusion protocol. Transfus Apher Sci. 2008;38:57–63.

Klein HG, Spahn DR, Carson JL. Red blood cell transfusion in clinical practice. Lancet. 2008;370:415–26.

Mannucci PM, Levi M. Prevention and treatment of major blood loss. N Engl J Med. 2007;356:2301–11.

Mirza SK, Deyo RA, Heagerty PJ, Konodi MA, Lee LA, Turner JA, et al. Development of an index to characterize the "invasiveness" of spine surgery: validation by comparison to blood loss and operative time. Spine. 2008;33:2651–61.

Muñoz M, García-Erce JA, Villar I, Thomas D. Blood conservation strategies in major orthopaedic surgery: efficacy, safety and European regulations. Vox Sang. 2009;96:1–13.

Chapter 31
Coagulopathy in Spinal Surgery

Andrew H. Milby, Casey H. Halpern, and James M. Schuster

Overview

More than 500,000 spinal operations are performed annually in the USA. Unanticipated coagulopathy during spine surgery is fortunately not a common occurrence. However, substantial blood loss is certainly possible, given the increasing complexity of spine surgery, longer durations of surgery, the size of incisions, instrumentation near large vascular structures, as well as vascular spinal metastatic lesions. Significant intraoperative coagulopathy, defined as recurrent microvascular bleeding despite electrocautery and/or suture or decreased clot formation of blood pooled within the surgical field, has been reported in up to 16% of patients undergoing major spinal surgery. This bleeding can result in serious consequences including early termination of the procedure, postoperative hematoma formation, and increased in-hospital mortality. Therefore, it is imperative to identify risk factors for coagulopathy during preoperative assessment and take appropriate preventative action (Table 31.1).

While congenital bleeding disorders cannot be overlooked, those with severe manifestations are likely to be detected prior to adulthood. As the vast majority of patients will have undergone routine preoperative evaluation of PT, aPTT, and platelet count, coagulopathy during spinal surgery is generally due to some preexisting platelet dysfunction (i.e., known or unidentified use of platelet inhibitors) or an acquired problem with coagulation during the surgery such as dilutional coagulopathy.

A.H. Milby, BS
Department of Orthopaedic Surgery, University of Pennsylvania School of Medicine, Philadelphia, PA, USA

C.H. Halpern, MD (✉)
Department of Neurosurgery, Hospital of the University of Pennsylvania, Philadelphia, PA, USA
e-mail: Casey.Halpern@uphs.upenn.edu

J.M. Schuster, MD, PhD
Department of Neurosurgery, University of Pennsylvania School of Medicine, Philadelphia, PA, USA

A.M. Brambrink and J.R. Kirsch (eds.), *Essentials of Neurosurgical Anesthesia & Critical Care*, DOI 10.1007/978-0-387-09562-2_31,
© Springer Science+Business Media, LLC 2012

Table 31.1 Risk factors and prevention strategies for coagulopathy in spine surgery

Risk factor	Prevention strategy
Common preexisting pharmacotherapy	Aspirin/NSAIDs/Plavix: discontinuation 5–7 days prior to surgery
Blood loss and fluid/blood product replacement	"Goal-directed" resuscitation (see text), use of colloid-containing fluids
Operative time and/or hypothermia	Fluid warmers, humidifiers, hot air blankets, serum calcium levels

Other comorbid conditions with systemic impacts on coagulation may include hepatic or renal failure and malignancy. In addition, there is evidence to suggest that spinal diseases, such as idiopathic scoliosis, may be associated with intrinsic platelet dysfunction.

An acquired problem with coagulation during surgery, such as a dilutional coagulopathy, can contribute to significant bleeding. Blood loss in large instrumented spine cases or resections of vascular spinal metastases can approach the patient's estimated blood volume. This loss is typically replaced with a combination of crystalloid, colloid, intraoperative autotransfused blood, allogenic blood and blood products. Continuing crystalloid administration without appropriate replacement of clotting factors and/or platelets can lead to severe coagulopathy over the course of long procedures. Coagulation factors typically remain functional down to concentrations approximately one-third of normal. However, this threshold is reached upon replacement of an entire blood volume. Of note, though coagulopathy may occur secondary to dilution of either coagulation factors or platelets, there is evidence suggesting that coagulation factor dilution and disturbed fibrin polymerization are of greater concern than thrombocytopenia.

It is extremely important to prevent hypothermia, especially in the setting of a concurrent acidosis, as both factors are strongly associated with coagulopathy. Other severe but uncommon causes of coagulopathy include allergic and immunologic reactions (e.g., transfusion, drug reaction), or disseminated intravascular coagulation (DIC). DIC is of particular concern in patients with multiple traumatic injuries, especially severe head injury, and in patients with widespread metastases. During spine surgery, exposed bone may act as a source of tissue plasminogen activator and urokinase which may lead to activation of the fibrinolytic system and subsequent DIC.

Possible platelet dysfunction as a cause of coagulopathy is often difficult to assess preoperatively and is even more difficult to assess intraoperatively. Platelet aggregation studies and bleeding times have variable predictive value preoperatively and are not useful in the intraoperative setting. Assessment of surgical bleeding by measuring the viscoelastic properties of whole blood by techniques such as thromboelastography (TEG) have not been well described other than in cardiac and liver transplant surgery, though they have potential for application in spine surgery. This technique measures the entire clotting process from fibrin formation to fibrinolysis. Because whole blood is used, the plasmatic coagulation system interacts with platelets and red cells, providing useful information on platelet function at the patient's temperature. However, there is a difference between in vitro and in vivo coagulation as viscoelastic coagulation tests measure coagulation under static conditions (no flow) in a cuvette (not an endothelialized blood vessel).

A certain percentage of coagulopathy cannot be anticipated or avoided. Significant intraoperative bleeding mandates rapid assessment and treatment. This requires close communication between the anesthesia and surgery teams, including the decision to "pack things off" and delay or abort further surgery for resuscitation as necessary.

Prevention

A complete review and reassessment, including obtaining a past medical history, current and recent medication use, family history, surgical and anesthesia history, is essential to avoid intraoperative bleeding difficulties. Excessive bruising and/or unusual bleeding with attempts at intravenous or arterial access may suggest the possibility of clotting difficulties. Baseline studies typically include coagulation labs (PT/INR, aPTT), hemoglobin (Hb) levels, and platelet count. Bleeding times and other studies of platelet aggregation are of questionable utility in the preoperative setting. There must also be direct discussion between the surgical and anesthetic team prior to beginning complex cases, as the consent or booking description may not completely convey the complexity, length, or potential for blood loss. This discussion will help determine the need for large bore vascular access, arterial line monitoring, blood products, and/or cell-saver. Consideration should also be given to staging procedures, especially if anterior and posterior approaches are planned.

Intraoperative fluid replacement strategies are highly controversial. Restrictive, "goal-directed" fluid administration has been increasingly advocated as a means to prevent dilutional coagulopathy, as opposed to a solely formula-based approach. Suggested parameters include a rate of 4 mL/kg/h, with additional goal-directed boluses of 250 mL (up to a total of 1,500 mL) given for periods of hypotension and tachycardia and for urine output dropping below 0.5 mL/kg/h for 2 or more hours. Vasopressors and/or furosemide may be used in patients not responding to these boluses. There is controversy regarding the value of administering fluids as colloid or crystalloid. Concerns exist over an increased risk of coagulopathy with the use of hetastarch in normal saline. Regardless of the fluid replacement strategy employed, the use of warming devices and the exclusive infusion of warmed fluids are recommended to maintain normothermia in long cases.

Further measures can be taken preoperatively and intraoperatively to help minimize the risk of significant blood loss. When positioning a patient prone, it is important to avoid abdominal compression that may cause engorgement of epidural veins, potentially exacerbating blood loss and contributing to a coagulopathy. It is advisable to have patients with vascular spinal metastases such as renal cell carcinoma undergo preoperative embolization to potentially reduce intraoperative blood loss. In these patients it is our practice to place the pedicle screws and pre-contoured rods before attempting tumor resection. This is done in case massive bleeding requires premature termination of the case. With large incisions it is also important to control local bleeding in portions of the incision not immediately being addressed to avoid continuous blood loss. The use of vasopressor agents during surgery for the purpose of maintaining cord perfusion in cases of spinal cord compression, for example, may mask reduced intravascular volume. Indirect measures of adequate perfusion such as urine output and possibly lactate levels should be assessed. Regular reassessment of hemoglobin levels is advised, as a loss of RBC mass may have adverse effects on coagulation due to altered blood rheology. Periodic monitoring of electrolytes may also be necessary, as coagulopathy can occur in the setting of electrolyte derangements. Of these, hypocalcemia is of particular concern given the complex interactions between ionized calcium and the negatively charged Vitamin K-dependent clotting factors. Hypocalcemia may also be worsened by volume replacement with colloid solutions or infusion of citrated blood products.

Crisis Management

Once an intraoperative bleeding issue is identified, it is imperative that there is rapid assessment and treatment (Table 31.2). This requires close communication between the anesthesia and surgical teams.

Pathophysiology and Clinical Presentation

Rapid blood loss can be both the cause and result of coagulopathy. Intraoperative emergencies such as laceration of a large artery or vein can be life threatening and require immediate packing and vascular repair. Rapid blood loss can lead to hypotension and possibly DIC. Blood loss with vascular spinal lesions such as renal cell metastasis can be substantial despite preoperative embolization. Nevertheless, aggressive fluid resuscitation can cause a dilutional coagulopathy. Strong consideration should be given to aborting the originally intended procedure even if the injury is rapidly repaired and the patient is physiologically stable.

The development of excessive bleeding in complex cases can also be a gradual process with the development of recurrent microvascular bleeding. Sometimes, this is a subjective response by the surgical teams that comes with experience as "things just seem oozy." Well-established communication between anesthesia and surgery teams will allow early identification and intervention in such circumstances. New-onset bleeding in previously hemostatic areas is most frequently dilutional in nature. Paradoxically, this is may be more likely to occur in cases where large-volume resuscitation has been required following rapid bleeding from other etiologies, such as a vascular injury. In these situations it is often advisable to stop and reassess before continuing.

General anesthesia masks symptoms of end-organ dysfunction, and many signs (hypotension, tachycardia, oliguria/hemoglobinuria) may be wrongly explained by

Table 31.2 Diagnostic and therapeutic approach to intraoperative coagulopathy during spine surgery

Initial presentation	Potential etiology	Assessment	Treatment response
Mildly increased microvascular bleeding from case onset (esp. in emergent cases)	Preexisting use of platelet-inhibitor or anticoagulant medication	Clinical impression	– Platelet transfusion regardless of platelet count – FFP administration if anticoagulation with warfarin suspected
Gradual-onset microvascular bleeding in previously hemostatic areas	Dilutional coagulopathy	PT/INR	– FFP administration (cryoprecipitate if additional volume undesirable and/or fibrinogen < 80–100)
		aPTT	– Platelet transfusion if < 50,000/μL
		Hemoglobin (Hb) Platelet count Fibrinogen	
Severe bleeding and/or evidence of end-organ dysfunction (changes in vital signs, urine output)	Hypoperfusion with or without DIC	(Above), plus: ABG	(Above), plus: – Correction of acidosis, hypothermia, electrolyte abnormalities
		Lactate	– RBC transfusion if Hb < 10 g/dL[a]
		D-dimer	– Consider termination of procedure to allow for stabilization of patient – Consider administration of rFVIIa if unstable and refractory to above measures

[a]Higher Hb than typical transfusion threshold may be necessary to restore clotting function during ongoing bleeding

other causes. DIC should be suspected at the first potential sign of end-organ dysfunction, as clinically apparent bleeding is a late manifestation that occurs only after consumption of coagulation factors. While exceedingly rare, consideration must also be given to the possibility of a transfusion reaction in all patients receiving blood products.

Patient Assessment

Any response to an intraoperative bleeding crisis must begin with an airway, breathing, and circulation assessment. Sites of intravenous or arterial access should be examined for evidence of new-onset bleeding and extremities examined for possible signs of ischemia or thrombosis. There should also be a simultaneous assessment of patient's intake and output balance, especially with regard to estimated blood loss and volume replacement. Initial laboratory evaluation should include Hb level, platelet count, and coagulation labs (PT/INR, aPTT). While PT and aPTT may often be mildly abnormal, values in excess of 1.5 times controls are most sensitive for clinically evident coagulopathy.

Periods of hypoperfusion or hypotension (i.e., patient requiring pressor agents to maintain blood pressure) should prompt an immediate blood gas to check for acidosis. Lactate levels may be useful in the assessment of systemic hypoperfusion, as lactic acidosis can preclude the restoration of normal coagulation. Additional laboratory evaluation may require levels of lactate dehydrogenase (LDH), fibrinogen, and fibrin split-products (D-dimer) to evaluate for hemolysis or DIC. While elevations are nonspecific, a D-dimer within normal limits along with a normal platelet count renders DIC highly unlikely. An adequate concentration of fibrinogen is critical for clot formation. Concern for a transfusion reaction should prompt retesting and cross-matching of blood samples for major incompatibility.

Intervention/Treatment

Treatment decisions must be based on the extent and etiology of coagulopathy. Temporary suspension of surgical activity is advised in order to achieve adequate hemostasis and resuscitation before proceeding with the operation.

All homeostatic parameters affecting coagulation must be addressed. Buffering to physiologic pH is required at a pH less than 7.1 or a base deficit of 12.5. Optimal Hb for restoration of coagulation is higher than the one required for oxygen delivery, and transfusion to values of 10–11 g/dL may be necessary to support platelet function. Aggressive warming must also be pursued for core temperatures less than 34°C.

Administration of fresh frozen plasma (FFP) is indicated for active bleeding following massive blood transfusion (more than one blood volume). The extent of PT and/or aPTT elevations may be used to guide coagulation factor replacement, as they have been found to positively correlate with volumes of FFP required to maintain hemostasis. Cryoprecipitate or packed factor concentrates may be used, when available, if additional volume is undesirable, or at fibrinogen concentrations less than 80–100 mg/dL. Platelets are often given prophylactically with normal counts even without documented coagulopathy on the presumption of altered platelet function; however, consideration must be given to the added expense, infectious risk, and risk of developing antibodies which could affect future transfusions.

Recombinant factor VIIa (rVIIa) has been increasingly applied in military and civilian trauma resuscitation, but systematic indications and dosing remain highly controversial. One clinical trial of rVIIa in spine surgery has shown its efficacy and safety in reducing blood loss and number of transfusions, but there are only case reports of its use in response to coagulopathic crisis situations. Thus, there is insufficient evidence to define the role of rVIIa in spine surgery, though its use may be considered in the "rescue" treatment of highly refractory coagulopathy.

Termination of the procedure to allow for optimal medical management of the coagulopathy is a complex decision that must be made in collaboration between the surgeon and the anesthesiologist. Factors to be considered include the patient's overall medical condition, acuity of the condition for which the patient is undergoing surgery, anticipated length of remaining procedure, response to treatment thus far, and availability of critical care services in the immediate postoperative period. This decision will be highly individualized to the clinical scenario, and requires communication between both teams to arrive at the best decision for the overall health and safety of the patient.

Key Points

- Preoperative clinical and laboratory assessment, as well as close communication between the surgical and anesthetic teams, are essential to avoiding coagulation difficulties, as well as dealing with them effectively when they arise.
- Early recognition of intraoperative bleeding difficulties should prompt a simultaneous and systematic evaluation and initiation of therapy and may require either temporarily or permanently stopping the surgical procedure to allow re-establishment of physiologic homeostasis.

Suggested Reading

Drews RE. Critical issues in hematology: anemia, thrombocytopenia, coagulopathy, and blood product transfusions in critically ill patients. Clin Chest Med. 2003;24:607–22.

Lier H, Krep H, Schroeder S, et al. Preconditions of hemostasis in trauma: a review. The influence of acidosis, hypocalcemia, anemia, and hypothermia on functional hemostasis in trauma. J Trauma. 2008;65:951–60.

Ornstein E, Berko R. Anesthesia techniques in complex spine surgery. Neurosurg Clin N Am. 2006;17:191–203, v.

Practice guidelines for blood component therapy: a report by the American Society of Anesthesiologists Task Force on Blood Component Therapy. Anesthesiology. 1996;84:732–47.

Shen Y, Silverstein JC, Roth S. In-hospital complications and mortality after elective spinal fusion surgery in the United States: a study of the nationwide inpatient sample from 2001 to 2005. J Neurosurg Anesthesiol. 2009;21:21–30.

Chapter 32
Postoperative Visual Loss Following Spinal Surgery

Lorri Lee

Overview

Incidence and Epidemiology

Postoperative visual loss (POVL) is a catastrophic perioperative complication that has come to the forefront of anesthesiologists' attention in the last 10–15 years. The extent of visual loss from POVL can be minimal unilateral visual field loss loss to complete blindness in both eyes. The incidence of symptomatic POVL varies from 0 to 4.5% depending on the institution and the type of cases studied. The highest reported incidence of symptomatic visual loss is 4.5% in cardiac cases and 0.2% in spine surgery. The most common types of surgical procedures associated with POVL include prone spine surgery, cardiopulmonary bypass procedures, head and neck procedures, and major vascular procedures. Radical prostatectomy is emerging as a new high-risk procedure for ischemic optic neuropathy (ION), particularly with the robotic prostatectomies that utilize an exaggerated steep Trendelenburg position. A wide variety of miscellaneous procedures have been associated with POVL including cholecystectomy, liposuction, supine spine surgery, nephrectomy, thoracotomy, and many others. Moreover, visual loss is known to occur in the critically ill in the absence of any surgical procedure, and it can affect any age of patient. Given this heterogeneous group of procedures and patients, it is not surprising that there are many different ophthalmologic diagnoses possible with POVL (Table 32.1) and many different suspected etiologies, most of which remain unproven (Table 32.2). The most common ophthalmologic diagnoses associated with POVL are central retinal artery occlusion (CRAO), cortical blindness, and anterior and posterior ischemic optic neuropathy (AION, PION).

L. Lee, MD (✉)
Department of Anesthesiology and Pain Medicine, University of Washington School of
Medicine, Seattle, WA, USA
e-mail: lorlee@u.washington.edu

A.M. Brambrink and J.R. Kirsch (eds.), *Essentials of Neurosurgical
Anesthesia & Critical Care*, DOI 10.1007/978-0-387-09562-2_32,
© Springer Science+Business Media, LLC 2012

Table 32.1 Postoperative visual loss (POVL) diagnoses and associated procedures/events

Ophthalmologic diagnosis	Associated procedures/events
Central retinal artery occlusion (CRAO)	Prone spine surgery, nasal and sinus procedures, cardiac bypass
Cortical blindness	Cardiac bypass, profound circulatory shock, emboli, major vascular surgery
Anterior ischemic optic neuropathy (AION)	Cardiac bypass, prone spine surgery, major vascular procedures, radical prostatectomy, abdominal compartment syndrome, liposuction, bilateral radical neck dissection
Posterior ischemic optic neuropathy (PION)	Prone spine surgery, bilateral radical neck dissection, cardiac bypass, nasal and sinus procedures
Acute angle closure glaucoma	Stress – no associated anesthetic technique or surgical procedure many suggested drugs utilized in the perioperative period
Retrobulbar hemorrhage	Nasal or sinus procedures

There is significant overlap in the procedures and the type of POVL. This table represents the most commonly associated procedures with each POVL diagnosis, respectively

Table 32.2 Suggested associated factors with most common types of postoperative visual loss (POVL)

Ophthalmologic diagnosis	Suggested associated factor (most common)
Central retinal artery occlusion (CRAO)	Globe compression, emboli
Cortical blindness	Emboli, profound hypotension, cerebral artery thrombosis
Anterior ischemic optic neuropathy (AION)	Hypotension, anemia, atherosclerosis, major blood loss, large fluid resuscitation, high-dose vasopressors, patient-specific anatomic/physiologic aberrancies
Posterior ischemic optic neuropathy (PION)	Venous congestion/elevated venous pressure, prolonged duration in prone position, major blood loss, large fluid resuscitation, hypotension, anemia, high dose vasopressors, patient-specific anatomic/physiologic aberrancies

Etiology

Each type of POVL can be associated with more than one etiology. Globe compression with periorbital trauma is the most common cause of perioperative CRAO, though embolic causation is also possible. Cortical blindness can be caused by either emboli or profound circulatory shock. (Table 32.2).

The etiologies of AION and PION remain unknown and may be multifactorial with both intrinsic and extrinsic risk factors. AION is more commonly associated with patients with atherosclerotic risk factors and their related surgical procedures in the supine position (e.g., cardiac bypass surgery and major vascular surgery). PION is more commonly associated with procedures with elevated venous pressure (e.g., prone position, bilateral radical head and neck surgery) and frequently occurs in relatively healthy patients. However, there is significant crossover with diagnoses, patient populations, and suggested risk factors.

The relatively low incidence of ION (both AION and PION) suggests that the patients themselves may have some unique anatomical or physiologic differences that promote its development. A small cup to disk ratio on fundoscopic exam has been described as an anatomic risk factor for spontaneously occurring AION. Many ophthalmologists believe that the small cup to disk ratio correlates with a narrow passage for the optic nerve and vessels as they pass through the semi-rigid sieve-like connective tissue (lamina cribrosa) on the way to the retina. Any swelling in this area in these individuals would impede flow through the blood vessels supplying the optic nerve. A recently published case–control study (Holy S et al. 2009) of perioperative ION did not demonstrate a small cup to disk ratio as a risk factor, but this study was limited by a small number of affected cases from a wide range of different surgical procedures and a mixture of both AION and PION diagnoses. Pillunat demonstrated that 20% of healthy volunteers have a reduced ability to autoregulate blood flow in the anterior optic nerve with an intraocular pressure of 25 mmHg – a value typically reached during prolonged prone spine surgery. Other studies in humans suggest that the ophthalmic artery may behave extracranially with respect to carbon dioxide reactivity and its ability to reverse flow with tight carotid stenoses. Because of the location and size of the optic nerve and its vasculature, definitive studies in humans regarding autoregulation, vasoreactivity, and the effect of various physiologic perturbations on optic nerve blood flow are not technically feasible at this time.

Atherosclerotic-related diseases have been associated with spontaneously occurring AION. However, certain high-risk surgical procedures such as cardiopulmonary bypass and major vascular procedures have concomitant coexisting atherosclerotic disease, making it unclear whether the atherosclerosis is contributory to the ION complication or not in these cases. In contrast, the American Society of Anesthesiologists (ASA) Postoperative Visual Loss Registry demonstrated that two-thirds of 83 patients with ION after spine surgery were relatively healthy (ASA Physical Status I–II). Perioperative ION after spine surgery has also been reported in 10–16-year-old children. These findings suggest that ION after spine surgery is more likely associated with prolonged physiologic perturbations in the prone position, rather than an atherosclerotic-induced disease. Anesthetic duration was ≥6 h in 94% of the ASA POVL Registry cases and estimated blood loss was ≥1,000 ml in 82% of cases. Animal studies indicate that the optic nerve is more sensitive to physiologic perturbations than the brain. Clinically, perioperative ION rarely occurs in association with cerebral infarction. Unfortunately, there is no reliable intraoperative monitor of optic nerve function to guide therapeutic interventions at this time.

Currently there are four case–control studies on POVL. Two of these studies with detailed data collection failed to demonstrate any association with POVL and lowest blood pressure or lowest hematocrit, though numerous case reports and case series frequently speculate that these two factors are causative. These studies were limited by either cases with different ophthalmologic diagnoses or by cases from multiple different types of surgical procedures. The remaining two studies utilized the nationwide Inpatient Sample to examine POVL associated with spine surgery. Patil's study on spinal fusion surgery found an association between ION and hypotension (OR 10.1), peripheral vascular disease (OR 6.3), and anemia (OR 5.3). Without detailed data consistently available from cases and controls, it is unclear that how hypotension and anemia were defined in this study and when it occurred in the perioperative course. Accuracy of data cannot be validated. Further, the Nationwide Inpatient Sample database is maintained for administrative purposes and cannot be used for comparison of non-routinely collected data between cases and controls. For example, the presence of perioperative hypotension is not routinely evaluated unless there is a complication. Therefore, the control group (without complication) is unlikely to have hypotension diagnosed. Roth's study ultilizing the same database for all procedures examined variables found more consistently in cases and controls. They found a significant multivariable association between ION and male sex, age > 50 years old, non-fusion orthopedic surgery, spinal fusion surgery, and cardiac surgery. The lack of detailed perioperative data such as operative duration, blood loss, and type of fluid administered prevented assessment of potential confounding factors.

Other suggested, but unproven, risk factors are use of high-dose vasopressors and excessive administration of crystalloid fluid replacement. It is unclear if these findings differ from patients with similar procedures.

Prevention

Given the short list of known etiologies and the relatively long list of suspected but unproven etiologies (Table 32.2), prevention of POVL is somewhat limited and speculative (Table 32.3). The POVL diagnosis most easily prevented is CRAO caused by globe compression. This complication is most commonly associated with prone spine operations and can be prevented by frequent checking of the eyes to ensure that they are free from direct pressure. Although all headrests have been associated with CRAO, devices that have a narrow margin between the eyes and the headrest edge (e.g., horseshoe headrest) may make checking of the eyes problem-

Table 32.3 Prevention of postoperative visual loss (POVL)

Ophthalmologic diagnosis	Preventative measures	Suggested (unproven) preventative measures
CRAO	1. Frequent eye checks 2. Avoid headrests with narrow margin between eyes and headrest	
Cortical blindness	1. Devices or maneuvers that reduce emboli 2. Avoid extreme hypotension	
AION and PION	Unknown	1. Avoid prolonged duration in the prone position with major blood loss 2. Use of colloid along with crystalloid 3. Keep the head at or above the heart level to minimize venous congestion

Table 32.4 The American Society of Anesthesiologists Practice Advisory for perioperative blindness associated with spine surgery[a]

For patients undergoing major spine surgery:
1. Consider consenting patients undergoing major spine surgery for the risk of POVL
2. Continually monitor blood pressure
3. Keep head at or above the heart level
4. Use colloids along with crystalloids for volume replacement
5. Consider staging procedure
Transfusion threshold and the use of deliberate hypotension have not been shown to be associated with postoperative visual loss

[a]Note that the Practice Advisory does not advocate the use of deliberate hypotension or extreme anemia, but did not find evidence that these factors were causative for postoperative blindness. Because of the low incidence of postoperative visual loss after spine surgery, prospective clinical trials are not currently feasible. With the lack of class I evidence, this Practice Advisory was based primarily on expert opinion, case reports, case report series, and one case–control study "(American Society of Anesthesiologists Task Force on Perioperative Blindness, Anesthesiology 2006)

atic. Emboli caused by cardiopulmonary bypass may be decreased with the use of special filters and epiaortic scanning but are not completely eliminated. Emboli from major orthopedic procedures are not currently preventable.

Other preventative measures are speculative as the etiology is unclear. Conditions which promote extreme physiologic stress (e.g., prone position, deliberate hypotension, severe anemia, etc.) for prolonged periods should be assessed with careful consideration of the risk to benefit profile, as their effect on optic nerve blood flow remains undetermined.

In the absence of class I evidence, the ASA has developed an advisory for the prevention of blindness associated with major spine surgery (Table 32.4), based on expert opinion, case reports, case series, and one case–control study. Briefly, it recommends to consider consenting patients for the risk of POVL, continually monitor blood pressure use of colloids along with crystalloids for fluid replacement, maintaining the head equal to or higher than the heart, and consider staging very prolonged procedures.

Crisis Management

Pathophysiology and Clinical Presentation (Table 32.5)

CRAO is most commonly associated with physical compression of the globe and typically has ipsilateral signs of periorbital trauma. In the absence of periorbital trauma, embolic causation is a possibility as CRAO can also occur spontaneously in the community in individuals who are hypercoagulable. The most common type of operation associated with CRAO is prone spine surgery, and specific head support devices that leave little room between the eyes and the headrest support margin (e.g., horseshoe headrest) may predispose to this injury. A complaint of visual loss is typically immediate on awakening from anesthesia. It is almost always unilateral and without a pupillary

Table 32.5 Patient findings for postoperative visual loss diagnoses

Diagnosis	Symptom onset	# Affected eyes	Pupillary light reflex	Visual fields	Visual acuity	Fundus	Diagnostic tests	Recovery
CRAO	Immediate	Unilateral (usually signs of ipsilateral periorbital trauma)	Absent in affected eye	Absent in affected eye	Usually blind in affected eye	Cherry red spot at macula; ischemic retina; attenuated retinal arteries	Fundoscopic exam alone is diagnostic; ERG and VEP abnormal (flattened)	Poor
Cortical blindness	Immediate	Bilateral	Normal	Usually absent; may have hemianopsia	Usually blind; may be normal in unaffected area with hemianopsia	Normal	CT, MRI to evaluate infarct; VEP abnormal (flattened); ERG normal	Good (~2/3 patients get good recovery)
AION	Immediate to several days postoperatively – can be progressive over several days	Usually bilateral; can be unilateral	RAPD or absent	Altitudinal field cut or scotoma; may be blind	Usually decreased to blind; may be normal in unaffected area	*Early exam*: edema/swelling of the optic disk, peripapillary flame-shaped hemorrhages; *late exam*: optic nerve pallor after several weeks to months	VEP abnormal (flattened); ERG normal	Poor
PION	Immediate	Usually bilateral; can be unilateral	RAPD or absent	Altitudinal field cut or scotoma; may be blind	Usually decreased to blind; may be normal in unaffected area	*Early exam*: normal; *late exam*: optic nerve pallor after several weeks to months	VEP abnormal (flattened); ERG normal	Poor

CRAO central retinal artery occlusion, *AION* anterior ischemic optic neuropathy, *PION* posterior ischemic optic neuropathy, *RAPD* relative afferent pupillary defect, *ERG* electroretinogram, *VEP* visual evoked potential, *CT* computed tomography, *MRI* magnetic resonance imaging

Findings noted above are for typical presentations of postoperative visual loss. An ophthalmology consultation is an essential component of the diagnostic workup where rarer causes of postoperative visual loss or those cases with atypical presentations can be evaluated

light reflex. It has a fundoscopic finding of a cherry red spot at the macula. This cherry red spot represents an island of well-perfused blood supply to the macula from the choriocapillaris, made prominent by the surrounding pale, ischemic retina that is devoid of blood supply from the central retinal artery. It may occur in association with AION, whose optic nerve pallor may not manifest until months later. There is no known beneficial treatment for CRAO, and recovery of vision is typically poor.

Cortical blindness is typically associated with emboli (air or particulate) or severe physiologic derangements. The most common procedure associated with the release of large numbers of emboli is cardiopulmonary bypass, but major orthopedic procedures such as femoral nailing and spinal fusion with instrumentation are also known to release large embolic loads. Because the retina has high blood flow, it serves as a repository for emboli that can be easily detected if emboli are suspected on the arterial side. Profound hypotension, as seen in cardiopulmonary resuscitation, has also been associated with cortical blindness. Patients will typically have bilateral involvement with a normal light reflex and fundoscopic exam. Recovery from cortical blindness is much better than either CRAO or ION with some significant improvement reported in approximately two-thirds of cases.

ION that occurs perioperatively is typically nonarteritic and consists of two types, AION and PION. Arteritic AION (e.g., temporal arteritis) almost never arises perioperatively. Patients most commonly complain of visual loss from PION immediately upon awakening or when they are first cognizant and able to communicate. It does not typically worsen from the time of the initial complaint. In contrast AION can present either immediately on awakening or up to several days postoperatively. It can have a more progressive onset and may worsen over the course of several days. Both AION and PION have an abnormal light reflex with either a relative afferent pupillary defect or absent light reflex. For ION cases with incomplete visual loss, there is either an altitudinal field cut and/or scotoma in one or both eyes, while visual acuity may be relatively normal in the unaffected portion of the visual field. Two-thirds of the ASA POVL Registry patients with ION had bilateral involvement, consistent with the theory that this injury is caused by systemic physiologic perturbations. The fundoscopic exam in PION is completely normal, whereas AION will demonstrate optic disk edema with or without peripapillary flame-shaped hemorrhages. The edema in AION eventually resolves and the peripheral heme gets absorbed. AION and PION are identical several months after the onset with only optic disk pallor. Recovery from perioperative ION is very poor. Some patients may get some mild improvement in vision but rarely return to baseline.

Patient Assessment

For any complaint of visual loss, consultation with the ophthalmology service should be obtained as soon as possible, preferably by a neuro-ophthalmologist if available. The ophthalmologic diagnosis is primarily based on physical exam, pupillary light reflexes, and dilated fundoscopic findings. It may be helpful in eliminating specific etiologies. Acute angle closure glaucoma is a very rare cause of POVL. It is typically painful, but this finding may be blunted with residual anesthesia and narcotics. It can be ruled out by the measurement of the intraocular pressures and is easily treatable with a lateral canthotomy. It is less common than the other four types of ophthalmologic diagnoses perioperatively, but is the only complication that has a defined and effective treatment. Computed tomography or magnetic resonance imaging (MRI) is frequently used to eliminate the possibility of cortical infarction or other intracranial pathology. Small punctuate lesions on these studies are consistent with embolic events. Larger strokes in watershed areas from hypoperfusion may also be detectable for cases with profound circulatory shock.

Diagnosis of CRAO can be made by the cherry red spot on fundoscopic exam. Electroretinograms (ERGs) in the presence of CRAO will be highly abnormal but are superfluous in the presence of an absent pupillary light reflex and a cherry red spot. ERGs will be normal in the presence of ION and cortical blindness, as the retina maintains normal function. Visual evoked potentials will be abnormal in CRAO, ION, and cortical blindness. Definitive diagnosis of ION can be made several months later with the appearance of a pale optic disk though the ability to distinguish AION from PION will be lost.

Intervention/Treatment

Because the incidence of each of these causes of POVL is low, randomized trials with proven benefit are lacking. Further, there is no proven effective treatment for the spontaneously occurring forms of CRAO or ION. Experimental selective thrombolysis for spontaneous CRAO has had mixed results. Case reports of hyperbaric oxygen therapy, mannitol, and steroids have also had inconsistent results. Normalization of the blood pressure and transfusion to a hematocrit of 30% or more is frequently recommended by consultants and also lacks proven efficacy.

Key Points

- POVL can occur after a wide variety of surgical procedures but is most commonly associated with prone spine surgery, cardiac bypass surgery, and head and neck operations.
- The most common POVL diagnoses are CRAO, cortical blindness, AION, and PION.
- CRAO is most commonly caused by pressure on the globe, and this cause of CRAO is preventable with frequent eye checks.
- The etiologies of AION and PION are unknown but are associated with operations and positions that impart significant physiologic perturbations for prolonged durations. Patient specific risk factors may also contribute to this complication.
- Consent for POVL should be considered for high-risk procedures.

Suggested Reading

American Society of Anesthesiologists Task Force on Perioperative Blindness. Practice advisory for perioperative visual loss associated with spine surgery. A report by the American Society of Anesthesiologists Task Force on Perioperative Blindness. Anesthesiology. 2006;104: 1319–28.

Holy SE, Tsai JH, McAllister RK, Smith KH. Perioperative ischemic optic neuropathy: a case control analysis of 126,666 surgical procedures at a single institution. Anesthesiology. 2009;110:246–53.

Lee LA, Nathens AB, Sires BS, McMurray MK, Lam AM. Blindness in the ICU: possible role for vasopressors? Anesth Analg. 2005;100:192–5.

Lee LA, Roth S, Posner KL, Cheney FW, Caplan RA, Newman NJ, et al. The American Society of Anesthesiologists' Postoperative Visual Loss Registry: analysis of 93 spine surgery cases with postoperative visual loss. Anesthesiology. 2006;105:652–9.

Lee LA, Deem S, Glenny R, Townsend I, Moulding J, An D, et al. The effects of anemia and hypotension on porcine optic nerve blood flow and oxygen delivery. Anesthesiology. 2008;108: 864–72.

Myers MA, Hamilton SR, Bogosian AJ, Smith CH, Wagner TA. Visual loss as a complication of spine surgery: a review of 37 cases. Spine. 1997;22:1325–9.

Patil CJ, Lad EM, Lad SP, Ho C, Boakye M. Visual loss after spine surgery: a population based study. Spine. 2008;33:1491–6.

Roth S. Postoperative blindness, Anesthesia, 6th edition. Edited by Miller RD. New York, Elsevier/ Churchill Livingstone 2005:2991–3020.

Shen Y, Drum M, Roth S. The prevalence of perioperative visual loss in the United States: a 10-year study from 1996 to 2005 of spinal, orthopedic, cardiac, and general surgery. Anesth Analg 2009;109:1534–45.

Part VI
Critical Situations During Anesthesia for Other Procedures Directly Affecting the Central Nervous System

Chapter 33
Perioperative Challenges During Diagnostic and Perioperative Magnetic Resonance Imaging (MRI)

Peter A. Farling and Richard C. Corry

Overview

The majority of patients with a neurological condition will undergo magnetic resonance (MR) imaging at some stage of their clinical management. MR imaging is non-invasive, but the patient is required to lie motionless in a narrow noisy tunnel with the body part to be imaged encased in a receiver coil. Therefore, several patient groups will require the services of the anaesthesia team (Table 33.1).

Anaesthetists may not be familiar with terminology used in MR so terms in *italics* are defined in the glossary at the end of this chapter. This chapter focuses on two main areas:

- The risks of MR procedures
- Crisis management in anaesthesia for MR.

The Risks of MR Procedures

MR images are produced when body tissues, in response to strong physical forces, emit energy depending on their different chemical make-up and water content. The timing and amount of emitted energy are detected and mapped by measuring coils within the scanner and the data is then processed to generate high-resolution, detailed images. The strong physical processes required are:

P.A. Farling, MB, BCh, FRCA (✉)
Department of Anaesthesia, Royal Victoria Hospital, Belfast, UK
e-mail: peter.farling@dnet.co.uk

R.C. Corry, MB, ChB, FRCA
Department of Anaesthesia, Royal Victoria Hospital, Belfast, UK

A.M. Brambrink and J.R. Kirsch (eds.), *Essentials of Neurosurgical Anesthesia & Critical Care*, DOI 10.1007/978-0-387-09562-2_33,
© Springer Science+Business Media, LLC 2012

- An intense **static magnetic field** – generated by superconductor magnets that are cooled by liquid helium.
- Pulses of **radiofrequency (RF) energy** – generated by a power delivery unit.
- Application of superimposed **gradient magnetic fields** for spatial encoding.

Each of these forces has the potential for patient injury.

Static Magnetic Field Hazards

The static magnetic field in MR systems is the most important hazard because it poses a constant invisible danger as the magnet remains switched on at all times. The major risks of the static magnetic field are:

- Pacemaker malfunction.
- Projectile effect.
- Implant dislodgement.
- Medical equipment malfunction.

Magnetic field strength is measured in units of *Tesla* (T) or *Gauss* (G). (1 T = 1,000 mT = 10,000 G). The magnetic field strength of the MR system is maximal at the bore of the magnet, with the field strength of most modern scanners in clinical use being between 1 and 3 T (10,000–30,000 G). This field strength reduces exponentially with increasing distance from the magnet, so the danger posed by the magnetic field increases as one moves closer to the magnet (Fig. 33.1).

Cardiac pacemakers may malfunction and fail within magnetic fields above 5 G (0.5 mT). For this reason, a safety line at a level of 5 G is usually specified and access for unscreened personnel is restricted. The area within this boundary is termed the *controlled area*. The magnetic field strength within the MR scanning room, containing the magnet, is obviously much higher and is called the *inner controlled area*. Pacemakers that are *MR conditional* have been developed. The radiographer and radiologist should ascertain the safety of medical implants and a number of databases are available (see http://www.mrisafety.com; Table 33.2; Fig. 33.2).

Hazards from RF Pulses and Gradient Magnetic Fields

During MR imaging, pulses of RF energy and *gradient magnetic fields* are superimposed on the strong static magnetic field for the generation of spatial images. The additional risks are summarised in Table 33.3.

Table 33.1 Patients requiring anaesthesia or sedation for MR Imaging
- Children
- Patients with learning difficulties
- Claustrophobic adults
- Patients with movement disorders
- Patients in which positioning is difficult, for example, severe back pain or sciatic nerve root irritation
- Intensive care patients

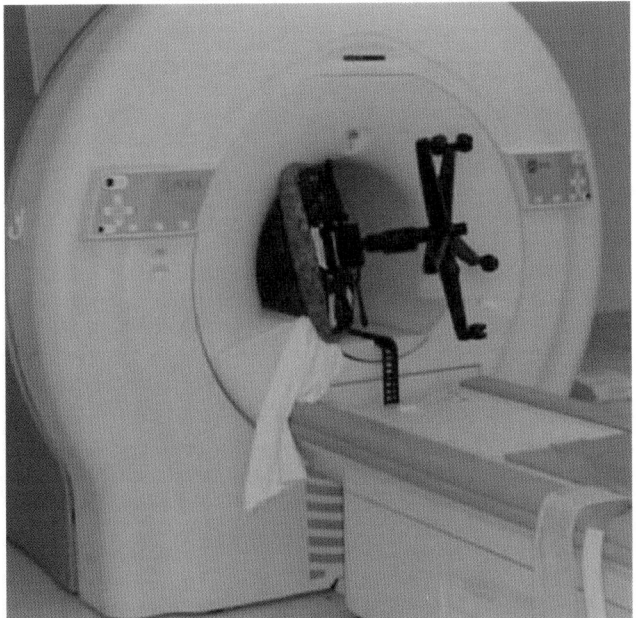

Fig. 33.1 Non-MR conditional chair attracted to magnet

Table 33.2 Risks of the intense static magnetic field in MR anaesthesia

Risk	Precaution
Projectile or "missile" effect	
• Ferromagnetic objects in the *inner controlled area* are attracted by the strong magnetic field and rendered projectile. Collisions can result in injury and death to patient and staff, as well as potential for damage to the scanner	• Access to the *controlled area* is restricted and all persons must be medically screened before admission
• Ferromagnetic objects include many pieces of essential anaesthetic equipment, e.g., laryngoscopes, gas cylinders, defibrillators, pulse oximeters	• A dedicated area adjacent to the magnet room and outside the strong magnetic field is provided for anaesthesia
• There are several case reports of both death and severe injury from the missile effect. For example, a small child died during MR imaging when struck by a projectile oxygen cylinder	• Only non-ferromagnetic (*MR safe* or *MR Conditional*) equipment is permitted within the *inner controlled area*, e.g., fibre-optic pulse oximeter, aluminium gas cylinders
	• In emergency, resuscitation equipment must not enter the *inner controlled area*; the patient should be immediately removed from the magnet room for treatment
Pacemaker malfunction	
• Pacemakers malfunction within the *controlled area*, where magnetic field strength exceeds 5 G, with reported fatalities	• A robust screening procedure is required to identify and prohibit persons with pacemakers and defibrillators entering the *controlled area*

(continued)

Table 33.2 (continued)

Risk	Precaution
Implant dislodgement	
• Ferromagnetic objects implanted in the patient may dislodge with potential for devastating internal injury	• A robust screening procedure is essential. Ferromagnetic implants are a contra-indication to MR procedures
• Medical implants include aneurysm clips, stents, prosthetic heart valves, internal defibrillators, intrauterine contraceptive devices and cochlear implants	• Non-ferromagnetic implants are safe e.g., general surgical clips, many joint prostheses, artificial heart valves and sternal wires
• Metal shrapnel and intra-ocular foreign bodies from welding or penetrating eye injury	• Radiographer checks database, e.g., http://www.mrisafety.com
	• Access to the *controlled area* is denied in the event of any uncertainty
Equipment malfunction	
• Standard equipment may malfunction within the strong magnetic field with potential harm from device failure, dysfunction or MR image distortion. A malfunctioning infusion device could result in incorrect drug delivery	• Standard equipment should only be used outside the strong magnetic field
	• Only equipment designated *MR safe* or *MR conditional* is safe to use within the *inner controlled area*
Teratogenicity	
• The long-term effects of strong magnetic fields on the developing foetus are unknown	• MR imaging should be deferred until after the first trimester whenever possible
	• Female staff of childbearing age should be aware of potential teratogenicity

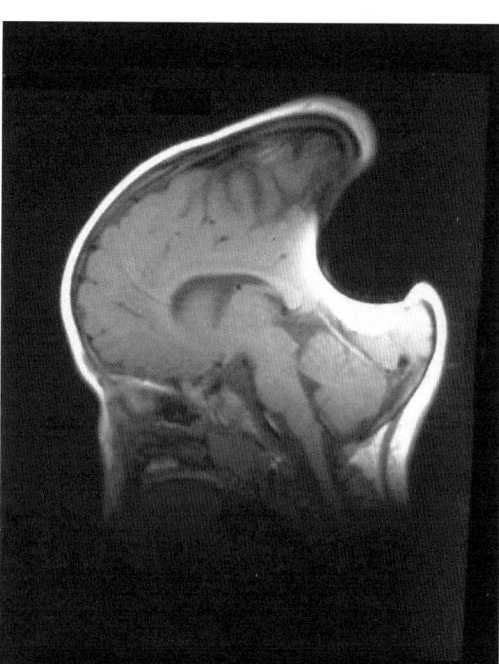

Fig. 33.2 Void artefact caused by ferromagnetic hair band

Table 33.3 Risks from RF energy and *gradient magnetic fields*

Risk	Precaution
Current induction and the heating effect	
• RF energy and oscillating magnetic fields induce currents in electrical conductors, such as monitoring cables and blood flowing in the thoracic aorta, producing ECG artefacts • Current flow is induced in metal objects in contact with the patient; this causes heating with potential thermal injury to surrounding tissues. Heating may also occur with metal pigments in tattoos or permanent make-up	• A robust screening procedure is essential to identify the presence and nature of patient-implanted objects • Only *MR safe* or *MR conditional* equipment should be used in the *inner controlled area* • Vigilance is required to ensure that metal objects or cables are not placed in direct contact with the patient
Noise	
• The generation of *gradient magnetic fields* causes mechanical vibrations and extremely loud noises (up to 100 dB) with potential for auditory damage	• Ear protectors or earplugs are essential for all patients and staff remaining within the *inner controlled area*

Intravenous MR Contrast

Gadolinium-based (GAD) intravenous contrast agents are used in MR for enhancement and diagnosis of pathology. In comparison with other radiological contrast agents, GAD is relatively safe with a high therapeutic ratio and low incidence of anaphylaxis (approximately 1:100,000). The side effects of GAD are generally mild and include headache, nausea and vomiting, local burning, skin wheals, itching, sweating, facial swelling and thrombophlebitis. Patients with renal failure who receive GAD are at risk of developing a rare, potentially life-threatening condition called nephrogenic systemic fibrosis (NSF). Glomerular filtration rate (GFR) should be estimated in all patients with kidney disease to identify those at risk of developing NSF. If the GFR is estimated at less than 30 ml min^{-1} m^{-2} then the risk should be balanced against the benefit and a minimal dose of GAD only administered if an unenhanced scan proves insufficient.

Practical Risks in MR Anaesthesia

There are several risks during anaesthesia for MR unrelated to the physics of involved (Table 33.4).

Ideal equipment for use within the *inner controlled area* meets the following three criteria:

1. It poses no hazards to the patient within the strong magnetic field.
2. It functions normally within the strong magnetic field.
3. Its presence does not degrade respective MR images.

The distinction between equipment designated *MR safe* and *MR conditional* is important. *MR safe* equipment only meets the first criterion above; it is free of

Table 33.4 Practical risks in MR anaesthesia

Risk	Precaution
Isolated environment	
• The MR Suite is often distant to intensive care unit and operating theatres. In the event of an emergency anaesthetic help is unlikely to be at hand immediately. New MR units should be built within radiology departments	• The MR suite is no place for the unsupervised novice anaesthesiologist. All anaesthetic, nursing and technical staff, involved in MR anaesthesia, should have formal training
Patient access	
• Access to the patient during MR imaging is physically and "magnetically" restricted. Once the patient is stable the anaesthesia team may remain outside the *inner controlled area*	• The anaesthesiologist must have confidence in the security of the airway • Remote monitors should be available
Movement of patient	
• The patient will require transfer to and from the *inner controlled area* and the table will move within the MR system. Dislodgement of LMA and IV access is possible and there will be periods where monitoring is disconnected	• The LMA, ET tubes and IV lines must be well secured and vigilance maintained to prevent dislodgement • The patient must be reconnected to monitoring as soon as possible

magnetic hazards but may still malfunction and cause image artefact. *MR Conditional* equipment meets all three of the above criteria and is, therefore, ideal; it must be appreciated, however, that equipment manufacturers may only guarantee compatibility up to a particular field strength limit. Anaesthetic equipment used within the MR Suite is often different from the standard equipment used elsewhere in the hospital. Practitioners of MR anaesthesia should be fully familiar with the local MR equipment in use.

Paediatric MR Anaesthesia

Children are the most common patient group requiring anaesthesia for MR. In paediatric lists, it is imperative that the anaesthesia team is adequately trained, equipped, and prepared for the challenges of paediatric anaesthesia. Some practical points relevant to paediatric anaesthesia for MR are summarised in Table 33.5.

Intensive Care Patients

MR imaging has superseded computed tomography as the investigation of choice in certain neurological conditions that require critical care. The most common indications in this population are suspected cord compression and undiagnosed coma. The principal concerns are:

- Cardiovascular instability and deterioration.
- Management of essential infusions.
- The risk of micro-shock.

MR procedures for intensive care patients are a significant undertaking, requiring planning and time (Table 33.6).

Table 33.5 Paediatric anaesthesia for MR procedures

- Young infants (<3 months) often sleep through short MR scans if well fed and wrapped
- Intravenous access must be secured for all anaesthetic cases
- Spontaneous ventilation technique avoids the pitfalls of IPPV via extended tubing
- There are several important pitfalls with IPPV and long tubing:
  - Patient airway pressures may be quite different to pressures measured at the machine
  - The increased compliance of long tubing can "absorb" much of a set tidal-volume breath; pressure-control ventilation will partially compensate for compliance losses
  - Leak at LMA or uncuffed ETT will further reduce the delivered breath
  - Resistance to expiration increases with increased tubing length and fresh gas flow
- LMA anaesthesia is convenient for uncomplicated children
- The valve in LMA/ETT pilot balloons may contain metal with potential for MR image degradation; the balloon should be secured outside the receiver coil in head scans
- With long tubing, breathing systems that deliver fresh gas at the patient end are appropriate; for example, an Ayre's T-piece for young children (<15 kg) and Bain's circuit for older children and adults
- T-piece systems require an adequate fresh gas flow to prevent re-breathing
- *MR conditional* temperature probes are available
- Ear protectors must be used

Table 33.6 Practical considerations for MR anaesthesia in critical care patients

- MR imaging is a potentially dangerous procedure for the intensive care patient. The balance of risk and benefit should be considered for each case
- A full screening procedure is essential. This may require family involvement for an unconscious patient. Plain radiography should be used to detect implanted foreign bodies. Metal implants, including ICP "bolts" and incompatible monitoring equipment must be removed. *MR conditional* ICP monitors are available
- MR imaging is contraindicated in the unstable patient
- Infusion pumps malfunction in the strong magnetic field with potential for devastating over- or under dose. Planning is essential for safe infusion delivery:
  - Only essential infusions are continued during MR imaging, e.g., vasopressors
  - A common strategy is the use of long infusion lines from standard pumps situated outside the magnet room
  - The patient should be stable, with any fresh infusions established, before transfer to the magnet room
- Current induction in lines or wires in direct contact with heart muscle may cause micro-shock; ventricular fibrillation and cardiac arrest will ensue. Temporary pacing wires and pulmonary artery catheters should be removed for MR procedures

Crisis Management in Anaesthesia for MR Procedures

Safe practice in the MR environment requires robust screening, adequately trained staff, multidisciplinary teamwork and eternal vigilance. Table 33.7 summarises the immediate management of some potential complications in MR anaesthesia.

Screening

A robust and thorough screening procedure, to protect vulnerable patients and staff from the hazards of MR, is essential. Contraindications to MR imaging are directly related to the major risks discussed in Table 33.2. The role of screening cannot be understated as fatalities have been reported in MR when the presence of an implanted

Table 33.7 The management of possible complications in MR anaesthesia

Complication	Assessment	Intervention
Cardio-respiratory arrest	• Airway • Breathing • Circulation	• Commence basic life support • Immediate removal of patient from the *inner controlled area* before beginning advanced life support • *Do not* allow the cardiac arrest team to enter the *inner controlled area*
Object stuck in MR scanner	• Assess patient safety	• Remove patient *inner controlled area* • Removal of object
"Quenching" emergency • See below	• Hypoxic alarm • Helium present	• Evacuation of patient and staff from *inner controlled area* • Quenching procedure
Contrast reaction	• ABC • Consider anaphylaxis	• Stop administration immediately • Assess patient and remove from *inner controlled area* for resuscitation • Institute anaphylaxis protocol – oxygen, adrenaline, IV fluids, etc. • Referral to an allergy clinic
Airway fault • Regurgitation, hypoxia, disconnection	• Confirm airway position and patency • Assess breathing • Circulation	• Correct abnormality • If not immediately remediable remove patient from *inner controlled area* • Do not bring anaesthetic equipment into *inner controlled area*, e.g., laryngoscope

pacemaker was not elicited by screening. Screening and access authorisation are ultimately the responsibility of the radiology staff. The anaesthesia team shares a common obligation to safe practice for patients and staff at all times. Multidisciplinary teamwork in MR procedures is vital.

Emergency Shutdown

It should be appreciated that emergency shutdown of the magnetic field is a risky and expensive process. Emergency shutdown causes *quenching*, where the liquid helium of the magnet cooling system rapidly boils to the gaseous state. For safe *quenching*, the resulting helium gas must be successfully vented from the scanner. Any failure of venting from the MR scanner is an emergency; helium gas will spill into the *inner controlled area* rendering the atmosphere hypoxic and at high pressure. Persons in the *inner controlled area* are at immediate risk of asphyxia or hyperbaric injury. Such an eventuality may occur with, for example, fracture of the venting quench pipe.

Staff should be aware of systems and protocols in place for the detection and management of a *quenching* emergency. The MR suite should be fitted with hypoxia alarms, and, in the event of *quenching*, procedures to open and evacuate the *inner controlled area* are instituted; this may include breaking the window between control room and *inner controlled area*. The potential danger of *quenching* is one reason why, in the event of a patient emergency, the patient must be removed from the magnetic field rather than causing an emergency magnet shutdown. *Quenching* may also occur sporadically as a system fault.

Interventional MR Procedures

Advances in technology mean MR image-guided surgery is now possible, providing the surgeon with dynamic high-resolution images during intricate stereotactic neurosurgery.

Various MR systems have been configured, including "doughnut" shaped magnets permitting surgery with real-time concurrent imaging, and portable systems set up to allow easy and rapid interchange between scanning and surgery.

All the complications associated with diagnostic MR also apply to interventional procedures. There are additional risks from patient repositioning, contamination of the sterile field, and the proximity of ferromagnetic surgical instruments, including scalpels, to the magnetic field. Some units employ staff, with metal detectors, to prevent personnel entering the MR theatre with ferromagnetic objects (Fig. 33.3).

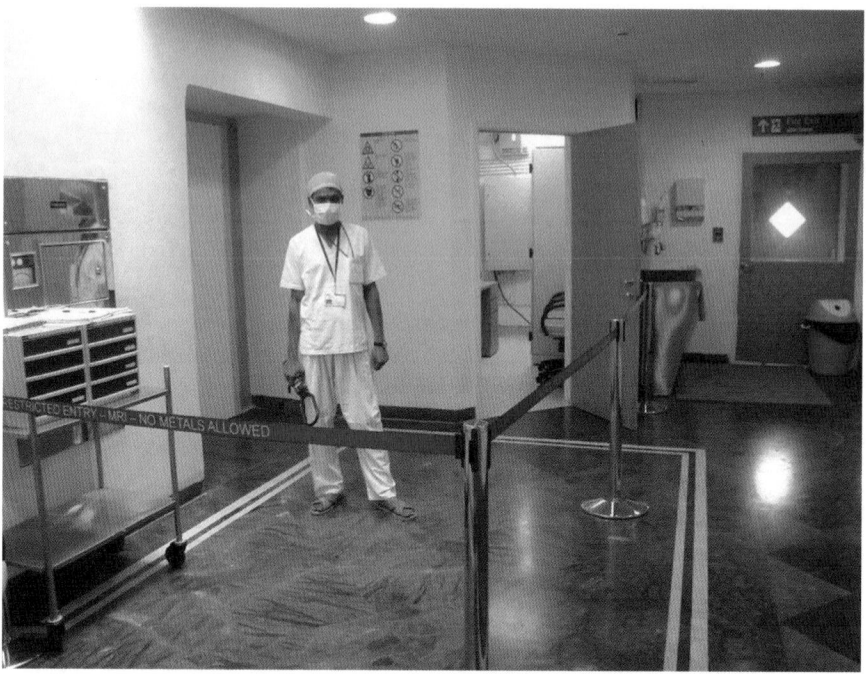

Fig. 33.3 Staff with metal detector employed to prevent anyone entering with ferromagnetic objects

Key Points

- Robust screening procedures must be in place to confirm that patients and staff are safe to enter the *controlled area.*
- Provision of anaesthesia within MR units presents unique challenges to the anaesthesia team. Practitioners in MR anaesthesia must be adequately trained, experienced, and aware of the risks, complications, and emergency procedures relevant to magnetic resonance imaging (MRI).
- During imaging, access to the patient is restricted.
- All anaesthetic intervention and resuscitation takes place in a designated area outside the strong magnetic field.
- In the event of deterioration, a patient must be removed from the *inner controlled area* for resuscitation. Essential anaesthetic equipment, including laryngoscopes, is ferromagnetic and subject to the potentially fatal projectile effect.
- Emergency magnet shutdown in a patient crisis is potentially dangerous and not advised. The patient should be removed from the magnet room.
- Equipment that is used in the *inner controlled area* should be *MR conditional* and familiar to the anaesthesia team.
- Minimum monitoring standards for conventional anaesthesia apply equally to MR anaesthesia.
- Multidisciplinary teamwork and eternal vigilance are essential.

Glossary

Controlled area	The controlled area wholly contains the 0.5 mT magnetic field contour. Self-locking doors with coded locks control access to the controlled area. Only authorised personnel have unsupervised access to the controlled area. All patients, visitors and non-authorised staff should be medically screened before entering the controlled area.
Gauss	Gauss is a unit of magnetic field strength (the correct term is magnetic flux density). The SI Unit, Tesla, has mostly superseded it. 1 Gauss = 0.1 milliTesla (mT). 1 Tesla = 10,000 Gauss. The cardiac pacemaker field contour is often referred to as the 5 Gauss line.
Gradient magnetic fields	The technique of MRI uses magnetic field gradients to localise and encode the MR signals with spatial information to generate an image. The gradient fields are superimposed onto the static field but are only switched on for short periods (typically just a few milliseconds). The fast switching of the gradient fields generates rapidly varying magnetic fields. This may cause interference on the patient's electrocardiogram and, on higher performance MR systems, may cause peripheral nerve stimulation. The electromagnet coils that generate the switched gradient fields vibrate, generating acoustic noise, which is often in excess of 100 dB. Hearing protection should always be provided to patients whether conscious or unconscious.
Inner controlled area	The inner controlled area is a term that is often used to describe the MR examination room that contains the MR system magnet. The attractive force of the fringe field is at its greatest in this room presenting a significant projectile hazard. The inner controlled area is always contained within the controlled area.
MR conditional	An item that has been demonstrated to pose no known hazards in a specified MR environment with specified conditions of use.
MR safe	Equipment is designated as MR safe if it presents no safety hazard to patients or personnel when it is taken into the MR examination room, provided that instructions concerning its use are correctly followed. This does not, however, guarantee that it will function normally and not interfere with the correct operation of the MR imaging equipment, with degradation of image quality.

| Quenching | Quenching refers to the rapid, almost explosive, boil-off of liquid helium and the accompanying loss of super-conductivity. The magnetic field is lost and a large volume of helium gas is generated and should normally be vented to the outside atmosphere through a quench pipe. If this pipe were to fracture it would present a potentially lethal hazard caused by the rapid build-up of helium gas in the MR examination room, leading to asphyxiation. Quenches can be spontaneous, usually occurring when the magnet is being powered up or down during installation or services, or can be deliberately activated in an emergency, such as fire. |
| Tesla | Tesla is the SI unit of magnetic field strength (the correct term for field strength is magnetic flux density). The cardiac pacemaker field contour is often referred to as the 0.5 mT line. Typical nominal field strengths of commercial MR systems are 0.5, 1.0 and 1.5 T. Higher field strength (e.g., 3 T) systems are becoming commercially available. |

Suggested Reading

Association of Anaesthetists of Great Britain and Ireland. Provision of anaesthetic services in magnetic resonance units. The Association of Anaesthetists of Great Britain and Ireland. 2002. http://www.aagbi.org/publications/guidelines/docs/mri02.pdf.

Farling PA, McBrien ME, Winder RJ. Magnetic resonance compatible equipment: read the small print! Anaesthesia. 2003;58:86.

Safety guidelines for magnetic resonance imaging equipment in clinical use. Section 4.17 Training. MHRA, London. 2007. http://www.mhra.gov.uk/Publications/Safetyguidance/DeviceBulletins/CON2033018.

Safety in magnetic resonance units: an update. Association of Anaesthetists of Great Britain and Ireland. Anaesthesia. 2010;65:766–70.

Shellock FG, Spinazzi A. MRI safety update 2008: Part 2, screening patients for MRI. AJR Am J Roentgenol. 2008a;191:1140–9.

Shellock FG, Spinazzi A. MRI safety update 2008: Part 1, MRI contrast agents and nephrogenic systemic fibrosis. AJR Am J Roentgenol. 2008b;191:1129–39.

Chapter 34
Perioperative Challenges During Electroconvulsive Therapy (ECT)

Carrie C. Bowman and James G. Hilliard

Since 1938, electroconvulsive therapy (ECT) has been used in the treatment of severe and refractory depression, catatonia, schizophrenia, and suicidal ideation. Although ECT was conducted without anesthesia for almost 30 years, the collaboration between anesthesia practitioners and our psychiatric colleagues has resulted in safer techniques, improved patient comfort, and more efficacious therapy. To be safe, the anesthesia practitioner must understand the physiologic response to the electrical stimulus and the effect of anesthetic drugs on the treatment to decrease the risks and increase the effectiveness of ECT.

The risks of ECT are well documented (see Table 34.1). In recent years, a peri-treatment mortality rate of 0.002% has been published. The most frequent causes of morbidity and mortality related to ECT are cardiovascular events including, arrhythmia, myocardial infarction, congestive heart failure, and cardiac arrest. This chapter will focus on the cardiovascular complications associated with ECT, along with pulmonary, neurological, and musculoskeletal consequences of ECT.

Cardiovascular Complications

Overview

Electroconvulsive therapy (ECT) stimulates the parasympathetic and sympathetic branches of the autonomic nervous system. Following application of the electrical current to the brain, a vagal reflex occurs and parasympathetic dominance is generally

C.C. Bowman, MS, CRNA
Department of Anesthesiology, Georgetown University School of Medicine, Washington, DC, USA

J.G. Hilliard, MS, CRNA (✉)
Department of Anesthesiology and Perioperative Medicine, Oregon Health & Science University, Portland, OR, USA
e-mail: hillarja@ohsu.edu

A.M. Brambrink and J.R. Kirsch (eds.), *Essentials of Neurosurgical Anesthesia & Critical Care*, DOI 10.1007/978-0-387-09562-2_34, © Springer Science+Business Media, LLC 2012

Table 34.1 Complications
associated with ECT

- Pulmonary
  - Aspiration
  - Obstruction
  - Laryngospasm
  - Pulmonary edema
- Cardiovascular
  - Dysrhythmia
  - Hypertension
  - Myocardial infarction
  - CHF
  - Cardiac arrest
- Neurological
  - Pretreatment anxiety
  - Status epilepticus
    (a) Convulsive
    (b) Nonconvulsive
  - Delirium and agitation
  - Inadequate seizure length
  - Headache
  - Intracranial hemorrhage
- Musculoskeletal
  - Long bone fractures
  - Dislocations
  - Dental damage
  - Oral lacerations
  - Myalgia
- Other
  - PONV
  - Recall

observed for approximately 10–60 s. The patient's hemodynamic profile then quickly changes as catecholamines are released from postganglionic sympathetic nerves and the adrenal medulla. The hemodynamic impact of this sympathetic stimulation is generally observed for approximately 5–10 min, with peak heart rate and systemic blood pressure readings observed 3–5 min after the electrical stimulation. Profound bradycardia, and asystole have been observed during the parasympathetic phase, and cardiac rhythms ranging from transient sinus tachycardia to ventricular tachycardia have been reported in the sympathetic phase. In addition, hypertension is common with the average increase in systolic blood pressure around 30–40%. While studies have demonstrated that most patients experience impairment in left ventricular systolic and diastolic function for up to 6 h following ECT, the majority of patients tolerate the cardiovascular alterations well. Patients at increased risk for the development of life-threatening cardiovascular complications during ECT and respective associated prevention strategies are summarized in Table 34.2.

Table 34.2 Prevention of cardiovascular complications during ECT

Patient risk factors	Potential complications	Prevention strategies
• Cardiovascular disease • Previous myocardial infarction • LVEF <50% • >10 PVC an hour	• Myocardial ischemia • Myocardial infarction • Arrhythmias • Ventricular tachycardia • Cardiac rupture	• Pretreatment w/beta-blockers • Optimize outcomes by controlling hypertension, diabetes mellitus, CHF, angina, and arrhythmias
• Monoamine oxidase inhibitor therapy	• Hypertensive Crisis • Arrhythmias	• Consult psychiatrist for risk/benefit analysis of discontinuing for 2 weeks before ECT • Avoid meperidine • Avoid indirect sympathomimetics
• Tri-cyclic antidepressants	• Arrhythmias • Synergistic with anticholinergic drugs • Synergistic with sympathomimetic drugs	• Consult psychiatrist for risk/benefit analysis of discontinuing for 2 weeks before ECT • Titrate sympathomimetic drugs carefully • Avoid preemptive anticholinergic drugs
• Hyperkalemia	• Arrhythmia w/ Succinylcholine administration	• Avoid succinylcholine • Consider small dose of atracurium or *cis*-atracurium
• Atrial fibrillation	• Thromboembolism following conversion to sinus rhythm with ECT stimulation	• Recommend anticoagulation therapy prior to ECT for all patients with concurrent atrial fibrillation
• Cerebral aneurysm	• Enlargement or rupture of aneurysm from increased wall stress	• Complete pharmacologic suppression of sympathetic nervous system response • In patients with known coronary artery disease, reduced ejection fraction or aortic insufficiency consider nitroprusside 30 mcg/min IV with atenolol 50 mg PO and arterial line monitoring
• Hypertension	• Intracerebral hemorrhage	• Maintain BP within 20% of patient's baseline. See Table 34.3 for preferred agents and ECT-related considerations
• Brady arrhythmias and cardiac conduction delays	• Profound bradycardia • Asystole	• Pretreat with anticholinergic agent • Avoid repeat dosing of succinylcholine

Prevention

Patients should be pretreated with an anticholinergic agent. Standard monitors are generally sufficient during anesthesia for ECT procedure. Hemodynamic and respiratory derangement requires prompt intervention to prevent cardiovascular crisis with ECT. Hypoxemia secondary to compromised airway patency can be a confounding

Table 34.3 Antihypertensive agents and effect on seizure duration

Preemptive medication	Effect on seizure duration	ECT-related considerations
Esmolol 1–1.3 mg/kg	Mildly decreased	Short duration of action desirable
Labetalol 0.1–0.2 mg/kg	Decreased	Effect on seizure duration controversial
Nicardipine 1.25–2.5 mg IV	No change	Used in combination w/labetalol to avoid rebound ↑ HR
Diltiazem 10 mg IV	Decreased	Nicardipine preferred for ECT
Nitroglycerin 3 mcg/kg IV	No change	Advised if at risk for myocardial ischemia
Nitroprusside 0.1–5 mcg/kg/min	No change	Advised for co-existing aneurysms, and aortic stenosis; Arterial line required
Trimethaphan 5–15 mg	No change	Studies demonstrates minimal side effects when used for ECT

[a]Based on current evidence, opioid analgesics, lidocaine, and alpha-2 agonists such as clonidine and dexmedetomidine appear relatively ineffective in blunting the hyper dynamic response associated with ECT

variable if bag-mask ventilation is provided during the procedure. Patients may benefit from pretreatment with an anticholinergic agent if the psychiatrist is using subthreshold stimuli or repeated stimuli to determine the seizure threshold, if the patient is taking a beta-adrenergic antagonist medication, or if there is a history of failure to induce a seizure following electrical stimulation. In any of these situations there is a much higher risk of clinically significant bradycardia and asystole because the sympathetic response may be diminished or absent and the patient remains under unopposed vagal discharge following the induced seizure. Glycopyrrolate may be superior to atropine in this context because it offers a stronger antisialagogue effect with less tachycardia and does not have central nervous system side effects.

In high-risk patients, additional suppression of the hyperdynamic response is desirable to prevent cardiovascular crisis such as myocardial infarction arising from tachycardia, other significant arrhythmias, and hypertension. Table 34.3 summarizes agents that have been effectively used to minimize autonomic nervous system effects of ECT and their effect on seizure duration. When using antihypertensive agents during ECT one must be cautious that cerebral perfusion pressure is maintained. Adequate cerebral blood flow is crucial during ECT because the induced seizure will increase cerebral oxygen demand by 200%.

Crisis Management

In the event of a life-threatening cardiovascular complication, the anesthesia provider must be prepared intervene with ACLS protocols. Emergency medications and resuscitative equipment must be immediately available.

If myocardial ischemia is suspected, oxygenation and hemodynamic parameters should be optimized immediately following current evidence-based protocols. The patient should be admitted to a monitored bed with continuation of supportive therapies. Serial cardiac markers including troponin should be followed to quantify myocardial damage.

Key Points

- Following electrical brain stimulation with ECT, patients will predictably experience a vagal reflex followed 15–60 s later by sympathetic discharge.
- Patients at risk for cardiovascular complications from ECT-related autonomic nervous system stimulation include those with coronary artery disease, cerebral vascular disease, hypertension, congestive heart failure, aneurysms, and pre-existing arrhythmias or those currently taking TCA or MAOI.
- Premedication with an anticholinergic agent is recommended particularly if the patient is taking beta-adrenergic antagonists or in cases where repeated electrical stimulation or subthreshold stimulation is being used.
- Premedication to attenuate the hyperdynamic responses to ECT can be considered for patients at high risk for cardiovascular complications.
- Cardiovascular complications are the leading cause of ECT-related mortality. Complications include: bradycardia, asystole, severe hypertension, severe sinus tachycardia, ventricular tachycardia, myocardial ischemia, and infarction.
- Anesthesia for ECT, as any other anesthetic can only be administered in an environment which is equipped and trained for immediate delivery of ACLS.

Pulmonary Complications

Overview

Commonly, ECT regimens require patients to receive treatments 3–4 times per week. The frequent treatments coupled with their short duration make the mask anesthetic the technique of choice, unless contraindicated because of known difficult ventilation, significant gastroesophageal reflux disease or late-term pregnancy.

Most of the pulmonary complications associated with ECT are similar to those of any mask anesthetic: aspiration, laryngospasm, and hypoxia or hypoventilation resulting from an obstructed airway. While the incidence of aspiration is rare (1 out of 2,000 patients), the event can be life threatening.

Lastly, pulmonary edema has been known to be a rare complication of ECT. The sympathetic output after the stimulus increases after load dramatically over a short period of time. In patients with compromised myocardium, this results in decreased flow through the pulmonary circuit causing increased hydrostatic pressure and capillary leak.

Table 34.4 Treatment strategies for pulmonary complications during ECT

Complication	Treatment	Potential adverse effects
Aspiration of gastric contents	Support oxygenation and ventilation Trendelenburg position and suction oral pharynx Secure airway	Injury to teeth and soft tissue structures; sore throat
Laryngospasm	Positive pressure ventilation Succinylcholine	Bradycardia
Obstruction	Reposition airway Insert oral/nasal airway Call for assistance Consider LMA or ETT	Epistaxis
Pulmonary edema	Support oxygenation and ventilation Confirm diagnosis Restrict IV fluids and consider diuretics	Hypovolemia, hypotension

Prevention

The prevention of pulmonary complications begins with a thorough preoperative assessment. Gastric reflux disease can be stratified and optimized with timely aspiration prophylaxis. Proper positioning of the patient with the head of bed elevated 15–30° reduces the chance of passive aspiration and improves pulmonary compliance.

Preparation of airway resuscitation equipment is imperative. The anesthesia provider must be able to support oxygenation and ventilation quickly and effectively.

Patients at risk for pulmonary edema should be identified early. Tight control of hemodynamics can be achieved with beta-adrenergic antagonists or direct acting vasodilators. These agents can be administered throughout the procedure.

Crisis Management

Treatment strategies for pulmonary complications are summarized below in Table 34.4.

Key Points

- A thorough preoperative assessment and preparation of airway equipment is paramount.
- Patients at risk for aspiration should receive prophylaxis and endotracheal intubation should be considered.

Neurological Complications

Overview

Neurological complications result from the effects of the electrical stimulus on extracranial and intracranial structures, as well as mental status changes associated with the postictal state.

Headaches (HA) are a common complaint after ECT, occurring in about 45% of patients. When the electrodes deliver a direct stimulus, the muscles of the head and face contract for the duration of the stimulus. The contraction of the temporal is and masseter muscles, along with ECT-related vascular changes are proposed etiologies.

Intracranial hemorrhage is a reported complication of ECT; however, it is extremely rare. While there is no scientific evidence to support neuronal changes after ECT, the impact of the acute hyperdynamic response can cause transient neurologic deficits, cortical blindness and damage to vascular structures.

Tonic-clonic seizures of adequate length are consistent with efficacious treatment. Some medications can cause prolonged seizure length resulting in convulsive or nonconvulsive status epilepticus (SE). Convulsive SE is characterized by continued myoclonus. Nonconvulsive SE requires EEG to confirm diagnosis and may present like emergence delirium or delayed emergence. Patients who may be tapering their antipsychotic medications or patients currently on aminophylline are at risk for this complication. Propofol and Thiopental can inhibit the ECT seizure, rendering it ineffective. Most sedatives or anxiolytics will decrease the efficacy of the ECT.

While most patients recover quickly, some patients develop confusion, agitation, and violent behavior postprocedure. These patients may require premedication (see below), increased vigilance in the recovery room or sedation post – ECT.

Prevention

A thorough preoperative assessment is crucial to reducing the incidence of neurological complications during ECT. A careful examination of the patient's current medications and a history of epilepsy may reveal a potential cause for prolonged or attenuated seizures. Tailoring the anesthetic to optimize therapy can also prevent shortened seizure length.

Patients who report HA can receive pretreatment in the form of oral NSAIDS unless contraindicated.

The incidence of postprocedure agitation can be reduced with premedication of benzodiazepines; however, these agents may also reduce the efficacy of treatment. Administration of a half dose of the induction agent (typically methohexital) after the stimulus has also been described. Efforts by the staff to reduce stimulation and provide reassurance may be helpful.

Table 34.5 Crisis management for neurological complications during ECT

Complication	Treatment	Potential adverse effects
Headache	NSAIDs	Gastric ulcers Renal failure Platelet inhibition
Intracranial hemorrhage	Support oxygenation and ventilation Maintain MAP to ensure adequate CBF Monitor for signs of intracranial hypertension Reduce ICP: • Hyperventilation • Osmotic diuresis • HOB elevated • Ventriculostomy Consult neurosurgeon • Confirm diagnosis (STAT head CT) • Consider emergency surgery	Cerebral vasoconstriction and reduced flow through collateral vasculature
Status epilepticus • Convulsive • Nonconvulsive	Support oxygenation and ventilation Administer benzodiazepines, barbiturates or propofol Consider administration of other anticonvulsants (e.g., phenytoin) Confirm diagnosis with EEG Administer benzodiazepines or other anticonvulsants as necessary (consult neurologist)	Sedation, respiratory depression, and airway obstruction Bradycardia Sedation, respiratory depression, and airway obstruction
Agitation and delirium	Reduce stimulation during the postictal phase Provide verbal reassurance Administer benzodiazepines or antipsychotics as needed	Sedation, respiratory depression, and airway obstruction

Crisis Management

Crisis management for neurological complications of ECT is summarized in Table 34.5.

Key Points

• Headaches are common and can be avoided by premedicating with NSAIDS.
• Intracranial hemorrhage is an important differential diagnosis if LOC is inadequate following ECT.
• Status epilepticus results in increased cerebral metabolic demand and an unprotected airway. Pharmacologic and nonpharmacologic methods can be employed to reduce post-ECT agitation.

Musculoskeletal Complications

Overview

Musculoskeletal injuries caused by ECT were commonplace prior to the application of anesthesia to the procedure. Now long bone fracture and dislocations are extremely rare. These complications can be a result of inadequate dosing of muscle relaxants or delivery of the stimulus prior to complete paralysis. Patients with a history of osteoporosis are at greater risk for skeletal injury.

Damage to the teeth and soft tissues of the mouth remain a concern. Direct electrical stimulation causes sustained contraction of the masseter muscle despite profound muscle relaxation. Anesthesia and psychiatric personnel must take measures to prevent injury to the teeth, tongue, and lips.

Myalgia continues to be a relatively common complication. The etiology is unclear; both the fasciculations from succinylcholine and the motor activity during convulsions may be responsible.

Prevention

Accurate dosing of muscle relaxants and careful timing by the psychiatrist can prevent long bone fractures and dislocations. Deep tendon reflexes are a reliable indicator of muscle tone and can be used to determine the optimal time for stimulation. Meticulous care and vigilance ensure minimal injury to the teeth and mouth. Two gauze rolls placed between the teeth from molars to incisors provide adequate protection. The lips are at risk for laceration and should be free of the teeth prior to the stimulus.

The prevention of myalgias remains controversial. Success has been reported with reduced succinylcholine doses, defasciculation with nondepolarizing muscle relaxants and premedication with NSAIDS. Administration of enteric-coated aspirin (650 mg orally) or acetaminophen (650 mg orally) consistently provides relief from post-ECT myalgia. Other practitioners provide ketorolac (30 mg iv) with good success if no contraindications are present.

Crisis Management

Crisis management for musculoskeletal complications of ECT is summarized in Table 34.6.

Table 34.6 Crisis management for musculoskeletal complications during ECT

Complication	Treatment	Potential adverse events
Long bone fractures and dislocations	Stabilize fracture Control pain with opioids Administer IV fluids Consult orthopedics	Fat embolism Respiratory depression, nausea, vomiting, pruritus
Dental damage and oral lacerations	Remove any broken teeth to prevent aspiration Consult oral surgery	
Myalgia	IV NSAIDS (Ketorolac 30 mg)	Gastric ulcers Renal failure Platelet inhibition

Key Points

- Accurate dosing of muscle relaxants and a well-timed electrical stimulus reduce the incidence of fractures and dislocations.
- Structures of the mouth require careful attention in order to prevent damage and aspiration of foreign bodies.
- Two soft, gauze bite blocks provide adequate protection for the teeth and lips.
- Premedication with NSAIDS can reduce to incidence of myalgia.

Suggested Reading

Chanpattana W. Anesthesia for ECT. German J Psychiatry. 2001;4:33–9.

Ding Z, White PF. Anesthesia for electroconvulsive therapy. Anesth Analg. 2002;94:1351–64.

Folk JW, Kellner CH, Beale MD, Conroy JM, Duc TA. Anesthesia for electroconvulsive therapy: a review. J ECT. 2000;16(2):157–70.

Kadar AG, Caleb HI, White PF, Wakefield CA, Kramer BA, Clark K. Anesthesia for electroconvulsive therapy in obese patients. Anesth Analg. 2002;94:360–1.

Saito S. Anesthesia management for electroconvulsive therapy: hemodynamic and respiratory management. J Anesth. 2005;19:142–9.

Tecoult E, Nathan N. Morbidity in electroconvulsive therapy. Eur J Anaesthesiol. 2001;18:511–8.

Chapter 35
Perioperative Challenges During Carotid Artery Revascularization

Ursula Schulz and Peter Rothwell

Introduction: Carotid Revascularization Procedures

Carotid stenosis is an important cause of ischemic stroke. About 10–15% of patients with carotid territory strokes and transient ischemic attacks (TIA) have a carotid stenosis >50%. On best medical treatment, these patients have a high risk of further, potentially disabling, cerebral ischemic events of up to 10% in the first week, and 15% in the first month after the initial event. Urgent treatment of the carotid stenosis to prevent recurrent strokes is therefore mandatory.

The most widely used procedure to treat carotid stenosis is carotid endarterectomy (CEA), which very effectively reduces the long-term risk of stroke. A pooled analysis of the largest trials showed that the 5-year absolute risk of any stroke or death was reduced by 15.3% (95% CI 9.8–20.7) in patients with 70–99% stenosis, and by 7.8% (3.1–12.5) in patients with 50–69% stenosis. Surgery has no benefit in patients with <50% stenosis. Because the risk of recurrent stroke is highest in the first few days after the initial event, this is also when the benefit from CEA is highest. Benefit from surgery rapidly diminishes over time, and surgery within 2 weeks after the initial event is recommended in patients with a TIA or nondisabling stroke who are neurologically stable and medically appropriate.

While the benefit of surgery for recently symptomatic carotid stenosis is uncontested, there is more debate about the benefit from surgery for asymptomatic carotid stenosis. The risk of stroke from an asymptomatic carotid stenosis is lower than

U. Schulz, MD, D.Phill (✉) • P. Rothwell, MD
Senior Research Fellow, Nuffield Department of Neurosciences,
University of Oxford, Oxford, UK
e-mail: ursula.schulz@clneuro.ox.ac.uk

A.M. Brambrink and J.R. Kirsch (eds.), *Essentials of Neurosurgical
Anesthesia & Critical Care*, DOI 10.1007/978-0-387-09562-2_35,
© Springer Science+Business Media, LLC 2012

from a recently symptomatic stenosis, and the benefit from surgery therefore smaller. Two large trials showed an absolute risk reduction of about 5% over 5 years. As medical treatment has become more aggressive since these trials were done, and, as the risk from surgery in the trials was probably lower than in "real life," the actual benefit from CEA in asymptomatic stenosis may well be lower. It may still be beneficial in selected patients, and further research to identify patients with asymptomatic stenosis who would benefit from surgery is ongoing.

In recent years, carotid artery angioplasty and stenting (CAS) has been increasingly used as an alternative to CEA. While it is generally more convenient, may avoid some of the complications associated with open surgery, and the hospital stay may be shorter, there are also specific risks of CAS. These include stroke caused by dislodged atherothrombotic debris, arterial wall dissection, arterial rupture and, in the longer term, restenosis. CAS is currently recommended for patients in whom CEA would be risky and difficult, for example, in the presence of past neck irradiation or when the stenosis is surgically inaccessible. Some practitioners favor CAS if no contra-indications exist, leading to considerable differences between institutions regarding the indication of CAS versus CEA. However, in patients with low surgical risk, it is still unclear if endovascular treatment is as safe and as durable as surgery, and, in this setting, its use is only recommended within clinical trials.

One other revascularization procedure, which is far less commonly used, is *extra-intracranial bypass surgery*, in which a branch of the superficial temporal artery is anastomosed with a cortical branch of the middle cerebral artery via a cranial burr hole. This surgery is sometimes used in recurrently symptomatic carotid occlusion or in stenosis of the distal carotid or middle cerebral artery. There has only been one randomized trial, which showed no benefit. The results of recently available trials (International Carotid Stenting Study – ICSS and the Carotid Revascularization Endarterectomy vs. Stenting Trial – CREST) are still subject of discussion, and while the FDA has approved carotid stenting as an acceptable alternative to CEA, in many European countries CEA is still regarded as the safer option.

Complications of Carotid Revascularization Procedures

Complications arising during and after carotid revascularization can be classified as follows:

- General complications arising from general anesthesia and from cerebral angiography.
- Complications arising from manipulation and recanalisation of the carotid artery.
- Procedure-specific complications associated with CEA or CAS.

The complications arising from general anesthesia and neuroradiological interventional procedures are dealt with elsewhere in this book (Sect. 3.5 and 5.2). In this chapter, we focus on complications specifically associated with carotid revascularization procedures.

Stroke Associated with Carotid Revascularization Procedures

Background

Periprocedural stroke is the main neurological risk associated with both CEA and CAS. The reported risks vary widely, but in patients with symptomatic stenosis are generally about 5–6% for CEA and 4–8% for CAS. During surgery, ischemic stroke may occur from embolisation of atheromatous material or low flow associated with temporary vessel occlusion and insufficient collateral vessels. Surface thrombus or atheromatous material may also be dislodged during CAS, but in addition stroke may be caused by vessel wall dissection with subsequent thrombus formation and embolisation, thrombus formation on the guide wire or air embolism. Postprocedural stroke may occur from thrombus formation on the endarterectomized surface, on suture lines, on the inserted stent or from embolisation from residual atheromatous plaque.

Prevention of Periprocedural Stroke

Carotid endarterectomy

- Antiplatelet therapy: Patients should be on Aspirin before and, for secondary stroke prevention, indefinitely after the procedure. There is evidence that treatment with a combination of Aspirin and Clopidogrel reduces the number of emboli from a recently symptomatic carotid plaque. However, the combination of these two drugs also increases the overall risk of hemorrhage, and there is currently insufficient evidence to recommend the use of this antiplatelet combination after CEA.
- Anticoagulation: A heparin bolus is usually given before clamping the carotid artery.
- Shunting during surgery maintains blood flow through the internal carotid artery while it is clamped. However, this procedure carries a risk of dislodging thrombus, and routine shunting has not been found to be associated with a reduced risk of stroke, although it may be helpful in individual cases.
- Intraoperative monitoring: If done under local anesthetic, the patient's functional state can be assessed during the procedure and shunting can be performed if the neurological status deteriorates after clamping of the carotid artery. Under general anesthetic, other monitoring methods, such as transcranial Doppler (TCD), EEG, or sensory-evoked potentials have been used to help decide if shunting should be used.

Carotid artery angioplasty and stenting

- Antiplatelet therapy: Generally patients should be on dual antiplatelet therapy (Aspirin and Clopidogrel) at least 3 days prior to the procedure, and this should be continued for 1–3 months postprocedure. Indefinite antiplatelet therapy for secondary stroke prevention then continues according to local guidelines.

- Anticoagulation: Patients are generally anticoagulated with Heparin throughout the procedure to prevent thrombus formation on the catheter and guidewire. Anticoagulation is not routinely used after the procedure.
- Protection devices: These are deployed prior to angioplasty and stenting to prevent any debris that may be dislodged during the procedure from embolising distally. Even though the use of these devices is recommended as standard in some countries, they also have inherent risks. There have been no randomized trials comparing CAS with and without the use of protection devices, and it is still unclear if their use is beneficial.

How to Recognize and Investigate a Periprocedural Stroke

Consider a periprocedural stroke if the patient develops a new focal neurological deficit during or after the procedure, or – less frequently – becomes restless and develops a decreased level of consciousness.

During the Procedure

If done under local anesthetic, exclude other possible causes for agitation, for example pain or urinary retention. Assess the patient's vital signs, neurological status and blood sugar. If the patient is undergoing a stenting procedure and the angiography catheter is still in place, the neuroradiologist will be able to check blood vessels for patency and – if a vessel occlusion is present – it may be appropriate to give intra-arterial thrombolysis or to perform clot retrieval. The latter might also be feasible if a stroke occurs during endarterectomy and the patient can quickly be transferred to an angiography suite.

After the Procedure

After a general anesthetic, the patient may awake with a new neurological deficit. In this case, the therapeutic options will depend on the care provider's best estimate of time of onset of the deficit. In addition, a patient may develop a neurological deficit several hours or days after the procedure. In this situation proceed as follows:

- Try to ascertain as precisely as possible when the deficit developed.
- Quickly assess the patient to determine the extent of the deficit (vital signs, quick neurological examination).
- Urgently contact the responsible neurologist/stroke unit physician and the neuro-radiologist for further assessment, brain imaging (intracerebral hemorrhage after

Table 35.1 General management of acute ischemic stroke

Blood pressure (Hyper- and hypotension)
- Hypertension in acute stroke usually settles spontaneously and should not be treated unless systolic BP is >220 mmHg or diastolic BP is >120 mmHg
- Causes of hypertension, such as pain, anxiety or urinary retention should be treated
- If systolic BP >220 mmHg or diastolic BP >120 mmHg, lower BP very cautiously, for example, with Labetalol 10–20 mg iv over 1–2 min
- Hypotension after stroke is rare. Any causes should be sought and corrected. Treatment includes volume replacement, correction of arrhythmias, and the use of vasopressors

Blood glucose
- Hyperglycemia is associated with a poorer outcome after stroke
- Blood glucose should be kept at <10 mmol/l

Body temperature
- A raised temperature may lead to a poorer outcome in ischemic stroke
- Temperature should be kept within normal limits

Oxygen saturations
- Maintaining adequate tissue oxygenation is important to prevent hypoxia and worsening of brain injury. Maintain O_2-saturations in the normal range, aiming for >92%

Prophylaxis of venous thromboembolism
- Early mobilization and use of compression stockings
- Low-dose heparin is safe in patients with ischemic stroke and should be used

Adequate hydration and nutrition, swallowing assessment
- Stroke patients are at increased risk of aspiration and require a swallowing assessment before they can be allowed to eat and drink
- Adequate hydration will improve cerebral perfusion and help prevent venous thrombosis
- Stroke patients are at high risk of malnutrition and may require enteral feeding

carotid revascularization is not uncommon) and repeat vascular imaging. In case of a recent ischemic event, intervention may be appropriate (e.g., intra-arterial thrombolysis/clot retrieval).

The potential for salvaging brain tissue after vessel occlusion decreases rapidly with increasing time since onset even within the first few hours, and intra-arterial intervention might only be feasible within the first 6 h after onset. However, this will have to be decided on an individual basis, so urgent discussion with the stroke team and neuroradiologist or surgeon who has done the procedure is mandatory.

Treatment of a Periprocedural Stroke

Any interventional treatment will be done by the stroke team/neuroradiologist.

Any further treatment will follow the general guidelines for treatment of ischemic stroke outlined in Table 35.1.

Cerebral Hyperperfusion Syndrome

Background

Cerebral hyperperfusion syndrome (CHS) is a complication that occurs in 0–3% of patients following carotid revascularization. It usually occurs within a few hours or days after revascularization, but may occur up to 28 days later. The exact pathophysiology is incompletely understood. Generally, it is thought to be due to sudden restoration of blood flow in a chronically hypoperfused area of the brain. Autoregulation in that part of the brain is impaired, and the cerebral blood vessels fail to constrict fully in response to increased perfusion, which is therefore markedly increased compared to before the revascularization procedure. Generally, cerebral perfusion increases by at least 100%, although more recently CHS has also been reported in patients showing perfusion increases of only 40–60%.

Clinical Presentation

- Headache, usually ipsilateral, often throbbing, frontal or periorbital
- Seizures: focal with secondary generalization
- Focal neurological deficits
- Hypertension
- Cerebral hemorrhage

Investigations

One of the main diagnostic questions in a patient who develops a new neurological deficit after a revascularization procedure is whether the patient has had an ischemic event due to vessel occlusion or embolisation from the procedure site, or has CHS. The main investigations are therefore

- *Brain imaging*: CT or preferably MRI. MRI should be done with diffusion and perfusion-weighted imaging (DWI and PWI). The aim is to look for new infarction or for a cerebral hemorrhage. CHS may show diffuse cerebral edema in one hemisphere, and, if severe, may show an intracerebral hemorrhage.
- *Vascular imaging*: to rule out re-stenosis or occlusion of the operated vessel. In CHS the carotid arteries are patent.
- *Perfusion imaging*: with SPECT, MRI, or CT. This should show markedly increased perfusion ($\geq 100\%$) in the affected hemisphere compared to baseline or, perhaps to a lesser extent, in comparison to the contralateral hemisphere. Transcranial Doppler (TCD) shows a flow velocity increase of 150–300% in the ipsilateral middle cerebral artery and may be the most convenient way of monitoring the patient's progress.

Table 35.2 Management of cerebral hyperperfusion syndrome

Blood pressure control
- There are no trial data to give the optimum blood pressure range for patients with CHS. General recommendations are that systolic blood pressure should not exceed 90–140 mmHg. Blood pressure control may be very difficult to achieve
- Recommended drugs for blood pressure lowering are labetalol and clonidine. Vasodilating antihypertensive agents and ACE-inhibitors should be avoided, because they can lead to further increases in cerebral blood flow and worsening of CHS

Seizures
- If a patient develops seizures, these should be treated with anticonvulsants, for example, Phenytoin
- There is no evidence that prophylactic anticonvulsants are helpful

Cerebral edema
- There are no specific data on how this should be managed in CHS. Reduction in perfusion pressure remains the main aim of treatment

Monitoring of treatment
- Monitoring of treatment effect is clinical
- Monitoring of flow velocities in the middle cerebral artery with transcranial Doppler may be helpful

Duration of treatment
- Tight blood pressure control is recommended until cerebral autoregulation is restored, which can be checked with transcranial Doppler. As all patients will have atheromatous disease, close blood pressure control should continue indefinitely as a secondary prevention measure for further vascular events

Treatment

This should occur in a Neuro Intensive Care Unit or High Dependency Unit. The mainstay of treatment is aggressive blood pressure management with the goal of reducing cerebral hyperperfusion. Management is outlined in Table 35.2.

Prognosis

The few studies that are available suggest that mortality may be as high as 50%, and that 30% of the surviving patients remain disabled.

Cardiovascular Complications

Hypotension and Bradycardia

Carotid plaque is usually located close to the carotid baroreceptors. Manipulation during surgery or distension of the artery during angioplasty and stenting may therefore produce a hypotensive response. The reported incidence varies widely between

12–60%. This tends to be more frequent and more prolonged after CAS and can rarely also occur with a delay of several hours after the procedure. It may be associated with an increased risk of stroke and is of concern in ischemic heart disease, which is highly prevalent in patients with carotid atheromatous disease. More rarely, in 10–15% of cases, patients may also develop a hypertensive response.

Prevention

- Some centers withhold the patient's usual antihypertensives before the procedure and for 12 h afterwards. However, because hypertension may be associated with a higher risk of CHS and perioperative stroke, this is not a generally accepted practice.
- Before CAS some centers premedicate with atropine or glycopyrrolate.
- Before CEA some surgeons inject the area around the carotid baroreceptors with local anesthetic.

Myocardial Infarction

Myocardial infarction during, or in the early days after surgery, occurs in 1–2% of patients, more often if there is a history of symptomatic coronary heart disease, and particularly if myocardial infarction has occurred in the previous few months or if the patient has unstable angina. Perioperative myocardial infarction can be painless so clues to the diagnosis are unexplained hypotension, tachycardia, and dysrhythmias. Congestive cardiac failure, angina, and cardiac dysrhythmias are also occasional concerns following surgery.

Management of Cardiovascular Complications (See Table 35.3)

Table 35.3 Cardiovascular complications after carotid revascularisation

Cardiovascular complication	Management
Hypotension	• Intravenous fluids • Consider starting vasopressors if BP is persistently <90 mmHg systolic
Bradycardia	• Atropine or glycopyrrolate • Temporary pacing is only rarely required
Hypertension	• No specific antihypertensives are recommended. Given the danger of bradycardia, beta-blockers should probably be avoided. Continuous infusion of Calcium antagonists, for example, nicardipine, has been used

Cranial Nerve Injuries

Cranial nerve injuries may occur in up to 20% of patients following CEA and are caused by traction, pressure, or transection of a cranial nerve. These injuries tend to recover spontaneously and rarely have any long-term consequences, but may cause short-term complications, particularly if a bilateral endarterectomy is done and bilateral damage occurs. Because of the danger of serious bulbar dysfunction with bilateral cranial nerve damage, if a patient has symptoms referable to both severely stenosed carotid arteries which require bilateral CEA, it is probably safer to do the operations a few weeks apart. Furthermore, a permanent nerve injury may be as disabling as a mild stroke, which needs to be taken into account when considering the risks and benefits of surgery. Table 35.4 shows which cranial nerves may be damaged during endarterectomy and which deficits this may cause.

Table 35.4 Cranial nerve damage after carotid endarterectomy

Affected cranial nerve	Deficit caused by nerve damage
Recurrent and superior laryngeal nerve, vagus nerve	• Change of voice quality, hoarseness, difficulty coughing and sometimes dyspnoea due to vocal cord paralysis • Bilateral damage during a bilateral endarterectomy may cause airway obstruction and require temporary airway support
Hypoglossal nerve	• Ipsilateral tongue weakness, leading to dysarthria, dysphagia, and difficulty chewing. Bilateral damage may lead to airway obstruction
Spinal accessory nerve	• Shoulder and neck pain and stiffness • Weakness of sternomastoid and trapezius muscles
Facial nerve (marginal mandibular branch)	• Mild weakness of the corner of the mouth
Greater auricular nerve	• Numbness of ear lobe and angle of jaw
Transverse cervical nerves	• Numbness of scar area

Key Points

- CEA and CAS are the two most commonly used carotid revascularization procedures. While endarterectomy is still the established standard procedure, stenting is increasingly used, particularly in patients with high surgical risk or a poorly accessible stenosis.
- While the benefit of revascularization in recently symptomatic stenosis ≥70% is well established, the benefit of intervention in asymptomatic stenosis is less clear.
- The main risks specific to carotid revascularization procedures are periprocedural stroke and CHS. Cardiovascular complications, especially hypotension and bradycardia, and, in endarterectomy, cranial nerve injuries may also occur.

(continued)

- In periprocedural ischemic stroke, it is important to determine the time of onset as accurately as possible. Urgent discussion with the responsible stroke team and neuroradiologist are mandatory, as endovascular intervention to treat a new vessel occlusion may be possible.
- CHS is thought to be due to sudden restoration of blood flow in a hypoperfused area of the brain. It presents with headache, seizures, focal deficits, and hypertension. Mainstay of treatment is aggressive blood pressure control.
- Manipulation and stretching of the carotid baroreceptors may cause hypotension and bradycardia during the procedure.
- Cranial nerve injuries mainly occur after endarterectomy. They rarely have long-term consequences, but may be problematic in the short term, especially if bilateral.

Suggested Further Reading

Adams HP, Adams RJ, Brott T, del Zoppo GJ, Furlan A, Goldstein LB, et al. Guidelines for the early management of patients with ischemic stroke. A scientific statement from the Stroke Council of the American Stroke Association. Stroke. 2003;34:1056–83.

Adams HP, Adams RJ, Del Zoppo GJ, Goldstein LB. Guidelines for the early management of patients with ischemic stroke. 2005 guidelines update. A scientific statement from the Stroke Council of the American Heart Association/American Stroke Association. Stroke. 2005;36:916–23 (The last two papers give a good overview over current recommended management of ischemic stroke).

Arnold M, Fischer U, Schroth G, Nedeltchev K, Isenegger J, Remonda L, et al. Intra-arterial thrombolysis of acute Iatrogenic intracranial arterial occlusion attributable to neuroendovascular procedures or coronary angiography. Stroke. 2008;39:1491–5 (i.a. thrombolysis after angiography associated stroke may be helpful).

Chambers BR, Donnan G. Carotid endarterectomy for asymptomatic carotid stenosis. Cochrane Database Syst Rev 2005, 4. Art. No. CD001923. (Cochrane review of carotid endarterectomy in asymptomatic stenosis.)

Dangas G. Editorial comment–hypotension after carotid revascularization. Stroke. 2003;34:2581–2 (Editorial to Reference 7).

Howell SJ. Carotid endarterectomy. Br J Anaesth. 2007;99:119–31 (Review of carotid endarterectomy with a specific view to anesthetic problems).

International Carotid Stenting Study investigators. Carotid artery stenting compared with endarterectomy in patients with symptomatic carotid stenosis (International Carotid STenting Study): an interim analysis of a randomised controlled trial.

Mantese VA, Timaran CH, Chiu D, Begg RJ, Brott TG. CREST Investigators. The Carotid Revascularization Endarterectomy versus Stenting Trial (CREST): stenting versus carotid endarterectomy for carotid disease. Stroke. 2010;41(10 Suppl):S31–4.

McKevitt FM, Sivaguru A, Venables GS, et al. Effect of treatment of carotid artery stenosis on blood pressure: a comparison of hemodynamic disturbances after carotid endarterectomy and endovascular treatment. Stroke. 2003;34:2576–82 (Trial investigating cardiovascular changes after CEA and CAS. Associated editorial with a good review in Dangas G. See 2 references above).

Ricotta JJ, Malgor RD. A review of the trials comparing carotid endarterectomy and carotid angioplasty and stenting. Perspect Vasc Surg Endovasc Ther. 2008;20:299–308 (Review of the currently available trials comparing carotid endarterectomy and stenting).

Rothwell PM, Eliasziw M, Gutnikov SA, et al. Analysis of pooled data from the randomised controlled trials of endarterectomy for symptomatic carotid stenosis. Lancet. 2003;361:107–16 (Individual patient data meta-analysis of the carotid endarterectomy trials for symptomatic stenosis).

van Mook WNKA, Rennenberg RJMW, Schurink GW, van Oostenbrugge RJ, Mess WH, Hofman PAM, et al. Cerebral hyperperfusion syndrome. Lancet Neurol. 2005;4:877–88. Good review of cerebral hyperperfusion syndrome.

Part VII
Specific Perioperative Concerns in Adult Neuroanesthesia

Chapter 36
Venous Air Embolism During Neurosurgery

Liping Zhang, Min Li, and Chris C. Lee

Overview

Venous air embolism (VAE), the entrainment of air into the venous system, is a complication that develops during some types of neurosurgical procedures. Symptomatic VAE results in injury to pulmonary vasculature, circulation obstruction, and decreased cardiac output. In rare cases, it leads to hemodynamic collapse and even death.

The reported incidence of VAE in neurosurgery varies according to the sensitivity of detection methods, the type of the procedures, and the positioning of the patients. The surgeries in the sitting position have the highest rate of occurrence of VAE, with an incidence of 10–80%. The air from the operative field may enter the venous vasculature whenever the open vein is above the level of the right side of the heart. This is the reason why VAE is most often associated with sitting position. VAE may also occur in neurosurgical procedures performed in the lateral, prone, or supine positions with reported incidence from 10 to 25%. Table 36.1 lists the neurosurgical procedures with VAE risk.

Besides the type of surgery, there are other contributing factors, both procedure-related and patient-related, which may have an impact on the occurrence of air entrainment during neurosurgery (Table 36.2).

L. Zhang, MD (✉) • M. Li, MD
Department of Anesthesiology, Peking University Health Science Center, Beijing, China
e-mail: lipingzhang01@yahoo.com.cn

C.C. Lee, MD, PhD
Department of Anesthesiology, Washington University School of Medicine in St. Louis, St. Louis, MO, USA

A.M. Brambrink and J.R. Kirsch (eds.), *Essentials of Neurosurgical Anesthesia & Critical Care*, DOI 10.1007/978-0-387-09562-2_36,
© Springer Science+Business Media, LLC 2012

Table 36.1 Neurosurgical procedures associated with venous air embolism (VAE)

Procedure	Known incidence (%)	Relative risk
Sitting position craniotomies	9.3, 27.4, 43	High
Posterior fossa procedures	76	High
Craniosynostosis repair	8, 82.6	High
Cervical laminectomy	23	Medium
Posterior spinal fusion	10	Medium
Peripheral denervation	2	Low
Torticollis corrective surgery		Low
Deep brain stimulator placement		Low

Table 36.2 Factors contributing to the occurrence of venous air embolism (VAE)

Factors
Procedure-related
• Surgical site relative to the level of right heart
• Extensive operation field exposure
• Investigational procedures which requires injection of gas
• Decompression of the abdomen
• Hydrogen peroxide for wound irrigation
Patient-related
• Preexisting hypovolemia
• Spontaneous respiration

Prevention

Since VAE can be lethal, its prevention and having a high index of suspicion are crucial in clinical practice. Various measures have been taken to reduce the incidence of VAE in neurosurgery (Table 36.3).

Positioning

Avoid sitting position if possible. In fact, with the awareness of the VAE risk associated with sitting position and the improvement of surgical technique, the popularity of the sitting position has greatly declined. If sitting position is strongly recommended, try to place the patient in a more semi-recumbent position than sitting up. The legs elevated to the level of heart can also help to reduce the pressure gradient between the right atrium and the surgical site.

Hydration

Ensure adequate intravascular volume to maintain the right atrial pressure. This method can not only reduce the negative pressure gradient between the wound and the

Table 36.3 Prevention of venous air embolism (VAE)

- Avoid sitting position if possible
- Elevate the legs/Wrap the legs
- Maintain adequate intravascular volume
- Controlled positive pressure ventilation
- Avoid nitrous oxide
- Avoid drugs that dilate the venous capacitance vessels, such as nitroglycerin (NTG)

right heart but also reduces the right–left atrial pressure gradient, which is then beneficial in reducing the incidence of VAE and paradoxical air embolism. It has been proposed that the right atrial pressure be maintained between 10 and 15 cm H_2O. However, hydration should be applied cautiously in patients with elevated intracranial pressure or those with either preexisting or borderline cardiopulmonary disease.

Controlled Ventilation

Since spontaneous inspiration is related to the increased negative intrathoracic pressure and greater pressure gradient between the surgical site and right atrium, general anesthesia with controlled positive pressure ventilation is recommended in high-risk surgery. The advocating mechanical ventilation with positive end-expiratory pressure (PEEP) during anesthesia is controversial. Some studies state that PEEP induces a reliable and sustained increase in right atrial pressure, which is sufficient to increase venous pressure above atmospheric level. Others suggest that PEEP may facilitate the occurrence of paradoxical air emboli in a patient with a patent foramen ovale (PFO) and also potentially result in hemodynamic deterioration by impeding venous return and reducing right ventricular preload. Therefore, PEEP should not be routinely used in craniotomies unless there is a strong indication.

Avoiding the Use of Nitrous Oxide

Since nitrous oxide expands the size of embolized air bubbles tremendously, it is reasonable to avoid its use in high-risk surgeries and patients at high risk, especially those with known intracardiac septal defects.

Crisis Management

Pathophysiologic Manifestation of VAE

If the embolism is large (>5 ml/kg), the obstruction to the right ventricular outflow tract may immediately occur and subsequently result in acute right heart failure and cardiovascular collapse. The lethal dose of intravascular air in adult has been estimated

Table 36.4 Clinical
presentations of venous air
embolism (VAE)

Clinical presentations
Respiratory (Early signs)
Awake patient
• Coughing
• Chest pain
• Dyspnea
• Tachypnea
Anesthetized patient
• Decreased $P_{ET}CO_2$
• Hypercarbia
• Hypoxemia
• Wheezing
Cardiovascular (Late signs)
• EKG: Tachycardia or bradycardia, arrhythmias, ST-T changes, and myocardial ischemia
• Hypotension
• Elevated PAP or CVP
• Jugular venous distension (JVD)
• "Mill-wheel" murmur
• Acute right heart failure
• Cardiac arrest
Neurological
• Altered mental status (in awake patients)
• Neurological deficit

as 200–300 ml or 3–5 ml/kg. Small amount of air can be dissipated and absorbed by the lungs. The embolization of pulmonary circulation may cause pulmonary vaso-constriction, pulmonary hypertension, V/Q mismatch, and the release of inflamma-tory mediators (e.g., endothelin 1 and platelet activator inhibitor). This, in turn, may result in pulmonary capillary injury, bronchoconstriction, and pulmonary edema. The V/Q mismatch is characterized by decreased $P_{ET}CO_2$, decreased PaO_2, and increased $PaCO_2$.

The release of vasoactive mediators, such as thromboxane, leukotrienes, and 5-HT, into systemic circulation will cause vasoconstriction and thromboembolism of other organs. In a patient with a PFO, right to left shunting may develop, leading to a paradoxical air embolus with catastrophic cardiac and cerebral events.

Clinical Presentation

The clinical manifestation and the severity of the pathophysiologic effects of a VAE are directly proportional to the rate of air entrainment and volume of accumulation of air in the right atrium. A small amount of air entrained may be of little conse-quence. However, if the air is entrained rapidly or if the cumulative volume is large, hypoxemia and acute right heart failure may be present (Table 36.4).

Respiratory system: The awake patients may experience coughing as the first symptom, followed by chest pain, dyspnea, tachypnea, and a sense of "impending doom." A "gasp" leads to further decrease of intrathoracic pressure, resulting in more air entrainment. For anesthetized patients under mechanical ventilation, the major changes in respiratory system are the decreased $P_{ET}CO_2$, decreased PaO_2, and increased $PaCO_2$. If patients develop bronchoconstriction, wheezing may be present.

Cardiovascular system: There may be several EKG changes, including sinus tachycardia or bradycardia, arrhythmias, right heart strain pattern, ST-T changes, and myocardial ischemia. Other hemodynamic responses include hypotension, elevated CVP or PA pressure, and jugular vein distension. In the most devastating cases, cardiac arrest may occur. The "mill-wheel" murmur may be detected by auscultation, indicating a significant amount of air has entered the right heart.

Central nervous system: Low cerebral perfusion may result from hypotension and hypoxemia. Altered mental status, convulsion, and even coma may develop in awake patients. The brain damage is exacerbated by cerebral (arterial) air embolism with possible long-term neurologic deficits.

Patient Assessment

In neurosurgical procedures with high VAE risk, routine monitoring such as EKG, SpO_2, $P_{ET}CO_2$, direct measurement of arterial pressure and arterial blood gases are essential. In addition, specific monitoring such as transesophageal echocardiography and precordial Doppler has enabled earlier diagnosis of VAE. The current available monitoring devices for VAE are listed in Table 36.5.

Transesophageal echocardiography (TEE). TEE is currently the most sensitive monitoring device for VAE. It can detect as little as 0.02 ml/kg of air given by bolus injection. However, TEE has to be inserted orally, which may cause injury. Also, it is expensive and requires expertise for continuous monitoring, limiting its use in neuroanesthesia.

Precordial Doppler. Precordial Doppler is the most sensitive noninvasive monitor for VAE, and is able to detect as little as 0.05 ml/kg of air. The performance of the Doppler is related to the correct placement of the transducer. Placing the probe over the right side of the sternum may provide better detection than along the left sternal border. In high-risk neurosurgical procedures, precordial Doppler is strongly recommended. It is the most cost effective and relatively easy to use. However, precordial Doppler is nonquantitative and can be difficult to place in obese patients and those in prone or lateral positions.

Capnography. End-expiratory CO_2 ($P_{ET}CO_2$) is an effective and convenient method of detecting VAE. Its use is required as a standard intraoperative monitor by ASA, and it can be used in any position. However, it is less sensitive than precordial Doppler and a decreased $P_{ET}CO_2$ may have alternative etiologies. Nevertheless,

Table 36.5 Monitors for detection of venous air embolism (VAE)

Monitor	Advantages	Disadvantages
TEE	• High sensitivity (0.02 ml/kg) • High specificity	• Moderate invasive • Expensive • Need experienced operator to monitor continuously
Precordial Doppler	• High sensitivity (0.05 ml/kg) • Noninvasive	• Correct placement of the probe can be hard in obese patients and those in prone or lateral positions • The auditory signal gives no indication of the size of the bubble • Subjective, false-negative rate reported to be 3%
Capnography	• Noninvasive • Most convenient • Routinely used for any surgery	• Less sensitive (sensitivity as 0.5 ml/kg) • Not specific for air embolism
Pulmonary artery catheter	• Provide intensive hemodynamic monitor for patients with significant cardiopulmonary comorbidities	• Less sensitive (sensitivity as 0.5 ml/kg) • Invasive

a sudden decrease in $P_{ET}CO_2$ with hypotension in high-risk patients should always alert the anesthesiologist to the diagnosis of VAE.

Pulmonary artery catheter (PAC). VAE results in an increase in pulmonary arterial pressure. The degree of the increase is proportional to the amount of air entrainment. PA pressure monitoring has a sensitivity similar to $P_{ET}CO_2$. It can measure the pressure gradient between the left and right atria, which may be useful in assessing the risk of paradoxical air embolism. Nevertheless, it is an invasive procedure and should not be used as a routine monitor.

Transcranial Doppler: Transcranial Doppler has demonstrated its ability in detecting air bubbles in the cerebral artery with a sensitivity of 91.3% and specificity of 93.8%. Transcranial Doppler is suitable for monitoring intracranial VAE in a patient with a PFO.

Treatment

Early diagnosis and rapid intervention is the key element in improving the patient's outcome. If possible, the entrapped air should be aspirated as much as possible. Fortunately, most cases of VAE are clinically mild. Table 36.6 lists the elements of treatment.

Table 36.6 Treatment of
venous air embolism (VAE)

Minor: Inform surgeon
Flood the wound
Close open vein
Discontinue nitrous oxide if used
Start controlled ventilation if the patient is spontaneously breathing
Moderate: Switch to 100% O_2
Aspirate air from a CVP or PA catheter
Hemodynamic support
Severe: Abandon surgery
Resuscitation

Prevent further air entrainment. If a VAE is suspected, then the surgeon should be immediately informed to inspect the possibility of air entrainment into the open veins. The field should be flooded with saline or covered by saline-soaked dressings. Closing the open vessels as soon as possible should stop the source of the gas embolism.

Reposition the patient. Immediate change to Trendelenburg position will increase venous pressure at the operative site and reduce air entrainment. Rotating the patient to the left side with head-down position helps to localize air into the right heart, which prohibits the air entering the orifice of pulmonary artery and facilitates the aspiration through a central catheter. However, it may be difficult to change the position of the patient in some situations.

Institute 100% oxygen. Nitrous oxide should be turned off immediately if used. Controlled positive ventilation enhances the intrathoracic pressure which is beneficial for both oxygenation and prevention of further air entrainment.

   If a central venous catheter is in place, aspirating air from the right atrium should be attempted promptly. This maneuver is diagnostic and therapeutic. It has been reported that air could be best aspirated with multiorificed catheter placed with the tip at or 2 cm below the sinoatrial node. Blood should be withdrawn until no air bubbles are seen. Emergent catheterization takes time, and is not routinely recommended to date.

Hemodynamic support. IVF, ephedrine, dobutamine, norepinephrine, and/or epinephrine have been recommended.

   If cardiac arrest occurs, ACLS protocol should be followed and cardiopulmonary resuscitation (CPR) initiated immediately. A thoracotomy may be necessary to aspirate the air from the right ventricle.

   If possible, the patient should be taken to a hyperbaric chamber and the treatment should be started as soon as possible to prevent severe and possible long-lasting brain damage. For VAE patients, especially for those with cerebral embolism, the hyperbaric oxygenation therapy has many advantages. The best outcome results from early recognition and prompt treatment.

Key Points

- Venous air embolism (VAE) is most commonly seen in neurosurgeries in sitting position.
- Prevention from its occurrence and having a high index of suspicion are crucial in clinical practice.
- Constant vigilance and inclusion of VAE in the differential diagnosis of intraoperative cardiovascular collapse, especially in the high-risk procedures and patients at high risk, are the best preparation for this lethal complication.
- Early diagnosis with prompt intervention is the key element in improving the patient's outcome.
- Capnography ($P_{ET}CO_2$) and precordial Doppler are the most convenient and practical detection methods for VAE. Their combination is the current standard of care.
- Once the diagnosis is made, prevention of further air entrainment and expansion of the air embolus with nitrous oxide, 100% O_2, lowering the height of surgical site, aspiration of air from right heart, and maintenance of cardiac output are essential.

Suggested Reading

Archer DP, Pash MP, MacRae ME. Successful management of venous air embolism with inotropic support. Can J Anaesth. 2001;48:204–8.

Gale T, Leslie K. Anaesthesia for neurosurgery in the sitting position. J Clin Neurosci. 2004;11:693–6.

Leslie K, Hui R, Kaye AH. Venous air embolism and the sitting position: a case series. J Clin Neurosci. 2006;13:419–22.

Miller RD. Venous Air Embolism. In: Miller RD, editor. Miller's Anesthesia. 6th ed. New York: Elsevier Churchill Livingstone; 2005. p. 2138–43.

Mirski MA, Lele AV, Fitzsimmons L, Toung TJ. Diagnosis and treatment of vascular air embolism. Anesthesiology. 2007;106:164–77.

Palmon SC, Moore LE, Lundberg J, Toung T. Venous air embolism: a review. J Clin Anesth. 1997;9:251–7.

Rozet I, Vavilala MS. Risks and benefits of patient positioning during neurosurgical care. Anesthesiol Clin. 2007;25:631–53.

Chapter 37
Arterial Hypotension and Hypertension During Neurosurgical Procedures

Kirstin M. Erickson and Daniel J. Cole

During ordinary clinical circumstances, cerebral/spinal autoregulation maintains a constant blood flow across wide variations in perfusion pressure. However, as a function of neurologic pathology, surgical risk, or comorbidities, many neurosurgical scenarios are anything but ordinary, and "tight" but strategic control of blood pressure is warranted. Intraoperative arterial blood pressure that is either too high or too low can cause or indicate serious complications for neurosurgical patients. This section addresses three clinical settings in which arterial blood pressure is a common and critical management challenge.

Overview

Carotid Endarterectomy

Atherosclerosis is a systemic disease, and, accordingly, patients with carotid plaque also often have coronary artery disease. Long-standing essential hypertension is also a frequent comorbidity along with its effects on cardiac function (e.g., diastolic dysfunction or left ventricular hypertrophy). Therefore, both hypertension and hypotension are common in patients with atherosclerosis.

In patients with poorly controlled hypertension, the blood pressure range for normal cerebral autoregulation is shifted to the right (Fig. 37.1). Moreover, in patients with advanced carotid artery disease, cerebral autoregulation is often impaired, making regional cerebral blood flow (CBF) exquisitely sensitive to perfusion pressure. Carotid sinus baroreceptor manipulation can cause bradycardia and hypotension.

K.M. Erickson, MD (✉)
Department of Anesthesiology, Mayo Clinic, Rochester, MN, USA
e-mail: Erickson.Kirstin@mayo.edu

D.J. Cole, MD
Department of Anesthesiology, Mayo Clinic, Scottsdale, AZ, USA

A.M. Brambrink and J.R. Kirsch (eds.), *Essentials of Neurosurgical Anesthesia & Critical Care*, DOI 10.1007/978-0-387-09562-2_37,
© Springer Science+Business Media, LLC 2012

Fig. 37.1 The relationship between cerebral perfusion pressure (CPP) and mean arterial pressure (MAP) shows autoregulation of CPP across a range of MAP. The curve is shifted to the right in patients with chronic hypertension

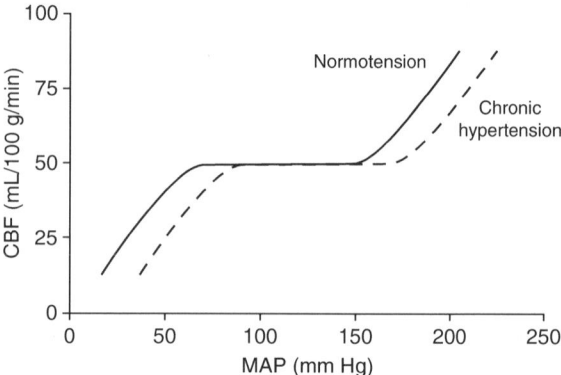

Severe hypertension (>180/110 mmHg) increases overall morbidity and mortality. The most common complication of hypertension is myocardial ischemia. Hypotension can lead to or worsen ischemic neurologic deficits. Active blood pressure management is essential in the perioperative setting.

Prevention

Hypertension and Hypotension in Carotid Endarterectomy (CEA)

Chronic hypertension should be well controlled before carotid endarterectomy (CEA). Ordinary intraoperative alterations in the level of stimulation should be anticipated and treated early with small doses of therapeutic medication. Invasive arterial blood pressure monitoring is recommended for beat-to-beat assessment and precise control.

Blood pressure is maintained at pre-operative, awake values until the carotid artery is cross-clamped. Blood pressure is then increased as much as 20% during cross-clamping to improve perfusion via collateral vessels. Small doses of phenylephrine or ephedrine are appropriate. Careful phenylephrine infusion is often used although it is associated with a higher risk of myocardial ischemia compared to lightened anesthesia. Coughing and other causes of blood pressure spikes during emergence should be averted to minimize stress on the freshly repaired artery.

Crisis Management

Hypertension and Hypotension in CEA

Table 37.1 summarizes intraoperative events requiring blood pressure management, signs or indications for treatment, and suggested therapy for hypertension and hypotension during CEA.

Table 37.1 Intraoperative events requiring blood pressure management, signs or indications for treatment, and suggested therapy for hypertension and hypotension during CEA

Event/Pathology	Signs/Indications for treatment	Suggested therapy
Direct laryngoscopy, intubation, incision	Hypertension, tachycardia	Deepen anesthetic Lidocaine Fentanyl Esmolol/metoprolol Nicardipine Nitroglycerin
Post-induction	Hypotension	Lighten anesthetic Phenylephrine Ephedrine
Chronic untreated hypertension	Severe or refractory intraoperative hypertension	Nitroprusside Nitroglycerin Esmolol
Intravascular volume depletion, hemorrhage	Hypotension, tachycardia, systolic pressure variation	Intravenous fluid Blood Phenylephrine Ephedrine
Carotid cross-clamping	Blood pressure low or low-normal	Increase baseline blood pressure by 20% (phenylephrine, decrease anesthetic dose)
Carotid sinus baroreceptor manipulation	Hypotension, bradycardia	Vagolytic (atropine, glycopyrrolate)
Decrement in neurologic monitoring (e.g., EEG slowing)	Hypotension	Raise blood pressure w/ phenylephrine, ephedrine, lighten anesthetic
Emergence, coughing	Hypertension	Beta-blocker (labetolol, esmolol) Lidocaine

Key Points
Hypertension and Hypotension in CEA

- The autoregulation curve is shifted to the right in patients with chronic hypertension.
- Prevention of blood pressure lability is achieved by anticipating stimuli and using small doses of therapeutic drugs.
- Normotension is the goal during CEA before and after cross-clamping of the carotid artery. During cross-clamping, blood pressure should be mildly elevated from baseline (by approximately 20% is appropriate).

Overview

Aneurysm Repair

Tight control of blood pressure during cerebral aneurysm repair is essential. Hypertension increases transmural pressure and risks vessel rupture, brain edema, and postoperative cerebral hyperperfusion. Conversely, hypotension lowers cerebral perfusion pressure (CPP) and risks ischemia, especially in areas of vasospasm. Moreover, acute hypertension may be a sign of aneurysm rupture and intracranial hypertension.

Prevention

Hypertension and Hypotension in Aneurysm Repair

Anticipation of stimulating events prevents abrupt blood pressure changes. Placement of invasive arterial pressure monitoring is routinely used. The decision regarding placement of the monitor prior to or following induction of general anesthesia must take into consideration the possibility that placement may cause pain that results in hypertension and cerebral vessel rupture. Intravenous administration of small doses of vasopressors guard against marked reductions in blood pressure following induction of anesthesia. Dramatic blood pressure increases may occur with laryngoscopy, pinion placement, incision, dural opening, and surgical manipulation. Lidocaine, esmolol, or short-acting opioids will diminish hemodynamic stimulation from these events.

Crisis Management

Hypertension and Hypotension in Aneurysm Repair

If an aneurysm ruptures intraoperatively, immediate temporary proximal occlusion by the surgeon is necessary. Maintaining cerebral perfusion should continue to be the goal while the surgeon gains control.

If vasospasm develops, more aggressive therapy combining hemodynamic augmentation ("triple-H therapy"), angioplasty, and intra-arterial infusion of vasodilator drugs are used. In the presence of an unclipped cerebral aneurysm, excessive hypertension risks rebleeding.

Table 37.2 summarizes intraoperative events requiring blood pressure management, goal of intervention, and suggested therapies.

Table 37.2 Intraoperative events requiring blood pressure management, goal of intervention, and suggested therapies

Event	Goal of blood pressure management	Suggested therapy
Dissection, manipulation of the aneurysm, placement of temporary clips on the parent vessel, aneurysmal clip ligation and closure	Normotension	Deepen anesthetic Lidocaine Fentanyl Labetalol, esmolol Nicardipine Phenylephrine Ephedrine
Following temporary clipping of parent artery	Normotension, or may need to increase blood pressure by approximately 20% to maintain CPP	Phenylephrine Ephedrine
Rupture	Normotension; may need to increase blood pressure to maintain adequate CPP if intracranial pressure rises, balance with need to control hemorrhage	Maintain intravascular volume Phenylephrine Ephedrine
Vasospasm	Induced hypertension as part of "triple-H" therapy (hypervolemia, hypertension, and hemodilution)	Volume expansion Phenylephrine Dopamine

Key Points
Hypertension and Hypotension in Aneurysm Repair

- Strict maintenance of normotension minimizes abrupt changes in transmural pressure and optimizes collateral circulation.
- Anticipation of stimulating events is key to optimal blood pressure management.
- If rupture occurs, blood pressure should be kept in the high normal range to maintain CPP and minimize ischemia.
- Inducing mild hypertension following subarachnoid hemorrhage after the aneurysm is secured improves neurologic outcome. Marked hypertension in the context of an unsecured cerebral aneurysm increases the risk of rebleeding.

Overview

Traumatic Brain Injury

Traumatic brain injury (TBI) per se is associated with hypertension either due to increased circulating catecholamines or as a response to intracranial hypertension. Cerebral autoregulation is impaired which increases the risk that systemic hypertension, may cause hyperemia, vasogenic edema, and intracranial hypertension. In the setting of intracranial hemorrhage (ICH), minimizing hypertension has been shown to reduce hematoma growth. Hypotension can develop when TBI is severe or accompanied by systemic injuries and significant blood loss.

Prevention

Hypertension and Hypotension in Acute TBI

Intra-arterial pressure monitoring is customary, although catheters may need to be placed during or after surgical incision to facilitate immediate surgical intervention and thereby limit secondary brain injury.

Hypotension is usually a sign of hypovolemia. Hypovolemia is best assessed by clinical signs including arterial blood pressure, and systolic pressure variation. Urinary output may be confounded as a guide if mannitol has been given at the request of the surgeon to allow for brain relaxation.

Hemorrhage should be treated with immediate and aggressive volume resuscitation. Glucose-containing solutions should be avoided because hyperglycemia is associated with worsened neurologic outcomes. To prevent hypotension in the patient receiving large amounts of mannitol, diuresed fluid should be replaced. Iso-osmolar and colloid solutions should be used as appropriate. Intravenous administration of vasopressors may be appropriate for blood pressure management, if fluid administration leads to worsening of cerebral edema. Control of bleeding and volume resuscitation takes precedence over immediate surgical intervention, as systolic pressure of less than 80 mmHg leads to poor outcomes.

Crisis Management

Hypertension and Hypotension in Acute TBI

Targets for lowering arterial pressure are based on intracranial pressure (ICP) and CPP. Although controversial, CPP should be 70 mmHg or greater. Overaggressive fluid administration may worsen intracranial edema and ICP.

Hematoma growth is reduced if blood pressure is lowered within hours of onset. 2007 guidelines set a systolic blood pressure target of less than or equal to 180 mmHg. Recent data suggest that a lower systolic pressure of 140 mmHg reduces hemorrhagic growth without adverse effect. No specific agents have been shown to outperform others.

Table 37.3 summarizes differential diagnoses and suggested therapeutic approaches to hypertension and hypotension in TBI.

Table 37.3 Differential diagnoses and suggested therapeutic approaches to hypertension and hypotension in TBI

Sign	Differential diagnosis	Therapeutic approach
Hypertension, tachycardia	Catecholamine release Increasing ICP Inadequate anesthesia Coughing, bucking	1. Lower ICP 2. Ensure adequate anesthesia, oxygenation, ventilation 3. Avoid hypocapnea unless herniation evident 4. Beta-blocker (avoid vasodilators in a closed cranium)
Hypertension, bradycardia, irregular respiration	Impending herniation (Cushing phenomenon)	Manage blood pressure based strictly on direct ICP monitoring

Hypotension, tachycardia	Hypovolemia
	  – Hemorrhage from systemic injuries
	  – Acute mannitol diuresis
	  – Central diabetes insipidus
	  – Chronic diuretic therapy
	Severe traumatic brain injury (variable heart rate)
		1. Iso-osmolar colloid or crystalloid solutions
		2. Transfusion
		3. Vasopressor or inotrope
		4. Vasopressin for diabetes insipidus

Key Points
Hypertension and Hypotension in Acute TBI

- TBI alone is associated with increased catecholamines and arterial hypertension.
- Arterial hypertension may be a marker of intracranial hypertension and impending herniation.
- Limiting hypertension after ICH reduces hematoma formation.
- Hypotension should be treated as hypovolemia, until proven otherwise.

Suggested Reading

Carotid Endarterectomy

Biller J, Feinberg WM, Castaldo JE, et al. Guidelines for carotid endarterectomy: a statement for healthcare professionals from a special writing group of the Stroke Council, American Heart Association. Stroke. 1998;29(2):554–62.

Herrick IA, Gelb AW. Occlusive cerebrovascular disease: anesthetic considerations. In: Cottrell JE, Smith DS, editors. Anesthesia and neurosurgery. 4th ed. St. Louis, MO: Mosby; 2001. p. 459–72.

Yastrebov K. Intraoperative management: carotid endarterectomies. Anesthesiol Clin N Am. 2004;22(2):265–87.

Aneurysm/Arteriovenous Malformation Repair

Drummond JC, Patel PM. Neurosurgical Anesthesia. In: Miller RD, editor. Miller's Anesthesia. 6th ed. Philadelphia, PA: Elsevier Churchill Livingstone; 2005. p. 2127–73.

Lam A. Cerebral aneurysms: anesthetic considerations. In: Cottrell JE, Smith DS, editors. Anesthesia and Neurosurgery. 4th ed. St. Louis, MO: Mosby; 2001. p. 367–96.

Morgan, GE, Mikhail, MS, Murray, MJ. Anesthesia for neurosurgery. In Clinical anesthesiology. 4th ed. New York, NY: McGraw-Hill; 2006:631–46.

Traumatic Brain Injury

Anderson CS, Huang Y, Wang JG, et al. for the INTERACT Investigators. Intensive blood pressure reduction in acute cerebral haemorrhage trial (INTERACT): a randomized pilot trial. Lancet Neurol. 2008;7:391–9.

Gopinath SP, Robertson CS. Management of severe head injury. In: Cottrell JE, Smith DS, editors. Anesthesia and neurosurgery. 4th ed. St. Louis, MO: Mosby; 2001. p. 663–91.

Tenenbein P, Kincaid MS, Lam AM. Head trauma – anesthesia considerations and management. In: Smith CE, editor. Trauma anesthesia. New York, NY: Cambridge University Press; 2008. p. 172–86.

Chapter 38
Hyperthermia and Hypothermia During Neurosurgical Procedures

Akiva Leibowitz, Evgeni Brotfain, and Yoram Shapira

Overview

Humans are euthermic beings, that is, critical physiologic functions must be maintained within a fixed temperature range. Any shifts from a body core temperature of $36.6°C \pm 0.2°C$ results in either hyperthermia or hypothermia, causing pathophysiologic reactions. Normal thermoregulation is a highly complex positive and negative feedback system depending on input and feedback from nearly every tissue of the body, and several well-identified response mechanisms. While the hypothalamus and skin are identified as having the major role in thermal regulation, nearly every tissue of the body is involved in the process. More frequently, intraoperative thermal dysregulation results in hypothermia. However, when hyperthermia occurs it must also be quickly addressed, particularly in patients with neurological injury or disease. Processing of thermoregulatory information occurs in three phases:

- Afferent input: Temperature-sensitive cells fire in response to excessive cold and heat. Information is transmitted in distinct neural fibers via multiple spinal tracts to the hypothalamus where it is then processed.
- Central control: Most of the processing takes place in the hypothalamus, where input from different sites is compared and integrated, and responses are regulated when deviation from threshold appears. Many factors influence the absolute

A. Leibowitz, MD (✉) • E. Brotfain, MD • Y. Shapira, MD, PhD
Department of Anesthesiology and Critical Care, Soroka University Medical Center,
Ben Gurion-University of the Negev, Beer-Sheva, Israel
e-mail: akival@exchange.bgu.ac.il

A.M. Brambrink and J.R. Kirsch (eds.), *Essentials of Neurosurgical Anesthesia & Critical Care*, DOI 10.1007/978-0-387-09562-2_38,
© Springer Science+Business Media, LLC 2012

Table 38.1 Factors influencing the threshold

Factor		Effect
Drugs and substances	Norepinephrine, dopamine, 5-hydroxytryptamine, acetylcholine, prostaglandin E1, neuropeptides, alcohol, sedatives, nicotine	Mediation of absolute threshold
Sex	Female > male	Female core temperature up to 1°C > male
Menstrual cycle		Further rise in second half of menstrual cycle
Circadian rhythm	Daily variation in core temperature	Lowest temperatures in mornings
Systemic disease	Hypothyroidism, hyperthyroidism, infection	

Table 38.2 Response mechanisms

Response	Mechanism	Other effects
Cutaneous vasoconstriction/ vasodilation	Metabolic heat is lost primarily through convection and radiation from the skin surface, and vasoconstriction reduces this loss. Thermoregulatory skin blood flow is comprised primarily of the arteriovenous shunt component and is relatively insensitive to circulating catecholamines. Active vasodilation is not blocked by any known drugs	Variation in BP up to 15 mmHg
Sustained shivering	Augments heat production by 50–100%. Not fully developed in infants	Blocked by anesthetics and neuromuscular blocking agents
Nonshivering thermogenesis	Increases metabolic heat production without producing mechanical work	Activated by circulating norepinephrine. Blocked by β-blockers
Sweating	Dissipation of heat mediated by postganglionic cholinergic nerves	Blocked by anticholinergics (e.g., Atropine)

threshold and normal core temperatures in humans. Distinguishing normal deviations from pathological states is of major importance. Table 38.1 lists some of the major contributors to threshold and core temperature variation. The inter-threshold range is range bounded by sweating on the upper end and shivering on the lower end where perturbations of 0.2°C from threshold do not typically trigger an autonomic response.

- Efferent response: Thermal perturbations from normal limits activate effector responses that increase metabolic heat production or alter environmental heat loss. Each thermoregulatory effector has its own threshold and gain, so there is an orderly progression of responses and response intensities in proportion to need. Aside from autonomic responses, behavioral responses play an important role, and the lack of this response in anesthetized patients should be taken into account. Table 38.2 summarizes the major autonomic effector responses.

Thermoregulation During Anesthesia

Thermoregulation during anesthesia – general or regional – is often significantly impaired. Anesthetics may modulate thermoregulatory thresholds and influence effector responses. Other factors prevalent in the OR environment and in surgical procedures, such as cold surroundings, exposed body surface, cold IV fluid replacement, and mechanical ventilation further contribute to the difficulty in maintaining normothermia. Incidence of perioperative hypothermia is reported to be as high as 70% and is of major concern particularly in lengthy procedures. Hyperthermia is a less frequent intraoperative complication, but when occurring – may have devastating effects in the context of central nervous system injury. Later in this section mild hypothermia will be discussed as a controversial treatment modality in neurosurgery (see Table 38.3).

Prevention: Hypothermia

Body heat redistribution following anesthesia follows a specific pattern, extensively studied by Sessler et al. A gross summary of this pattern is represented in Fig. 38.1.

The physician's role is crucial in intervening in each of these phases, minimizing the development and extent of hypothermia.

Phase 1: Redistribution hypothermia, once initiated, is extremely difficult to treat, since it is a result of heat flow from core to periphery (rather than cutaneous heat loss) and warming the core compartments is a lengthy procedure. Nevertheless, this phenomenon may be prevented (but is not necessarily required) by following means:

- Increasing body heat content by prewarming the patient 1° preoperatively.
- Pharmacologic vasodilation preoperatively, inducing redistribution prior to anesthesia.
- Phenylephrine-induced vasoconstriction during the first hour of anesthesia has been shown to decrease the extent of redistribution hypothermia.

Table 38.3 Summary of thermoregulatory alterations during general anesthesia

Influences of anesthesia on thermoregulation	
Behavioral responses	Abolished
Thermoregulatory threshold	Significantly altered. Reduced from 37 to 34.5°C, interthreshold range widened to ±4°C, sweating threshold slightly elevated, and vasoconstriction threshold markedly lowered
Vasoconstriction	Impairment of vasoconstriction response, primarily in AV shunts, affects redistribution of body heat
Shivering thermogenesis	Impaired by all general anesthetics, even without muscle blockade
Nonshivering thermogenesis	Primarily affects infants who depend on this mechanism. In adults, an insignificant mechanism

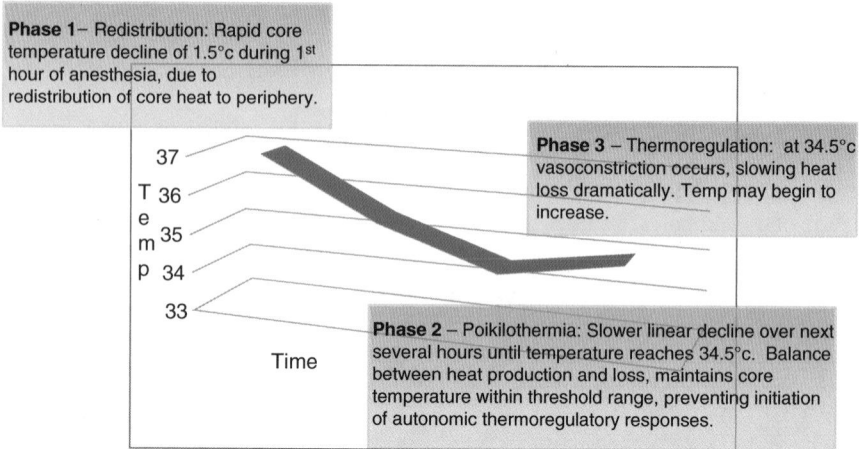

Fig. 38.1 Phases of intraoperative heat loss

Phase 2: Most of the heat lost during this stage is due to radiation or convection. Thus, effectively interrupting these pathways has been found to be effective in minimizing heat loss. Approximately 90% of body heat is lost via the skin surface. Another 10% is lost via surgical incisions and cold IV fluid administration. Another negligible amount of heat is lost through respiration. In neurosurgical cases involving large incisions or massive fluid shifts, heating IV fluids has a greater significance. Cutaneous insulation and warming remain the mainstay of preventing perioperative hypothermia and include the following:

- Raising ambient temperature: This minimizes heat lost to radiation. Often, controlling ambient temperature may be impractical, as the ambient temperature necessary may reach levels to high to be tolerated by the scrubbed-in surgical team (e.g., 23–26°C for an infant patient).
- Cutaneous warming: Passive insulation is highly effective. A single layer of cotton blankets or surgical drapes reduces heat loss by as much as 30%, while the effectiveness of subsequent layers decreases. Heat preservation is proportional to the body surface area insulated. This is important with respect to infants whose proportions are different from those of adults (i.e., covering the head may be of significance.).
- Active warming: Two main methods – forced warm air and circulating heated water – are clinically used for active warming. Since 90% of heat loss is via skin surface, cutaneous heating is an efficient way of elevating core body temperature. Thermoregulatory vasoconstriction impairs heat flow from the periphery to core and poses a difficulty in warming unanesthetized hypothermic patients efficiently. Therefore, active warming is best when applied to vasodilated anesthetized patients. Numerous studies have shown use of forced warm air to be superior to circulating hot water systems, albeit some studies demonstrate quicker heating with circulating water systems. When used, circulating hot water systems should

be applied on top of the patient rather than underneath, as most foam mattresses provide good insulation and patient weight impairs cutaneous blood flow and increases risk of burns.

- Heated IV fluids: Heated IV fluids (limited to 40°C) are not sufficient to maintain normothermia in anesthetized patients. Nevertheless, in cases involving large fluid shifts, extensive blood loss or extremely long procedures, heated IV fluids provide some protection against development of hypothermia associated with cool IV fluid administration.
- Warmed and humidified gasses: As this route of heat loss is negligible in adults, there is no significant benefit of warming inspired gasses. Infants might have some benefit, as this route is somewhat more significant for them.

Crisis Management: Hypothermia

Managing hypothermia, once initiated in the intraoperative period, includes temperature monitoring and adequate warming. Complications of hypothermia should be sought and treated as indicated.

Monitoring Sites

Five monitoring sites reliably provide core temperature – pulmonary artery (which is the gold standard), distal esophagus, nasopharynx, tympanic membrane, and bladder. Other sites may be both inaccurate and misleading, recording temperatures other than core temperature. Table 38.4 summarizes the different temperature-monitoring sites.

Complications of Perioperative Hypothermia

Perianesthetic hypothermia produces potentially severe complications. The controversial benefits of mild hypothermia in the neurosurgical setting will be discussed further below.

Wound infection and healing: Wound infection and impairment of healing are among the most common serious complications of anesthesia and surgery, known to increase morbidity and lengthen hospital stay, and have been shown to be reduced when normothermia is maintained.

Coagulation: Coagulation is impaired in hypothermic patients and is thought to be mainly a result of a decrease in activity of clot-activating factors. Other mechanisms shown to be impaired include platelet function and the fibrinolytic system. Two points should be kept in mind:

Table 38.4 Major temperature monitoring sites

Monitoring site	Reliability	Advantages	Disadvantages
Pulmonary artery catheter	Gold standard. Reflects core blood temperature	Accurate	Highly invasive Impractical in most clinical scenarios
Distal esophagus	Reliable, accurate	Reliable, easy to use, accessible	Sensitive to site of placement. Malpositioning leads to false recordings
Nasopharynx and tympanic membrane	Reflects core brain temperature. *Infrared aural canal thermometers inaccurate*	If properly placed – reflects temperature reliably. Accessible	Tympanic membrane thermometer must be in direct contact with tympanic membrane. Positioning might be difficult. Risk of eardrum perforation
Bladder	Close approximation to core temperature	Tolerable by awake patients	Accuracy varies with urine output
Rectal	Close approximation to core temperature	Tolerable by awake patients. Highly accessible site	Presence of stool and bacteria may falsely elevate temperature. Temperature changes lag behind core temperature changes
Skin	Inaccurate. Many confounding conditions	Simple, accessible	Confounded by: ambient temperature, redistribution, and vasomotor tone

Table 38.5 Effect of hypothermia on drug metabolism

Drug class	Effect
Neuromuscular blocking agents	Mainly pharmacokinetic effect. Onset of action delayed. Prolonged duration. Recovery minimally affected. Vecuronium affected more than Atracurium. Efficacy of neostigmine not altered
Inhaled anesthetics	Pharmacodynamic effect. Solubility increases. Decrease in MAC of 5% for every °C
Propofol	Increase in plasma concentration of 30% when temperature decreased by 3°C

- Platelet count is not affected
- Routine coagulation studies will usually result in normal coagulation function, as these tests are performed routinely in an environment of 37°C

Adverse myocardial events: Mild hypothermia has been shown in some studies, to increase the risk of postoperative adverse myocardial events threefold. Particular care should be taken with patients suffering from preexisting cardiac ischemic disease, and elderly patients.

Drug metabolism: Drug metabolism is decreased by perioperative hypothermia, and postanesthetic recovery is prolonged. The effect of hypothermia differs from drug to drug, and is listed in Table 38.5.

Postoperative shivering: Patients report shivering and thermal discomfort as their worst experience of the perioperative period, even worse than surgical pain. Of particular interest in neurosurgery – shivering increases ICP and intraocular pressure, in addition to stretching surgical incisions, and interrupting monitoring devices. Incidence is as high as 40%, but decreases when patients are kept normothermic and larger doses of opioids are used intraoperatively. Shivering may increase metabolic rate and oxygen consumption by 200%, but currently is not thought to contribute significantly to the adverse myocardial events.

The approach to postoperative shivering should include the following:

- Skin surface warming: Shivering threshold is dependent on core and mean skin temperature. Thus, aside from heating, this augments cutaneous warm input, allowing more core hypothermia, decreasing the shivering threshold. Skin warmers increase mean skin temperature by only a few degrees, thus it is important to raise core temperature >35°C, for augmentation of warm input to be efficient and to prevent shivering.
- Drugs: Meperidine (25–75 mg IV) is considerably more effective in treating shivering than equianalgesic doses of other µ-agonists, and this may be attributed to its effect on κ receptors and other non-opioid sites of action. Other proposed treatments include clonidine (75–150 µg IV, most probably by reducing vasoconstriction and shivering thresholds), ketanserin (10 mg IV), tramadol (1–2 mg/kg), physostigmine (0.04 mg/kg), magnesium sulfate (30 mg/kg).

Therapeutic Hypothermia in Neurosurgery

The decrease in metabolic rate and oxygen demand has led researchers and clinicians to postulate that hypothermia might have beneficial effects on neurological outcomes, in a vast array of situations involving cerebral ischemia and brain trauma. While numerous studies have shown mild hypothermia to provide protection against cerebral ischemia and hypoxemia in animal species, the only benefit unequivocally proven in humans is on the neurological outcomes following cardiac arrest/ventricular fibrillation.

Global ischemia: Several studies have shown improved neurological outcome and reduced mortality in comatose survivors after cardiac arrest treated with mild hypothermia (32–34°C) for a period of 12–72 h.

Intracranial aneurysms: Human-controlled studies have not shown clear-cut beneficial effects of hypothermia. A number of studies show some possible benefit of hypothermia as a last resort treatment for carefully selected subgroups of patients suffering cerebro-vascular spasm (CVS) following subarachnoid hemorrhage (SAH). Nevertheless – complications are often severe and should be closely monitored.

Traumatic brain injury: Hypothermia as a protective mechanism in traumatic brain injury is under debate. It has been shown to decrease ICP. Some studies have been able to show some benefit in particular subgroups of the study. Recent investigations show no overall beneficial effect of hypothermia on outcomes of traumatic brain injury. If a decision to induce hypothermia does occur – several factors must be taken into consideration:

- Opposing thermoregulatory responses to hypothermia: This means providing anesthesia/sedation and preventing shivering.
- Cooling techniques: There is a wide variety of techniques, invasive and noninvasive. The most appropriate technique should be selected.
- Rewarming: There is no consensus on the ideal time or rate for rewarming patients. Common practice is 0.5–1°C/h. When hypothermia is prolonged, rewarming may be as gradual as 1°C/day.

Key Points

- Shifts from a body core temperature of 36.6°C±0.2°C results in hyperthermia or hypothermia, causing pathophysiologic reactions, setting off a variety of response mechanisms. General anesthesia impairs normal regulation significantly.
- Effector mechanisms preventing hypothermia include: Vasoconstriction, Shivering, and Nonshivering thermogenesis.
- Factors contributing to hypothermia which may be modified include OR ambient temperature, drugs, exposure, and duration.

(continued)

- Core body temperature monitoring is extremely important, and is reliable when monitored in one of five sites – pulmonary artery, distal esophagus, nasopharynx, tympanic membrane, and bladder.
- Intervention in three phases of hypothermia is crucial: Phase 1 – minimizing redistribution hypothermia. Phase 2 – minimizing heat loss due to radiation or convection. Phase 3 – monitoring and prevention of hyperthermia in the vasoconstriction phase.
- Passive insulation and active warming are the mainstay of maintaining normothermia.
- Perioperative hypothermia causes a variety of systemic complications and should be avoided. Evidence advocating permissive hypothermia in neurosurgery is limited.
- Meperidine is the Opiate of choice for treatment of postoperative shivering.

Overview: Hyperthermia

Even a mild elevation in brain temperature may be detrimental to the hypoxic, ischemic, and injured brain. Hyperthermic states may be caused by a wide variety of clinical disorders which are divided into two major groups: (1) controlled hyperthermia – resulting from a deviation of thermoregulatory set points and thresholds, (2) uncontrolled hyperthermia – resulting from impaired thermoregulatory responses or excessive heat production. Table 38.6 lists major causes of hyperthermia.

Numerous studies have found pyrexia to be associated with increased mortality and morbidity after stroke. Early fever is associated with a poor Glasgow Coma Scale score in traumatic brain injury patients. Patients with subarachnoid hemorrhage are at increased risk for cerebral ischemia due to vasospasm. Hyperthermia may potentially worsen this vasospasm-mediated brain injury. Several studies have shown hyperpyrexia to be an independent risk factor, predicting worse outcomes in TBI, SAH, and ischemia. Blood in the cerebrospinal fluid induces fever in experimental models, and temperature is thus a likely marker for the primary severity of the hemorrhage. The major damage of hyperthermia is a result of direct cellular toxicity, i.e., deterioration of mitochondrial activity and, alterations of enzymatic reactions and cell membrane instability. Cellular effects may progress to widespread organ pathophysiologic reactions. *Muscle* damage, degeneration, and necrosis are direct results of extreme heat production and are associated with significant elevation in muscle enzymes. *Cardiovascular* effects caused by elevated core body temperature are associated with high cardiac output due to an increase in demand and diminished peripheral vascular resistance (secondary to vasodilation and dehydration), and tachyarrhythmias (sinus tachycardia, SVT, and also VT/VF). High-output cardiac failure and heat-induced myocardial damage often lead to various degrees of systemic hypotension.

Table 38.6 Major causes of hyperthermia

Increased heat production	Impaired heat loss	Surgical and medical conditions	Drugs
• ↑Metabolic rate	• High ambient	• Hypothalamic	• Anticholinergics
• Fever	temperature	bleeding	• Monoamine
• Heat stroke	and humidity	• Fourth ventricle	oxidase
• Thyrotoxicosis,	• Excessive	bleeding	inhibitors
thyroid storm	heating	• CNS lesions	• Serotonin releasers
• Pheochromocytoma	• Cardiovascular	• Hemispherectomy	• Serotonin reuptake
• Drugs: amphet-	disease	• Infectious causes	inhibitors
amines,	• Hypokalemia	• Meningitis	• Amphetamines
halucinogens	• Dehydration	• Encephalitis	• Ecstasy
• Malignant	• Old age	• Cerebral abscess	• LSD
hyperthermia	• Skin disease	• Subdural empyema	• Tricyclic
• Neuroleptic	• Cystic fibrosis	• Medullary abscess	antidepressants
malignant		• Sepsis	• Analgesics
syndrome			• Antihistamines
			• Phenothiazines
			• Butyrophenones
			• Thiothixenes
			• Barbiturates
			• Anti-Parkinsonian
			agents
			• Diuretics
			• β-Blockers
			• Alcohol

CBF and CMR are increased by elevated body temperature (between 37 and 42°C), but above 42°C cerebral oxygen consumption decreases due to cellular enzymatic degradation. Uncoupling of CNS metabolism may lead to further damage if CBF is compromised, and may have deleterious effects on the noncompliant brain by raising ICP. Other effects of hyperthermia on the injured and ischemic brain include direct brain and spinal cord toxicity associated with cell death, alterations in membrane stability, enzyme function and neurotransmitter release, BBB disruption, cerebral edema and local hemorrhage, epileptic activity, and increased peritumoral edema. These processes may lead to profound stupor, coma, and seizures. In conscious patients – ataxia, dysmetria, and dysarthria may be seen. *CSF* analysis may reveal increased protein levels, xanthochromia, and slightly elevated lymphocyte count. Any underlying pathological condition of the central nervous system (traumatic brain injury, ischemic stroke, intracranial hemorrhage) may be adversely affected by hyperthermia, and clinical outcomes may be worse. Coexisting hyperthermia and impaired brain autoregulation in brain injury may put patients at risk for cerebral hypoperfusion during periods of low blood pressure, whereas they may be prone to the development of vasogenic edema, vascular engorgement, and worsening of intracranial hypertension during periods of high blood pressure.

Hyperthermic reactions may cause acute renal failure (incidence 5%) secondary to dehydration, hypotension, and muscle damage. Acute tubular necrosis with

Table 38.7 Clinical and laboratory manifestations of hyperthermia

Clinical manifestations	
Cardiovascular effects	Tachyarrhythmia, various degree of systemic hypotension
Neurologic effects	Ataxia, dysmetria, dysarthria, profound stupor, coma and seizures
Respiratory	Pulmonary edema, ARDS
Renal failure	Acute tubular necrosis, renal failure
Muscle	Degeneration and necrosis, rhabdomyolysis
Gastrointestinal	Bleeding, elevated liver enzymes, cholestasis, and hepatic necrosis
Laboratory tests	
White blood cell count	Elevated
Coagulation	DIC
Electrolytes, chemistry, hormones	Hyperglycemia, elevated serum cortisol, growth hormone, and aldosterone levels
	Hypokalemia, mild hypophosphatemia, and hypocalcemia

moderate proteinuria is more common. In the gastrointestinal tract, hyperthermia frequently leads to ischemic ulcerations that may result in bleeding, elevated liver enzymes, cholestasis and hepatic necrosis.

White blood cell count is frequently elevated in hyperthermic patients. In cases of fatal hyperthermia DIC may evolve, leading to bleeding diathesis and multiple organ failure. Laboratory blood tests will reveal hyperglycemia, elevated serum cortisol, and elevated growth hormone and aldosterone levels. Electrolyte disorders include decreased serum potassium, mild hypophosphatemia, and hypocalcemia. Pulmonary thermal injury may cause cor-pulmonale and ARDS. Pulmonary edema is also common. Table 38.7 summarizes the major clinical and laboratory manifestations of hyperthermia.

Prevention: Hyperthermia

Core body temperature should be measured continuously throughout the entire perioperative period. Core temperature is best reflected by measurements in five sites: tympanic membrane, pulmonary artery, distal esophagus, nasopharynx, and bladder. Rectal temperature tends to lag behind core body temperature.

Crisis Management: Hyperthermia

Hyperthermia is suggested by recording above normal core temperature. The diagnosis is confirmed by history and physical examination of the patient. A thorough examination and diagnostic evaluation for all vital signs (pulse, blood pressure, oxygenation, $ETCO_2$, arterial blood gas analysis) should be conducted to identify the particular cause of hyperthermia. Differential diagnosis must include most common causes of hyperthermic state (Table 38.6). The most common cause of intraoperative hyperthermia is passive hyperthermia caused by excessive insulation and heating.

Hypothalamic tumors or intraoperative brain hemorrhage may produce hyperthermia by elevating core body temperature and may be distinguished from heat stroke or severe infection, by noting associated clinical conditions such as diabetes insipidus and anhydrosis. Central nervous system infections are characterized by relevant history, clinical signs, and elevated enzyme and white cell count in CSF.

While the underlying cause of hyperthermia should be sought, symptomatically correcting fever in the brain-damaged patient is warranted, minimizing damage and improving outcomes. The ideal method (physical cooling or pharmacologic) for treating hyperpyrexia is not yet clear. Disadvantages of physical cooling include patient discomfort, limited effectiveness, and elevation of CMR and catecholamine levels – particularly in instances of "controlled" fever. Some evidence exists, demonstrating advantages in pharmacologic control of hyperpyrexia in brain-injured patients. Nevertheless, the benefits of pharmacologic antipyretic therapy, compared with associated risks, have not been clearly established.

Malignant hyperthermia is a rare but fatal phenomena encountered in anesthesia. Most commonly, it occurs under severe stress and after administration of triggering anesthetic agents (most notable – volatile anesthetics and succinylcholine). Several reports have associated brainstem hemorrhage with MH like symptoms. Hyperthermia is usually a late sign, and is preceded by masseter muscle contraction, tachyarrhythmia, combined respiratory and metabolic acidosis, muscle rigidity, and hypertension. Aberrations in calcium homeostasis may contribute to increased neuronal damage. The cerebellum has been noted to be particularly vulnerable. Neuroleptic malignant syndrome may be diagnosed by history of use of neuroleptic agents (butyrophenones, phenothiazines, thioxanthenes, dopamine-depleting agents, and others). A wide variety of other drugs not included in this category have been suspected to cause hyperthermia as well. The use of Haloperidol for treatment of agitation in TBI patients is increasing. Several reports have shown TBI patients to have greater risk of developing NMS following this treatment, and particular attention should be given to early detection. If malignant hyperthermia is suspected, Dantrolene (IV Dantrolene Sodium 1–10 mg/kg) must be administered as soon as possible. Forced diuresis and hemodialysis may be indicated to treat rhabdomyolysis and renal failure. Supportive therapy aimed at treating systemic disturbances (tachyarrhythmias, hypotension, decreased urine output, and metabolic acidosis) associated with hyperthermia should be initiated. Continuously monitoring arterial blood gas analysis, urine output, and serum electrolytes are critical in the management of the acute crisis.

Treatment of hyperthermic disorders depends on the etiology of underlying cause. The following approach is suggested (Fig. 38.2).

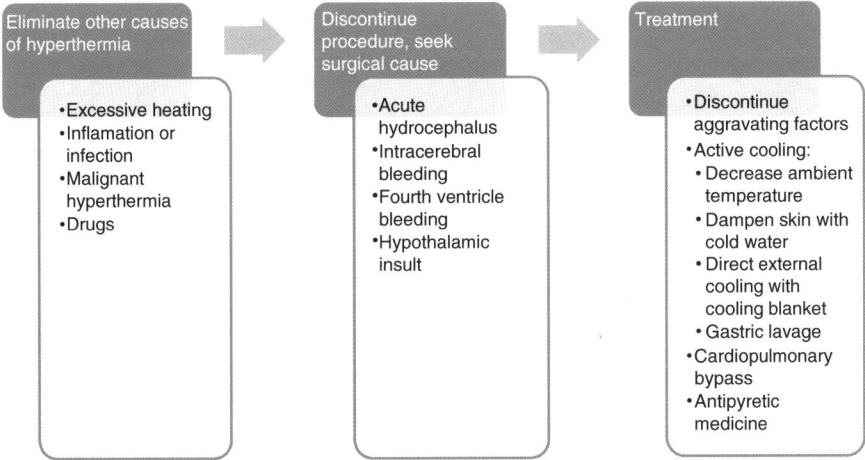

Fig. 38.2 Treatment approach for hyperthermia

Key Points

- Hyperthermia is caused by a variety of clinical states. It is important to differentiate controlled and uncontrolled hyperthermia and evaluate the underlying cause.
- Continuous temperature monitoring is essential, and may be an indicator of a life-threatening syndrome.
- Malignant hyperthermia is life threatening and should be treated promptly. Elevated core temperature lags behind other signs and symptoms. When suspected, discontinue causative agents, treat with IV Dantrolene, cool patient, and provide support.
- Surgical intraoperative causes of hyperthermia include acute hydrocephalus, fourth ventricle bleeding, hypothalamic insult, and intracerebral bleeding.
- Treatment depends on etiology, and includes active cooling and pharmacologic antipyretic therapy, and is warranted particularly in the injured brain.

Suggested Reading

Hypothermia

Hutchison JS, Ward RE, Lacroix J, Hebert PC, Barnes MA, Bohn DJ, et al. Hypothermia therapy after traumatic brain injury in children. N Engl J Med. 2008;358:2447–56.

Kurz A. Thermal care in the perioperative period. Best Pract Res Clin Anaesthesiol. 2008;22:39–62.

Marion DW. Moderate hypothermia in severe head injuries: the present and the future. Curr Opin Crit Care. 2002;8:111–4.

Matsukawa T, Sessler DI, Sessler AM, Schroeder M, Ozaki M, Kurz A, et al. Heat flow and distribution during induction of general anesthesia. Anesthesiology. 1995;82:662–73.

Sessler DI. Temperature monitoring and perioperative thermoregulation. Anesthesiology. 2008;109:318–38.

Sessler DI, McGuire J, Sessler AM. Perioperative thermal insulation. Anesthesiology. 1991;74:875–9.

Seule MA, Muroi C, Mink S, Yonekawa Y, Keller E. Therapeutic hypothermia in patients with aneurysmal subarachnoid hemorrhage, refractory intracranial hypertension, or cerebral vasospasm. Neurosurgery. 2008;64(1):86–92. discussion 92–3.

Todd MM, Hindman BJ, Clarke WR, Torner JC. Mild intraoperative hypothermia during surgery for intracranial aneurysm. N Engl J Med. 2005;352:135–45.

Hyperthermia

Cairns CJ, Andrews PJ. Management of hyperthermia in traumatic brain injury. Curr Opin Crit Care. 2002;8:106–10.

Cormio M, Citerio G, Portella G, Patruno A, Pesenti A. Treatment of fever in neurosurgical patients. Minerva Anestesiol. 2003;69:214–22.

Grogan H, Hopkins PM. Heat stroke: implications for critical care and anaesthesia. Br J Anaesth. 2002;88:700–7.

Lenhardt R, Grady M, Kurz A. Hyperthermia during anaesthesia and intensive care unit stay. Best Pract Res Clin Anaesthesiol. 2008;22:669–94.

Roth J, Rummel C, Barth SW, Gerstberger R, Hubschle T. Molecular aspects of fever and hyperthermia. Neurol Clin. 2006;24:421–39.

Washington DE, Sessler DI, Moayeri A, Merrifield B, McGuire J, Prager M, et al. Thermoregulatory responses to hyperthermia during isoflurane anesthesia in humans. J Appl Physiol. 1993;74:82–7.

Chapter 39
Challenges Associated with Perioperative Monitoring During Neurosurgery

Osama Ahmed and Claudia Robertson

Invasive neuromonitoring in the perioperative period includes monitoring of intracranial pressure (ICP) and brain oxygenation. In some circumstances, the patient will already have these monitors preoperatively. Alternatively, the monitors may be placed as a part of the operative procedure or postoperatively. Other types of neuromonitoring are performed in the perioperative period, including electroencephalography, near-infrared spectroscopy, and transcranial Doppler. These procedures are noninvasive and have minimal risk of complications.

ICP monitoring provides information about the volume of intracranial contents. An increase in any intracranial compartment or development of a mass lesion will raise ICP. Normally, resting ICP is less than 10 mmHg. A sustained ICP greater than 20 mmHg is clearly abnormal. An ICP between 20 and 40 mmHg is considered moderate intracranial hypertension. An ICP greater than 40 mmHg represents severe, usually life-threatening, intracranial hypertension. These thresholds for severity of intracranial hypertension assume a normal blood pressure. When a temporal mass lesion is present, however, herniation can occur at ICP values less than 20 mmHg.

Measures of cerebral oxygenation, such as jugular venous oxygen saturation ($SjvO_2$) or brain tissue pO_2 ($PbtO_2$) are used as a surrogate for cerebral perfusion, because they give an indicator of the adequacy of cerebral blood flow (CBF) relative to cerebral metabolic requirements. Since cerebral metabolic requirements may be reduced in neurological disorders, normal CBF values may not apply. When CBF is low (25–30 ml/100 g/min), it can be difficult to decide if this is an appropriate response to lower cerebral metabolic requirements or whether the brain is hypoperfused. A measure of cerebral oxygenation can be helpful in making this distinction.

O. Ahmed, MD (✉)
Department of Neurosurgery, Louisiana State University Health Sciences Center Shreveport, Shreveport, LA, USA

C. Robertson, MD
Department of Neurosurgery, Baylor College of Medicine, Houston, TX, USA

A.M. Brambrink and J.R. Kirsch (eds.), *Essentials of Neurosurgical Anesthesia & Critical Care*, DOI 10.1007/978-0-387-09562-2_39,
© Springer Science+Business Media, LLC 2012

If the brain is hypoperfused, brain oxygenation will be reduced. If CBF is appropriate for the brain's metabolic requirement, then brain oxygenation will be normal. Often this information is more clinically useful than the absolute CBF values.

Intracranial Pressure Monitoring

Overview

Although several new types of monitors have become commercially available, the ventriculostomy catheter remains the best device for monitoring ICP in most circumstances. The ventriculostomy catheter is positioned with its tip in the frontal horn of the lateral ventricle and is coupled by fluid-filled tubing to an external pressure transducer that can be reset to zero and recalibrated against an external standard. This arrangement provides the most reliable measurement of ICP throughout the normal and pathologic ranges. In addition, a ventriculostomy catheter allows treatment of an elevated ICP by intermittent drainage of cerebrospinal fluid. However, the risk of ventriculitis and of intracranial hemorrhage is highest with ventriculostomy, and proper placement of the catheter tip in the lateral ventricle can be difficult in patients with small, compressed ventricles.

When the ventricle cannot be cannulated, alternative devices that incorporate a miniaturized transducer at the tip of the catheter can be used. These miniature pressure transducer-tipped catheters can be inserted in the subdural space or directly into brain tissue. The main advantage of these monitors is the ease of insertion, especially in patients with compressed ventricles. They provide more reliable measures of ICP than subarachnoid bolts and fluid-coupled catheters in the subdural space because they have no lumen to become obstructed. The transducers, however, cannot be reset to zero after they are inserted into the skull, and they exhibit drift over time.

Prevention

The two major complications of ICP monitoring are ventriculitis and hemorrhage. Infection may be confined to the skin wound, but in 1–10% of cases, ventriculitis occurs. Factors that predispose to ventriculitis are: intraventricular hemorrhage, subarachnoid hemorrhage, cranial fracture with CSF leak, craniotomy, systemic infections, catheter manipulation, leak, and irrigation. Duration of catheterization is correlated with an increasing risk of CSF infections during the first 10 days of use. Prophylactic catheter exchange does not reduce risk of infection. Systemic prophylactic antibiotics are ineffective in reducing infections, but antibiotic-impregnated ventriculostomy catheters have been shown to reduce the risk of CSF infection from 9.4 to 1.3%. The best strategies for reducing the risk of ventriculitis associated with ICP monitoring are the use of meticulous aseptic technique with the catheter insertion, the use of antibiotic-impregnated catheters, and minimization of the duration of the monitoring.

The second major complication of ICP monitoring is intracerebral hemorrhage. Although the risk of hemorrhage has been shown to be consistently low (1–2%), it is an important complication to recognize and treat. Patients with coagulopathies are at a greater risk of developing this complication. Some evidence suggests that an INR ≤ 1.6 has a very low risk of hemorrhage, if a parenchymal catheter is placed.

Crisis Management

Ventriculitis is diagnosed by culture of the cerebrospinal fluid, and clinical findings of fever, altered mental status, headache. Treatment of catheter-related ventriculitis is removal of the catheter, when possible, and appropriate antibiotics.

Treatment of catheter-induced hemorrhage depends on the size. If small, the hemorrhage can be observed. If large or associated with significant ICP elevation or neurological deterioration, then the hematoma will usually need surgical evacuation.

Key Points About ICP Monitoring

- Ventriculostomy catheters are preferred in many circumstances because of greater accuracy, and because ICP can be treated by draining CSF.
- Miniature transducer tipped catheters are an alternative to the ventriculostomy catheter and are easier to insert, have lower risk of complications, but measurements can drift over time.
- The rate of ventriculitis can be up to 10% with ICP monitoring.
- Factors that reduce the risk of developing ventriculitis include meticulous aseptic technique in placing the catheter, use of antibiotic-impregnated catheters, and minimizing the duration of monitoring.
- Practices that do not reduce the risk of developing ventriculitis include prophylactic changing of the catheter and prophylactic antibiotics.
- Treatment of catheter-induced ventriculitis is the removal of catheter when that is feasible and appropriate antibiotics.
- The risk of intracranial hemorrhage from ICP monitor placement is low (1–2%) but may require surgical evacuation if the hematoma is large.

Jugular Venous Oxygen Saturation Monitoring

Overview

To monitor $SjvO_2$, a fiberoptic oxygen saturation catheter is placed percutaneously in the jugular vein with the tip positioned in the jugular bulb. Because there may be incomplete mixing of cerebral venous blood before the sagittal sinus divides into the right and left transverse sinuses, significant differences in oxygen saturation values may exist between the two internal jugular bulbs. One strategy for deciding which internal jugular vein to cannulate is to select the dominant side. This can be determined directly by ultrasound or indirectly by assessing the ICP rise to temporary compression of the internal jugular vein. The side with the dominant flow will have the greatest ICP rise during compression.

Prevention

Potential complications of $SjvO_2$ monitoring can be divided into those associated with insertion of the catheter, including carotid artery puncture, injury to nerves in the neck and pneumothorax, and those associated with the catheter remaining in the jugular vein, including infection, an increase in ICP and venous thrombosis.

Carotid puncture is the most common complication associated with internal jugular vein catheterization. However, it rarely has serious consequences, and the risk can be minimized by making certain that the puncture is lateral to the carotid pulsation and through the use of ultrasound to guide insertion. Most arterial punctures can be managed conservatively by applying local pressure for 10 min. Other insertion complications, such as pneumothorax, are rare when inserting jugular bulb catheters.

Line sepsis is a complication that is commonly associated with all types of indwelling catheters. Most studies have reported an overall rate of 0–5 episodes of infection per 100 catheters. Proper sterile technique in the placement and maintenance of the jugular bulb catheter should be observed to minimize this risk.

ICP can be increased by maneuvers that obstruct venous return from the brain, and concern that a catheter in the jugular vein might raise ICP has been addressed. The 4F or 5F catheter used for $SjvO_2$ monitoring is quite small relative to the lumen of the internal jugular vein, especially when the dominant vein is cannulated, and does not significantly raise ICP.

Nonobstructive, subclinical thrombus in the internal jugular venous has been observed in up to 40% of patients undergoing bulb catheterization. Symptomatic thrombosis of the internal jugular vein is very uncommon with jugular bulb catheters but could have serious consequences. Depending on the normal flow to the thrombosed internal jugular vein, the obstruction could impair venous return from the head and elevate ICP.

> **Key Points About SjvO$_2$ Monitoring**
>
> - SjvO$_2$ monitoring provides a continuous measure of the adequacy of cerebral perfusion relative to cerebral metabolic requirements.
> - The dominant internal jugular vein should be cannulated for SjvO$_2$ monitoring.
> - Insertion complications, such as carotid puncture and pneumothorax, are uncommon but can be minimized by the use of ultrasound guidance.
> - Insertion of a jugular bulb catheter does not obstruct venous flow sufficiently to raise ICP.
> - Nonocclusive thrombosis of the internal jugular vein occurs in up to 40% with jugular bulb catheters but is rarely symptomatic.

Brain Tissue pO$_2$ Monitoring

Overview

Local cerebral oxygenation can be monitored continuously using an intraparenchymal Clark-type pO$_2$ sensitive catheter. The catheter measures pO$_2$ over a surface area of 13 mm^2 and, therefore, gives an average tissue pO$_2$ value for the brain around the tip of the catheter. The location of the catheter tip is, therefore, critical in interpreting the PbtO$_2$ values. When the catheter is placed in relatively normal brain, trends of PbtO$_2$ generally represent global brain oxygenation. When the catheter is placed in an area of injured brain, the PbtO$_2$ values reflect the local pO$_2$ in that area of the brain. This can be an advantage in heterogeneous disorders like traumatic brain injury.

Prevention

The complications associated with PbtO$_2$ monitoring are similar to that with ICP monitoring and include infection and hemorrhage. Since the PbtO$_2$ catheter is smaller in diameter than ICP catheters, the risk of hemorrhage is probably much lower. Prevention strategies are similar to those associated with ICP monitoring and include aseptic technique when placing the catheters and limiting the duration of monitoring.

Key Points About PbtO$_2$ Monitoring

- PbtO$_2$ catheters give a local measure of tissue pO$_2$ in the brain around the tip of the catheter.
- When the PbtO$_2$ catheter is in relatively normal brain, the pO$_2$ values reflect global cerebral oxygenation.
- When the PbtO$_2$ catheter is in injured brain, the pO$_2$ values reflect the local tissue oxygenation near the tip of the catheter.
- Complications of PbtO$_2$ catheters are similar to ICP catheters, but the risk of hemorrhage is probably lower because of the smaller diameter of the catheter.

Suggested Reading

Bratton SL, Chestnut RM, Ghajar J, Connell Hammond FF, Harris OA, Hartl R, et al. Guidelines for the management of severe traumatic brain injury. VII. Intracranial pressure monitoring technology. J Neurotrauma. 2007;24 Suppl 1:S45–54.

Coplin WM, O'Keefe GE, Grady MS, Grant GA, March KS, Winn HR, et al. Thrombotic, infectious, and procedural complications of the jugular bulb catheter in the intensive care unit. Neurosurgery. 1997;41:101–7.

Davis JW, Davis IC, Bennink LD, Hysell SE, Curtis BV, Kaups KL, et al. Placement of intracranial pressure monitors: are "normal" coagulation parameters necessary? J Trauma. 2004;57:1173–7.

Stiefel MF, Spiotta A, Gracias VH, Garuffe AM, Guillamondegui O, Maloney-Wilenshky E, et al. Reduced mortality rate in patients with severe traumatic brain injury treated with brain tissue oxygen monitoring. J Neurosurg. 2005;103:805–11.

Zabramski JM, Whiting D, Darouiche RO, Horner TG, Olson J, Robertson C, et al. Efficacy of antimicrobial-impregnated external ventricular drain catheters: a prospective, randomized, controlled trial. J Neurosurg. 2003;98:725–30.

Chapter 40
Unintended Wake-Up During Neurosurgery

Jeffrey Yoder and Chris C. Lee

Overview

Unintended wake-up during neurosurgery is a potentially catastrophic complication that can be limited with appropriate vigilance. Light anesthesia may present as movement, coughing, and/or hemodynamic response. Intraoperative arousal can lead to hypertension, increased surgical bleeding, cardiopulmonary complications, and risk of recall. Special concerns in neurosurgical patients also include risk of increased ICP and/or herniation, increased cerebral edema, and potential injury from movement while in pins.

These patients are at increased risk for the occurrence of light anesthesia for several reasons. Many procedures wax between minimal and intense stimulation, given that the scalp, dura, and cranial nerves carry pain fibers while the brain itself is insensate. Due to the desire for a prompt awakening, longer-acting agents and high dosages of anesthetic/analgesics are often avoided. However, these patients may also be at increased risk due to tolerance (from chronic benzodiazepine or opioid use) and/or enzymatic induction of the P450 system, such as caused by anti-epileptic medications. Therefore, effect and duration of action of muscle relaxants, opioids, and other agents may be decreased.

The anesthesia provider must pay close attention to anesthetic depth, administration of analgesics, and level of stimulation in order to avoid unintended patient arousal. Prevention is key; however, early recognition and treatment of light anesthesia is important to minimize complications.

J. Yoder, MD (✉)
Saint Anthony's Hospital, Denver, CO, USA
e-mail: jyoder8@gmail.com

C.C. Lee, MD, PhD
Department of Anesthesiology, Washington University School of Medicine in St. Louis,
St. Louis, MO, USA

A.M. Brambrink and J.R. Kirsch (eds.), *Essentials of Neurosurgical Anesthesia & Critical Care*, DOI 10.1007/978-0-387-09562-2_40, © Springer Science+Business Media, LLC 2012

Prevention

Attention to anesthetic depth is critical. The provider must ensure that the patient is adequately anesthetized and has appropriate analgesia for the procedure being performed. Intraoperative hypertension and/or tachycardia should prompt an immediate reassessment of the patient with consideration toward light anesthesia.

Stimulating events must be anticipated. Examples include:

- Laryngoscopy and intubation
- Pinning
- Surgical incision, manipulation of scalp wound
- Surgical manipulation of dura
- Manipulation of cranial nerves
- Request from surgeon for Valsalva maneuver.

Special care should be taken to confirm that the patient has adequate anesthesia and analgesia prior to these events. It is prudent to deepen the anesthetic and/or give a bolus of opioid (e.g., IV fentanyl 50–100 mcg or alfentanil 10 mcg/kg) prior to events such as pinning and start of surgery.

Depth of anesthesia monitors are poorly predictive of the risk of patient arousal as these quantitative measures lag behind changes in the level of stimulation. As movement by anesthetized patients in response to surgical stimulus is primarily mediated via the spinal cord, cortical EEG-based monitors are unable to effectively predict patient movement. However, these monitors may have some use in following trends, particularly when a total intravenous anesthetic is performed. These monitors, for example, can aid in the detection of inadvertent discontinuation of anesthetic infusion, such as IV disconnect or infiltration.

Adequate analgesia is essential for the prevention of hemodynamic responses, coughing/straining, and other movement. Short-acting opioids (remifentanil, alfentanil, and fentanyl) may be preferable for allowing a rapid emergence at the conclusion of surgery or a planned intraoperative wake-up. Continuous infusion of remifentanil has been demonstrated to decrease movement in non-paralyzed patients during craniotomy in a dose-dependent manner. Dexmedetomidine (0.2–0.7 mcg/kg/h) can also be a useful anesthesia adjunct for its sedative, sympatholytic, and opioid sparring properties. Dexmedetomidine has been demonstrated to improve perioperative hemodynamic stability in patients undergoing craniotomy.

Pharmacologic paralysis with non-depolarizing muscle relaxants is preferred for patients when pinned, especially for intracranial surgery, unless precluded by neuromonitoring techniques such as transcranial motor evoked potentials, EMG, or planned intraoperative wake-up. Due to the risk to the patient from coughing and movement in pins, paralytic drugs can provide an additional margin of safety. When paralytics must be avoided, adequate analgesia is imperative as is strict attention to detail. For non-paralyzed patients, especially while pinned, an intravenous anesthetic (such as a syringe of propofol) should be immediately available to deepen the plane of anesthesia.

Conclusion of surgery and emergence from anesthesia require special attention to timing to prevent an early wake-up. This is of particular importance when the patient is in pins, positioned other than supine, and/or the anesthesia provider has limited access to the patient's airway. Premature discontinuation of anesthetics and/or administration of neuromuscular reversal, especially before pins are removed, can place patients at risk.

Crisis Management

Pathophysiology and Clinical Presentation

Neurosurgical patients are at increased risk for complications secondary to unintended wake-ups due to multiple reasons:

- Positioning – Movement while in pins can result in cervical spine injury or dislocation of pins. Change in position can also interfere with neuroimaging/navigation systems such as STEALTH or intraoperative MRI. As the anesthesia provider often has limited access to the patient after surgery start, patient movement can risk loss of airway, lines, or monitors.
- Increased ICP – Coughing and straining result in increased ICP by the transmission of increased venous pressures. Increased ICP may lead to herniation syndromes within the closed skull, or produce a bulging brain or frank herniation through a craniotomy.
- Bleeding – Perioperative hypertension has been shown to be associated with intracranial hemorrhage following craniotomy. Bulging or herniation through a craniotomy may also result in a hemorrhagic brain. Coughing/straining and hypertension can all increase the danger of aneurysmal rupture in at risk patients.
- Cerebral hyperemia – Hypertension and tachycardia contribute to cerebral hyperemia which may worsen cerebral edema and contribute to bleeding risk.
- Direct tissue injury by in situ surgical instruments during unexpected movement.
- Cardiovascular complications.
- Intraoperative awareness.

Patient Assessment

Light anesthesia typically presents as hypertension, tachycardia, and possibly movement in patients without significant pharmacologic paralysis. The occurrence of any of the above should prompt an immediate reassessment of the patient and should be directed toward rapid differentiation of light anesthesia from other potential causes. As many patients receive beta-blockers and other anti-hypertensives, these early signs of light anesthesia may not be present in some patients, making it very difficult to predict when a patient may move. Other patients have exaggerated hemodynamic responses to anesthesia and may not maintain a reasonable blood pressure at target values of either intravenous or inhaled agents.

Differential Diagnoses

- Light anesthesia/pain
- Increased ICP (hypertension)
- Cerebral ischemia
- Drug effect
- Volume depletion/blood loss and anemia (tachycardia)
- Essential – hypertension
- VAE (tachycardia)
- Seizure
- Electrical stimulation of motor cortex.

Clinical suspicion of light anesthesia should trigger an assessment of the current anesthetic regimen/dosage, opioids administered, and level of stimulation.

- Check the vital signs. Hypertension and tachycardia generally accompany light anesthesia but should be limited due to risk of complications.
- Check that the patient is receiving the planned anesthetic regimen: vaporizer full and appropriate ET agent concentration for current setting, IV lines running and intravenous anesthetics being received.
- Check progress of surgical procedure with attention toward recent changes in the level of stimulation, and likelihood of intracranial hypertension and/or ischemia.
- Check train-of-four ratio or other assessment of neuromuscular blockade.

Intervention/Treatment

- Ask for temporary cessation of surgical stimulation and removal of surgical instruments (if possible).
- Intermittent mandatory ventilation can exacerbate coughing in a light patient. Consider changing to a synchronous breathing mode or briefly discontinue the ventilator and open the pop-off valve.
- Deepen the anesthetic. This can be most rapidly accomplished with a bolus of an intravenous agent (e.g., propofol 50 mg).
- Ensure adequate analgesia. Consider additional fast-acting opioid administration, (e.g., fentanyl 100–200 mcg).
- Control hemodynamic response. Intravenous esmolol is well suited to this purpose as it is short acting, and does not increase cerebral blood flow. Exercise caution with coadministration of anti-hypertensives and anesthetic bolus to avoid hypotension.

- After the patient is reanesthetized, consider redose of non-depolarizing muscle relaxant.
- In procedures where neuromuscular blocking agents would be contraindicated, the anesthesia provider may need to administer an infusion of a vasopressor (e.g., phenylephrine) so that a deeper plane of anesthesia may be achieved, in patients who become hypotensive from subanesthetic concentrations of inhaled or intravenous agents.
- Recheck patient positioning with specific attention to pressure points, airway, monitors, and IV access.
- Evaluate and treat for potential neurologic sequelae.
- Assess the patient postoperatively for recall. Intraoperative awareness has the potential to cause prolonged psychological and emotional distress. When intraoperative recall is deemed likely, it is important to provide explanation and reassurance. Follow-up and consider referral to a psychologist.

Key Points

- Prevention is key. Maintain an adequate plane of anesthesia and anticipate stimulating events
- Anticipate higher anesthetic requirements in at-risk patients
- Ensure adequate analgesia for the procedure being performed
- Pharmacologic paralysis is preferred for craniotomies and patients in pins
- Rapid intervention in cases of light anesthesia can limit complications from movement, coughing, and hypertension
- Support hemodynamics pharmacologically when patient's blood pressure will not tolerate target concentrations of inhaled or intravenous anesthetic agents.

Suggested Reading

Basali A, Mascha EJ, Kalfas I, Schubert A. Relation between perioperative hypertension and intracranial hemorrhage after craniotomy. Anesthesiology. 2000;93(1):48–54.

Bekker A, Sturaitis M, Bloom M, Moric M, Golfinos J, Parker E, et al. The effect of dexmedetomidine on perioperative hemodynamics in patients undergoing craniotomy. Anesth Analg. 2008;107:1340–7.

Grillo P, Bruder N, Auquier P, Pellissier D, Gouin F. Esmolol blunts the cerebral blood flow velocity increase during emergence from anesthesia in neurosurgical patients. Anesth Analg. 2003;96:1145–9.

Jameson LC, Sloan TB. Using EEG to monitor anesthesia drug effects during surgery. J Clin Monit Comput. 2006;20:445–72.

Rose JC, Mayer SA. Optimizing blood pressure in neurological emergencies. Neurocrit Care. 2004;1:287–99.

Chapter 41
Cardiac Arrest/Code

Michael Bernhard, Jürgen Knapp, and Bernd W. Böttiger

Overview

It is not known how many patients suffer cardiocirculatory arrest and need to be resuscitated while in the hospital. However, we do know that fewer than 20% of patients who suffer cardiocirculatory arrest in the hospital survive and leave the clinic again. We also know that during and around surgery 2 out of 1,000 patients develop myocardial infarction – which is one of the most important causes of cardiocirculatory arrest (Table 41.1). For major surgery or surgery associated with a high loss of blood, the risk of cardiovascular complications is as high as 2%. Successful cardiopulmonary resuscitation (CPR) requires intensive practical instruction and training and good teamwork as well.

Prevention

There is no sure means of preventing cardiocirculatory arrest. Thus, it is all the more important to preoperatively identify those patients who are at risk of developing cardiocirculatory arrest due to previous diseases (e.g., coronary heart disease, diabetes associated with renal insufficiency) or who present with risk factors (e.g., perioperative myocardial infarction, electrolytic disturbance, Table 41.1) and to monitor these individuals intensively and give appropriate treatment.

M. Bernhard, MD (✉)
Emergency Department/Emergency Admission Unit, University Hospital of Leipzig,
Leipzig, Germany

J. Knapp, MD
Department of Anesthesiology, University of Heidelberg, Heidelberg, Germany

B.W. Böttiger
Department of Anesthesiology and Intensive Care Medicine,
University of Cologne School of Medicine, Cologne, Germany

A.M. Brambrink and J.R. Kirsch (eds.), *Essentials of Neurosurgical Anesthesia & Critical Care*, DOI 10.1007/978-0-387-09562-2_41,
© Springer Science+Business Media, LLC 2012

Table 41.1 Causes of cardiocirculatory arrest

Etiology	Cause
Cardiac: 70–90%	– Myocardial infarction
	– Cardiac arrhythmia
	– Pericardial tamponade
	– Pulmonary embolism
Noncardiac: 10–30%	– Bleeding
	– Intoxication
	– Metabolic lapse/electrolytic disturbance
	– Suffocation
	– Central respiratory depression
	– Tension pneumothorax
	– Severe hypovolemia
	– Anaphylaxia

Crisis Management

Patients undergoing surgery and intensive care patients who are intubated and ventilated comprise special circumstances. In the following we present procedures for standard situations. Particularly in the operating room and in the intensive care unit; however, patients are often being monitored continuously so that cardiocirculatory arrest is detected sooner and the appropriate treatment can be implemented earlier. In Europe CPR measures are carried out according to the Guidelines of the European Resuscitation Council (ERC) (Fig. 41.1).

Clinical Presentation of Cardiac Arrest

- After 10–15 s patient is unconscious (collapse).
- After 15–45 s cerebral convulsions may develop.
- After 30–120 s pupils are dilated and the skin color is pale to cyanotic.
- Patient may show symptoms of the underlying disease (Table 41.1).

Patient Assessment

Checking State of Consciousness, If the Patient Is Not Intubated

- Speak loudly and clearly to the patient (if the patient is not sedated or anesthetized).
- Use tactile stimulation (e.g., shake, pain stimulus).
- Call additional personnel for help.

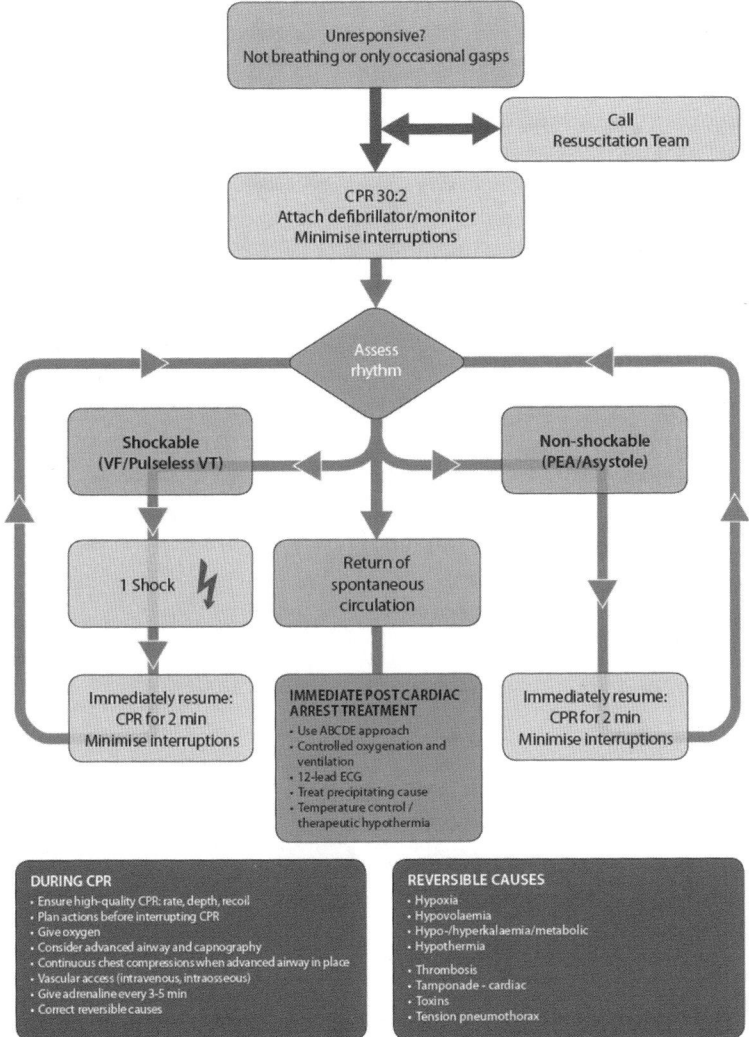

Fig. 41.1 CRP Algorithm of the Guideline of the European Resuscitation Council

Check Breathing

- Check breathing for no longer than 10 s.
- Do not mistake gasping for adequate breathing.
- When in doubt, assume that breathing is inadequate and start resuscitation.
- If the patient is intubated: check the ventilation, airway patency, and the respirator.

Checking the Pulse

- Look for "signs of life" (e.g., coughing, pressing, and spontaneous movement).
- At the same time manually palpate the carotid artery (total time for checking the pulse, max. 10 s). Never palpate the two carotid vessels at the same time.
- If cardiocirculatory arrest is diagnosed: immediately start chest compression and face mask ventilation (compression–ventilation ratio: 30:2).
- If a pulse can be felt: secure airways and measure blood pressure.
- If the patient has invasive arterial blood pressure monitoring: check monitor and arterial access.

Medical History from Third Party

- Without delaying resuscitation measures obtain the patient's medical history from a third party in order to gain additional information that may reveal potentially reversible conditions [electrolytic disorder, intoxication (Table 41.2)].
- Review the ICU documentation, check for recently performed interventions (e.g., central venous catheter placement).

Treatment

- Call for additional help (optimize manpower).
- Immediately start chest compressions.
- Treat potentially reversible causes.

Table 41.2 Potentially reversible causes and specific treatment options during CPR

Cause	Treatment option
Hypoxia	Intubation and ventilation with 100% oxygen, check position of the tube and exclude malpositioning
Hypovolemia	Blood volume support and possibly surgical repair of the cause of bleeding
Hyperkalemia	Administration of glucose and insulin (while monitoring serum glucose concentration and electrolytes), administration of calcium (while monitoring electrolytes)
Hypokalemia	Administration of potassium (while monitoring electrolytes)
Hypocalcemia	Administration of calcium (while monitoring electrolytes)
Acidosis	Administer sodium bicarbonate buffer (while monitoring electrolytes and blood gases)
Severe hypothermia	CPR and immediate extracorporeal circulation
Tension pneumothorax	Relieve, thoracic drainage
Pericardial tamponade	Pericardiocentesis (ultrasonographically guided)
Pulmonary embolism and myocardial infarction	Thrombolysis and/or PTCA, if necessary
Intoxication	Administration of antidote, gastric lavage, hemodialysis, etc.

Table 41.3 Ventilation for resuscitation

Ventilation parameters	
Tidal volume	Goal: "visible chest movement"
Duration of inspiration	1.0 s
Ventilation frequency	10/min
Concentration of inspired oxygen (F_iO_2)	1.0

ECG Diagnosis

As soon as an ECG/defibrillator is available, the heart rhythm should be analyzed. When circulatory collapse occurs in the operating room or intensive care unit, monitoring is already established and the check can be performed immediately. Four different forms of cardiocirculatory arrest are considered:

- *Ventricular fibrillation* (VF) is marked on the ECG by chaotic electrical activity and not clearly identifiable QRS complexes of alternating amplitude and frequency.
- *Pulseless ventricular tachycardia* (pulseless VT) is marked by tachycardia with wide QRS complexes but no palpable pulse because there is no cardiac ejection.
- *Asystole* is marked by the complete lack of QRS complexes on the ECG. Artifacts may be mistaken for VF. Lead defects must be excluded by changing leads, controlling amplitude, and controlling the cables and electrodes.
- *Pulseless electrical activity* (PEA) is characterized by presence of QRS complexes on the ECG and absence of palpable pulses (cardiac ejections).

Airways and Ventilation

- Open the airways by tilting the patient's head back and using the Esmarch maneuver (head tilt, chin lift maneuver).
- Remove any foreign bodies and regurgitated fluid from the mouth and throat.
- Perform synchronized face mask ventilation: after compressing the chest 30 times ventilate twice.
- Intubate the patient endotracheally as soon as possible to secure the airways and prevent aspiration. The time for endotracheal intubation should not be any longer than 30 s; if the procedure exceeds 30 s it should be aborted and face mask ventilation should resume. Endotracheal intubation can be attempted again at the earliest after another 2 min CPR cycle. If the second attempt is also unsuccessful, alternative methods to secure the airways should be chosen, e.g., laryngeal mask, laryngeal tube.
- The basic parameters for ventilation can be found in Table 41.3.

- Immediately after endotracheal tube placement chest compression should be resumed, and the position of the tube should be verified by auscultation, capnometry/ capnography, or by using an esophageal detector device. If there is any doubt that the tube is in the correct position, it should be removed ("If in doubt, take it out!") and face mask ventilation should continued.
- Secure the endotracheal tube properly.

Circulation

Chest Compression

Only if chest compressions are continuously performed adequate cerebral and myocardial perfusion is achieved (Table 41.4).

Because chest compression is a physically very strenuous activity, helpers should switch with one another every 2 min.

Defibrillation

Defibrillation represents the only effective treatment if the electrocardiogram indicates VF or pulseless VT. While a defibrillator is retrieved, applied and charged, CPR must be performed. Defibrillation should be commenced as soon as the defibrillator is available.

It is important that the mechanical CPR is resumed immediately after defibrillation and that the heart rhythm is not analyzed until after a subsequent 2 min cycle of CPR has been performed. The defibrillator should be charged at the end of the 2 min cycle of CPR, so that delivery of another shock would be possible with only

Table 41.4 Chest compression

Compression parameters	
Compression frequency	100–120/min
Pressure point	Center of the chest
Depth of chest compression	5–6 cm
Compression–decompression ratio	1:1
Compression–ventilation ratio for face mask ventilation	30:2 synchronized = interrupted for ventilation
Compression–ventilation ratio after intubation of the trachea or securing the airways using an alternative method (LT, CT, LM)	30:2 nonsynchronized

a very brief interruption of chest compressions (<5 s) if VF/pulseless VT persist. During defibrillation, the person who is defibrillating must ensure that no one touches the patient ("clear – all clear").

Administering Medications

When emergency medications are injected intravenously each dose of drug should be followed by a bolus injection of 20 ml of a 0.9% saline solution ("flush").

Drug Administration During Resuscitation

For CPR a venous access should be established as quickly as possible. In intensive care patients or in patients undergoing an intervention, a venous access has often already been placed before cardiac arrest ensued and this access can be used to administer any necessary medication during CPR. If a central venous access is not available, a secure peripheral vascular access is sufficient.

If only an intraosseous access is available, administration of CPR medications follows the same guidelines that are established for the intravenous route. An intraosseous access (medial proximal tibia or distal tibia) is preferred particularly in infants and young children if an intravenous access cannot be established. The rate of successfully placing this access in pediatric patients is very high and in rare cases an intraosseous access may be the only viable option in an adult patient. The endotracheal application of drugs is not recommended. Subcutaneous or intramuscular administration of drugs is obsolete during CPR secondary to the profoundly reduced regional blood flow.

Medications

Oxygen is the most important medication. An overview of the most common emergency drugs for CPR is presented in Table 41.5.

In general, blood volume substitution or fluid resuscitation is not indicated, except for hemorrhagic or anaphylactic shock, diabetic coma, or in patients with burns.

In case of cardiovascular collapse or cardiac arrest secondary to an intoxication with local anesthetics an initial intravenous bolus of 1.5 ml/kg 20% lipid emulsion is recommended in addition to standard advanced life support. The bolus dose can be repeated up to three times at 5 min intervals and can be followed by an infusion of 15 ml/kg/h until ROSC is achieved or the patient has received the maximum of 12 ml/kg.

Table 41.5 Emergency mediations for resuscitation

Medication	Effect	Dosage	Special features
Adrenaline	Sympathetic mimetic, α- and β receptors, increases coronary and cerebral perfusion pressure	1 mg every 3–5 min i.v. or i.o.	Can be administered for all forms of cardiocirculatory arrest
Amiodarone	Class III antiarrhythmic	300 mg once i.v., possibly repeated at 150 mg i.v. and subsequent chronic infusion at 900 mg/24 h	First-line anti arrhythmic drug for VF and pulseless VT
Lidocaine	Class Ib antiarrhythmic	1–1.5 mg/kg body weight i.v.	Max, dosage 3 mg/kg body weight. Higher doses decrease possibility to defibrillate. Use only when amiodarone is not available. Do not use when amiodarone was given to start with
Magnesium	Membrane stabilization	8 mmol = 2 g 50% magnesium sulfate solution i.v.	Administration for hypomagnesemia (e.g., diuretic treatment and torsade-de-pointes tachycardia)
Sodium bicarbonate	Chemical alkalization and buffer for acidic valence	50 mval (=50 ml sodium bicarbonate 8.4%)	Consider for hyperkalaemia and triglycyric overdose. In case of prolonged resuscitation use only based on blood gas analysis. Catecholamine flakes with concomitant administration via an infusion system and is inactivated. Thus a separate venous access is needed
Calcium	Calcium replacement	2–4 mg/kg body weight i.v.	Generally, administration of calcium is not recommended for CPR and only suitable in special circumstances. Administration for hypocalcemia, hyperkalemia, and intoxication with calcium antagonists
Thrombolytics (e.g., urokinase, rt-PA, tenecteplase)	Lysis for a thromboembolic event	Depending on the thrombolytic drug	Administer to treat pulmonary embolism and other thromboembolic events on a case-by-case basis. For thrombolytic treatment under CPR, continue CPR for 60–90 min

Key Points

During cardiocirculatory arrest we distinguish fundamentally between ECG rhythms with a defibrillation indication (VF/pulseless VT) and without a defibrillation indication (asystole/PEA). The former require defibrillation and administration of antiarrhythmic drugs to reestablish a survivable heart rhythm. Otherwise, the two groups are managed in the same way.

- Perform chest compression continuously and preferably without interruption.
- Push hard and fast: 5–6 cm of compression depth and 100–120 chest compressions per minute.
- Secure the airways and ventilate the patient.
- Establish venous access.
- Administer adrenaline.
- Search for reversible causes for cardiocirculatory arrest.

For patients in whom pulmonary embolism is the suspected cause of cardiac arrest, thrombolysis can be indicated if the intra- or postoperative situation permits this.

Resuscitation Protocol for Ventricular Fibrillation and Pulseless Ventricular Tachycardia

For ventricular fibrillation (VF) and pulseless ventricular tachycardia (pulseless VT) defibrillation represents the key therapeutic measure in addition to chest compression and ventilation (30:2). CPR measures for VF and pulseless VT should be carried out in the following order (Fig. 41.2):

- Primary check.
- Call for assistance and, if not readily available, a defibrillator.
- Perform chest compression and ventilation (30:2).
- Analyze heart rhythm as soon as a defibrillator is available.
- Perform single biphasic defibrillation at 150–200 J, alternatively single monophasic defibrillation at 360 J.

  - Position the defibrillator paddle on the left above the cardiac apex and on the right above the second intercostal space along the medioclavicular line.
  - Contact pressure for the paddle on the chest should be about 12 kg.
  - Use contact gel.

- After defibrillation, chest compression and ventilation should be initiated again immediately and performed for 2 min; then the heart rhythm is analyzed again.

Perform primary check.
Call for assistance and defibrillator.
Perform chest compression and ventilation (30:2)

Analyze heart rhythm (as soon as possible, if defibrillator is available).
If VT/pulslessVT is present: perform single defibrillation:
150-200 Joule (biphasic) or 360 Joule (monophasic)
Defibrillator paddle: left above the cardiac apex and right above the
second intercostal space along the MCL.Contact pressure 12 kg. Use contact gel

After defibrillation: chest compression and ventilation for 2 min,
then analyze the heart rhythm.

If VF/pulseless VT persist:
Perform single defibrillation: 150-200 Joule (biphasic) or 360 Joule (monophasic).
After defibrillation: perform chest compression and ventilation for 2 min,
then analyze the heart rhythm.

If VF/pulseless VT persist: perform third defibrillation at 200 (biphasic) or
360 Joule (monophasic).

After defibrillation: perform chest compression and ventilation for 2 min,
administer 1 mg adrenaline and 300 mg amiodarone during that time,
then analyze heart rhythm.

If VF/pulseless VT persist: perform fourth defibrillation at 200 (biphasic)
or 360 Joule (monophasic).
After defibrillation perform chest compression and ventilation for 2 min,
then analyze heart rhythm.

If VF/pulseless VT persist: perform defibrillation at 200 (biphasic)
or 360 Joule (monophasic).
Continue the CPR measures and administer 1 mg adrenaline every 3-5 min.

Fig. 41.2 CPR measures for VT and pulseless VT

- If VF/pulseless VT persist, a second single biphasic defibrillation at 200 J,
  alternatively single monophasic defibrillation at 360 J is performed.
- After defibrillation chest compression and ventilation should be initiated again
  immediately and performed for 2 min, then the heart rhythm is analyzed again.
- If VF/pulseless VT continue to persist: perform a third single defibrillation at
  200 or 360 J.
- After chest compressions have restarted administer 1 mg adrenaline.

- 300 mg amiodarone is also given after the third shock.
- After each defibrillation, chest compression and ventilation should be initiated again immediately and performed for 2 min, then the heart rhythm is analyzed again.

If VF/pulseless VT still continue to persist, administer 1 mg adrenaline every 3–5 min, i.e., immediately after every other additional defibrillation attempt. If a rhythm potentially indicating perfusion develops during the heart rhythm analysis, check the pulse. If a pulse cannot be felt, perform another 2 min CPR cycle followed by another rhythm analysis and, if necessary, pulse check. When a pulse clearly can be identified, the patient's blood pressure is measured and the cardiovascular system stabilized; furthermore, electrolytes and blood pH should be optimized. If the rhythm changes to asystole/PEA, manage this accordingly.

Resuscitation Protocol for Asystole and PEA

Asystole and PEA represent the two ECG manifestations of cardiocirculatory arrest without an indication for electrical defibrillation.

Proceed as follows for both asystole and PEA (Fig. 41.3):

- Perform chest compression and ventilation (30:2).
- Establish iv-access and administer 1 mg adrenaline as quickly as possible.
- Secure the airways.

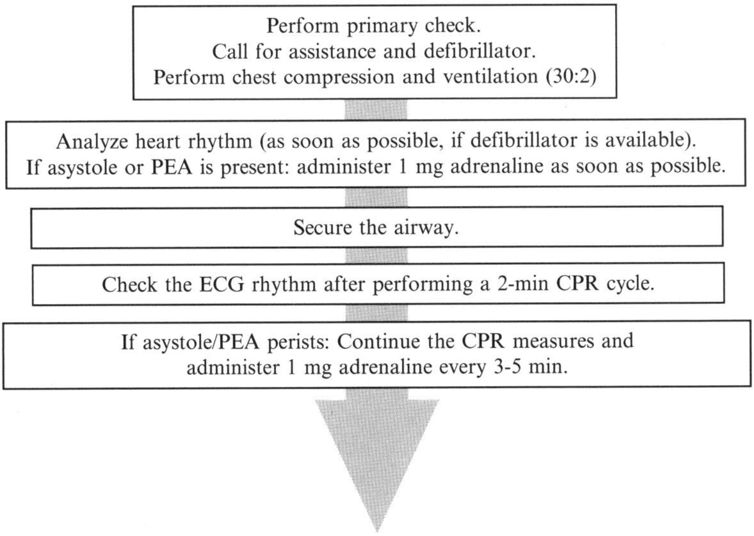

Perform primary check.
Call for assistance and defibrillator.
Perform chest compression and ventilation (30:2)

Analyze heart rhythm (as soon as possible, if defibrillator is available).
If asystole or PEA is present: administer 1 mg adrenaline as soon as possible.

Secure the airway.

Check the ECG rhythm after performing a 2-min CPR cycle.

If asystole/PEA perists: Continue the CPR measures and
administer 1 mg adrenaline every 3-5 min.

Fig. 41.3 CPR measures for asystole and PEA

- Check the ECG rhythm after performing a 2 min CPR cycle.
- If asystole/PEA persists, continue CPR.
- Administer 1 mg adrenaline every 3–5 min.

If an ECG rhythm is detected that could be associated with cardiac ejection check for a pulse, but no longer than 10 s. If no pulse can be detected, perform another 2 min CPR cycle followed by another check of the ECG and, if indicated, of the pulse. If a pulse is detected without doubt, the patient's blood pressure is measured and the cardiovascular system stabilized; furthermore, electrolytes, and blood pH should be optimized. If the rhythm changes to a VF/pulseless VT, proceed accordingly.

If there is doubt from the ECG as to whether asystole or a subtle VF is present, assume asystole and do not defibrillate.

Postresuscitation Care

After ROSC all comatose patients should be treated with therapeutic hypothermia (32–34°C core body temperature) for 12–24 h aimed at improving the neurological outcome [1, 2]. Postresuscitation care on the basis of standardized protocols including coronary intervention and hypothermia may be beneficial after successful resuscitation.

References

1. Deakin CD, Nolan JP, Soar J, et al. European Resuscitation Council Guidelines for Resuscitation 2010. Section 4. Adult advanced life support. Resuscitation. 2010;81:1305–52.
2. Hypothermia after Cardiac Arrest Study Group. Mild therapeutic hypothermia to improve the neurologic outcome after cardiac arrest. N Engl J Med. 2002;346:549–56.

Suggested Reading

Böttiger BW, Arntz HR, Chamberlain DA. Thrombolysis for resuscitation during out-of-hospital cardiac arrest. N Engl J Med. 2008;359:2651–62.
European Resuscitation Council Guidelines for Resuscitation 2010. Section 1. Executive Summary. Resuscitation. 2010;81:1219–76.
Sandroni C, Ferro G, Santangelo S, et al. In-hospital cardiac arrest: survival depends mainly on the effectiveness of the emergency response. Resuscitation. 2004;62:291–7.
Zipes DP, Wellens HJ. Sudden cardiac death. Circulation. 1998;98:2334–51.

Chapter 42
Arousal from Anesthesia
After Neurosurgical Operations

W. Scott Jellish

Introduction

Prolonged emergence after a neurosurgical procedure is a very disconcerting problem for both the surgeon and anesthesiologist. Delayed emergence may lead to expensive neuroradiologic testing that would otherwise not be done. Failure to emerge from anesthesia after a neurosurgical procedure may be multifactorial in nature and may be affected by the type of anesthesia used, the area of the brain traumatized by surgery, the size of the tumor, and medications administered to the patient prior to surgery (see Fig. 42.1).

Overview: Surgical Area and Size of Tumor

The effects of the surgical excision, brain retraction, frontal pathology and abnormal elastance have been blamed for delayed emergence after intracranial surgery. Frontal brain resection and posterior fossa tumors are associated with the highest incidence of delayed emergence.

Mass effect of intracerebral lesions will also affect emergence with >30 mm tumor size or a midline shift of >3 mm, with cerebral edema being predictive for delayed emergence after surgery. Likewise, surgical retraction used to remove a large tumor may cause ischemia to adjacent tissue and present with delayed emergence. In addition, infarction or tumor resection in close proximity to the ascending reticular activating system will be associated with preoperative lethargy and delayed

W.S. Jellish, MD, PhD (✉)
Department of Anesthesiology, Loyola University Medical Center, Stritch School of Medicine, Maywood, IL, USA

A.M. Brambrink and J.R. Kirsch (eds.), *Essentials of Neurosurgical Anesthesia & Critical Care*, DOI 10.1007/978-0-387-09562-2_42,
© Springer Science+Business Media, LLC 2012

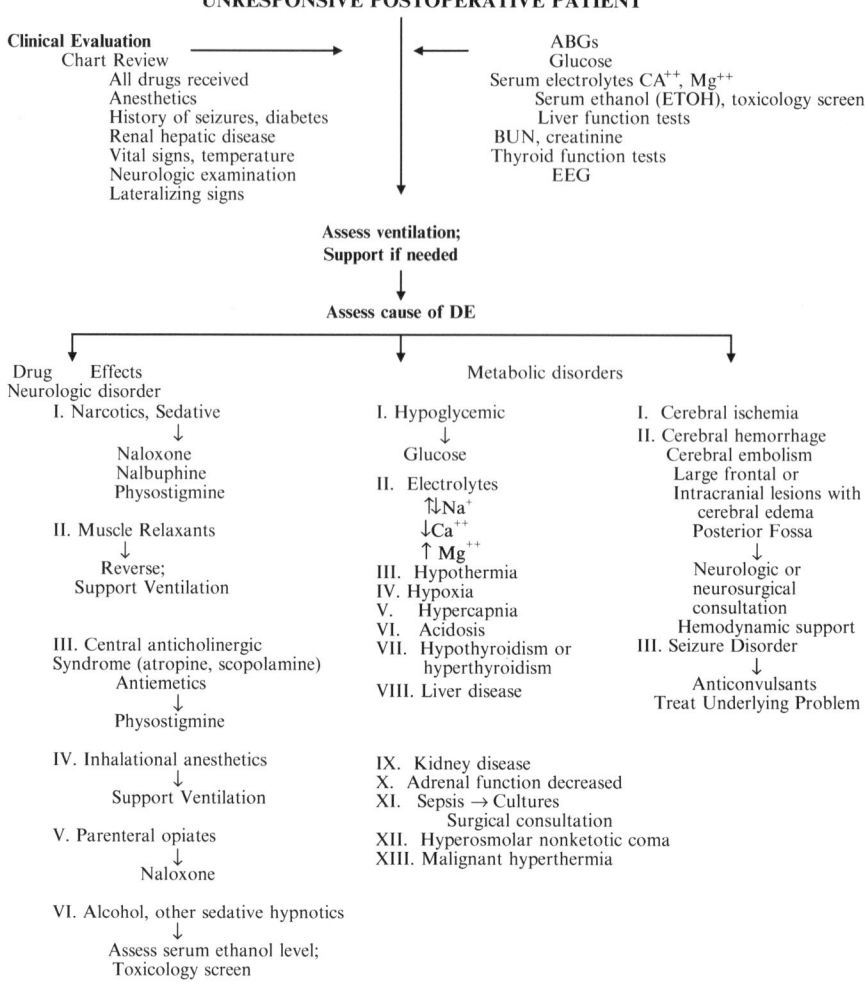

UNRESPONSIVE POSTOPERATIVE PATIENT

Clinical Evaluation
Chart Review
All drugs received
Anesthetics
History of seizures, diabetes
Renal hepatic disease
Vital signs, temperature
Neurologic examination
Lateralizing signs

ABGs
Glucose
Serum electrolytes CA++, Mg++
Serum ethanol (ETOH), toxicology screen
Liver function tests
BUN, creatinine
Thyroid function tests
EEG

Assess ventilation;
Support if needed

Assess cause of DE

Drug   Effects
Neurologic disorder
I. Narcotics, Sedative
Naloxone
Nalbuphine
Physostigmine

II. Muscle Relaxants
Reverse;
Support Ventilation

III. Central anticholinergic
Syndrome (atropine, scopolamine)
Antiemetics
Physostigmine

IV. Inhalational anesthetics
Support Ventilation

V. Parenteral opiates
Naloxone

VI. Alcohol, other sedative hypnotics
Assess serum ethanol level;
Toxicology screen

VI. Other drugs

Metabolic disorders
I. Hypoglycemic
Glucose

II. Electrolytes
$\uparrow\downarrow Na^+$
$\downarrow Ca^{++}$
$\uparrow Mg^{++}$
III. Hypothermia
IV. Hypoxia
V. Hypercapnia
VI. Acidosis
VII. Hypothyroidism or
hyperthyroidism
VIII. Liver disease

IX. Kidney disease
X. Adrenal function decreased
XI. Sepsis → Cultures
Surgical consultation
XII. Hyperosmolar nonketotic coma
XIII. Malignant hyperthermia

I. Cerebral ischemia
II. Cerebral hemorrhage
Cerebral embolism
Large frontal or
Intracranial lesions with
cerebral edema
Posterior Fossa
Neurologic or
neurosurgical
consultation
Hemodynamic support
III. Seizure Disorder
Anticonvulsants
Treat Underlying Problem

Fig. 42.1 A systematic approach to assess delayed emergence (DE)

emergence from anesthesia. Finally, if temporary occlusion of cerebral arteries is required to affect surgical repair, the patient could develop ischemic/reperfusion cerebral injury after restoration of blood flow. As with brain tumors, mass effect from a cerebral hematoma (regardless of the cause) exceeding 2–3 cm in diameter or large lobar hematomas often will produce coma and require surgical evacuation.

Prevention

Little can be done to prevent the effects of tumor size or the area of resection on emergence from anesthesia after the surgical procedure. However, meticulous control of fluids and blood pressure are important to avoid cerebral edema and possible postoperative hematoma formation. Control of emergence hypertension is complex but key to reducing the possibility of postoperative cerebral edema, bleeding, or increased ICP. The size of the lesion is important in producing emergence hypertension, with a shift in midline structure of more than 5 mm on cerebral imaging an independent risk factor for hypertension at the end of the procedure. Coughing, bucking, or straining on the endotracheal tube may also cause increased ICP and postoperative bleeding. Thus, an anesthetic technique should be used with antitussive effects to reduce the incidence of this occurrence.

Other causes of delayed emergence with major brain resection must also be anticipated and prevented. Possible cerebral thromboembolism and related neurological dysfunction is highest with vascular procedures involving the carotid or cerebral vasculature.

In addition, maintenance of cerebral perfusion and elevation of blood pressure should always be optimized in cases where temporary disruption of blood flow occurs during resection of vascular tumors, aneurysms, or ablation of arteriovenous malformations.

Crisis Management

If delayed emergence is suspected and believed to be secondary to postsurgical cerebral edema or hemorrhage, hemodynamic perturbations must be limited and meticulous control of blood pressure maintained. Preventing hypertension with short-acting beta blockers (e.g., esmolol) or calcium channel blockers (e.g., nicardipine), administered by bolus or infusion, have been utilized with success. If the patient is hypotensive from a large loss of blood, hemodynamic support should be initiated with fluids (colloid or crystalloid) and vasopressors, such as ephedrine or neosynephrine. Hypotension, due to an arrhythmia, should be corrected pharmacologically or by cardioversion, depending on the urgency of the situation. If postsurgical cerebral ischemia is suspected secondary to vasospasm, nicardipine treatment has been shown to reduce neurologic impairment if started in less than 6 h after onset. Cerebral perfusion can also be improved by reducing blood viscosity with hemodilution and pharmacologically supporting blood pressure.

On an emergent basis, intracranial hypertension is quickly treated by reducing cerebral blood volume by acute hyperventilation. However, attention must be paid to not hyperventilate to an extreme because of the possible risk of cerebral ischemia. If hyperventilation is needed to reduce ICP, FIO_2 should be increased to 100%.

Mannitol and hypertonic (e.g., 3%) saline are also used to reduce brain volume by osmotically removing water from the uninjured brain. Furosemide may also be added to reduce brain volume and also inhibit the formation of CSF.

Key Points

- Frontal brain resection and posterior fossa procedures have a higher incidence of delayed emergence.
- A tumor >30 mm in size with a midline shift of >3 mm with cerebral edema preoperatively is a good predictor of delayed emergence.
- The size of the cerebral lesion is important in producing emergence hypertension with a midline shift >5 mm an independent risk factor for hypertension. Blood pressure control is a key during emergence from anesthesia.

Overview: Anesthetic Effects

Rapid emergence from anesthesia is paramount when devising a neuroanesthetic plan. Patients with larger intracranial lesions may have procedures that last for prolonged periods of time. This could result in prolonged administration of opioids or inhalational agents which could delay emergence, depending on the agent or opioid used. Hyperventilation during the procedure to reduce brain size and improve surgical resection may also result in prolonged emergence from anesthesia. An increase in pH may result in a higher total volume of distribution and longer elimination half-life for sufentanil. Similarly, fentanyl brain concentrations may also be prolonged in hyperventilated individuals presumably because of reduced brain washout from a change in the drug lipid/plasma distribution. In addition, intraoperative hypocapnia has also been linked to postoperative impairment in reaction time and short-term memory.

Opioids are frequently implicated in producing a prolonged state of unconsciousness with the degree and duration of postoperative sedation related to the timing, route, and total dosage of the drug administered. Prolonged depression is especially common after intraoperative administration of long-acting opioids such as morphine, meperidine, or hydromorphone. Shorter-acting opioids, such as fentanyl or sufentanil, may also exhibit a prolonged sedative effect when given in high doses or infusions for prolonged periods of time. Remifentanil, with its metabolism linked to plasma cholinesterase, has the shortest half-life and is the least likely contributor to postoperative unconsciousness. Some opioids, like meperidine, are metabolized to active metabolites, which prolong and add to central neural depression. In addition, these drugs will also decrease spontaneous minute ventilation slowing the washout of residual inhalational anesthetics prolonging sedation. The intense analgesic component of opioids also minimizes the arousal generated by postoperative pain.

The administration of sedative premedications to achieve anxiolysis or amnesia may also contribute to prolonged unconsciousness, particularly if long-acting sedatives (hydroxyzine, promethazine, or lorazepam) were administered. The administration of certain antiemetics or anticonvulsants, as part of an anesthetic regimen, may have a profound effect on depression of consciousness in the PACU, especially if they are given toward the end of surgery. Antiemetics such as droperidol, prochlorperazine, or scopolamine have sedative side effects that can augment sedation from anesthesia. Other parenteral medications such as propofol, short-acting barbiturates, or etomidate, especially if used as a continuous infusion during the surgery, could result in redistribution of high concentrations of drug into the tissue and accentuate delayed awakening.

Both the length of exposure to the volatile agent and the solubility of the agent must be considered to prevent build-up of agent in tissues that have lower perfusion, which would lead to a prolonged washout of anesthetic after discontinuation. Obese patients may be particularly prone to prolonged emergence after extensive intracranial procedures because of their relatively high proportion of body fat. Lower solubility agents such as sevoflurane or desflurane are unlikely to cause prolonged emergence after anesthesia because they are eliminated rapidly after discontinuation. However, if these agents are combined with other longer-acting parenteral medications, sedation may be prolonged.

Finally, the patient who appears to have delayed emergence could have residual paralysis from an infusion of neuromuscular blocking agents and be unable to move or respond to commands but be completely awake. The use of atropine intraoperatively, for treatment of bradycardia, could produce a central anticholinergic syndrome causing somnolence and unconsciousness, especially in older individuals.

Prevention

To prevent the possibility of delayed emergence after intracranial procedures related to anesthetic agents or medications, the practitioner should review the drugs that were administered perioperatively over the last 24 h period. Nonanesthetic drugs such as reserpine, methyldopa, clonidine, lidocaine, antihistamines, certain antiemetics, and anticonvulsants have sedative properties that may prolong emergence. Antiemetics such as droperidol, prochlorperazine, and scopolamine should only be used with great caution when delayed emergence would be of concern following intracranial procedures. If hyperventilation to reduce brain size is needed, the anesthesia provider must consider how this will change the pharmacokinetics of opioids, producing higher brain opioid concentrations. Ideally the patient should be as normocarbic as possible after dural closure.

A procedure estimated to last for a prolonged period of time should utilize a less soluble inhalation anesthetic. In addition, combination inhalational and opioid-based anesthetics reduce the overall concentration of inhalational anesthetics used and produce an early emergence. A fentanyl infusion in the presence of low-dose isoflurane has been noted to produce a more rapid emergence with much less hypertension when compared to a propofol total intravenous anesthetic. Desflurane, with similar effects as isoflurane on cerebral vasculature, can be used for prolonged intracranial procedures with minimal cumulative effect. Use of a scalp block with a long-acting local anesthetic (e.g., ropivacaine) in preference to opioid administration will obviate the concern that opiates have added to the cause for delayed emergence.

If opioids are administered, longer-acting ones should be avoided. In addition, IM administration, which leads to slower uptake and prolonged action, should also be avoided. Remifentanil may be used for many neurosurgical procedures to avoid a delay in emergence, but postoperative management of pain and emergence hypertension is a key factor that must be considered with its use. Opioid premedication should also be avoided to prevent preoperative hypoventilation, especially in patients with large intracranial masses where increased ICP could be a factor.

If propofol infusions are added to an opioid/inhalational anesthetic to improve neurophysiologic monitoring, discontinuation of the infusion should occur as soon as possible to avoid the accumulative effect of propofol on emergence from anesthesia. If antiemetics are to be used as part of the anesthetic regimen, dexamethasone and serotonin-blocking agents (i.e., ondansetron, dolasetron), which do not have sedative effects, should be administered. In many instances, neuromuscular blocking agents are not needed for intracranial procedures and, in some instances, (facial nerve or other cranial nerve monitoring) should be avoided altogether. If muscle relaxants are used, appropriate titration of intermediate neuromuscular blocking agents will avoid the prolonged paralysis that may occur with multiple boluses or infusions of long-acting agents such as pancuronium. Finally, if bradycardia occurs during the intracranial procedure, glycopyrrolate can be substituted for atropine to increase heart rate. This drug does not cross the blood–brain barrier and will not produce a central anticholinergic syndrome.

Crisis Management

When determining the reason for prolonged unresponsiveness after intracranial surgery, the initiation of analgesia and sedation regimens should be delayed until the source of the unconsciousness is identified. Generally, a patient demonstrating signs of pain will also exhibit some degree of consciousness. To determine whether prolonged unconsciousness is related to residual opioids, small incremental doses of Naloxone 40 mcg IV can be administered. Careful titration can reverse both ventilatory depression and sedation without precipitating excessive sympathetic activity which may result from rapid reversal of narcosis. If benzodiazepines are suspected, flumazenil can be given in titrated incremental doses of 0.1 mg IV q 2 min to reverse the sedative effect. Its duration of action is short, however, and repeated doses may be needed to maintain consciousness.

There is no specific reversal for barbiturates, propofol, phenothiazines, or butyrophenones. However, the administration of physostigmine 1.25 mg generates a degree of arousal that may counter, but not reverse, depression from sedatives, antiemetics, and other CNS depressants. Physostigmine can also be used to reverse the central nervous system effects associated with central anticholinergic syndrome.

Finally, unconsciousness or prolonged sedation after anesthesia could be simulated by a paralyzed patient. If the patient is totally unresponsive after the neurosurgical procedure and muscle relaxants were utilized, the patient's neuromuscular integrity should be assessed with the use of a nerve stimulator. If no twitches are observed or if a minimal train of four is realized, the patient should be supported and antagonizing agents (neostigmine with glycopyrolate) administered.

Key Points

- Hyperventilation and extreme hypocapnia could alter opioid pharmacokinetics and reduce brain washout of the drug, prolonging emergence from anesthesia.
- Long-acting sedatives should not be administered preoperatively for anxiolysis as they could prolong postoperative emergence.
- The administration of certain antiemetics and anticonvulsants, as part of an anesthetic regimen, may have a profound depressant effect at the end of surgery.
- Residual paralysis from neuromuscular blocking agents – as well as central anticholinergic syndrome, if atropine is used – should be considered in neurological procedures with delayed emergence.

Overview: Patient Factors

Individual patient factors, not related to the anesthetic or surgical procedure, could also affect emergence from anesthesia after an intracranial procedure. Physiologic abnormalities could exist in patients that would cause a prolonged return to consciousness. For example, patients on high doses of steroids may be hyperglycemic which could interfere with consciousness by increasing serum osmolarity. In the other extreme, patients may also be hypoglycemic if overtreated with bolus or insulin infusion, which results in unconsciousness because of the loss of essential substrates necessary for neuronal function.

The level of consciousness can also be impacted by an acute hypo- or hyperosmolar state. These changes in osmolar state may be iatrogenic in cause (choice of fluid administration) or from changes in antidiuretic hormone secretion levels. Serum sodium levels below 125 meq/L are especially troublesome and could lead to seizures or prolonged postoperative unconsciousness. Unconsciousness due to hypernatremia is rare but could occur if urine output and intake are not carefully monitored during the intraoperative period.

A reduction in core body temperature will decrease the level of arousal and increase the effect of anesthetics and muscle relaxants. Body temperatures below 34°C impair consciousness, and extremely low body temperatures will produce fixed pupils and areflexia. Hypothermia is rarely the primary cause of postoperative unconsciousness. However, a moderately decreased body temperature will certainly augment the depression of consciousness or impair the clearance of anesthetic agents and muscle relaxants.

Preexisting patient conditions should also be ascertained since some could contribute to a prolonged emergence after anesthesia. Patients with porphyria will exhibit a prolonged state of unconsciousness with the use of barbiturates, propofol, and other medications. Hunter's syndrome and other mucopolysaccharide disease states may also produce prolonged unconsciousness. Patients who are hypothyroid, especially if not properly medicated, may be especially slow to emerge from anesthesia.

Finally, the postcraniotomy patient could be postictal, having had an unrecognized seizure under anesthesia or during emergence. It is a common practice to give anticonvulsant therapy to patients undergoing a supratentorial craniotomy. Seizures in the early postoperative period are not common if the patient has been administered the correct level of anticonvulsants. However, seizures have been noted to occur on emergence from anesthesia and may go undetected.

Crisis Management

Alterations in patient physiologic parameters that could alter emergence from anesthesia after an intracranial procedure must be recognized quickly and treated appropriately to avoid neurologic injury. If unconsciousness is suspected from hypoglycemia, an empiric trial of intravenous 50% dextrose solution should be initiated. It is inappropriate to delay the administration of dextrose until serum glucose is corroborated. If acute hyperglycemia is demonstrated with hyperglycemic hyperosmolar coma, hydration should be immediately initiated with saline and titration of IV regular insulin either in small incremental doses or by an infusion. During insulin infusion potassium replacement (as potassium moves into cells) and serial blood glucose measurements are essential.

Acute hypoosmolar states can occur (<260 mOsm/L) by a sudden increase in antidiuretic hormone secretion, especially in cases involving the pituitary or hypothalamus. If severe hyponatremia is recognized, care should be taken to restore the serum sodium gradually. Replacement of fluids with normal saline and IV administration of furosemide to promote renal wasting of free water in excess of sodium should be initiated. Infusions of hypertonic saline may be necessary, but care should be taken to avoid rapid overcorrection of electrolyte levels, which could predispose to the development of central pontine myelinolysis. Unconsciousness due to a hypernatremic, hyperosmolar state is rare in postoperative patients. If diminished antidiuretic hormone is secreted due to neurosurgical injury, the patient will develop hypernatremia with high output dilute urine. The treatment of diabetes insipidus consists of the administration of an isotonic crystalloid solution and infusion of aqueous ADH (100–200 milliunits/h). Serum sodium and plasma osmolarity are measured on a regular basis and therapeutic changes are made accordingly.

Hypothermic patients should be treated by rewarming with warm ambient air and the use of heated IV fluids. Covering the patient's head will also help retain heat. Surface or radiant warmers and humidification of inspired gases will also reduce heat loss. Patients with a temperature below 35°C should be rewarmed using radiant lighting, heating blankets, warmed forced air, reflective coverings and heated nebulized air. As the temperatures rise, patients should be carefully monitored for hypotension related to increasing venous capacitance. Resolution of metabolic acidemia usually accompanies re-warming.

Key Points

- Physiologic abnormalities could occur during intracranial neurosurgical procedures which could lead to extremes in glucose concentrations, sodium levels and serum osmolarity, all of which could affect emergence from anesthesia.
- Body temperature, especially hypothermia, could lead to prolonged anesthetic effects with delayed emergence from anesthesia.
- Always consider the possibility that the postcraniotomy patient may have had an intraoperative seizure and are in a postictal state, which could delay wakening after an intracranial procedure.

Suggested Reading

Bhagat H, Dash HH, Bithal PK, Chouhan RS, Pandia MP. Planning for early emergence in neurosurgical patients: a randomized prospective trial of low-dose anesthetics. Anesth Analg. 2008;107(4):1348–55.

Bruder NJ. Awakening management after neurosurgery for intracranial tumours. Curr Opin Anesthesiol. 2002;15(5):477–82.

Grover VK, Tewari MK, Mahajav R. Cranial surgery: impact of tumour size and location on emergence from anaesthesia. J Anesth Clin Phamacol. 2007;23(3):263–8.

Himmelseher S, Pfenninger EB. Anesthetic management of neurosurgical patients. Curr Opin Anaesthesiol. 2001;14(5):483–90.

Schubert A, Mascha E, Bloomfield EL, DeBoer FE, Gupta MK, Ebrahim ZY. Effect of cranial surgery and brain tumor size on emergence from anesthesia. Anesthesiology. 1996;85(3):513–21.

Zelcer J, Wells DG. Anesthetic-related recovery room complications. Anaesth Intensive Care. 1996;15:168.

Chapter 43
Communication Challenges During the Perioperative Period

David Murray

Overview

Risk, Incidence and Epidemiology

Effective communication on the part of the physician is an intrinsic component of high-quality medical care. The ability to "listen and communicate effectively" is recognized by the Association of American Medical Colleges (AAMC) as an essential skill, yet only recently has the need for training and assessment of communication been recognized for encounters beyond the physician–patient setting. In the hospital environment, interactions with nurses, peers, and various members of a health-care team are central to patient care. As the acuity of patient care increases, particularly in the specialized, high-acuity operating room and ICU environments, the consequences of ineffective communication among members of the health-care team pose a greater threat to patient safety.

The Joint Commission has reported that ineffective communication led to 70% of all preventable errors resulting in death or serious injury from 1995 to 2003. A number of recent studies have explored the communication effectiveness of team members, including anesthesiologists, surgeons, and operating room nurses. Several authors have demonstrated significant opportunities for improved communication in the OR and ICU.

D. Murray, MD (✉)
Department of Anesthesiology, Washington University School of Medicine in St. Louis,
St Louis, MO, USA
e-mail: mailto:murrayd@anest.wustl.edu

A.M. Brambrink and J.R. Kirsch (eds.), *Essentials of Neurosurgical Anesthesia & Critical Care*, DOI 10.1007/978-0-387-09562-2_43,
© Springer Science+Business Media, LLC 2012

Etiology of Communication Failure

Communication failure is ubiquitous in human relationships, so the finding that miscommunication occurs in the perioperative period should not be surprising. The relationship between team function and communication is essential in determining how communication failure leads to perioperative complications. Strategies to improve communication are based on improving overall team function. Teams are defined as two or more individuals who share a common goal. Communication, whether explicit or implicit, is how teams exchange information. The exchange of information is essential to accomplish their common team goals. Each team member has specific roles, tasks, and responsibilities. The quality of the teamwork determines how well the team accomplishes their goal. In the perioperative period, team function and the associated communication of essential information to accomplish an operation is crucial to success. Based on the requirements for team function, individual expertise may not translate to effective team performance. In the team setting, a combination of expertise and teamwork are needed for effective team performance.

Salas et al. define teamwork as including five associated components. These team functions or components include leadership, mutual performance monitoring, backup behavior, adaptability, and orientation. The relative importance and the activity of these team components vary during team-related activities. In a health-care professional team composed of multiple experts, the expectation is that leadership may shift among the team members at various times in order to achieve the goal. Team members must coordinate activities and often manage tasks in a sequential and interdependent manner. In the perioperative routine, the steps to reach the goal occur in a relatively predictable and predetermined manner. Often limited communication is observed or required, as team members are cognizant of the team goal as well as engaged in specialized activities demanding their full attention.

In highly functional teams, progress toward the desired goal may be "on track" even in the absence of explicit communication. The team is monitoring mutual performance with multiple shifts in leadership among team members in order to achieve the goal. Even though in the routine situation communication is not relevant and potentially distracting to team members, when a circumstance or event leads to a change, then communication becomes imperative. When team members share a common understanding of the expected and usual, then team members more easily accomplish "backup" behaviors and adapt to avert or manage a crisis. For example, in the operating room, an air embolus occurs during a craniotomy, the anesthesiologist asserts leadership by alerting the operating room team. The scrub nurse and neurosurgeon, who understand the backup behavior, immediately flood the operative field with saline. Once the crisis is resolved, the neurosurgeon evaluates the surgical field to determine the source of air entrainment. The team monitors and adapts to the change in circumstances. Similarly, if a ventricular catheter is inserted and brisk continuous bleeding results, the neurosurgeon asserts leadership and indicates the need for immediate craniotomy. The team members (anesthesia provider and OR nurses) would be expected to adopt backup behaviors, adapt to the changing circumstances, and assume leadership for various activities that are needed to convert the operative procedure from ventricular catheter placement to craniotomy. In these examples, the team recognizes the "abnormal" and responds to correct the crisis either averting or mitigating an unfavorable outcome. An awareness of the roles and responsibilities of various team members, mutual performance monitoring, backup behaviors and adapting to a changing clinical situation by team members results in prompt recognition of deviations and obstacles to achieving team goals.

Communication Assessment and Teamwork Complications

Communication and teamwork are widely recognized as important factors in patient safety. Effective teamwork, however, is not automatic. In order to deliver safe care, experts must possess task work skills and coordinate the delivery of these skills and activities with other team members. Such task interdependence, where tasks performed by one member are dependent on tasks performed by other members, is characteristic of medical teams and requires effective communication and a shared understanding of conditions and goals. This is particularly evident when a deviation from the "usual" occurs due to an acute, uncommon, or infrequent event. The knowledge, skills, and attitudes expected in team settings become crucial. Some of the potential causes of team failure include

- Roles and responsibilities are not understood by team members both by profession and discipline (nursing, physician) and specialty (surgeon, anesthesiologist, internist).
- Few contingency plans are in place when a critical event occurs during the perioperative period.
- Team members unable or unwilling to support or crossover to help other team members when a work overload exists.
- Team members fail to recognize crisis or adapt to a changing situation.
- Changing expectations about performance exist among team members, and many of the actions are not clearly designated to individual members of the team (e.g., assuring donated blood is readily available for administration).

Crisis Management

Clinical Presentation

The causes of communication breakdown are often multifaceted primarily because expert teams require both expertise and teamwork to accomplish goals. Many teamwork failures attributed to communication are due to expertise factors associated such as insufficient experience, inadequate team knowledge, poor judgments or failure to take responsibility. The resulting teamwork failures that result from communication and expertise are major sources of patient morbidity and mortality.

Some of the most striking examples of morbidity attributed to communication failure are operative procedures conducted on the patient's wrong side. Despite the relatively low frequency of this obviously preventable and egregious error, this type of error is often perceived by the lay public that medical practice is flawed and in serious need of more effective oversight. This type of "wrong operation" error is now attributed to the hospital and operating room team, rather than individual members of the team. A key reason for these types of errors related to behaviors that are perhaps related to a combination of teamwork and communication failure. A "silo" approach to specialty training and an absence of interdisciplinary training often is the root cause of these errors. The use of a "time-out" procedure is a current Joint Commission recommendation to encourage information exchange and shared responsibility for the operative goal.

In order for a team to accomplish a shared goal, one of the teamwork roles is to assume responsibility for understanding the goal and the expected requirements to achieve the goal. In anesthetic practice, this includes understanding the nature of the patient's illness. A "wrong"-sided operation would be less likely in an operating room with an anesthesia provider who had participated in the patient care throughout taking the preoperative anesthetic history, inducing anesthesia, positioning of the patient and surgical preparation. There are a number of these types of teamwork failures that result in "preventable" morbidity including

Examples of perioperative adverse events related to team or communication failure:

- Operations on the wrong side/level
- Operation guided by wrong MRI
- Error in preparing operative site (none, toxic solution for preparation)
- Contaminated OR equipment (sterilization failure)
- Positioning morbidity (position or equipment to position)
- Solutions on the surgical field

    - Concentration of epinephrine
    - Neurotoxicity from irrigation (formalin/chlorhexidine/alcohol/antibiotic irrigation instead of saline)
    - Flammable substances on the field (collodian/alcohol)

- Prophylactic antibiotic administration errors

    - Allergic, dosage, timing, susceptibility

- Blood transfusion errors
- Pathologic specimen discarded/mislabeled

Intervention/Prevention

Current training methods place too much emphasis on training individuals as specialists with limited training in team performance. In the perioperative neurosurgical environment, an operative team is convened to manage patients.

The experts, who participate in these teams, by necessity, acquire the complex skills to manage these events during specialty training. This specialty training, whether during residency or advanced training in nursing, most commonly occurs with limited, if any, interaction with future team members. This training results in experts who have the knowledge and skills to accomplish the cognitive and technical skills expected but may not result in efficient and effective competence in teamwork skills.

There are a variety of strategies that are used to improve the function of teams in medical settings. One of the global strategies applied by hospitals is through the use of surveys of the safety culture of the health-care professional team. The responses by the health-care professional team correlate with measures of patient safety. In hospitals that are perceived by health-care professionals as "safer" in terms of the environment and commitment to patient care, the measures of patient safety in terms of outcome are improved. Studies that have observed these differences in morbidity and mortality have resulted in a Joint Commission initiative for hospitals to measure their safety environment. In hospitals with a safety climate that is not favorable to safe patient care, the strategy to improve the environment is not clearly defined, but the majority of research suggests some form of team training. The nature of the team-training curriculum may not be as important as the involvement of the entire health-care professional team.

A variety of team-training curriculum and strategies are available that potentially improve teamwork. The adaptations from the military and aviation industry (frequently referred to as "Crew Resource Management" strategies) are relatively directive in terms of the conduct of training and team member expectations. One example, the Team Strategies and Tools to Enhance Performance and Patient Safety (TeamSTEPPS) program includes an interactive curriculum for teaching teamwork concepts can be divided into four modules: communication, situation monitoring, mutual support, and leadership. In terms of communication between team members, the participants are instructed to use defined communication skills and structured opportunities for information exchange. The use of a pneumonic such as Situation, Background, Assessment and Recommendation (SBAR) to convey communication about relevant patient information is applied to communication training.

Overview of Communication in Teamwork (TeamSTEPPS) Curriculum

- SBAR eponym for communication of relevant patient information (*s*ituation, *b*ackground, *a*ssessment, *r*ecommendation)
- DESC eponym indicates *d*escribe the behavior, *e*xpress concerns, *s*pecify a course of action, and assure *c*onsensus
- Two-challenge (the action of verbalizing a safety concern twice if no action is taken)

- Check back (closed loop communication between the sender to ensure that the receiver has heard and understands the message correctly)
- Call out (calling out loud to staff important decision for anticipating next steps)

Implications of improvements in teamwork and communication,

- Enhanced coordination of care
- Better initial as well as more comprehensive patient care plans
- Fewer adverse patient outcomes
- Increased patient satisfaction
- A reduction in frequency of medico legal cases and decreased magnitude of claim settlements

Key Points

- Communication failure and miscommunication among health-care professional teams are serious, preventable causes of patient morbidity and mortality.
- Communication is a key component of teamwork. Health-care teams are ubiquitous in medicine, so concepts of teamwork are essential in patient care.
- The cumulative expertise of the health-care professional team does not necessarily translate into expert patient management. While the medical team requires individuals to possess the knowledge, skills, experiences and attitudes to perform essential tasks, teamwork is essential. Teamwork is not automatic.
- A commitment to the principles of team effectiveness is required to improve patient outcome.
- Training can improve teamwork.

Suggested Reading

Burke CS, Salas E, Wilson-Donnelly K, Priest H. How to turn a team of experts into an expert medical team: guidance from the aviation and military communities. Qual Saf Health Care. 2004;13(Suppl):i96–104.

Helmreich RL, Davies JM. Human factors in the operating room: interpersonal determinants of safety, efficiency and morale. In: Aitkenhead AR, editor. Quality assurance and risk management in anaesthesia, Bailliere's clinical anaesthesiology international practice and research. London: Bailliere Tindal; 1996. p. 277–95.

Institute for Healthcare Improvement. 100,000 Lives Campaign. 20 Mar 2005. http://www.ihi.org/IHI/Programs/Campaign/Campaign.htm.

JCAHO. Sentinel Event Statistics. 2004. http://www.jcaho.org/.

Joint Commission on Accreditation of Healthcare Organizations (JCAHO). 2008 National Patient Safety Goals. http://www.jointcommission.org. Accessed 15 Jan 2009.

Lindgard L, Espin S, Whyte S, Regehr G, Baker GR, et al. Communication failures in the operating room: an observational classification of recurrent types and effects. Qual Saf Health Care. 2004;13:330–4.

Makary MA, Sexton JB, Freischlag JA, et al. Operating room teamwork among physicians and nurses: teamwork in the eye of the beholder. J Am Coll Surg. 2006;202:746–52.

Murray D, Enarson C. Communication and teamwork: Essential to learn but difficult to measure. Anesthesiology. 2007;106:895–6.

Salas E, Sims DE, Burke CS. Is there a "Big Five" in teamwork? Small Group Res. 2005;5:555–99.

TeamSTEPPS. http://dodpatientsafety.usuhs.mil/index.php.

Part VIII
Fundamentals of Pediatric Neurosurgery and Neuroanesthesia

Chapter 44
Anatomy and Physiology
of the Central Nervous System in Children

Stuart Friess, Todd J. Kilbaugh, and Mark Helfaer

Overview

The pediatric patient brings unique challenges to the neuroanesthesiologist and neurointensivists. Anatomy and physiology of the pediatric central nervous system has substantial differences to the adult patient. Further challenges are presented by the fact that there are rapid changes in the anatomy and physiologic responses of the central nervous system as the pediatric patient grows and matures.

- The pediatric cranial vault is much softer and more pliable than the adult due to the higher content of cartilage.
- The bone of the cranial vault also has a rich vascular supply, especially in the youngest of pediatric patients.

The Fontanels

Infants at birth have two fontanels, and understanding their natural course is critical to recognizing possible challenges for the practitioner.

- Posterior fontanel usually measures 1–2 cm and closes by 2 months of age
- Anterior fontanel measures 4–6 cm and closes between 4 and 26 months of life

S. Friess, MD (✉) • T.J. Kilbaugh, MD
Department of Anesthesiology and Critical Care Medicine,
The Children's Hospital of Philadelphia, Philadelphia, PA, USA
e-mail: FRIESS@email.chop.edu

M. Helfaer, MD
Departments of Anesthesiology and Critical Care, Pediatrics and Nursing,
Perelman School of Medicine at the University of Pennsylvania,
Philadelphia, PA, USA

A.M. Brambrink and J.R. Kirsch (eds.), *Essentials of Neurosurgical Anesthesia & Critical Care*, DOI 10.1007/978-0-387-09562-2_44,
© Springer Science+Business Media, LLC 2012

Fig. 44.1 Cranial vault
compliance. Note the
increased compliance of
the infant cranial vault
(dash line)

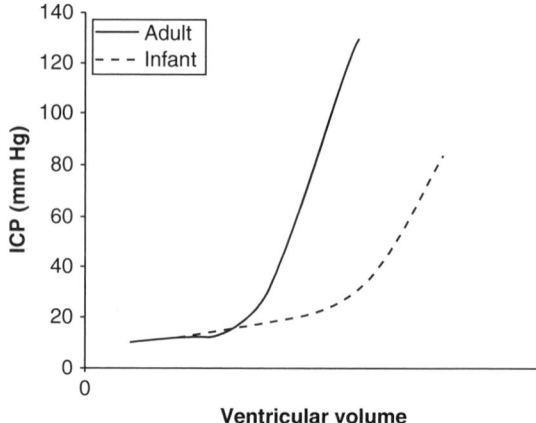

- Fontanel should be examined with the patient in the upright position and on palpation should feel slightly concave and a pulse may be palpable
- A slightly full fontanel can occur during vagal maneuvers such as crying, coughing, or emesis, but a full fontanel may be a sign of increased intracranial pressure
- A full fontanel may be the result of an obstructed or poorly functioning ventriculo-peritoneal shunt
- A depressed fontanel can be sign of dehydration
- A depressed fontanel may be the result of over draining of a ventriculo-peritoneal shunt
- Infants with severe dehydration are at risk for sinus thrombosis which may lead to increased intracranial pressure. In this specific case, a full fontanel may be observed in the presence of severe dehydration.

There are noninvasive trend monitors to assess the fullness of the fontanel due to increased intracranial pressure. Delayed or early closure of sutures and the fontanels can be signs of systemic disease or genetic syndromes, such has hypothyroidism and craniosynostosis.

Intracranial Compartments

The intracranial compartments of the pediatric brain are similar to the adult, with volume accounted for as follows:

- Brain and interstitial fluid 80%
- Cerebrospinal fluid (CSF) 10%
- Blood 10%.

The presence of unfused sutures and an open fontanel alters the Monroe–Kellie doctrine as it is applied to children (Fig. 44.1). The increased compliance of the cranial vault decreases the slope of the curve, allowing for larger increases in intracranial volume before rapid increases in intracranial pressure are observed.

It is important to note that unfused sutures and open fontanels do not preclude the pediatric patient from herniation during rapid increases in intracranial volume and pressure.

Cerebrospinal Fluid

CSF occupies similar percentage of the intracranial volume in adults and children. Although actual CSF volume is smaller in the children, CSF daily production can be similar to adults. CSF is produced by the choroids plexus located in the ventricular system (lateral, third, and fourth ventricles). It then circulates and is absorbed by the arachnoid villi into the venous system. Hydrocephalus can be the result of three different conditions related to CSF regulation.

- Increased CSF production (choroids plexus papillomas)
- Obstruction to circulation through the ventricular system (aqueductal stenosis)
- Impaired absorption by the arachnoid villi (intracranial blood).

Cerebral Blood Flow and Autoregulation

Cerebral blood flow has been observed to be age-dependent. Infants have been found to have cerebral blood flow rates similar to adults (50 mL/100 g of brain tissue). Cerebral blood rises with age and peaks around 70 mL/100 g of brain tissue between 3 and 8 years. It then decreases to adult levels by mid to late adolescence. Although cerebral blood flow rates are similar in infants and adults, it should be noted that a much higher percentage of cardiac output is directed to the brain in the child (25%) compared with the adult (15%).

The maintenance of cerebral blood flow to meet the metabolic needs of the brain is called autoregulation. There are several aspects to autoregulation. Pressure autoregulation refers to the maintenance of cerebral perfusion over a range of mean arterial pressures to meet brain metabolism.

- In adults, this range is between 50 and 150 mmHg. The pressure limits of autoregulation vary with age and the thresholds are lower in the younger pediatric population. In the healthy newborn, this mean is below 48 mmHg and is lower in premature children.
- The exact lower limit of autoregulation is not well known, and, in fact, premature infants may have a flow passive pattern of cerebral blood flow.
- This must be taken into account when utilizing cerebral perfusion pressure-directed therapy in the pediatric patient with severe brain injury.

Chemical autoregulation describes the relationship between partial pressures of arterial carbon dioxide and oxygen with cerebral blood flow.

- Rises in arterial carbon dioxide cause decreases in cerebral interstitial pH which results in cerebral vessel dilation and increases in cerebral blood flow and cerebral blood volume.
- In general, otherwise healthy children will tolerate the systemic effects of hypercarbia better than adults. The cerebral vascular effects in children, however, follow the same principles as in adults.
- Arterial oxygen does not affect cerebral flow until it reaches levels less than 50 Torr, below which, cerebral vessel dilation occurs.

It must also be noted that anesthetics may alter cerebral autoregulation. In these circumstances, cerebral blood flow becomes dependent on perfusion pressure (flow passive) and chemical autoregulation can be modified in critical illness. In general, the potent inhalational anesthetics affect autoregulation more than intravenous agents. Most, but not all, fentanyl derivatives preserve autoregulation.

Spinal Cord

The spinal cord anatomy also changes during childhood development. The conus medullaris (terminal end of the spinal cord) is lower in infants (L3) and does not reach the adult stage (L1) until 1 year of life. In children, the sacrum is narrower and flatter allowing a much more direct approach to the subarachnoid space. A sacral dimple may be a sign of underlying spinal cord abnormalities requiring furthering diagnostic testing (ultrasound and magnetic resonance imaging). Children are also more prone to neck and cervical spinal cord injuries due to their weaker neck musculature.

Implications for the Neurosurgical Patient

In the pediatric patient, the mass ratio of head to body is much higher than adults. This, in combination with the weaker neck musculature, places the child at greater risk for head injuries than the adult. Due to the incomplete myelination of axons and the smaller astrocyte and oligodendrocyte populations, the pediatric brain also has a higher water content and different viscoelastic properties compared with the adult brain. These properties along with the more elastic skull and rich vascular supply of the subarachnoid space lead to predominance of diffuse axonal injury and subarachnoid hemorrhage in the younger pediatric population following traumatic brain injury. As the central nervous system matures, mass lesions such as epidural, subdural, and intraparenchymal hematomas, become more prevalent following traumatic brain injury. Special consideration must be taken for the prematurely born infant, where the blood–brain barrier has not completely matured, and its fragility places the premature neonate at higher risk for intraventricular hemorrhage.

Besides increased head to body mass ratio, pediatric patients also have higher body surface area to mass ratios. This has important implications in the operating room, where pediatric patients are at higher risk for hypothermia, and care must be taken to regulate temperature carefully. Cooled cleaning solutions such as iodine and chlorhexidine can produce significant drops in body temperature in the pediatric patient compared with the adult.

Concerns and Risks

The increased vascularity of the cranial vault provides unique challenges to care of the pediatric patient. Large blood replacement requirements may be observed during cranial vault reconstructions. When the dura is breached and the blood–brain barrier is compromised, a disseminated intravascular coagulation cascade can be initiated intraoperatively and postoperatively requiring resuscitation with Fresh Frozen Plasma, Cryoprecipitate, and other component therapies. Cephalohematomas, which are subperiosteal hemorrhages, are common in infancy but when associated with linear skull fractures and/or coagulopathy may cause life-threatening hemorrhage.

Inflicted or non-accidental pediatric TBI (shaken-baby or shaken-impact syndrome) is a common cause of morbidity and mortality, especially in infants and young children. The practitioner must be familiar with the typical features of non-accidental head trauma and have a low threshold for further investigation.

- Non-accidental head trauma is most common in children under the age of 3 with the majority being less than 1 year.
- Typically the history is vague or varies over time and consists of a minor blunt impact of the head with a mechanism of injury that is not consistent.
- Presenting symptoms in the infant can also be vague. Lethargy, irritability, or poor feeding may be the initial complaint for seeking medical attention. Infants may also present with seizures, hyper- or hypotonia, or a full fontanel.
- Extracranial findings are not always present but may include bruising, burn marks, or fractures.
- Retinal hemorrhages are found in a majority of patients and may be unilateral or bilateral but are not specific for the diagnosis. For instance, vaginally delivered infants may have retinal hemorrhages up to 1 month after delivery.

Nontraumatic causes of retinal hemorrhages include sepsis, coagulopathy, galactosemia, and malignant hypertension which can be difficult to differentiate without considering the entire clinical picture. Intracranial bleeding should prompt a coagulation workup including fibrinogen, PT, INR, Platelet count, and PTT, although controversial retinal hemorrhages are not associated with CPR when there is no coagulopathy. If non-accidental TBI is suspected, a skeletal survey should also be performed since extra-cranial abnormalities are detected in a large percentage of cases. Likewise, there are conditions such as osteogenesis imperfecta that can mimic non-accidental fractures. In addition, other occult injuries, such as blunt abdominal trauma, should be investigated with laboratory data and/or a CT and surgical consultation. Once there is a concern for possible non-accidental trauma, social services should be consulted.

Key Points

- Central nervous system anatomy and physiology of the pediatric patient are not static and vary with age.
- Open fontanel and unfused sutures do not preclude the pediatric patient to herniation.
- Cerebral blood flow rates change with age and peak in school age children.
- The limits of pressure autoregulation vary with age and infants have lower pressure thresholds compare with adults.
- Children have a rich vascular supply to the subarachnoid space and more compliant skull predisposing them to subarachnoid hemorrhage and diffuse axonal injury following traumatic brain injury.
- Control of the cerebral circulation changes with age and critical illness.
- Inflicted head trauma must always be considered in the pediatric patient where there is no clear history or mechanism of accidental trauma.

Suggested Reading

Cheng MI, Khairi S, Ritter AM. Pediatric head injury. In: Reilly PL, Bullock R, editors. Head injury pathophysiology and management. 2nd ed. New York: Oxford University Press; 2005.

Duhaime AC, Christian CW, Rorke LB, Zimmerman RA. Nonaccidental head injury in infants-the "shaken baby syndrome". N Engl J Med. 1998;338(25):1822–9.

Odom A, Christ E, Kerr N, Byrd K, Cochran J, Barr F, et al. Prevalence of retinal hemorrhages in pediatric patients after in-hospital cardiopulmonary resuscitation: a prospective study. Pediatrics. 1997;99(6):E3.

Soul JS, Hammer PE, Tsuji M, Saul JP, Bassan H, Limperopoulos C, et al. Fluctuating pressure-passivity is common in the cerebral circulation of sick premature infants. Pediatr Res. 2007;61(4):467–73.

Udomphorn Y, Armstead WM, Vavilala MS. Cerebral blood flow and autoregulation after pediatric traumatic brain injury. Pediatr Neurol. 2008;38(4):225–34.

Urlesberger B, Müller W, Ritschl E, Reiterer F. The influence of head position on the intracranial pressure in preterm infants with posthemorrhagic hydrocephalus. Childs Nerv Syst. 1991;7(2):85–7.

Chapter 45
Pediatric Anesthetic Care Requirements

Gregory J. Latham and Donald Shaffner

Overview

The anesthesiologist involved in the neuro-anesthetic care of children needs to understand the anatomic and physiologic differences compared to the adult population (Chap. 44). Planning age-appropriate, perioperative, neuro-anesthetic care of children requires an understanding of both the neurologic and general maturational changes as well as an understanding of the neurosurgical procedure, the existing neurologic deficits, the underlying comorbidities, the presence of congenital defects, and the effects of anesthesia on all of these factors.

The risk of perioperative morbidity and mortality increases as age decreases; the risk to a child is similar to that of an adult, but the risk of anesthesia is increased for the infant and increased even more for the neonate. As with adults, the American Society of Anesthesiology (ASA) physical status predicts the risk of anesthesia for children. Children who are less than 2 years or critically ill generally receive anesthetic care by providers with special training in pediatric anesthesiology. This chapter highlights key differences in anesthetic care for children during their preoperative, intraoperative, and postoperative management.

General Preoperative Assessment of Children

The pediatric preoperative assessment should include knowledge of the procedure, diagnosis, history, physical examination, and NPO status. A list of highlights for the typical pediatric preoperative assessment is included in Table 45.1. A list of

G.J. Latham, MD (✉)
Department of Anesthesiology and Pain Medicine, Seattle Children's Hospital, Seattle, WA, USA

D. Shaffner, MD
Department of Anesthesiology and Critical Care Medicine, Johns Hopkins
The Medical Institutions, Baltimore, MD, USA

A.M. Brambrink and J.R. Kirsch (eds.), *Essentials of Neurosurgical Anesthesia & Critical Care*, DOI 10.1007/978-0-387-09562-2_45, © Springer Science+Business Media, LLC 2012

Table 45.1 General pediatric preoperative assessment

General	Developmental level, previous anesthetic problems, family history of MH
Birth	Prematurity: use of monitoring or oxygen at home, chronic lung disease (BPD), subglottic stenosis; congenital abnormalities (often more than one)
Cardiac	Congenital heart disease, murmur (need for SBE or bubble prophylaxis)
Pulmonary	Reactive airway disease, obstructive apnea (tonsillar hypertrophy)
Neurologic	Seizures, myopathies
Infectious	Upper respiratory infection (URI)
GI	Gastroesophageal reflux
Hematologic	Sickle cell disease, coagulopathy
Other	Renal, hepatic or endocrine problems

Table 45.2 General pediatric anesthetic preparation, equipment, and drugs

Airway equipment – in pediatric sizes	Masks
	Laryngeal mask airways (LMA)
	Endotracheal tubes
	Nasal and oral airways
	Laryngoscopes and blades
Pediatric positive pressure ventilator and circuit	
Temperature control	Patient warmers
	Fluid warmers
Fluid administration	Volumetric devices
	Pediatric size catheters
	Intraosseous needles
Monitors	Pulse oximetry probes – in pediatric sizes
	Blood pressure cuffs – in pediatric sizes
	ECG pads
	Temperature
	Capnography
Difficult airway equipment	Equipment for fiberoptic intubation and cricothyrotomy
Portable equipment for transport to ICU	To provide oxygenation and ventilation
	Portable monitoring
Resuscitation Cart	Defibrillator with pediatric paddles
	Vasoactive medications in dilutions appropriate for weight-based administration
	Dantrolene
	Pediatric dosing schedule

highlights for the preoperative assessment for the pediatric neurosurgical patient is included in Table 45.3.

Prematurity is often associated with multiple chronic problems. The presence of one congenital defect is often associated with other congenital defects. Patients with intracardiac connections may be at risk for subacute bacterial endocarditis (SBE), embolic events, cardiovascular instability, hypoxia, or arrhythmias. Children with upper respiratory infection (URI) or reactive airway disease may be at increased

Table 45.3 Preoperative assessment of the pediatric neurosurgical patient

Assessment	Rationale
Presence of neurologic deficits	Determine a change in postoperative period
Developmental level	Determine a change in postoperative period
Presence of elevated ICP	Cerebral perfusion, vomiting
Congenital abnormalities	Airway difficulty, SBE risk, embolism risk
Hydration status	Risk of hypotension, reduction of CPP
Use of diuretics or osmotic agents	Effect on volume status or electrolytes
Use of antiepileptic medications	Effect on platelets or coagulation factors, effect of large blood loss on blood levels, need for immediate postoperative continuation

CPP cerebral perfusion pressure, *ICP* intracranial pressure, *SBE* subacute bacterial endocarditis

risk of laryngospasm or bronchospasm. Children with myopathies or a positive family history may be at increased risk of malignant hyperthermia (MH) and should receive a non-triggering anesthetic. Children without any significant history or medications usually do not require any preoperative lab studies.

General Preoperative Sedation for Children

Parental separation and entrance into the operating room can provoke anxiety in a child. While many regimens exist for preoperative sedation, oral midazolam (0.25–1 mg/kg, maximum of 20 mg) is commonly used. If vascular access is in place, intravenous midazolam may be titrated to effect (IV dose is much less than oral dose). Preoperative sedation may be beneficial for children without elevated intracranial pressure (ICP) and especially for those at risk for intracranial bleeding (e.g., arteriovenous malformation and aneurysm) to decrease anxiety and hypertension during induction.

General Preparation of the Pediatric Operating Room

Much of the preparation of the operating room for the anesthetic care is dictated by the specific procedure to be performed. Pediatric-specific preparations for all anesthetics have been suggested and endorsed by the ASA and American Academy of Pediatrics (AAP). Anesthetic personnel need to be trained to administer anesthetics and medications in appropriate doses and volumes appropriate for pediatrics and have experience in the ventilation of infants and children. Equipment necessary for the pediatric environment is listed in Table 45.2. Discussion of specific monitoring for pediatric neurosurgical procedures can be found in Chap. 47.

General Induction of Anesthesia for Children

The choice between inhalation induction and intravenous induction is dictated by the presence or absence of intravenous access, the patient's neurological status, any coexisting disease processes, and the child's NPO status. While the majority of children coming from home to the operating room may receive an inhalation induction, those with full stomachs, loss of airway reflexes, vomiting, intracranial hypertension, decreased level of consciousness, or severe illness are best induced with a balanced technique of intravenous medications. For IV inductions in children, premedication with atropine IV (to prevent or treat bradycardia) is recommended for children less than 2 years, for children less than 6 years and receiving succinylcholine, or if bradycardia is present.

A rapid-sequence IV induction should be performed for patients with a decreased level of consciousness or other risk factors for aspiration. The US Food and Drug Administration (FDA) has issued a "boxed" warning about the use of succinylcholine in children. In summary, the use of succinylcholine for routine use in children has been abandoned except in cases of emergent airway management. High-dose rocuronium, 1.2 mg/kg, is an alternative for rapid sequence intubations. If succinylcholine is required (e.g., laryngospasm, suspected difficult airway, or concern that inadequate paralysis will cause a spike in ICP), then atropine 0.02 mg/kg IV/IM should precede succinylcholine.

Inhalation inductions in children are usually performed with sevoflurane with or without nitrous oxide. Sevoflurane is the least noxious and best tolerated potent inhalational agent for pediatric induction. Nitrous oxide is generally considered odorless and for the elective case may precede the application of sevoflurane to minimize the initial impact of the more noxious smell. Children then can be maintained on sevoflurane or switched to isoflurane or desflurane after induction.

It should be noted that the choice of induction and the agents used depends on a clear understanding of the child's physiology, neurological status, and the effect of the anesthetics on the disease process.

Implications for the Neurosurgical Patient

Preoperative Assessment of the Pediatric Neurosurgical Patient

Documentation of the preexisting neurologic deficits and the child's developmental level will help with postoperative assessment. The presence of elevated ICP and associated vomiting will have implications on the use of preoperative-sedation, induction technique, and intraoperative management. Lastly, the hydration status should be assessed prior to administering anesthetic agents that can cause hypotension and decrease cerebral blood flow (CBF) (Table 45.5).

No specific laboratory tests are required for pediatric neurosurgical patients. However, measuring preoperative electrolytes may be important in children with a history of vomiting or the use of osmotic diuretics. Platelet number or coagulation studies may be affected by the use of some anti-epileptic medications. In general, type and cross-matched blood should be available for craniotomies and large blood loss procedures.

Children with a history of chronic steroid treatment or replacement (hypopituitarism) may benefit from intraoperative replacement of stress dose steroid (1–2 mg/kg of hydrocortisone [Solu-Cortef] IM/IV or an equivalent dose of dexamethasone IV [0.05–0.1 mg/kg]). More than 3 weeks of exogenous corticosteroid therapy (>20 mg/day prednisone or equivalent) can produce measurable suppression and inability to mount a stress response for up to a year.

Preoperative Pediatric Neurosurgical Sedation

Over sedation can lead to respiratory depression, hypercarbia, hypoxia, and resultant increases in ICP. Sedative premedications should never be given to children with symptomatic intracranial hypertension or central nervous system depression, unless directly monitored by the anesthesiologist. Calm reassurance or parental presence through the time of induction may be the better approach for such children.

Preparation of the Pediatric Neurosurgical Operating Room

If warranted for the specific patient and procedure, equipment for ICP monitoring, for detection of venous air embolism (VAE), and for evoked potentials may be needed. Mannitol and hypertonic solutions may be needed. Blood products may need to be in the room if large or sudden blood loss is likely.

Induction of Pediatric Neurosurgical Anesthesia

In children with intracranial hypertension, the goals of induction are protection of the airway, hemodynamic stability, and avoidance of precipitous swings in CBF and ICP. Maintaining hemodynamic stability during induction will entail frequent measurement of blood pressure, calculation of cerebral perfusion pressure (CPP), if ICP monitoring is available, careful titration of anesthetic agents, and the availability of appropriately diluted vasoactive drugs to tightly control blood pressure and CPP. Typical medications for intravenous induction are listed in Table 45.4.

Table 45.4 Pediatric induction drug dosages

Type of induction agent	Drug	IV dosage	Notes
Sedative/hypnotic	Propofol, or	3–4 mg/kg	Titrate to avoid systemic and
	Thiopental	5–8 mg/kg	cerebral hypotension
Blunt hyperdynamic	Fentanyl, or	1–5 mcg/kg	Watch ventilation and BP
response	Lidocaine	1 mg/kg	2–3 Min prior to laryngoscopy
Paralysis	Vecuronium, or	0.1 mg/kg	Vecuronium and pancuronium
	Pancuronium	0.1 mg/kg	avoid histamine release
Paralysis for rapid-	Rocuronium, or	1.2 mg/kg	
sequence induction	Succinylcholine	1–2 mg/kg	Consider contraindications
Vasoactive drugs to treat	Phenylephrine	3–10 mcg/kg	Titrate to effect
changes in CPP	Thiopental	1–2 mg/kg	
	Sevoflurane	1–2%	

A rapid-sequence induction should be performed for patients with a decreased level of consciousness or other risk factors for aspiration. When the rapid-sequence induction technique is used, increases in ICP will occur if hypoventilation is prolonged and hypercarbia develops. Lidocaine IV, 1 mg/kg, is an additional adjunct to laryngoscopy that is tolerated well in children to prevent ICP increases during laryngoscopy or suctioning of the trachea. Lidocaine works best if given 2–3 min before laryngoscopy.

If an inhalational induction is chosen when there may be a risk of elevated ICP, then slight hyperventilation during the inhalation induction is believed to approximately offset the cerebral vasodilatory properties of sevoflurane during induction.

The use of Ketamine for an intramuscular induction of uncooperative children should be avoided when intracranial hypertension is a concern because it increases cerebral metabolism, CBF, and ICP.

Maintenance of Pediatric Neurosurgical Anesthesia

No single anesthetic technique has been shown to be superior for maintenance of anesthesia for children undergoing neurosurgery. The most important factor in choosing an anesthetic technique is to understand the pharmacokinetics of the agents, the effects of the agents on ICP and CBF (Table 45.5), and the needs of the surgical procedure. For children, a balanced technique of opiate, paralysis, nitrous oxide, and low-dose volatile anesthetic is chosen to provide analgesia, amnesia, hemodynamic stability, motor paralysis, and quick postoperative emergence.

Factors considered in the choice of anesthetics for the maintenance of anesthesia include past experience, impression of impact on neuromonitoring, ability to titrate to rapid emergence, requirements of the specific surgical procedure, and cost. The volatile anesthetics isoflurane and sevoflurane vary in their use for induction, cost, rapidity of emergence, cerebral vasodilation, and autoregulation effect. Recent literature suggests that sevoflurane may lead to better preservation of CBF and

Table 45.5 Cerebral effects of anesthetic agents

Drug	CBF	CMRO$_2$	ICP	Autoregulation
Propofol	↓↓	↓↓	↓↓	Preserved
Opioids	↔	↔	↔	Preserved
Thiopental	↓↓	↓↓	↓↓	Preserved
Benzodiazepines	↓	↓↓	↓	Preserved
Ketamine	↑↑	↔	↑↑	Unknown
N$_2$O	↑	↔ or ↑	↑	Preserved
Sevoflurane	↑	↓↓	↑	Abolished[a]
Isoflurane	↑	↓↓	↑	Abolished[a]
Desflurane	↑	↓↓	↑	Abolished[a]
Halothane	↑↑	↓	↑	Abolished

↑, increase; ↑↑, significant increase; ↔, no change; ↓, decrease; ↓↓, significant decrease; CBF, cerebral blood flow; CMRO$_2$, cerebral metabolic rate; ICP, intracranial pressure; N$_2$O, nitrous oxide

[a]Abolished in a dose-dependent fashion

autoregulation than isoflurane and, especially, desflurane. Nitrous oxide is an adjunct that may help speed emergence. The use of nitrous oxide varies upon the user's experience with its effect on evoked potentials and upon the risk for expanding pneumocephaly or VAE.

Propofol can help preserve evoked potentials but may need to be titrated as the length of the case progresses because accumulation can lead to loss of signals. Because of concerns for propofol infusion syndrome, a continuous infusion must be limited to less than 6 h in children. Furthermore, the clinical duration of propofol after infusion is difficult to gage if a wake-up test or rapid emergence is planned.

The usual opioid choices for use during a case include the short-acting agents fentanyl and remifentanil. The rapid metabolism of remifentanil aids rapid emergence, but experience is helpful in knowing when and how to add longer acting opioids for postoperative pain relief. The greater cost of remifentanil is also a consideration.

Paralytics are often used to minimize motion during surgery, prevent injury to patients in head pins, and allow low dose anesthetic administration when critical for monitoring. Titration of paralytics may be needed if motor evoked potentials are being used.

Antiemetics may be administered intraoperatively to reduce the risk of postoperative nausea and vomiting, which may exacerbate any elevated ICP. Ondansetron is an effective antiemetic in children with a minimum of side effects and can be given as 0.15 mg/kg IV, 30 min before emergence. Dexamethasone is also used in children for antiemetic effects and may also be requested by the neurosurgeons to minimize vasogenic edema from operative manipulation. Dexamethasone has been found to have antiemetic properties in doses of 0.0625–1.0 mg/kg IV, with some studies showing low doses as effective as high.

Specific pediatric neurosurgical procedures may have specific intraoperative needs and are discussed in Sect. 4.2.

Table 45.6 Pediatric analgesic dosages

Analgesic	Dosage	Notes
Acetaminophen (oral)	10–15 mg/kg PO q 4 h	Maximum dose: lesser of 100 mg/kg/day or 4 g/day; 75 mg/kg/day in infants
Acetaminophen (rectal)	30 mg/kg PR × 1, then 20 mg/kg PR q 6 h	q 12 h dosing in neonates
Morphine	0.025–0.1 mg/kg increments IV in children > 2 months of age	Half life 2 ± 1.8 h after ~2 months of age
Hydromorphone	15–30 mcg/kg IV q 3 h 30–80 mcg/kg PO/PR q 3 h	
Fentanyl	0.5–1 mcg/kg IV	
Oxycodone	0.05–0.15 mg/kg PO	
Hydrocodone	0.05–0.15 mg/kg PO	
Morphine PCA	10–20 mcg/kg/dose, lock out 8–15 min, basal 0–30 mcg/kg/h, 250–400 mcg/kg 4 h limit	
Hydromorphone PCA	2–4 mcg/kg/dose, lock out 8–15 min, basal 0–5 mcg/kg/h, 50–80 mcg/kg 4 h limit	
Fentanyl PCA	0.5 mcg/kg/dose, lock out 6–10 min, basal 0–0.5 mcg/kg/h, 7–10 mcg/kg 4 h limit	

Pain Management for Pediatric Neurosurgical Procedures

Scalp incisions, even for minimally invasive neurosurgical procedures, cause postoperative pain. Commonly, parenteral opiates are used intraoperatively and postoperatively. However, acetaminophen and NSAIDs have less effect on neurologic examination and less respiratory depression and may be useful alone or as adjunct to opiates. The potential for bleeding, however, should be considered with NSAIDS. Typical postoperative analgesia pediatric dosages are listed in Table 45.6.

Scalp blocks may be used for supplemental analgesia of excisions of the scalp. These blocks usually need to be performed while children are anesthetized, and total dosages of local anesthetic need to be monitored to avoid neurologic or cardiovascular toxicity. Maximum recommended doses of commonly used local anesthetics include 7 mg/kg of lidocaine, 2.5 mg/kg of bupivacaine, and 3 mg/kg of ropivacaine; maximum doses should be decreased by 30% in infants younger than 6 months. Epinephrine is often included as a vascular marker because of the toxicity risk associated with inadvertent intravascular administration.

Supraorbital and supratrochlear nerve blocks provide analgesia of the anterior forehead and scalp, from the bridge of the nose to the apex of the head. Occipital nerve blocks provide analgesia to the occipital and temporal regions of the scalp, from the nuchal line to the apex of the head. Both blocks are easy to perform. The reader is directed to a textbook of pediatric regional anesthesia for further discussion of the technique of these blocks.

Postoperative Pediatric Neurosurgical Management

The PACU or PICU responsible for children that are recovering from a neurosurgical procedure should have the same pediatric capabilities mentioned in Table 45.2. In addition to being familiar with pediatric respiratory and hemodynamic physiology, the staff needs to be familiar with the pediatric neurologic examination. Units taking care of children should be familiar with weight-based dosing for patients less than 40 kg and with Pediatric Advanced Life Support for patients less than 12 years (intraosseous access technique, appropriate defibrillator paddles, etc.).

Because of the sensitivity of children to pain medications, titration of medications is recommended to avoid hypotension and hypoventilation. The same basic goals of avoiding hypotension, hypoxia, hypoventilation, hyper- or hypoglycemia, and hypo- or hyperthermia apply. The staff needs to be aware that even without neurologic problems, neonates are at risk for periodic breathing and hypoventilation/hypoxia in the postanesthetic period. Children with pharyngeal tonsil hypertrophy are at risk for postoperative obstructive apnea.

It is especially important for the postanesthetic staff to know the preoperative neurologic findings and the developmental level of the patient because postoperative neurologic changes may require immediate investigation and intervention. Some abnormalities may be age appropriate such as Babinski reflexes, Moro reflexes, Asymmetric Tonic Neck reflexes, and clonus in very young children. Additionally, a description of typical seizure patterns can be helpful to the postanesthetic care staff for recognition and appropriate response to post-procedure seizures. The postoperative neurologic examination in an ICU setting needs to be recorded serially and at regular intervals with age appropriate measures so that subsequent examiners can review for changes in examination.

In addition to close neurologic monitoring, the postoperative staff should look for related complications and also prevent subsequent problems. These related complications include fluid and electrolyte disturbances. Children need to have weight-based fluid administration and depending on age and health may need to have glucose added. The same postoperative disturbances in volume and sodium status can occur in children, such as syndrome of inappropriate antidiuretic hormone (SIADH), diabetes insipidus, or cerebral salt wasting. A common pediatric postoperative complication is hyponatremic seizures in a child who is NPO, having continuous CSF drained by ventriculostomy, and whose maintenance fluid only contains one-quarter normal saline.

Concerns and Risks

Preoperative Management

The hydration status should be assessed prior to administering anesthetic agents that can cause hypotension and decrease CBF. NPO guidelines must be followed (Table 45.7). If significant dehydration is a concern, preoperative intravenous hydration may be necessary.

Table 45.7 Pediatric NPO guidelines

Solids	8 h
Infant formula	6 h
Breast milk	4 h
Clear liquids	2 h

Table 45.8 Methodologies to reduce or prevent cerebral edema

Promote venous drainage
- Head elevation
  - Note: increased risk for VAE if burr holes or craniotomy underway
- Head midline
  - Reduces venous outflow obstruction but may not be possible for surgical positioning
- Minimize intrathoracic pressure

CPP maintenance – age appropriate
- No guidelines exist for a minimum CPP in children, either under anesthesia or not
- Maintain adequate age appropriate mean arterial pressure (MAP)
  - Note: while hypotension is bad, adult data in trauma implies complications more likely if MAP elevation is too great; no data exists for children
- Minimize ICP

Hyperventilation
- Avoiding hypoventilation is prudent ($PaCO_2$ 35–40 mmHg)
- Mild hyperventilation with problematic ICP/edema management ($PaCO_2$ 30–35 mmHg)
- More aggressive hyperventilation ($PaCO_2 < 30$ mmHg) has risks and if needed for a prolonged period, monitoring of SjO_2, PbO_2, or CBF is suggested

Osmolar therapy
- Mannitol
  - 0.25–1 g/kg raises serum osmolarity by 10–20 mOsm/L
- Furosemide
  - 1 mg/kg
- Hypertonic saline
  - 12 cc/kg of 3% NaCl should raise serum Na 10 mEq/L and serum osmolarity by 20 mOsm/L
- Urine output measurement
  - Urinary catheter helps monitor diuresis caused by diuretic agents and CVP helps monitor volume status; while increasing osmolarity may decrease edema, hypotension may decrease CBF and reduce CPP; volume shifts in children may be more dramatic than in adults

Barbiturate
- Useful to reduce ICP/edema by cerebral vasoconstriction and reduction in $CMRO_2$
- May impair neurologic examination and emergence from anesthesia

Dexamethasone
- Useful for peri-tumor or peri-abscess vasogenic edema
- Unclear if useful for vasogenic edema secondary to surgical manipulation
- Not useful for traumatic edema
- Complications include hyperglycemia and hypertension

Hypothermia
- May reduce ICP/edema by reducing $CMRO_2$
- Unclear if improves outcome from traumatic injuries

CSF drainage
- May be useful when shunt or ventricular drain is available

Pediatric Intraoperative Cerebral Resuscitation

The same general guidelines for cerebral resuscitation apply to children and adults. Hypotension and hypoxemia have been shown to have a negative effect on the outcome of children with neurologic injury. Other general factors may have an impact on outcome and should be considered in the intraoperative management: avoid hyperthermia, seizures, and hypo- or hyperglycemia. Specific responses to concerns about brain edema are included in Table 45.8. It should be noted that while ICP may fall when the dura is open, brain swelling may continue during this time.

Key Points

- Sedative premedications increase risk when given to children with symptomatic intracranial hypertension or central nervous system depression.
- Succinylcholine should be avoided in children, except in situations of emergent airway management.
- The choice of inhalation versus intravenous induction depends on several factors. Most importantly, patients with full stomachs, loss of airway reflexes, vomiting, intracranial hypertension, decreased level of consciousness, or severe illness are best induced with a balanced technique of intravenous drugs.
- No single anesthetic technique has been shown to be superior for maintenance of anesthesia for children undergoing neurosurgery. The most important factor in choosing an anesthetic technique is to understand the effects of the agents on ICP and CBF, intraoperative monitoring, rapidity of emergence, and the needs of the surgical procedure.
- It is imperative that the anesthesiologist is aware of the methodologies to reduce or prevent cerebral edema preoperatively, intraoperatively, and postoperatively.

Suggested Reading

Dinsmore J. Anaesthesia for elective neurosurgery. Br J Anaesth. 2007;99(1):68–74.

Hammer GB, Krane EJ. Perioperative care of the neurosurgical pediatric patient. Int Anesthesiol Clin. 1996;34(4):55–71.

McClain CD, Soriano SG, Rockoff MA. Pediatric neurosurgical anesthesia. In: Cote CJ, Lerman J, Todres ID, editors. A practice of anesthesia for infants and children. 4th ed. Philadelphia, PA: Saunders Elsevier; 2009. p. 509–34.

Soriano SG, Bozza P. Anesthesia for epilepsy surgery in children. Childs Nerv Syst. 2006;22(8):834–43.

Soriano SG, Eldredge EA, Rockoff MA. Pediatric neuroanesthesia. Neuroimaging Clin N Am. 2007;17(2):259–67.

Chapter 46
The Pediatric Airway in Neurosurgery

Debra E. Morrison and Zeev N. Kain

Overview

Characteristics of the Pediatric Airway

The pediatric airway is characterized by smaller size and developmental anatomical differences.

1. *Smaller size* implies increased likelihood of soft tissue obstruction and resistance to airflow, especially if edema is present, as well as less technology available for airway management. Smaller size also necessitates a more subtle technique and predicates more immediate and disastrous consequences for failure to manage the airway:

   - Rapid desaturation with bradycardia
   - Laryngospasm
   - Distention of the stomach with mask ventilation, making it difficult to expand the lungs.

2. *Developmental differences* include:

   - Relatively large occiput, which influences positioning
   - More pliable and collapsible tissue
   - Likely presence of relatively larger tongue and larger tonsils and adenoids, which contribute to airway obstruction
   - A more cephalad larynx, which makes a straight laryngoscope blade more practical

D.E. Morrison, MD (✉) • Z. N. Kain, MD
Department of Anesthesiology and Perioperative Care, University of California,
Irvine Medical Center, Orange, CA, USA
e-mail: dmorriso@uci.edu

A.M. Brambrink and J.R. Kirsch (eds.), *Essentials of Neurosurgical
Anesthesia & Critical Care*, DOI 10.1007/978-0-387-09562-2_46,
© Springer Science+Business Media, LLC 2012

- A shorter, narrower and angled epiglottis, which can be difficult to lift with a laryngoscope blade
- The possibility of transitioning dentistry (unanticipated loose teeth).

The airway examination is mostly external, including the entire head, and historical, and is either normal or probably abnormal, based on suspected or known syndrome or diagnosis.

Ventilation

The most effective technique for *mask ventilation*:

1. Gently place the mask below the lips over the open mouth and at the bridge of the nose with the thumb and forefinger using just enough pressure to create a seal.
2. The fourth and fifth fingers should grasp the angle of the mandible and gently pull the jaw upward into the mask (spare finger can also be used to manipulate cricoid cartilage).
3. The middle finger should be free or touching only the bony portion of the mandible to avoid compression of midline soft tissue.
4. A small roll may be placed under the shoulders to compensate for the large occiput, which may be stabilized by a small gel donut, or the entire body excluding the head may be elevated on a pad.
5. Gentle continuous positive airway pressure (CPAP) can be used to distend the pharynx and larynx during spontaneous or assisted ventilation, while maintaining low peak inspiratory pressures (at no more than 15 cm H_2O) to avoid gastric distension.
6. Use of CPAP is preferable to use of an oral airway, since the wrong size can compress or distort the anatomy and cause obstruction, trauma, or laryngospasm.
7. A lubricated nasal trumpet (if not contraindicated by choanal atresia, coagulopathy, neutropenia, or basilar skull fracture) approximately the diameter of the nasal opening can also be used to relieve airway obstruction during mask ventilation.
8. If mask ventilation is at all difficult despite simple maneuvers, it is best to move on rather than to waste time struggling.
9. The patient with uncorrected meningomyelocele can be elevated above the table for induction and intubation with a donut around the "cele," a large roll under the shoulders and support for the head adequate to maintain normal alignment of head and neck.

Alternative Methods of Ventilation If Difficult Mask

An appropriately sized, thermosoftened, *lubricated endotracheal tube (ETT)* placed nasally (if not contraindicated) can be used in lieu of mask ventilation.

The adult nasal passage can be vasoconstricted to minimize potential bleeding which could make fiberoptic intubation more problematic. It is hard to approximate a correct pediatric dose of nasal decongestant spray or to quickly dilute neosynephrine; thus, it is imperative that nasal ETT be placed with minimal trauma.

1. Use a suction catheter as an ETT stylet positioned just past the distal tip of the ETT to blunt the edges of the ETT and lubricate the distal tip with water-soluble gel before insertion. A 6 F suction catheter fits in a 2.5 ETT, an 8 F fits in a 3.0 ETT, a 10 F fits in 3.5–4.5 ETT, and a 14 F catheter fits in larger ETTs.
2. Introduce ETT nasally just past the nasal passage, then (after optional suctioning) remove the suction catheter, leaving ETT in place.
3. Other techniques have been described using an esophageal stethoscope as stylet (works only in ETT sizes 4.5 and larger) or a red rubber catheter placed over the ETT tip, but the esophageal stethoscope method is more elaborate and the red rubber catheter is made of latex.
4. A Parker Flex-Tip™ tracheal tube, which comes in sizes 2.5 and larger, can be placed with less trauma to the naris.
5. Gently occlude both mouth and other naris, attach circuit and ventilate.
6. If using lidocaine 1% to blunt response to intubation, use maximum of 1–2 mg/kg.
7. If considering use of phenylephrine 0.25%, use no more than 1–2 drops, maintain blood pressure at baseline with systemic vasodilation.
8. Nasal ETT should be positioned to avoid pressure-induced ischemia of the nasal ala.

A lubricated (with water-soluble surgical gel, not local anesthetic) *laryngeal mask airway* (LMA), such as either Dr. Brain's LMA Classic™ (best fit) or Dr. Cook's Air-Q™ (wide barrel) can also be used in lieu of mask ventilation and can be removed and replaced repeatedly.

The King Airway™ can always be placed in the esophagus, and both cuffs (a small one in the esophagus and a larger one in the oropharynx above the vocal cords) can be inflated using a single balloon. The single lumen connects to the anesthesia circuit and delivers respiratory gases through anterior vents to the space below the large cuff and above the vocal cords. The model currently available in the USA has a blind end in the esophageal lumen and is available in sizes 2 and above. A reusable model available elsewhere has a gastric suction port which leads to an esophageal lumen allowing placement of a gastric tube and comes in sizes 0 and above. The device can be useful for emergency CT or MRI in place of an LMA with less likelihood of insufflation of the stomach. A tube exchange device or small fiberoptic bronchoscope (FOB) can be passed into the trachea through the device to replace it with a definitive airway.

Both the nasal ETT and the LMA, with attached *double swivel connector with port* (DSC), can be used to introduce a small FOB without interruption of monitored oxygenation and ventilation.

Using either of these devices for ventilation and intubation allows easy ventilation even with the patient in a more upright position allowing compensation for increased intracranial pressure with the added benefit of allowing the epiglottis to fall forward away from the glottic opening to enhance exposure of the vocal cords during fiberoptic intubation.

Intubation

1. The *correct size of the ETT* is traditionally estimated for patients over 1 year by Cole's formula: Internal tube diameter (mm) = (16 + age in years)/4, but age does not always correlate with size, so the correct-sized ETT is usually about the same size as the tip of the child's fifth finger.
2. A slightly smaller high volume low pressure low-cuffed ETT can be used, inflating the cuff just enough, if at all, to minimize the leak appropriately.

In the normal pediatric airway, the *straight laryngoscope blade* should be inserted midline, approximately perpendicular to the patient, into the vallecula or used directly to lift the epiglottis to expose the vocal cords. Although the straight blade is the traditional blade, the Mac 2 blade, used in the normal manner, also works very well in many children greater than 1 year.

1. If there is a good view of the vocal cords but the approach is difficult, and the patient is large enough to accommodate a 3.0 or larger ETT, have an assistant discard the stylet and insert a *Cook Frova® intubating introducer* (bougie) several centimeters past the tip of the ETT.
2. Pinching the ETT tight to the bougie to prevent slippage, introduce the bougie through the vocal cords, and then slide the ETT over it into the trachea, all in one motion.
3. The bougie can alternatively be inserted without the ETT, even down the "barrel" of the blade, without obscuring the view of the vocal cords, but the bougie's adaptor must first be removed to allow the ETT to be placed over the proximal end of the bougie.

If the vocal cords cannot be seen with a conventional laryngoscope, there are some simple alternative strategies for which equipment is available.

Light-Assisted Blind Intubation

The Trachlight™ stylet and tracheal lightwand comes in 2 sizes, the smaller of which fits through ETT sizes 2.5–4.0 and the larger of which fits through ETT sizes 4.5 and above. The device, a malleable wire in a PVC sheath, attached to a reusable light handle, can aid in blind oral or nasal intubations.

Fiberoptic Oral Approach Through LMA

1. Insert LMA, inflate cuff, and demonstrate good $ETCO_2$ waveform.
2. Attach DSC to the LMA, place patient on positive pressure ventilation with low peak inspiratory pressure.
3. Remove connector from an appropriate sized ETT and slide it to the top of an appropriate sized FOB.

4. Introduce the FOB through the port of the DSC, down the LMA (through the center of the grid if there is a grid), through the vocal cords to just above the carina.
5. Disconnect the DSC from the LMA and slide it up over the ETT to the top of the FOB. With the Air-Q™, the connector can also be disconnected.
6. Slide the ETT down over the FOB until its top is level with the top of the LMA, at which point the tip will be past the vocal cords.
7. Remove the FOB.
8. Grasp the ETT with small tipped long grasping forceps (from ENT tray or cart) and hold it in place while sliding the LMA up over the forceps.
9. Attach the ETT connector, attach to the circuit and confirm that the ETT is appropriately placed in the trachea.
10. Alternatively, the LMA could be left in place during surgery if the risk of removing it (dislocation of ETT) with outweighs the benefit.

Fiberoptic Nasal Approach

1. The nasal approach to the airway is often the more direct approach in a pediatric patient.
2. Once an appropriate sized ETT is placed nasally just past the nasopharynx, occlude the other naris and the mouth and attach a DSC to the ETT.
3. Place patient on low positive pressure ventilation or allow patient to breathe spontaneously. Sedation or general anesthesia is possible with sevoflurane and/or intravenous propofol, with $ETCO_2$ monitoring.
4. Introduce the lightly lubricated FOB through the port of the DSC, down the ETT, and through the vocal cords to just above the carina.
5. Slide the ETT down the FOB through the vocal cords, remove the FOB, and confirm that the ETT is appropriately placed in the trachea.

"Fastrach™" Approximation (Blind, $ETCO_2$ Guided)

1. Insert LMA, inflate cuff, and demonstrate good $ETCO_2$ waveform.
2. Attach circuit to ETT and watch $ETCO_2$ waveform during either spontaneous ventilation or low positive pressure ventilation as ETT is advanced through LMA and then through vocal cords.
3. If patient is breathing spontaneously, and $ETCO_2$ waveform disappears, retract ETT slightly.
4. If $ETCO_2$ waveform does not return with retraction, consider laryngospasm, treat, and advance with $ETCO_2$ waveform as it returns.
5. If $ETCO_2$ waveform does return with initial retraction of the ETT, the LMA is probably not directing the ETT toward the vocal cords. Reposition LMA and reattempt or change technique.

Video Laryngoscope and Pediatric GlideScope

1. The Storz® video laryngoscope has a Miller 0 and a Miller 1 blade and can be used to intubate a smaller infant or child. The view in the fairly large screen is from the distal tip of the blade, not the proximal end.
2. Storz has also introduced the C-MAC® which consists of a laryngoscope that attaches directly to a portable LCD screen via a single cable. Everything needed is built directly into these two components and there are no fragile fiberoptic bundles. It is cheaper and has two associated pediatric blades.
3. The Verathon® GlideScope's curved disposable blade covers fit over a small pediatric wand which is part of a separate cable, come in two pediatric sizes, equivalent to Mac 2 and Mac 3 and can be used to intubate a larger infant or child. The view in the screen is from the distal tip of the blade, not the proximal end.
4. All three devices enable the vocal cords to be visualized easily, but the blade must be manipulated to place the vocal cords in the center of the screen so that the ETT, bougie or ETT-over-bougie (or lightwand) can approach the vocal cords.
5. If the vocal cords appear high or to the left of the screen, the blade should be withdrawn slightly and lifted, dropping the tip, not "cocking" the tip, enabling the vocal cords to drop lower into view.
6. The blade must be utilized such that the larynx is tilted with the arytenoids and interarytenoid fold more distal to the operator, so that the ETT does not slip behind the fold into the esophagus.

Video Laryngoscope or Pediatric GlideScope with FOB

1. If, despite manipulation of the blade, the tube cannot be made to approach the vocal cords, a second operator can introduce the ETT over an FOB, while the first operator is exposing the vocal cords with the video laryngoscope or GlideScope.

Implications for the Neurosurgical Patient

When the pediatric patient is a neurosurgical patient, implications include:

1. Urgency (intracranial hemorrhage)
2. Need to avoid stimulation or hemodynamic change during airway management (high ICP)
3. Need to avoid hypoventilation or apnea during airway management (rapid desaturation, high ICP)
4. Positioning issues such as known or possible spinal cord injury, meningomyelocele
5. Specific requirement or contraindication for an oral vs. nasal vs. special ETT

   (a) Wire reinforced tube might be necessary for an operation on the cervical spine when the position of the head may force the ETT to be compressed by the teeth or during a long operation where soft ETT may collapse (cranial synostosis) but would be contraindicated if the patient were anticipated to require an MRI

6. Possible full stomach and concerns regarding readiness for extubation.

In a worst-case scenario, consider a toddler patient with micrognathia who has fallen from a bed just after a meal and has diminished consciousness because of an intracranial bleed. The patient is a trauma patient, presumed full stomach, wearing a cervical collar (neck cannot be cleared), and requires an immediate operation. After preoxygenation, perform mask induction (if no IV) or IV induction, briefly maintaining, if possible and appropriate, spontaneous ventilation. At this point, an orogastric tube can be placed, exiting at the corner of the mouth and placed on suction; gentle cricoid pressure can, if desired, be utilized, and ventilation, if necessary, can proceed with mask, LMA or nasal ETT. Intubation can proceed with or without paralysis. Remember that an LMA can always be replaced and used in lieu of a mask for ventilation, with or without a gastric tube. The LMA ProSeal™ now comes in the full range of sizes, allowing a gastric suction device to be placed through the LMA.

Concerns and Risks

1. High oxygen flows may dilute $ETCO_2$ during mask ventilation, making it appear that ventilation is inadequate or that patient is being hyperventilated when this is not the case.
2. Low $ETCO_2$ waveform may also be caused by low cardiac output rather than by hyperventilation.
3. Positioning necessary for neurosurgical procedures can result in the ETT advancing to and stimulating the carina, advancing into the right main stem bronchus, withdrawing from the glottis, or being compressed by the teeth or gums. ETT position and patency should always be reconfirmed when the patient is in final position.
4. Insufflating the stomach with mask ventilation can lead to difficulty in ventilation and/or risk of aspiration.
5. An orogastric tube can be inserted and left in place during masking, before an LMA is placed, or through an LMA with a gastric vent.
6. Positioning necessary for neurosurgical procedures can increase the risk of accidental extubation. Prone position plus secretions can loosen tape. The weight of the ventilator tubing can pull out an ETT, especially when the head is resting on a frame instead of the bed (suspend the airway tubing or tie it to the Mayfield frame with umbilical ties to relieve weight). An ETT secured to the bed instead of to the frame can lead to accidental extubation when the patient is moved.
7. Regarding emergence and extubation: Do not rely on a twitch monitor to determine whether or not a pediatric patient is reversible. Assume a patient's muscle relaxant is reversible when the patient is making respiratory efforts. Lifting knees to chest can be considered the equivalent of head lift. Pediatric patients may be at high risk for postoperative apnea, thus a rush to extubate is not always appropriate.

Key Points

- Preparation for neurosurgical anesthesia on a range of pediatric patients includes assembling and handling an array of pediatric airway equipment and supplies (Table 46.1).
- Prepare for challenging patient by thinking through scenarios while practicing strategies in advance on normal patients (Table 46.2).

Table 46.1 Airway equipment

LMAs: LMA Classic or ProSeal, or Air-Q	Masks
Endotracheal tubes: Uncuffed, cuffed and reinforced (know in advance which size tube fits through which LMA)	Fiberoptic bronchoscopes Nasal trumpets Suction catheters and gastric tubes
Accordion connectors for patients with tracheostomy who must be positioned prone	Laryngoscopes and blades Double swivel connector with port
Long grasping forceps (from pediatric ENT cart)	Cook Frova® intubating introducer
Video laryngoscope/Pediatric GlideScope	Surgical lubricant
Nasal vasoconstrictor	1% Lidocaine/MADD adaptor
Trachlight	

Table 46.2 Syndromes, diagnoses, and scenarios associated with neurosurgical procedures with airway issues

Condition	Potential complications
Myemeninglocele/ myelodysplasia/Chiari malformations	Positioning Hydrocephalus Difficult intubation Latex avoidance Risk of postoperative apnea
Craniosynostosis	Difficult intubation Long operation Airway edema Head manipulation leading to right mainstem intubation or unintended extubation Need for intermittent suctioning
Intracranial masses	High ICP Positioning including sitting with risk of ETT kinking or compression Venous air embolism
Intracranial bleed	High ICP Emergency Positioning

(continued)

Table 46.2 (continued)

Condition	Potential complications
Spine surgery	Positioning
	Risk of venous air embolism
	Difficult intubation
	Risk of unintended extubation
	Airway edema
Vascular anomalies	Avoid stimulation
	Risk of intracranial bleed
Seizure surgery	Ease of emergence for neurological evaluation
	Intraoperative EEG
Encephalocele	Avoidance of nasal intubation
	Difficult intubation
	Positioning
Neuroradiologic procedures	Avoid metal in ETT
	Need to limit equipment or intubate outside MRI suite
	Limited access to patient even during induction
Trauma	Emergency
	Full stomach
	Many of above considerations

Suggested Reading

American Society of Anesthesiologists Task Force on Management of the Difficult Airway. Practice guidelines for management of the difficult airway: an updated report by the American Society of Anesthesiologists Task Force on Management of the Difficult Airway. Anesthesiology. 2003;98:1269–77.

Gregory GA. Classification and assessment of the difficult pediatric airway. Anesthesiol Clin North Am. 1998;16:729–41.

Markakis DA, Sayson SC, Schreiner MS. Insertion of the laryngeal mask airway in awake infants with the Robin sequence. Anesth Analg. 1992;75:822–4.

Seo KS, Kim J-H, Yang SM, Kim HJ, Bahk J-H, Yum KW. A new technique to reduce epistaxis and enhance navigability during nasotracheal intubation. Anesth Analg. 2007;105:1420–4.

Wheeler M. Management strategies for the difficult pediatric airway. Anesth Clin North Am. 1998;16:743–61.

Chapter 47
Specific Aspects of Positioning and Fluids, Glucose, and Temperature Management in Children Undergoing Neurosurgical Procedures

Gerhard K. Wolf, John H. Arnold, and Sulpicio G. Soriano

Overview

This chapter discusses the optimal strategies regarding patient positioning as well as intraoperative fluid, glucose, and temperature management as they pertain to children who have to undergo neurosurgical procedures.

Implications for the Neurosurgical Patient

Positioning

Patient positioning requires careful preoperative planning to allow adequate access to the patient for both the neurosurgeon and the anesthesiologist. Table 47.1 describes common surgical positions applied for pediatric neurosurgery and their physiologic sequelae. These issues should be considered because the duration of

G.K. Wolf, MD (✉)
Department of Anesthesiology, Perioperative and Pain Medicine, Children's Hospital Boston,
Harvard Medical School, Boston, MA, USA

J.H. Arnold, MD
Departments of Anaesthesia, Perioperative and Pain Medicine, and Respiratory
Care/ECMO/Biomedical Engineering, Children's Hospital Boston,
Harvard Medical School, Boston, MA, USA

S.G. Soriano, MD, FAAP
Department of Anaesthesia, Harvard Child Hospital, Boston, MA, USA

A.M. Brambrink and J.R. Kirsch (eds.), *Essentials of Neurosurgical Anesthesia & Critical Care*, DOI 10.1007/978-0-387-09562-2_47, © Springer Science+Business Media, LLC 2012

Table 47.1 Physiologic effects of patient positioning

Position	Physiologic effect
Head elevated	Enhanced cerebral venous drainage
	Decreased cerebral blood flow
	Increased venous pooling in lower extremities
	Postural hypotension
Head down	Increased cerebral venous and intracranial pressure
	Decreased functional residual capacity (lung function)
	Decreased lung compliance
Prone	Venous congestion of face, tongue, and neck
	Decreased lung compliance
	Increased abdominal pressure can lead to venocaval compression
Lateral decubitus	Decreased compliance of down-side lung

most neurosurgical procedures can lead to significant physiologic impairment or injury if positioning problems are left undetected. All pressure points should be padded and peripheral pulses checked to prevent compression or pressure injury. In addition to compression and stretch injuries, the prone position can compromise the respiratory and cardiovascular system. It is important to minimize pressure on the abdomen because increased intraabdominal pressure can impair ventilation, cause venocaval compression, and increase epidural venous pressure and bleeding during surgical intervention. Soft rolls are used to suspend the chest and abdomen to minimize any increase in abdominal and thoracic pressure. During prone procedures, the airway is often in a dependent position, which may lead to significant airway edema. This can lead to postextubation airway obstruction or croup.

Neurosurgical procedures are performed with the head slightly elevated to facilitate venous and cerebrospinal fluid drainage from the surgical site. However, superior sagittal sinus pressure decreases with greater head elevation, and this increases the likelihood of venous air embolism. Extreme head flexion can cause brainstem compression in patients with pathologic conditions of the posterior fossa, such as mass lesions or Arnold–Chiari malformations. It can also cause endotracheal tube obstruction from kinking or migration into the mainstem bronchus and head and tongue swelling due to impaired venous or lymphatic drainage. Extreme rotation of the head can hinder venous return through the jugular veins and lead to impaired cerebral perfusion, increased intracranial pressure, and cerebral venous bleeding.

Volume Status

Measurement of urine output as a surrogate for volume status should be interpreted with great caution in neurosurgical patients, as urine output may be profoundly influenced by changes in antidiuretic hormone (ADH) levels rather than by intravascular volume status and renal perfusion alone. Any neurosurgical patient with oliguria could have a component of syndrome of inappropriate vasopressin secretion (SIADH) and be volume overloaded; rather than additional volume boluses, this patient would benefit from fluid restriction until the SIADH resolves. On the other hand, a patient with polyuria could have diabetes insipidus (DI) and be volume depleted after uncontrolled urine losses. This patient would benefit from careful fluid resuscitation and administration of Vasopressin. Volume status should be assessed clinically, with emphasis on clinical exam and vital signs. Central venous pressures or echocardiography may provide useful additional information about left atrial pressures and left ventricular preload.

Glucose Control

Normoglycemia should be achieved in all patients. There is sufficient evidence that hyperglycemia contributes to secondary brain injury and is associated with worse outcome in patients with traumatic brain injury. Hyperglycemia may also be associated with an increased risk of wound infection. On the other hand, intensive glycemic control has not been shown to improve mortality in critically ill patients in general and in critically ill patients in the neuro-intensive care setting. Intensive glycemic control may lead to hypoglycemic episodes, which can be detrimental in neurosurgical patients.

Thermal Homeostasis

Infants and children are especially susceptible to hypothermia during any surgical procedure because of their large surface area to weight ratio. Active heating of the patient by increasing the ambient temperature and using radiant light warmers during induction of anesthesia, catheter insertion, and preparation and positioning of the patient are prophylactic measures against hypothermia. Mattress warmers, forced hot air blankets, and humidification of inspired gases can also prevent intraoperative temperature loss and postoperative shivering.

Induced Hypothermia

Induced hypothermia has been unequivocally shown to reduce neurological injury in laboratory studies. Its efficacy in the clinical setting has been controversial. Head cooling and mild hypothermia has been demonstrated to be protective in asphyxiated neonates. However, induced hypothermia in adult traumatic brain injury has mixed results. Recently, Adelson and colleagues demonstrated in a Phase II trial that induced hypothermia can be a safe therapeutic option in children with TBI.

An NIH sponsored Phase III trial is underway. Recently, an international multicenter trial of induced hypothermia in pediatric patients reported that hypothermia did not improve the neurologic outcome and may increase mortality.

Concerns and Risks

Intraoperative Diabetes Insipidus

The diagnosis of intraoperative DI in pediatric patients is straightforward and is – as in the adult – characterized by the presence of

- Urine output of 4 mL/kg/h
- Serum Na > 145 mEq/L
- Serum osmolality > 300 mOsm/kg
- Urine osmolality < 300 mOsm/kg
- Polyuria persisting > 30 min
- Other causes of polyuria must be ruled out (e.g., administration of mannitol, furosemide, osmotic contrast agents, and presence of hyperglycemia).

Once the diagnosis of DI is established, a Vasopressin infusion is commenced at 1 milliunit/kg/h and is increased every 5–10 min to a maximum of 10 milliunit/kg/h aimed at decreasing the urine output to <2 mL/kg/h. Total maintenance fluids (intravenous and oral fluids) should not exceed the insensible losses plus the obligate urinary losses. It is convenient to calculate the total intravenous fluids as 2/3 maintenance. The appropriate intravenous fluid for pediatric patients in the context of neurosurgery is 0–5% dextrose, 0.9% saline with 0–40 mEq of potassium chloride/L. Blood loss should be replaced with normal saline, Lactate Ringer's solution, or 5% albumin or blood products as appropriate. We view the antidiuretic effect of Vasopressin as an "all or none" phenomenon. Once the patient's urine output is less than 2 mL/kg/h, we regard the urine output as "captured."

The following clinical scenarios may occur intraoperatively:

The patient is not responding at all and the urine output remains high:
If the patient is not responding to the vasopressin infusion, the intravenous catheter must be checked for patency and the infusion preparation and rate should be checked.

The patient stops producing urine:
Even with a maximal dose of vasopressin, the kidneys will produce a minimal urine output. If a patient stops producing urine entirely, this may represent prerenal failure secondary to hypovolemia. Some degree of dehydration is to be expected in most patients after a period of uncontrolled urine output prior to establishing the diagnosis of DI. The diagnosis of hypovolemia has to be made using all clinical parameters

(clinical exam, vital signs, and central venous pressure) except the urine output. In this scenario, we confirm patency of the urinary catheter and give judicious (10 mL/kg) fluid boluses of normal saline until the urine output resumes. We do not recommend altering the vasopressin infusion rate in this setting. Reducing the vasopressin infusion rate to enhance urine output will result in unnecessary confusion about the patient's volume status.

Postprocedure, the vasopressin infusion should be continued and the child should be admitted to an intensive care unit. DI has been reported to occur in 8% of patients preoperatively and 70–90% of all patients presenting postoperatively from craniopharyngioma surgery. Of note, the onset of postoperative DI is usually 1–12 h after surgery. A triphasic response (DI-SIADH-DI) after craniopharyngioma resection has been described. The triphasic response is characterized by initial diabetes insipidus after resection of the pituitary gland, followed by a "honeymoon period" where ADH is thought to be released from necrotic cells in the pituitary stump. This phase of relative SIADH can last 3–6 days, and is usually followed by a definitive deficiency in ADH, resulting in permanent DI.

Cerebral salt wasting (*CSW*) is a disorder of excessive natriuresis in the presence of an intracerebral lesion. The pathophysiology of CSW is poorly understood, and there is no convincing animal model that explains the mechanism by which cerebral disease might lead to renal salt wasting. CSW can easily be confused with SIADH, as hyponatremia is a feature of both disorders. It is important to differentiate both diseases as may occur in brain injury: CSW is associated with volume depletion secondary to natriuresis; SIADH is a situation of volume overload secondary to free water overload. Some authors have speculated that CSW is an overdiagnosed entity; the same group of authors have also pointed out that in most cases where CSW is speculated, natriuresis is secondary to volume expansion and ADH levels are appropriately elevated. It is important to note that it is impossible to make the diagnosis of CSW in the absence of an intracerebral lesion. The therapy of CSW is volume repletion with isotonic saline. In severely hyponatremic patients or in patients with ongoing sodium losses, sodium repletion with 3% NaCl (513 mEq/L) may be required. Symptomatic patients (seizures) may require a 1 mL/kg 3% NaCl bolus over 30 min, which may be given more rapidly if the patient is actively seizing. As a rule of thumb, 1 mL/kg 3% NaCl will elevate the serum sodium by 1 mEq/L.

Hyponatremia is the most common electrolyte disorder in hospitalized patients. Iatrogenic induced hyponatremia suggests a surplus of water and a deficit of sodium in the extracellular fluid compartment. It is a common but dangerous practice to use hypotonic fluids such as half-normal saline (77 mEq Na/L) or 0.2 normal saline (31 mEq Na/L) as maintenance fluids in pediatrics. Children who have elevated levels of ADH such as children with pneumonia, sepsis, meningitis, and postoperative patients are at risk for hyponatremia, as their ability to excrete excessive free water may be impaired. Bohn and coworkers reported that hyponatremia occurred not uncommonly in the first 48 h of admission to the hospital. Catastrophic neurologic sequelae and death resulting from iatrogenic induced hyponatremia have been described. Hypotonic fluids must not be used in neurosurgical patients.

Key Points

- In pediatrics, patient positioning for surgery requires careful preoperative planning to allow adequate access to the patient for both the neurosurgeon and the anesthesiologist.
- Infants and children are especially susceptible to hypothermia because of their large surface area to weight ratio.
- Neurosurgical patients are at particular risk for electrolyte derangements.
- Normoglycemia should be achieved, but intensive glucose control can lead to potentially detrimental episodes of hypoglycemia.
- Hypotonic fluids must be avoided by all means.
- Volume status should be assessed clinically, as urine output can be influenced by SIADH, DI, and CSW.
- SIADH is characterized by free water retention, and ADH levels are inappropriately elevated.
- Cerebral salt wasting is probably a less common cause of hyponatremia than SIADH in patients with cerebral injury.
- Intraoperative diabetes insipidus is characterized by urine output greater than 4 mL/kg/h, low urine and high serum osmolality in the absence of other causes of polyuria.

Suggested Reading

Cochran A, Scaife ER, Hansen KW, Downey EC. Hyperglycemia and outcomes from pediatric traumatic brain injury. J Trauma. 2003;55(6):1035–8.

Grady MS, Bedford RF, Park TS. Changes in superior sagittal sinus pressure in children with head elevation, jugular venous compression, and PEEP. J Neurosurg. 1986;65(2):199–202.

Halberthal M, Halperin ML, Bohn D. Lesson of the week: Acute hyponatraemia in children admitted to hospital: retrospective analysis of factors contributing to its development and resolution. BMJ. 2001;322(7289):780–2.

Singh S, Bohn D, Carlotti AP, Cusimano M, Rutka JT, Halperin ML. Cerebral salt wasting: truths, fallacies, theories, and challenges. Crit Care Med. 2002;30(11):2575–9.

Van den Berghe G, Wilmer A, Hermans G, Meersseman W, Wouters PJ, Milants I, et al. Intensive insulin therapy in the medical ICU. N Engl J Med. 2006;354(5):449–61.

Wise-Faberowski L, Soriano SG, Ferrari L, McManus ML, Wolfsdorf JI, Majzoub J, et al. Perioperative management of diabetes insipidus in children [corrected]. J Neurosurg Anesthesiol. 2004;16(1):14–9.

Part IX
Critical Situations During Anesthesia for Pediatric Surgery

Chapter 48
Challenges During Surgery for Hydrocephalus

Inger Aliason and Jeffrey Koh

Overview

Hydrocephalus is caused by excessive ventricular cerebrospinal fluid (CSF), usually due to an obstruction (noncommunicating hydrocephalus) or inadequate CSF reabsorption (communicating hydrocephalus). In rare cases, hydrocephalus can result from a choroid plexus papilloma, which causes an overproduction of CSF. The most common causes of pediatric hydrocephalus are myelomeningocele (obstruction) and posthemorrhagic hydrocephalus of prematurity (inadequate reabsorbtion at the arachnoid granulations).

The prevalence of hydrocephalus is reported to be 0.63–1.2 cases per 1,000 children, [1] making it one of the most common neurosurgical problems encountered in both the adult and pediatric populations. Medical advances in the care of premature infants may be leading to an increased incidence of hydrocephalus due to the survival of infants with intraventricular hemorrhage.

I. Aliason, MD (✉)
Departments of Anesthesiology, The University of Oklahoma College of Medicine,
Oklahoma City, OK, USA

J. Koh, MD
Department of Anesthesiology and Perioperative Medicine, Oregon Health & Science University,
Portland, OR, USA

A.M. Brambrink and J.R. Kirsch (eds.), *Essentials of Neurosurgical
Anesthesia & Critical Care*, DOI 10.1007/978-0-387-09562-2_48,
© Springer Science+Business Media, LLC 2012

Congenital causes of hydrocephalus	Acquired causes of hydrocephalus
• Myelomeningocele • Dandy–Walker malformation • Arnold–Chiari malformation • Aqueductal stenosis • Cysts (arachnoid, interhemispheric) • Neoplasms • Encephalocele • Vascular malformations • Mucopolysaccharidoses • X-linked hydrocephalus • Maroteaux–Lamy syndrome • Congenital conditions affecting the skull (Crouzon, Pfieffer, achondroplasia)	• Prematurity (posthemorrhagic hydrocephalus) • Subarachnoid hemorrhage (trauma, aneurysm) • Neoplasm • Meningitis • Encephalitis

Symptoms that accompany pediatric hydrocephalus, range from mild headache to life-threatening lethargy, bradycardia, and ultimately brain herniation. Key factors that determine how symptomatic the child will be include intracranial compliance and the rate at which the hydrocephalus develops. Neonates have high intracranial compliance, therefore development of hydrocephalus is usually accommodated by increasing head circumference, and maintenance of near normal intracranial pressure (ICP).

Symptoms of *slowly* developing hydrocephalus in neonates	Signs and symptoms of *acutely* increased ICP in patients of all ages
• Enlarged head circumference • Full fontanelle • Separating sutures • Irritability • Vomiting	• Headache • Lethargy • Vomiting • Cranial nerve dysfunction • Papilledema • Decorticate or decerebrate posturing • Hypertension • Bradycardia • ECG changes due to brainstem compression • Irregular respirations • Eventual brain herniation and death

Hydrocephalus is usually treated with an intraventricular catheter or endoscopic ventriculostomy to relieve the obstruction to CSF flow. Intraventricular catheters shunt CSF to a variety of locations including the: peritoneal cavity (most common), pleural cavity, right atrium, or externally (temporary measure). Endoscopic ventriculostomy creates a path between the ventricular system (usually the third ventricle) and another intracranial space.

The remainder of this chapter discusses the preoperative and intraoperative complications that can occur in ventriculoperitoneal (VP) shunt placement, as well as the complications associated with ventriculostomy.

Preoperative	Intraoperative	Ventriculostomy

• Further increased ICP
• No IV access
• EVD dislodgement
   or acute change in height
	• Aspiration
	• Latex allergy
	• Surgical trauma
	   – Subdural hematoma
	   – Intrathoracic trauma
	• Venous air embolism
		• Arrhythmias, asystole
		• Hemorrhage
		• Hypothalamus or cranial
		   nerve injury

Prevention of Preoperative Problems in Children with Increased Intracranial Pressure

The preoperative period can be especially challenging for patients who require surgery for hydrocephalus. Potential preoperative complications include:

- Further increase in ICP
- Lack of IV access
- Problems with external ventricular drains (EVDs).

Premedication is usually avoided due to altered level of consciousness and/or respiratory depression. Careful observation should occur during the preoperative period to ensure that a symptomatic increase in ICP can be quickly identified and treated. It is important to secure or evaluate existing IV access as it may be needed for acute intervention or to facilitate a modified rapid sequence induction (RSI).

Child without IV access and acute hydrocephalus

Crisis	Management
No IV access in a young child with acute symptomatic hydrocephalus for urgent VP shunt placement	Attempt preoperative IV access Consider IO access if pt obtunded If IV access cannot be obtained, consider an inhalation induction with cricoid pressure. Take over ventilation as soon as possible and hyperventilate while IV access is being established

Some children will present to the operating room with EVDs. Prior to transport, it is important to close the EVD to avoid excess CSF drainage. The surgeon can determine how long the EVD can be safely closed; usually, 15 min is not a problem. If the EVD is open and the drainage bag is suddenly lowered, CSF can drain quickly from the patient and lead to collapse of ventricles and rupture of cortical bridging veins causing subdural hematoma (SDH). During patient transport, the EVD must also be carefully monitored to prevent the catheter from being dislodged from the patient's head.

EVD preoperative crises and management

Crisis	Management
External ventricular drain (EVD) dislodgement during transport	Elevate patient head slightly
	Evaluate patient for signs of increased ICP
	Notify surgeon
External ventricular drain (EVD) system falls from IV pole to the floor	Close the EVD if it is not already closed. Return to the proper height
	Evaluate patient's neurologic status for signs of subdural hematoma

Prevention of Intraoperative Problems in Children with Increased Intracranial Pressure

Although VP shunt and endoscopic ventriculostomy are common neurosurgical procedures, anesthesia providers must always be vigilant for a few rare but life-threatening complications including, aspiration risk, latex allergy, intrathoracic trauma, and venous air embolism (VAE).

Aspiration Risk

Often, these patients either have a full stomach or have been vomiting and are, therefore, at risk for aspiration. A modified RSI should be considered for tracheal intubation. To avoid further increase in ICP, blunting the stimulus of laryngoscopy and intubation will be necessary. Judicious use of opioids, lidocaine, and/or intravenous anesthetics can be considered. However over-administration of these agents can cause a decrease in BP, leading to inadequate cerebral perfusion pressure. Ketamine should be avoided since it can acutely increase ICP. Succinylcholine can slightly increase ICP; however, the ICP increase can usually be offset by an adequate dose of intravenous anesthetics combined with hyperventilation.

Aspiration

Causes of aspiration	Patient assessment	Treatment/intervention
• Full stomach • Increased ICP→vomiting, altered level of consciousness • Ineffective cricoid pressure	• Gastric contents in the oropharynx or with tracheal suctioning • Hypoxemia • Bronchospasm/increased PIPs • CXR can have infiltrates	If aspiration is seen at time of intubation • Suction trachea *before* positive pressure ventilation • Ventilate with 100% FIO$_2$ and use PEEP • Supportive care – ICU postop prn – Bronchodilators prn – Steroids and antibiotics have *not* been proven beneficial in the acute situation

Latex Allergy

Children with a history of myelomeningocele are at significantly increased risk for latex allergy. Many children with myelomeningocele also have hydrocephalus. The literature reports that the prevalence of sensitization to latex may be as high as 64% in children with spina bifida [2]. Allergy to latex is a type 1 IgE-mediated reaction clinically manifested as urticaria, angioedema, bronchospasm, and anaphylactic shock. The best way to prevent latex allergy is to prevent latex exposure.

Latex allergy

Causes of allergic response	Assessment	Treatment/intervention
Exposure to latex • Latex gloves • Tape • Medication vials • Blood pressure cuffs • Other latex-containing products	• Hypotension • Tachycardia • Bronchospasm • Flushing/urticaria	• Remove all latex or other triggering agents • Inform the surgeons • Secure the airway, FIO_2 100% • Epinephrine as needed • Reduce or discontinue volatile anesthetics as dictated by hemodynamics • IV fluid boluses to support blood pressure • Corticosteroids • Antihistamines

Surgical Trauma

The other intraoperative problems associated with hydrocephalus surgeries usually involve surgical trauma, either indirectly or directly. It is important to recognize the problem and be ready to manage it in the acute situation.

• *Rapid surgical decompression* of hydrocephalus can lead to rupture of the cortical bridging veins and SDH, or upward herniation of the brainstem causing bradycardia, irregular respirations, or ECG changes [3].

Subdural hematoma/upward herniation

Causes	Patient assessment	Treatment/intervention
• Rapid surgical decompression • Rapid lowering of open EVD	• Evaluate vital signs for bradycardia and/or ECG changes (herniation) • Evaluate neurologic status for signs/symptoms of SDH	• Notify surgeon • Evaluate neurologic status for signs/symptoms of SDH • Hemodynamic support as clinical situation dictates

• *Intrathoracic trauma* (heart, lung, and great vessels) can occur when the passer sheath is tunneled across the chest wall and toward the abdomen.

Intrathoracic trauma

Cause	Patient assessment	Treatment/intervention
• VP shunt passer sheath inadvertently tunneled into chest cavity	• Evaluate patient for signs of hemodynamic instability • Evaluate ability to oxygenate/ventilate patient	• Depending on which organ has been damaged, the anesthesiologist must be prepared to treat hemorrhage, tamponade, and pneumothorax

Venous Air Embolism

VAE can occur at any time, but especially during placement of a ventriculoatrial shunt. To help prevent VAE anesthesia providers can (1) keep the surgical site lower than the level of the heart (if possible), (2) mechanically ventilate the patient, (3) maintain high venous pressure, and (4) remove air from IV tubing and solutions.

Venous air embolism

Cause	Patient assessment	Treatment/intervention
• Surgical site higher than heart • Air in IV tubing	• Abrupt decrease in end-tidal CO_2 • Hypotension • Bradycardia/arrhythmias • Hypoxia • "Mill wheel" murmur on auscultation • Precordial Doppler	• Notify surgeon who will flood field or pack wound/bone • FIO_2 100% • Reduce or discontinue volatile anesthetics as dictated by hemodynamics • Aspirate air if central line is in situ • IVFs/vasopressors to maintain BP • Valsalva • Surgical site below the heart and LLD, if possible • CPR if cardiac arrest

Complications Associated with Endoscopic Ventriculostomy

Third ventriculostomy is performed to relieve noncommunicating hydrocephalus by making a perforation in the floor of the third ventricle with an endoscope. The benefit of ventriculostomy is that no foreign materials are left in the patient (i.e., VPS). In addition, ventriculostomy is minimally invasive and can be performed via a burrhole. However, endoscopic ventriculostomies carry risks that are mainly related to damage of structures near the floor of the third ventricle. Endoscopic ventriculostomy can be acutely complicated by arrhythmias, asystole, hypertension, and hemorrhage. Bradycardia can occur in up to 40% of patients during endoscopic ventriculostomy [4]. The hemodynamic instability that often occurs during these procedures is likely due to the local effects on the third ventricle floor (hypothalamus, pons, and medulla) [5]. Due to the potential risks, careful consideration should be given to monitoring (arterial line placement) based on the clinical scenario.

Arrhythmias or bradycardia/asystole during ventriculostomy

Cause	Patient assessment	Treatment/intervention
• Stimulation of the floor of the third ventricle by the endoscope • High speed irrigation fluid • Rapidly increasing ICP • Vagal response to surgical or other manipulation (i.e., pressure on eye) • Venous air embolism	• Evaluate cardiac output (ETCO$_2$, BP) • Evaluate for hypoxia and/or hypercarbia	• Notify surgeons, ask to stop stimulating floor of third ventricle and to stop irrigation fluid • If arrhythmia does not resolve after stimulation is stopped, then treat supportively according to rhythm disturbance • FIO$_2$ 100%

Hypertension during ventriculostomy

Cause	Patient assessment	Treatment/intervention
• Catecholamine release due to surgical stimulation • Local surgical effects on third ventricle floor • Increased ICP	• Evaluate for signs of light anesthesia (tachycardia, sweating, tearing, mydriasis) • Evaluate for hypoxia and/or hypercarbia • Evaluate for distended bladder	• Repeat BP measurement to verify accuracy • Deepen anesthesia if needed • Notify surgeons, ask to stop stimulating floor of third ventricle and to stop irrigation fluid • Raised ICP may require mannitol, furosemide, and/or hyperventilation • Urinary catheter if bladder is distended • Judiciously consider anti-hypertensive medication therapies

Hemorrhage

Hemorrhage has been reported during third ventriculostomy [6]. Although it is impossible to predict which patients may suffer this complication, anesthesia providers must always be prepared to respond. Patients undergoing ventriculostomy should have adequate IV access, an arterial line, and blood products readily available in the event of hemorrhage and emergent craniotomy.

Cause	Patient assessment	Management
• Trauma to the basilar artery or its branches	• Visualization of blood via endoscope • Hemodynamic instability	• Communicate with surgeons • Call for help • FIO$_2$ 100% • Decrease or D/C volatile anesthesia • IVFs and vasopressors as needed • Transfusion of blood products as needed • Manage elevated ICP until craniotomy

- Other structures at risk for trauma during endoscopic ventriculostomy include:

  - Hypothalamus

    (a) SIADH or DI (assess sodium levels, fluid status)
    (b) Temperature regulation problems – can be mistaken for malignant hyperthermia
    (c) Post-op "trance-like state" (differential postop agitation/delirium)

  - Cranial nerves

    (a) Third and sixth nerve palsies have been reported.

Key Points

- Carefully evaluate each patient to determine degree of increased ICP. This is important for making decisions about premedication, type of induction, and urgency of interventions.
- IV access is needed for RSI or rapid intervention for critical increases in ICP.
- If present, close the EVD prior to patient transport.
- Take precautions regarding latex exposure in patients with myelomeningocele or other susceptible patient populations.
- Always be vigilant for surgical trauma and venous air embolus, especially during the tunneling phase of VPS placement.
- Patients undergoing endoscopic ventriculostomy should have adequate IV access and possibly an arterial line in the event of hemorrhage or arrhythmia.

References and Suggested Reading

1. Garton H et al. Hydrocephalus. Pediatr Clin N Am. 2004;51:305–25.
2. Rendeli C et al. Latex sensitization and allergy in children with myelomeningocele. Child Nerv Syst. 2006;22:28–32.
3. In: Flisher LA ed. Anesthesia and Uncommon Disease. Elseiver. 2006.
4. El-Dawlatly A et al. The incidence of bradycardia during endoscopic third ventriculostomy. Anesth Analg. 2000;91:1142–4.
5. Baykan N et al. Ten years experience with pediatric neuroendoscopic third ventriculostomy. J Neurosurg Anesthesiol. 2005;17:33–7.
6. Drake J. Ventriculostomy for treatment of hydrocephalus. Neurosurg Clin North Am. 1993;4:657–66.
7. Gaba DM et al. Crisis management in anesthesiology. New York: Churchill Livingstone; 1994.
8. Hamid R, Newfield P. Pediatric neuroanesthesia: hydrocephalus. Anesthesiol Clin North America. 2001;19(2):207–18.

Chapter 49
Challenges During Surgery for Traumatic Brain Injury

Chinwe Ajuba-Iwuji and Dolores B. Njoku

Overview

In 2008, approximately 1.4 million people experienced traumatic brain injury (TBI). From this group, approximately 1 million people were treated in hospital emergency rooms, and required surgical intervention. This is not trivial since severe TBI carries a mortality of 30–50% although deaths have declined because of improved treatments and systems for managing trauma. Hence, approximately 230,000 people hospitalized for TBI will survive.

For persons under 45 years of age, TBI remains the number one cause of coma and the leading cause of death with a frequency that is twice as high in men when compared to women. In addition to sex bias, the incidence of TBI is greatest at the extremes of age where those most at risk for severe injury are children between the ages of 5–9 and adults over 80 years. However, individuals between the ages of 15–24 have the greatest number of TBI. Hence, TBI is the leading cause of death in children greater than 1 year of age, and approximately 10–15% of children with TBI suffer from severe TBI.

Since 2008, the National Institute of Neurological Injury and Stroke (NINDS) has defined TBI as brain damage induced by a sudden trauma, and pediatric TBI is defined as TBI occurring in those less than 18 years of age. TBI can result by one of two mechanisms: (1) closed head injury (CHI) from a sudden and violent hit with an object or associated with acceleration/deceleration or (2) penetrating head injury when an object pierces the skull and enters brain tissue

Despite the ability to define TBI, shocking statistics about this major condition remain. While TBI can occur in isolation, 75–85% of all children with multiple traumas will have TBI. This is not insignificant since 80% of all pediatric trauma

C. Ajuba-Iwuji, MD • D.B. Njoku, MD (✉)
Department of Anesthesiology and Critical Care Medicine, Johns Hopkins University
School of Medicine, Baltimore, MD, USA
e-mail: dnjoku@jhmi.edu

A.M. Brambrink and J.R. Kirsch (eds.), *Essentials of Neurosurgical Anesthesia & Critical Care*, DOI 10.1007/978-0-387-09562-2_49,
© Springer Science+Business Media, LLC 2012

deaths are associated with TBI. Motor vehicle and vehicle–pedestrian accidents remain the most common causes of TBI (40–50%) in pediatric patients. Falls, which are most common in the very young and the elderly, remain the second most common cause of TBI. In children <4 years old, 30–50% of TBI cases are attributed to falls and abuse. Hence, nonaccidental trauma (NAT) should always be a consideration and is the main cause of death in infants. Assaults, including firearms, are third (5–10%), and recreational accidents, i.e., sports related injuries, are the fourth most common cause of TBI (10%).

Clinical Implications/Anticipated Problems

The skull is a rigid structure containing tissue, blood, and CSF. An increase in any of these components increases intracranial pressure. Cerebral swelling can develop within hours of TBI with resultant intracranial hypertension. Intracranial hypertension can significantly decrease cerebral perfusion resulting in ischemia, swelling, possible herniation, and neurological impairment. Moreover, resultant neurological impairment demonstrated by altered arousal, alertness, or responsiveness may impair protective airway reflexes and increase the patient's risk for aspiration of oral secretions or gastric contents.

Young children possess certain anatomical characteristics which predispose them to TBI: (1) a large head-to-body ratio which alters their center of gravity, (2) thinner cranial bones, and (3) decreased myelination of neural tissue. Some of these individual characteristics or in combination may increase their likelihood of diffuse axonal injury (DAI) and cerebral edema. Moreover, while in infants slow increases in ICP can be accommodated by expansion of cranial suture lines, rapid shifts are less well tolerated due to little time for adaptation.

Prevention

Motor vehicle and vehicle–pedestrian accidents are the most common cause of TBI with alcohol, illicit drugs, and nonprescribed use of prescription medications being the most common contributing factors. Therefore, primary prevention of TBI involves basic safe driving, appropriate utilization of child and infant car seats, in addition to clear legislation to support those practices.

Crisis Management

Pathophysiology and Clinical Presentation

The pathophysiology of TBI includes both the primary and secondary events. However, there are few randomized controlled trials regarding the pathophysiology of TBI in children. Thus, a large amount of data in the pediatric population is obtained by extrapolation from adult studies:

- *Primary injury* – direct injury to brain parenchyma from tearing, compression, and stretching of tissues and blood vessels. Possible mechanisms include the following:
  - *Compressive stress* – deformation of the brain structure
  - *Tensile stress* – stretching as a result of pulling the axis of the brain in opposite directions
  - *Shear stress* – pushing in opposite directions perpendicular to the axis of the brain that can cause injury to the brain stem
  - *Acceleration/deceleration* – rapid acceleration or deceleration which occurs when the force from the site of impact sends waves through the skull. Since the head-to-torso ratio is large in infants and younger children, acceleration–deceleration injuries are more common in the pediatric population and can lead to diffuse brain and upper spine injuries
  - *Coup and contrecoup* – injury that occurs either in the portion of the brain under the site of impact (coup) or on the side opposite the impact (contrecoup)

- *Secondary injury* – indirect injury to brain parenchyma from hypoxia, hypotension, or biochemical and metabolic events that may occur minutes to days following the initial trauma. Possible mechanisms of secondary injury include the following:
  - Hypoperfusion
  - Increased metabolic demand
  - Damage to the blood–brain barrier
  - Free radical formation
  - Mitochondrial dysfunction
  - Release of neurotransmitters including acetylcholine, glutamate, and aspartate

Pediatric patients with TBI may present with diffuse or focal injuries. Diffuse Injury results from microscopic damage throughout many areas of the brain. Types of diffuse injury to brain parenchyma include the following:

- *DAI* – characterized by shearing of large nerve fibers and stretching of blood vessels in the brain. The most common manifestation is impaired cognitive function with resultant impairment in memory, concentration, and organization. Within the pediatric population DAI is often defined as a loss of consciousness for greater than 6 min without a specific focal lesion on imaging or exam. DAI is most common in the craniocervical junction in children as opposed to the frontotemporal lobes in adults.
- *Hypoxic-ischemic injury* – a consequence of cerebral swelling and resultant restriction in blood flow which limits delivery oxygen, glucose, and key nutrients to the brain. In infants this is the most common abnormality in NAT.

Focal Injury is confined to specific areas of the brain. Types of focal injury include the following:

- *Contusions* – bruises to brain parenchyma that causes swelling, bleeding, and/or damage to brain tissue. These usually occur in frontal and temporal lobes which house the memory and behavior centers. Hence, symptoms of brain contusion may include abnormal sensations, coordination, memory, or behavior.
- *Hemorrhage* – blood escapes damaged blood vessels and enters brain tissue. The magnitude and symptoms depend on the location of the hemorrhage.
- *Stroke* – local blood flow to tissues is compromised by injury to large cerebral arteries or even tissues. Cerebral edema further compromises delivery of oxygen and nutrients. Strokes associated with TBI mostly affect the posterior cerebral artery circulation; however, the symptoms depend upon the vascular distribution. Pediatric strokes typically occur in children with neck injuries.
- *Subdural hematoma* – results from damage to bridging vessels on the surface of the brain. Patients may present with loss of consciousness, confusion, drowsiness, asymmetric pupils, focal deficits, headache, and respiratory changes. In the pediatric population subdural hematomas >5 mm are often treated with surgical intervention.
- *Epidural hematoma* – results from damage to the middle meningeal artery or epidural veins. Hence, intracranial pressure can increase within minutes and with symptoms similar to subdural hematoma. When promptly diagnosed and treated children with epidural hematoma have an excellent prognosis.
- *Subarachnoid hemorrhage* – result of a small amount of bleeding within the subarachnoid space. Subsequent changes in the pupil, neurological and respiratory exam may occur as previously described. This occurs in children primarily from acceleration/deceleration injuries, however, may also result from NAT. In the pediatric population, SAH carries a high morbidity and mortality even when adequately treated.
- *Skull fracture* – more common within the pediatric population and often does not require surgical intervention except when depressed or open. Depressed, open skull fractures are often treated with immediate surgical debridement and fracture repair to lessen the risk of developing meningitis, CSF leak, and/or seizures. Remember, skull fractures can be associated with underlying brain injury.

The Glasgow Coma Scale (GCS) is often used to help to initially determine the severity of TBI:

- Mild (GCS score 13–15)
- Moderate (GCS score 9–12)
- Severe (GCS score <8)

Mild TBI often has few to no lasting consequences. Severe TBI can cause significant disability and possibly death. Most children with a GCS<5 have a dismal prognosis.

Patient Assessment/Diagnostic Tests

Children with severe TBI should be promptly recognized and stabilized to improve outcomes.

- *Primary survey* – identify and treat potentially life-threatening conditions which include airway compromise and hemorrhagic shock. Always assume cervical spine injury and stabilize the cervical spine using an immobilization collar. Approximately half of the patients with cervical spine injury have concomitant TBI.
- *Secondary survey* – identify secondary life-threatening conditions and perform an in-depth neurological assessment. Children with TBI often have concomitant blunt abdominal trauma and long bone fractures, such as femur fractures, which can serve as a major source of blood loss.
- *Patient history* – obtained from the patient, family members, and/or witnesses should include the mechanism of injury, duration of loss of consciousness, changes in mental status, headache, nausea, vomiting, and progression of symptoms. Past medical history should include birth history and documentation of any congenital abnormalities. Additionally, any history of prior injuries, seizures, learning disabilities, substance abuse, prior psychological or psychiatric problems as well as medication or food allergies should be ascertained.
- Physical examination of a pediatric patient with TBI includes the following:

  - Assessment of ABC's and prompt management of airway if indicated by exam or if GCS < 8. Prompt treatment of hypotension and hypoxia.
  - Vital signs: temperature, blood pressure, heart rate, pulse oximetry, and weight (actual or estimate).
  - Assessment for Cushing triad of hypertension, bradycardia, and irregular respirations may indicate impending herniation. This is a LATE SIGN.
  - Prompt neck immobilization and cervical spine examination.
  - Focused neurological examination including the following:

    (a) Level of consciousness.
    (b) Pupil examination.
    (c) Fundoscopic examination.
    (d) Brainstem reflexes.
    (e) Deep tendon reflexes.
    (f) Response to pain.

  - Pay attention to indicators of increased ICP and impending herniation:

    (a) Cushing's triad (LATE SIGN).
    (b) Signs of uncal herniation: third nerve palsy (at rest, the eye tends to look down and to the side; no upwards, downwards or inwards movement possible; in addition: drooping upper eyelid, i.e., ptosis) followed by hemiplegia.

  - GCS score (Table 49.1) – a 15-point scale that assesses the patient's ability to follow directions, move extremities, and speak.

Table 49.1 Glasgow Coma Score (GCS)

	Infant < 1 year	Child 1–4 years	4 Years – adult
Eyes			
4	Open	Open	Open
3	To voice	To voice	To voice
2	To pain	To pain	To pain
1	No response	No response	No response
Verbal			
5	Coos, babbles	Oriented speech, interacts	Alert and oriented
4	Irritable but consolable	Confused speech, disoriented but consolable	Disoriented
3	Irritable but inconsolable	Confused speech, inconsolable	Confused speech
2	Moans to pain	Incomprehensible, agitated	Moans, unintelligible speech
1	Nonverbal to pain	Unresponsive	Unresponsive
Motor			
6	Normal spontaneous movements	Normal spontaneous movements	Follows commands
5	Withdraws to touch	Localizes pain	Localizes pain
4	Withdraws to pain	Withdraws to pain	Withdraws to pain
3	Decorticate posturing to pain (flexion)	Decorticate posturing to pain (flexion)	Decorticate posturing to pain (flexion)
2	Decerebrate posturing to pain (extension)	Decerebrate posturing to pain (extension)	Decerebrate posturing to pain (extension)
1	Unresponsive to pain	Unresponsive to pain	Unresponsive to pain

Laboratory Studies

Obtain a hematocrit, electrolyte panel with blood glucose, type and screen, coagulation studies (PT/PTT, INR), urinalysis, with urine toxicology assessment.
Caveats:

- Hyperglycemia is a poor prognostic indicator for patients with severe TBI.
- Pediatric patients who sustain head injury are at increased risk of coagulopathy because of brain tissue thromboplastin release; therefore, it is imperative to correct any coagulopathy.

Diagnostic Tests

- *Computed tomography (CT) of the head* – will detect most lesions requiring emergent surgery such as focal brain injuries and skull fractures. Repeat CT scans often show secondary injury as a result of cerebral edema.
- *MRI of the head* – may add information regarding long-term outcome. MRI may not be as useful in an emergency setting.

- *Angiography* – will allow assessment of blood vessels in the brain. CT/MRI angiography as a combined modality often may detect and define blood vessel pathology.
- *Electroencephalograph (EEG)* – can be utilized to detect presence of seizure-like activity or absence of cerebral activity.
- *ICP monitor* – can be used to measure intracranial pressure.
- *Single photon emission computed tomography (SPECT) or positron emission tomography (PET)* – imaging techniques that measure brain cell metabolism and detect changes or injury that cannot be detected by standard imagining modalities.

Intraoperative Interventions/Treatment

Airway

- Optimize oxygenation and ventilation. Hypoxia and hypercarbia are both potent cerebral vasodilators which increase CBF and ICP. Hypoxemia in pediatric patients is predictive of increased morbidity.
- An oral airway will relieve airway obstruction even in an unconscious child with suspected cervical spine injury.
- Chin lift and jaw thrust maneuvers when performed correctly can relieve airway obstruction without risking cord injury.
- If endotracheal intubation is required, a rapid sequence technique should be used.

  – Nasotracheal intubation should not be performed in patients with basilar skull or mid-face fractures.
  – Succinylcholine should be avoided because of concerns of hyperkalemic cardiac arrests in healthy children with undiagnosed myopathy. For this reason it is recommended that succinylcholine should be reserved only for emergency intubations such as, laryngospasm, difficult airway, full stomach, or intramuscular use when IV access is unavailable.
  – Use positive end expiratory pressure (PEEP) with caution because it may impair cerebral venous return or increase ICP if greater than 10 cm H_2O.

Breathing

- Hyperventilation should be performed if acute signs of increased ICP and impending herniation are present.

  – Hyperventilation in the nonacute setting compromises cerebral perfusion by inducing vasoconstriction at a time when cerebral perfusion is already reduced.
- In the nonacute setting normoventilation with a goal end-tidal CO_2 of 30 mmHg is utilized.

Circulation

- Fluid resuscitation may occur with isotonic solutions, blood or blood products if necessary.
- Systolic blood pressure should be maintained at normal to slightly elevated levels as determined by the age of the patient.
- Utilization of hypertonic saline for fluid resuscitation for up to 72 h has suggested benefits in the pediatric population.

  – Serum sodium must be closely monitored when hypertonic saline is utilized with a goal Na of <155.

- Children <24 months are especially at risk for cerebral hypoperfusion post TBI.
- Arterial and central venous access may be required for close hemodynamic monitoring and to allow for rapid administration of vasoactive substances if needed.

Cervical spine immobilization should be maintained in pediatric trauma patients until cleared by radiological and clinical exam.

Maintain CPP

- CPP is defined as MAP – ICP or jugular venous pressure, whichever is higher.
- CPP goal of >70 mmHg is often utilized in adults. Given the paucity of data in children, a CPP of greater than 70 mmHg is targeted in children as well.

Minimize ICP

- Elevation of the head to a maximum of 30° promotes venous drainage and potentially decreases ICP.
- Administer hyperosmolar therapy such as mannitol and hypertonic saline to create an osmolar gradient that will assist in normalizing ICP.

  – More specifically, 3% saline may be effective for acute treatment of intracranial hypertension in pediatric patients with TBI.

- Intravenous lidocaine can be utilized to treat acute increases in ICP that occur with suctioning, movement, and laryngoscopy.
- Intravenous sedation-hypnotic agents are potent cerebral vasoconstrictors and decrease CBF and ICP.

  – Ketamine can increase CBF and ICP; therefore, it must be used with caution.

- Consider neuromuscular blockade to control increases in ICP associated with shivering.

- In pediatric patients with refractory increases in ICP, barbiturate coma with pentobarbital is often used. Adverse effects of pentobarbital include hypotension.
- A ventriculostomy may also be required to drain the ventricles in the setting of increased ICP.
- Anti-seizure prophylaxis may reduce early posttraumatic seizures. These seizures increase brain metabolic demands and ICP leading to secondary injury.

Avoid Hyperthermia and Hyperglycemia

- Hyperthermia increases cerebral metabolic oxygen demand.
- Hyperglycemia may worsen brain tissue lactic acidosis. Insulin infusions may be required with caution especially for blood glucose levels greater than 200 g/dl.

Electrolyte Disturbances

- Evaluate for electrolyte imbalances caused by diabetes insipidus or syndrome of inappropriate antidiuretic hormone that often occur post TBI.

Key Points

- 80% of all pediatric trauma deaths are associated with TBI.
- Extremes of age (5–9-year olds and >80 years of age) are at increased risk for TBI.
- The most common cause of pediatric TBI is motor vehicle and vehicle–pedestrian accidents. However, NAT is the main cause of TBI in infants.
- Diffuse brain injury includes DAI and hypoxic-ischemic injury. Focal injuries include contusions, hematomas, and hemorrhages.
- The primary survey should identify life-threatening injuries.
- GCS score should be computed and the initial imaging often includes a head CT. If the GCS is <8, urgent endotracheal intubation may be necessary.
- Management of TBI includes close management of ABCs. The head of the bed should be elevated 30° and neurosurgical consultation should be obtained.
- Hyperosmolar therapy should also be considered.
- Anticonvulsants may help prevent early posttraumatic seizures.
- Patients exhibiting signs of herniation should be emergently managed.

Suggested Reading

Comper P, Bisschop SM, Carnide N, et al. A systemic review of treatments for mild traumatic brain injury. Brain Injury. 2005;19(11):863–80.

Ghajar J. Traumatic brain injury. Lancet. 2000;356(9233):923–9.

Graham DI. Paediatric head injury. Brain. 2001;124(7):1261–2.

Langlois JA, Rutland-Brown W, Thomas KE. Traumatic brain injury in the United States: emergency department visits, hospitalizations, and death. Atlanta, GA: Centers for Disease Control and Prevention, National Center for Injury Prevention and Control; 2006.

Chapter 50
Challenges During Surgery for Meningomyelocele and Encephalomyelocele

Allison Kinder Ross

Neural tube defects, also referred to as spinal dysraphism, myelodysplasia, or spina bifida, result from incomplete fusion of midline structures with lack of covering over neural elements. Although introduction of the use of folic acid to potential mothers prior to conception has decreased the risk of having a fetus with an open neural tube defect, the incidence is not negligible at 0.5–1 per 1,000 live births. A *meningocele* involves protrusion of only the meninges through the dysraphic defect and spares the neural contents. However, a *myelomeningocele* refers to a defect with protrusion of neural elements along with their covering and has implications for the patient and the provider from infancy to adulthood. This chapter focuses on perioperative complications of myelomeningocele as follows: (1) damage to neural placode, (2) hydrocephalus, (3) CSF leak, and (4) latex allergy. A miscellaneous section (5) is also included.

The latter part of the chapter focuses on the complications that are more unique to an infant with an *encephalocele*, the failure of the proximal end of the neural tube to fuse.

Myelomeningocele

Damage to Neural Placode

Overview

The first issue that is often confronted in the infant who presents to the operating room for repair of a myelomeningocele is the challenge of positioning for induction and intubation prior to surgery. An infant with myelomeningocele is at risk of

A.K. Ross, MD (✉)
Departments of Anesthesiology and Pediatrics, Duke University School of Medicine,
Durham, NC, USA
e-mail: allison.ross@duke.edu

A.M. Brambrink and J.R. Kirsch (eds.), *Essentials of Neurosurgical Anesthesia & Critical Care*, DOI 10.1007/978-0-387-09562-2_50,
© Springer Science+Business Media, LLC 2012

damage to the exposed neural placode, if any pressure or weight is placed on the unprotected neural elements.

Prevention

To protect the neural placode after birth, the infant is typically kept in the prone position with a light sterile wrap over the affected area. Because the prone position is not conducive to smooth airway management for induction and intubation prior to surgical repair, steps need to be taken to protect the neural placode during that critical time. To put the infant into the supine position, a platform needs to be built that elevates the infant above the height of the bed so that the defect is suspended without any weight on the neural elements. Several methods have been described keeping in mind that the goal is to not only keep the neural tube defect protected from pressure but to also keep it sterile. The presence of hydrocephalus with relative increased head size adds to the difficulty of positioning the patient for optimal airway management.

A small defect may simply require that a sterile towel be unwrapped and then twisted to form a circle that will perfectly surround the defect and allow the skin around it to rest upon the towel itself, while the defect falls into the hole in the middle. For stability, the head and legs will also need to be supported with either towels or foam padding.

A larger defect will require a higher platform. A foam head ring can support the defect by allowing the skin to sit upon the foam while the defect falls to the center hole. Another head ring may be turned in its opposite direction to hold the head and upper body in place. If this fails to support the particularly large neural tube defect in the supine infant, intubation should occur in the left lateral decubitus position.

Similar to induction and intubation, upon emergence, if it is determined that the infant is to be extubated following repair, this may be done in the prone or lateral position as long as there is a backup elevated platform and extra help available if the infant needs to be put urgently into the supine position for airway issues.

Key Points

- Risk can be completely avoided with proper positioning
- Infant should remain in prone or lateral position even after repair.

Hydrocephalus

Overview

Hydrocephalus occurs from either overproduction of CSF, inability to absorb CSF effectively, or most commonly, obstruction to CSF flow. The cause of hydrocephalus in an infant with myelomeningocele is the presence of a Chiari II malformation. A Chiari II results in the partial or full obstruction of flow of CSF from herniation of the cerebellar vermis, brainstem and fourth ventricle into the upper cervical region of the spinal canal. In fact, complications from the Chiari II malformation are the leading cause of death in individuals with myelomeningocele who are less than 2 years, and many of these are due to the resulting hydrocephalus.

Prevention

There is no clear way to prevent hydrocephalus in an infant with myelomeningocele; however, it is possible to prevent the complications of hydrocephalus by shunting the CSF, most commonly using a ventriculoperitoneal shunt. Particularly those who have more caudal defects, not all infants with myelomeningocele defects will require a CSF shunt. Application of stringent guidelines for shunt placement may reduce the number of shunts that need to be inserted from 85 to 51% but does not reduce the actual risk of hydrocephalus. A promising practice may be the in utero closure of the myelomeningocele which has shown to decrease the incidence of hydrocephalus. Although fetal surgery may result in a reduced incidence of shunt-dependent hydrocephalus, long-term improved outcome has not yet been proven.

Crisis Management

Pathology and Clinical Presentation

It is not the hydrocephalus itself that is the complication leading to crisis. In fact, slowly developing hydrocephalus often does not require immediate attention. It is the increasing intracranial pressure with a defined brain mass in a limited, restricted skull that creates the crisis. Potential complications of hydrocephalus include oculomotor palsy, dysphagia, protracted vomiting, and failure of closure of cranial sutures. When the sutures have closed and the intracranial space is restrictive, increased intracranial pressure is a risk. Twenty percent of infants with myelomeningocele may present with stridor due to hydrocephalus from Chiari malformation. Infants may also develop nerve dysfunction with life-threatening hypoventilation or apnea, even in cases where pressure on the brainstem is relieved with appropriate shunting.

Children with myelomeningocele have sleep-disordered breathing at an incidence as high as 20%. In children with obstructive sleep apnea, nasal CPAP is more effective than adenotonsillectomy. Central apnea may be treated with methylxanthines and supplemental oxygen, but these are not 100% effective and the children may ultimately require positive pressure ventilation.

Patient Assessment

Although most children will receive a CT scan for monitoring of hydrocephalus, symptoms and physical findings are more commonly used for diagnosing the degree of insult from the enlarging ventricles (Table 50.1). In an infant with open sutures,

Table 50.1 Hydrocephalus signs and treatment

	Signs/symptoms	Treatment
Increased ICP-mild or chronic	Nausea/vomiting	Shunt placement
	Headache	Mild hyperventilation
	Lethargy	
Increased ICP-severe or acute	As above, plus:	– Emergent shunt or ventricular decompression
	Bradycardia and/or irregular respirations	– Mannitol 0.25–0.5 g/kg (max of 30 g)
		– Furosemide 0.5–1 mg/kg (max of 10 mg)
		– Moderate hyperventilation
Respiratory irregularity	Tachypnea	Secure airway or CPAP depending on severity/timing
	Apnea	
	Stridor	
Aspiration	Vomiting	Rapid sequence induction (modified)
	Pre-induction	Cricoid pressure

a large head with massive open fontanels may be present. Signs of increased ICP may occur late in the process as the head expands slowly with the increasing volume of CSF. A child with sutures that are beginning to fuse or are closed will present with signs of increasing ICP such as headache, vomiting, lethargy, ataxia, visual disturbances, and in extreme cases, bradycardia or cardiorespiratory arrest. Patient assessment should primarily determine the degree of compromise from the increased intracranial pressure that is present with the hydrocephalus so that appropriate steps in a timely fashion may occur.

Intervention and Treatment

Treatment for symptomatic hydrocephalus is placement of a shunt or ventriculos-tomy; however, these procedures are not without risk (see Table 50.1). Firstly, in a child with increased ICP, the anesthetic plan should take into consideration the desire to avoid any further increase in the ICP. Barbiturates for induction with little to no apneic period, thus avoiding a climbing CO_2, and rapid tracheal intubation are necessary. The infant or child who has recurrent vomiting is at risk for aspiration during anesthetic induction. One must weigh the risk of aspiration and need for rapid sequence induction against the risk of herniation and desire for a controlled, hemodynamically stable induction for neuroprotection. A modified rapid sequence induction may be a fair compromise in this circumstance. A combination of agents that allows for cardiovascular stability and, therefore, reduces the risk of increasing intracranial pressure should be used during induction with cricoid pressure applied and relatively small positive pressure breaths prior to intubation. Agents that are suitable in this circumstance are either propofol or thiopental as the induction agent, preceded by lidocaine 1 mg/kg and a narcotic to blunt the response to laryngoscopy, followed by a nondepolarizing muscle relaxant. Intubation should be gentle, and moderate hyperventilation to an end-tidal CO_2 in the mid to low 30s is acceptable while the patient is prepped waiting for shunting. Avoid extreme head flexion, as it may result in brainstem compression in the presence of Chiari malformation. Intraoperatively during the shunting procedure, the basilar artery or its branches may be violated. This can result in severe intracranial bleeding and emergency craniotomy.

Of note, in an infant or child with hydrocephalus who has had a ventriculostomy tube inserted and connected to a drainage bag, it is important to keep the bag at the height of the head (ideally tragus level) so that sudden changes in CSF flow and pressure do not occur. The tubing should be clamped or closed during transport and transfer of child to bed, if the period is brief so that large drainage of CSF does not occur suddenly with position changes.

Key Points

- Hydrocephalus in an infant with myelomeningocele is a result of a Chiari II malformation.
- Acute hydrocephalus that results in increased intracranial pressure requires rapid treatment.
- Anesthetic technique in an infant or child with symptomatic acute hydrocephalus should aim at reducing the effects of the increased ICP while protecting the lungs from potential aspiration events.

CSF Leak

Overview

Following repair of a myelomeningocele, there is risk of continued CSF leak, particularly in those infants who have ongoing hydrocephalus or increased pressures. In these infants, the path of least resistance for the "pop off" of fluid pressure is at the fresh suture line after repair.

Prevention

Prevention of a CSF leak is primarily through surgical intervention at the time of repair and avoidance of hydrocephalus or increased pressures that result in leakage. Simultaneous insertion of a ventriculoperitoneal shunt during neural tube repair may reduce the chance of CSF leak by avoiding progressive ventricular dilation and increased CSF pressure at the fresh operative site. From an anesthetic standpoint, it is conceivable that other maneuvers that may increase cerebral or spinal pressures should be avoided such as sustained high airway pressures, coughing, or straining on emergence.

Crisis Intervention

Typically, the infant or child with CSF leak will present with a history of fluid or soft, fluctuant bulge at the site of repair. The child may or may not have other signs or symptoms of complications from the leaking CSF; however, leakage of cerebral spinal fluid may present with findings of hypotension and/or electrolyte imbalance from the loss of fluid. Appropriate volume resuscitation must occur prior to bringing these infants back to the OR for repair of their leak only after a recent electrolyte panel has been drawn and attempts made to correct any abnormalities. Because of potential electrolyte abnormalities, risk of postoperative apnea may be increased and the infant may need to remain intubated postoperatively depending on the preoperative condition.

An additional risk in these infants with CSF leak is CSF infection and, ultimately, life-threatening sepsis. Antibiotic administration should be ongoing through the perioperative period to avoid meningitis or ventriculitis from infected CSF. Perioperative myelomeningocele repair infections are often polymicrobial with gram negatives and *Staphylococcus aureus*. A protective covering or flap firmly affixed caudal to the repair site helps to prevent fecal contamination of wound.

Latex Allergy

Overview

Infants who are to undergo the repair of a myelomeningocele are not necessarily at risk for latex allergy at the time of surgery. However, as they age, children with spina bifida, even in the absence of multiple surgical procedures, are at risk for developing latex sensitization. Children with myelomeningocele who require many urologic and orthopedic procedures have a higher association with the development of latex sensitization than those who do not. True latex allergy is a Type I IgE-mediated hypersensitivity reaction that may present as local urticaria or may lead to life-threatening anaphylaxis.

Prevention

The best way to avoid latex allergy is to manage children who have myelodysplasia in a latex-free environment. This includes not only the perioperative area but also all urinary catheters, syringes, band-aids, tourniquets, and any gloves that are used for other procedures in the children at risk. As of 1998, the FDA mandated that products that contain latex have a warning label. In addition, some antibiotics and certain foods (bananas, avocados, and kiwi are only a few examples) should be avoided because of cross-reactivity in the children with true latex allergy. The ASA recommends that patients who have latex allergy be posted as first case in the morning when latex allergens are at their lowest level. In addition, the room should be labeled as being a latex-free environment and a resuscitation cart should be immediately available. Medications should be drawn from glass vials if possible into syringes that are either glass or have latex-free plungers. Use stopcocks for intravenous injections rather than injection ports that may be made of latex.

The prophylactic administration of antihistamines, steroids, or H-2 blockers are not recommended as they may blunt the early signs of anaphylaxis such as urticaria or mild bronchospasm, thus, leaving cardiovascular collapse as the first sign of anaphylaxis.

Crisis and Intervention

Pathology and Clinical Presentation

In a child with myelodysplasia, despite all precautions taken, if there is evidence of anaphylaxis during a surgical procedure, latex allergy should immediately be suspected and treated. The pathology of latex allergy is the sensitization and production of IgE antibodies. The IgE binds to mast cells and blood basophils, and upon reexposure, degranulation of the sensitized mast cells and basophils occurs and the patient suffers a latex reaction. Under anesthesia, the most common manifestations detected intraoperatively are bronchospasm and cardiovascular instability. It is often difficult to detect cutaneous signs of allergy or anaphylaxis in a child who is under surgical drapes.

Patient Assessment

A rapid survey of the skin for urticaria (if possible), vital signs for hypotension and tachycardia, and auscultation of the lung fields for signs of bronchoconstriction should occur immediately upon suspicion. Serum tryptase levels should be sent once the patient is stabilized. Skin tests to confirm the diagnosis are performed at least 4–6 weeks after the event and caution should be used, as the test itself may induce anaphylaxis.

Intervention and Treatment

When latex reaction is suspected, all latex-containing items should be removed immediately and a sign posted on the operating room door so that other providers do not enter and risk spreading airborne latex from glove powder or other venues.

Table 50.2 Intraoperative latex allergy signs and treatments

Reaction	Treatment	Potential side effect
Bronchospasm	– 100% oxygen	
	– Epinephrine 0.1–10 mcg/kg	Dysrhythmias
	– Albuterol or levalbuterol neb via anesthetic circuit	Tachycardia (with albuterol)
Hypotension-mild	– Epinephrine 0.1–1 mcg/kg	Dysrhythmias
	– Saline or Ringer's lactate solution 10–20 ml/kg	Pulmonary edema
Hypotension-severe	– Epinephrine 10 mcg/kg	Dysrhythmias
	– Epinephrine infusion 0.01–0.1 mcg/kg/min if needed	
	– Saline or Ringer's lactate 20–50 ml/kg	Pulmonary edema
Tachycardia	– Saline or Ringer's lactate 10 ml/kg up to 50 ml/kg	Pulmonary edema

Although anaphylaxis may occur from other agents intraoperatively, the treatment is essentially the same and should be initiated when signs are present (see Table 50.2). 100% oxygen and fluid boluses should be delivered. Epinephrine may be required and is advantageous in children with anaphylactic reactions because of its alpha- and beta effects.

Secondary therapy includes the addition of intravenous antihistamines, H-2 blockers, and steroids. Dosing is as follows:

Diphenhydramine 1 mg/kg (max of 50 mg)
Ranitidine 1 mg/kg (max of 50 mg)
Hydrocortisone 5 mg/kg, then 2.5 mg/kg q 4–6 h
Methylprednisolone 1 mg/kg, then 0.8 mg/kg q 4–6 h.

Key Points

- Manage children at risk in a latex-free environment.
- Have a high index of suspicion of latex reaction intraoperatively if signs/symptoms of allergy or anaphylaxis present.
- Rapid treatment with epinephrine, fluid, and second-line agents should occur in the presence of an anaphylactic event.

Miscellaneous Complications

Blood Loss

Blood loss is typically not a major risk in the simple repair of a myelomeningocele but is more of an issue when an extensive flap or undermining of the skin is required for closure. A hemoglobin and hematocrit should be drawn, and a type and screen for blood should be available preoperatively in case products are required.

Hypothermia

Neonates have poor ability to maintain body temperature due to their large body surface area and inability to create thermogenesis in normal circumstances. In infants and children with myelomeningoceles, there is also the potential of having poor autonomic control below the level of the defect, thus, putting them at greater risk of hypothermia in the operating room. It is, therefore, important to warm the operating room prior to entry with the patient, use radiant warmers during line placement, intubation and positioning, and provide forced air warmers around the patient during the procedure.

Urinary Retention

Urinary retention may be thought of as a late complication in children with myelo-dysplasia; however, only 12% of neonates actually have normal bladder emptying after closure of myelomeningocele. The remaining 88% have urinary retention with a mean volume of 20 ml due to a clinical pattern that is similar to spinal shock. Although most infants will have resumption of near-complete emptying within 2 weeks after closure, many will require catheterization for up to 6 weeks postrepair.

Long-term myelomeningocele is the commonest cause of neurogenic bladder in children. Routine catheterization is typically required and these children often have a significant number of urologic procedures. Renal insufficiency or renal failure occurs in up to 30–40% due to vesicoureteral reflux despite routine clean intermittent catheterizations. In addition, ventriculoperitoneal shunt infection occurs more commonly in children who have undergone an intraperitoneal uro-logic procedure.

Other Considerations

Spina bifida occulta may exist with normal-appearing overlying skin. A sacral dimple that suggests a dermal sinus, a patch of hair, or a fatty swelling should alert the practitioner to the presence of possible abnormal underlying neural structures. In these patients, caudal anesthetic techniques should be avoided until workup has occurred to avoid accidental neural trauma.

Additional complications secondary to myelomeningocele that often lead to further operative intervention include the following:

- Tethered cord
- Poor to no ambulation
- Decubitus ulcers
- Scoliosis.

Suggested Reading

Adzick NS, Walsh DS. Myelomeningocele: prenatal diagnosis, pathophysiology and management. Semin Pediatr Surg. 2003;12:168–74.
Chakraborty A, Crimmins D, Hayward R, Thompson D. Toward reducing shunt placement rates in patients with myelomeningocele. J Neurosurg. 2008;1:361–5.
Fichter MA, et al. Fetal spina bifida repair-current trends and prospects of intrauterine neurosurgery. Fetal Diagn Ther. 2008;23:271–86.
Hamid RK, Newfield P. Pediatric neuroanesthesia. Hydrocephalus. Anesthesiol Clin North America. 2001;19:207–18.
Hepner DL, Castells MC. Latex allergy: An update. Anesth Analg. 2003;96:1219–29.
http://www.asahq.org/publicationsAndServices/latexallergy.pdf.
Kaufman BA. Neural tube defects. Pediatr Clin North Am. 2004;51: 389–419.
Muller T, Arbeiter K, Aufricht C. Renal function in meningomyelocele: risk factors, chronic renal failure, renal replacement therapy and transplantation. Curr Opin Urol. 2002;12:479–84.
Shaer CM, Chescheir N, Schulkin J. Myelomeningocele: a review of the epidemiology, genetics, risk factors for conception, prenatal diagnosis, and prognosis for affected individuals. Obstet Gynecol Surv. 2007;62:471–9.

Encephalocele

An encephalocele is a protrusion of cranial contents through a defect in the skull that may occur either posteriorly at the occiput or can also be found in the frontal area. Although the overall incidence is about 1 case per 5,000 births, occipital encephaloceles present most commonly. Occipital, or basal, encephaloceles are typically managed by neurosurgeons in the neonatal period. An encephalocele, although similar in embryologic origins to the myelomeningocele, has unique characteristics that present additional challenges not only upon presentation but also in the intraoperative period. Complications that are similar to the myelomeningocele include the following:

- Risk of damage to neural placode

    - Lateral position preferred due to difficulty in safely securing airway with large defect in occipital region.

- CSF leak

    - Risk of CSF leak is significant because due to the lack of normal tissue and disrupted fascial planes from the encephalocele itself.

- Blood loss
- Increased ICP.

The two latter problems tend to be more severe in the infant with encephalocele compared with the infant with myelomeningocele.

Blood Loss

Overview

An encephalocele may present in many locations, but an occipital encephalocele presents the practitioner with the risk of significant blood loss intraoperatively because of its proximity with the transverse sinus.

Prevention/Treatment

Blood loss can only be prevented if there is no entry into the larger venous sinuses during encephalocele repair. An MRI is typically performed preoperatively so that the location of blood vessels in relation to the encephalocele helps guide the surgeon with their dissection. Prevention of significant hemodynamic instability from blood loss can occur if blood is available in the room, appropriate vascular access is obtained, and the anesthesia team is aware of the risk of bleeding in this type of procedure. If blood loss is ongoing or significant, FFP and platelets should also be made available and delivered depending on laboratory or clinical evidence of clotting abnormalities from massive transfusion. DIC is a risk in these infants when this occurs.

Increased ICP

Overview

With manipulation of the encephalocele surgically increased intracranial pressure may occur and needs to be treated (see above treatment under section "Hydrocephalus"). To close an encephalocele, good brain relaxation must be present and ICP must be maintained within the normal range. Unfortunately, as ICP increases, blood loss also increases and requires additional volume resuscitation requiring a delicate balance between decreasing ICP and increasing intravascular volume.

Suggested Reading

Hunt JA, Hobar PC. Common craniofacial anomalies: facial clefts and encephaloceles. Plast Reconstr Surg. 2003;112:606–16.

Chapter 51
Challenges During Cranial Decompression

Todd J. Kilbaugh, Stuart Friess, and Mark Helfaer

Overview

Decompressive craniectomy can be used as a treatment modality for refractory intracranial hypertension secondary to traumatic and non-traumatic brain injury (non-TBI), as well as for treatment for congenital malformations of the posterior fossa termed: Chiari malformations. The Monro–Kellie hypothesis states that brain, blood, and cerebral spinal fluid (CSF) are bound by the skull in a nearly incompressible compartment. There is some degree of capacitance due to the compression of CSF, blood vessels, and an open fontanelle, but, once this capacitance is exhausted and maximal volume reached, intracranial pressure (ICP) increases dramatically. After brain injury, cerebral autoregulation can become "uncoupled" to the metabolic demands of the brain, and alterations in cerebral perfusion pressure (CPP) may result in fluctuations of CBF, which can lead to either cerebral oligemia or cerebral hyperemia. Although further studies need to be done to determine "age-appropriate" CPP, common target CPPs are greater than 40–50 mmHg in infants and toddlers, 50–60 mmHg in children, and greater than 60 mmHg in adolescents.

Decompressive craniectomy involves the removal of sections of the calvaria and, depending on the indication, dural resection and duraplasty. Although first described over a century ago in the early 1900s by Drs Kocher and Cushing, decompressive craniectomy has survived until today but with continued controversies on indication, approach, and timing. In this chapter, we focus on the anesthetic approach to patients undergoing a decompressive craniectomy for refractory intracranial hypertension, resulting from traumatic and non-TBI, and Chiari malformations.

T.J. Kilbaugh, MD (✉) • S. Friess, MD
Department of Anesthesiology and Critical Care Medicine, The Children's Hospital of
Philadelphia, Philadelphia, PA, USA
e-mail: kilbaugh@email.chop.edu

M. Helfaer, MD
Departments of Anesthesiology and Critical Care, Pediatrics and Nursing, Perelman School
of Medicine at the University of Pennsylvania, University of Pennsylvania School of Medicine,
Philadelphia, PA, USA

A.M. Brambrink and J.R. Kirsch (eds.), *Essentials of Neurosurgical
Anesthesia & Critical Care*, DOI 10.1007/978-0-387-09562-2_51,
© Springer Science+Business Media, LLC 2012

Posterior Fossa Decompressive Craniectomy for Chiari Malformations

Chiari malformations are a group of disorders characterized by the caudal prolapse of the medulla, cerebellum, and fourth ventricle through the foramen magnum into the cervical canal. This caudal prolapse is secondary to abnormalities of the brain and a small, malformed skull base. There are four classifications of Chiari malformations (CM), types I–IV, depending on anatomic compression. Symptoms can vary dramatically: headache, often described as tension, neck pain, myelopathy, and brainstem compromise (Cushing triad: bradycardia, hypertension, and abnormalities in breathing); all resulting from anatomic compression/crowding of the brain stem, cerebellum, lower cranial nerves, and spinal cord. The two most common types of CM are Type I and Type II. Chiari Malformation Type I (Chiari I) is the caudal displacement of the cerebellar tonsils less than 6 mm below the foramen magnum into the cervical canal. This displacement is often associated with the disruption of CSF flow, causing CSF to enter the spinal cord and create a fluid-filled cavity called a syrinx. The chronic expansion of a syrinx can cause compression of the surrounding spinal cord nerve fibers and lead to a constellation of symptoms, collectively referred to as syringomelia. Syringomelia can occur at any portion of the spinal cord, but, in association with Chiari I and other posterior fossa abnormalities, it is often communicating from the cervical region to the fourth ventricle. In combination with syringomelia or in isolation, Chiari malformations may also be associated with obstructive hydrocephalus due to fourth ventricular outflow obstruction or aqueductal stenosis, necessitating diversion of CSF. Traditionally, CSF diversion has been accomplished with the placement of a ventriculoperitoneal shunt; however, endoscopic third ventriculostomy has also been described with good results. Chiari Malformation Type II (Chiari II) is associated with myelomeningocele and often with cerebellar herniation and a malformed brain stem. Chiari malformations Type III and IV are rare and usually present with gross herniation of the cerebellum and severely malformed brain stem. Due to the complexity of the many forms of Chiari malformations and inter-patient variability, surgical approach varies, but the basic tenets address decompression and stabilization of the craniocervical junction, restoration of CSF flow, and ablation of syringomelia when applicable. A common approach is suboccipital decompression of the posterior fossa, with or without duraplasty, with occipitocervical fusion with autogenous bone graft or posterior stabilization via screw fixation with bone fragments.

Decompressive Craniectomy for Refractory Intracranial Hypertension

TBI is the leading cause of death and disability in children and adolescents in the USA. In the 2003, "Guidelines for the acute management of severe TBI in infants, children, and adolescents," there is primary focus on controlling ICP as a supportive

Table 51.1 Therapeutic interventions to control intracranial pressure (ICP)

Cerebral blood volume (CBV) reduction with reduction of cerebral metabolic rate (CMV)	• Hyperventilation • Head position (30°, midline) • CBF reducing drugs (i.e., mannitol, hypothermia) • CBV/CMR reducing drugs (barbiturates, benzodiazepines, etomidate, propofol) • Seizure control
Cerebral spinal fluid reduction	• CSF drainage (ventriculostomy, lumbar drain)
Induction of serum hyperosmolarity	• Mannitol • Hypertonic saline
Resection of dead/injured brain tissue	
Resection of nonneural masses/hematoma	• Tumor, foreign body • Epidural/subdural hematoma
Decompressive craniectomy	• Hemicraniectomy, bifrontal craniectomy, and posterior fossa craniectomy

measure, to maintain CPP, and adequate oxygen delivery to preserve viable brain tissue until the underlying process can resolve. Kofke and Stiefel define six tiers of therapy for intracranial hypertension (Table 51.1). Specific thresholds for refractory intracranial hypertension have not been well established; however, sustained elevation of ICP greater than 20 mmHg is linked to increased morbidity and mortality in the pediatric patient. Decompressive craniectomy is considered a second-tier therapy to treat intracranial hypertension refractory to medical therapy as a means to control ICP, maintain CPP, and prevent herniation. There are two current approaches: hemicraniectomy or bifrontal craniectomy. A hemicraniectomy is usually performed when there is a focal or unilateral insult, and bifrontal craniectomy with diffuse swelling. A section of the calvaria is removed, the dura is resected, and a duraplasty performed to relieve ICP and allow cerebral expansion. The section of bone that is removed can be stored in a bone freezer or surgically placed in the subcutaneous tissue of the abdomen until ICP issues have resolved. In adults, there have been mixed results, and a recent Cochrane review suggests that the procedure lacks firm evidence, and further information may be obtained in current randomized controlled trials for TBI and stroke. The data are even more limited in pediatrics and difficult to interpret. Certainly, decompressive craniectomy reduces ICP and, in some reports, increases cerebral oxygenation. However, the impact of patient selection and optimal timing have yet to be determined, with some case series suggesting better outcomes with surgical intervention within 24 h of ICP elevation. There are no randomized controlled trials in pediatrics, but the pediatric literature would suggest that decompressive craniectomy should be considered in the treatment of severe TBI and refractory intracraninal hypertension in infants and young children with nonaccidental head trauma or shaken-impact syndrome, as these patients had improved survival and neurologic outcomes compared with those undergoing medical management alone. There is also some limited data to suggest that decompressive craniectomy may be effective in treating nontraumatic intracranial hypertension.

Crisis Management

Chiari Malformation Pathophysiology and Clinical Presentation

Patients require a detailed preoperative assessment, focusing on history, physical, and diagnostic studies to detect craniocervical anomalies, autonomic instability, atlanto-occipital instability, and cerebellar/lower cranial nerve involvement. Chiari I may be associated with central sleep apnea syndrome, and there are case reports describing sleep apnea as the presenting symptom for Chiari I confirmed by polysomnography. Chiari I is also frequently associated with tethered cord and Klippel–Feil syndrome. Klippel–Feil is a rare disorder associated with fusion of any of the cervical vertebral, as well as, a low posterior hairline and short neck. Other associated anomalies with Klippel–Feil are: rib and vertebral anomalies, cardiac and renal defects, cleft palate, scoliosis, torticollis, deafness, and atlanto-occipital instability.

Chiari Malformation Patient Assessment

An anesthetic plan for a patient with Chiari and associated Klippel–Feil syndrome must anticipate a difficult airway and difficult bag mask ventilation secondary to limited neck movement due to cervical fusion, atlanto-occipital instability, scoliosis, and palate abnormalities. During intubation and positioning, particular attention should be paid to in-line stabilization of the cervical spine, if there is a suspicion or diagnosis of atlanto-occipital instability. Finally, prior to suboccipital decompression, the anesthetic plan must avoid further elevations in ICP that may precipitate herniation and further decompensation.

Chiari Malformation Intervention and Treatment

In the event of life-threatening intracranial hypertension, acute management should include hyperventilation, hyperosmolar therapy with either mannitol (1 g/kg which may be divided in smaller doses and titrated to effect) or hypertonic saline (3%) 4 ml/kg, discussion with neurosurgery about emergent placement of ventriculostomy. While this scenario may be a rare occurrence in patients with a thorough preoperative evaluation, many children with Chiari malformations undergoing surgical procedures for other than a decompressive craniectomy are at increased risk for intracranial hypertension during the perioperative period, especially patients undergoing neurosurgical or craniofacial surgery.

Decompressive Craniectomy for Refractory Intracranial Hypertension

Patient Assessment

Anesthetic management should focus on the management of ICP and maintaining CPP prior to decompressive craniectomy. Detailed discussions should occur during preoperative evaluation with neurosurgery, trauma surgery, and critical care to delineate current therapies as well as develop a detailed understanding of other injuries. Physical exam should focus on findings of impending herniation syndromes: pupil exam, cranial nerve abnormalities, posturing, and Cushing's reflex (hypothalamic response to ischemia secondary to poor cerebral blood flow, with resulting sympathetic discharge attempting to raise arterial blood pressure, with accompanied bradycardia). In the pediatric multi-trauma patient, particular attention must be paid to solid organ injuries that may be evolving during the perioperative period. Coagulopathy should be aggressively treated, and optimizing hemoglobin to maintain end organ oxygen delivery is critical to avoid worsening secondary brain injury.

***Decompressive Craniectomy for Refractory Intracranial Hypertention Intervention

Continual reassessment of an unstable multi-trauma patient during the intraoperative period is critical. Monitors should include: arterial access for blood pressure management and CPP optimization, central venous access for central venous pressure, vasoactive and hyperosmolar delivery. In addition, discussions should take place with neurosurgery for insertion of multi-modal intracranial monitoring including ICP (pressure monitoring or ventriculostomy for pressure monitoring and CSF drainage.) Other multi-modal intracranial monitoring may also include brain tissue oxygen monitoring (i.e., Licox.) There is limited data on the impact of anesthetic management on patient outcomes with intracranial hypertension. All volatile anesthetics can increase cerebral vasoldilation and CBF especially at high doses; however, in responsive cerebral vasculature these effects can be abolished with mild to moderate hyperventilation titrated according to repeated ABGs to avoid cerebral ischemia. However, in diffuse injury, cerebral vascular reactivity may be nonreactive and it may not matter which anesthetic drug is employed. In addition, there continues to be much debate on volatile anesthetics as neuroprotectants, and their potential for neuronal damage via apoptosis. In animal models, nitrous oxide increases neurotoxic/neuroexcitation mediators, ICP, and CBF and should be avoided in this patient population. Other anesthetic medications (barbiturates, propofol, etomidate) decrease cerebral metabolic rate coupled with CBF and decrease ICP. Opioids should be administered for antinociception to prevent ICP spikes from noxious stimuli. Intraoperative goal directed therapy for pediatric intracranial hypertension should include: ICP < 20 mmHg, PbO_2 > 25 mmHg, and age directed CPP of greater than 40–50 mmHg in infants and toddlers, 50–60 mmHg in children, and greater than 60 mmHg in adolescents. First tiered therapies for the reduction of ICP and improvement of PbO_2 include brief periods of hyperventilation, drainage of CSF via a ventriculostomy, sedation and paralysis, and hyperosmolar therapy. The optimal intraoperative approach to hyperosmolar therapy has yet to be determined; however, hyperosmolar therapy with hypertonic saline may have some theoretical advantage over mannitol. Mannitol causes a significant osmotic diuresis, resulting in a loss of preload and a potential rise in hematocrit (decreasing rheology) and ultimately hypotension (decreasing CPP). Mannitol may also result in rebound ICP. There are two potential mechanisms both resulting in an increased parenchymal reflection coefficient and subsequent cerebral edema with mannitol administration. One, mannitol moves across a disrupted blood brain barrier, and, two, mannitol administration triggers the production of idogenic osmoles within the brain parenchyma. Hypertonic saline administration is very effective in lowering ICP, avoiding the side effects of ultimate side effects of mannitol discussed above, as well as supporting preload by acting as an excellent peripheral volume expander which, in turn, may support CPP.

With any disruption of the blood brain barrier such as occurs with decompressive craniotomies, disseminated intravascular contamination can occur. Vigilance in monitoring and correcting PT, PTT, fibrinogen and platelets can prevent catastrophic bleeding in the perioperative period.

Key Points

- Decompressive craniectomy involves the removal, of sections of the calvaria and depending on the indication, dural resection and duraplasty.
- Chiari malformations may also be associated with obstructive hydrocephalus due to fourth ventricular outflow obstruction or aqueductal stenosis necessitating diversion of CSF.
- Intraoperative goal directed therapy for pediatric intracranial hypertension should include: ICP < 20 mmHg, PbO_2 > 25, and age directed CPP of greater than 40–50 mmHg in infants and toddlers, 50–60 mmHg in children, and greater than 60 mmHg in adolescents.
- Maintenance of physiologic parameters, including coagulation, is paramount to successful management in the perioperative period.
- Early decompressive craniectomy should be considered in the treatment of severe TBI and refractory intracranial hypertension in infants and children.

Suggested Reading

Adelson PD et al. Guidelines for the acute medical management of severe traumatic brain injury in infants, children, and adolescents. Chapter 19. The role of anti-seizure prophylaxis following severe pediatric traumatic brain injury. Pediatr Crit Care Med. 2003;4(3 Suppl):S72–5.

Cakmakkaya OS, Kaya G, Altintas F, Bakan M, Yildirim A. Anesthetic management of a child with Arnold-Chiari malformation and Klippel-Feil syndrome. Paediatr Anaesth. 2006;16(3):355–6.

Friess SH, Helfaer MH, Raghupathi R, Huh JH. An evidence-based approach to severe traumatic brain injury in children. Pediatr Emerg Med Pract. 2007;4(12):1–27.

Kofke W, Stiefel M. Monitoring and intraoperative management of elevated intracranial pressure and decompressive craniectomy. Anesthesiol Clin. 2007;25(3):579–603.

Pompucci A, De Bonis P, Pettorini B, Petrella G, Di Chirico A, Anile C. Decompressive craniectomy for traumatic brain injury: patient age and outcome. J Neurotrauma. 2007;24(7):1182–8.

Sahuquillo J, Arikan F. Decompressive craniectomy for the treatment of refractory high intracranial pressure in traumatic brain injury. Cochrane Database Syst Rev. 2006;(1):CD003983.

Soriano SG, Eldredge EA, Rockoff MA. Pediatric neuroanesthesia. Anesthesiol Clin North Am. 2002;20(2):389–404.

Chapter 52
Challenges During Surgery for Craniosynostosis and Craniofacial Surgery

Heike Gries and Jeffrey Koh

The following complications are commonly associated with craniosynostosis repair: (1) difficult airway, (2) blood loss and blood transfusion, (3) venous air embolism, (4) increased intracranial pressure (ICP).

Difficult airway management is also a main focus during other craniofacial surgeries.

Difficult Airway

Overview

About 20% of craniosynostosis patients are in the category of syndromic craniosynostosis. The most common syndromes that present with craniosynostosis are Apert's syndrome and Crouzon's syndrome. In these patients, craniosynostosis repair often involves difficult airway management. Craniofacial surgeries, such as mandibular osteomies and genioplasties, are often performed on patients with facial disproportion and other congenital anomalies (e.g., Crouzon, Pierre Robin, and Treacher Collins syndromes) and may lead to difficulties in airway management.

H. Gries, MD, PhD (✉)
Department of Anesthesiology and Perioperative Medicine, Oregon Health & Science University, Portland, OR, USA
e-mail: griesh@ohsu.edu

J. Koh, MD
Department of Anesthesiology and Perioperative Medicine, Oregon Health & Science University, Portland, OR, USA

A.M. Brambrink and J.R. Kirsch (eds.), *Essentials of Neurosurgical Anesthesia & Critical Care*, DOI 10.1007/978-0-387-09562-2_52, © Springer Science+Business Media, LLC 2012

Table 52.1 Intravenous induction

	Titration	Continuous infusion
Propofol	1–2 mg/kg	150–200 µg/kg/min
Dexmedetomidine	0.5–1 µg/kg	0.5–1 µg/kg/h
Ketamine	0.5–1 mg/kg	

Prevention

Identifying patients at risk for airway problems is the first step to successful airway management. Take a careful history (including any prior history of surgery or intubation), perform a thorough physical examination, and tailor the anesthetic plan to include appropriate back-up strategies. This will minimize the risk of being caught by surprise. When a potentially difficult airway is identified, appropriate preparation is the next step. All airway equipment should be available, checked, and ready prior to the induction of anesthesia. In addition to the usual intubation equipment, the difficult airway equipment should include at least a fiber-optic bronchoscope as well as appropriately sized laryngeal masks, a rigid bronchoscope, and equipment for tracheostomy and resuscitation.

Premedication may be varied to suit the patient's needs. Preoperative IV placement (consider topical anesthesia) is usually indicated when a difficult airway is anticipated. Glycopyrrolate (0.005–0.001 mg/kg) or atropine (0.01–0.02 mg/kg) is administered to block excessive secretions and to prevent unwanted autonomic vagal reflexes. An intravenous dose of corticosteroid (dexamethasone 0.4 mg/kg) can be given as prophylactic against airway edema. Finally, topical decongestant such as 0.05% oxymetazoline intranasally should be considered prior to the induction to prevent nasal bleeding. The decision regarding the use of anxiolysis either orally or intravenously should be balanced with the anticipated degree of airway compromise.

After communicating with the surgeon about the plan(s) and when the surgeon is in the operating room, inhalational or intravenous induction can be initiated. If an ENT surgeon is not already involved in the patient's care, consideration should be given to preoperative consultation and presence during induction in case emergency airway assistance is needed. If the ENT surgeon is not available, it is suggested to ask a second anesthesiologist to be available.

Inhalational induction with 100% oxygen and sevoflurane can be used safely with the goal of maintaining spontaneous ventilation. It is often necessary to use jaw thrust and place an oral/nasopharyngeal airway as the upper airway muscles start to relax. Alternatively, intravenous induction with careful titration of propofol, dexmedetomidine, or ketamine can be used (Table 52.1). As with an inhalational induction, the initial titration goal should be to maintain spontaneous ventilation, at least until the provider can confirm the ability to mask ventilate. Muscle relaxants should not be used until the airway is secured.

In a patient with a potentially difficult airway, it might be reasonable to try a direct laryngoscopy while the patient is breathing spontaneously; however, each attempt for direct intubation may cause trauma and will make a potential fiber-optic intubation more difficult.

If it is difficult to manage spontaneous breathing under anesthesia, a laryngeal mask airway (LMA) is often very useful. Although, in most cases, the LMA must be removed before surgery, it can be helpful to place an endotracheal tube exchanger (Cook Airway Exchange Catheter, Cook Critical Care, Bloomington, IN) before removing the LMA and use it to place the endotracheal tube. Alternatively, fiber-optic intubation can be performed through the LMA.

Crisis Management

Figure 52.1 shows an algorithm for the unexpected difficult airway in pediatric patients.

Key Points

- Thorough evaluation of the patient to identify a potentially abnormal airway is the first step in preventing difficult airway situations.
- Designing a tailored anesthesia plan with appropriate back-up strategies and preparation with attention to details followed by clear communication with the surgical team are essential for a safe and successful procedure.
- Call for help early in an emergency and use algorithms thoughtfully to manage the situation.

Blood Loss and Blood Transfusion

Overview

Blood loss during craniosynostosis repair is very common. This blood loss combined with the small blood volume of the young patients that typically undergo craniosynostosis repair makes transfusion of red blood cells often unavoidable. The need for additional blood products such as platelets and fresh frozen plasma (FFP) is much less common in sagittal and unicoronal suture repair where a blood loss of approximately 25% of the estimated blood volume has been described. However, FFP and platelets are frequently needed in bicoronal suture repair where blood loss of up to 65% has been described.

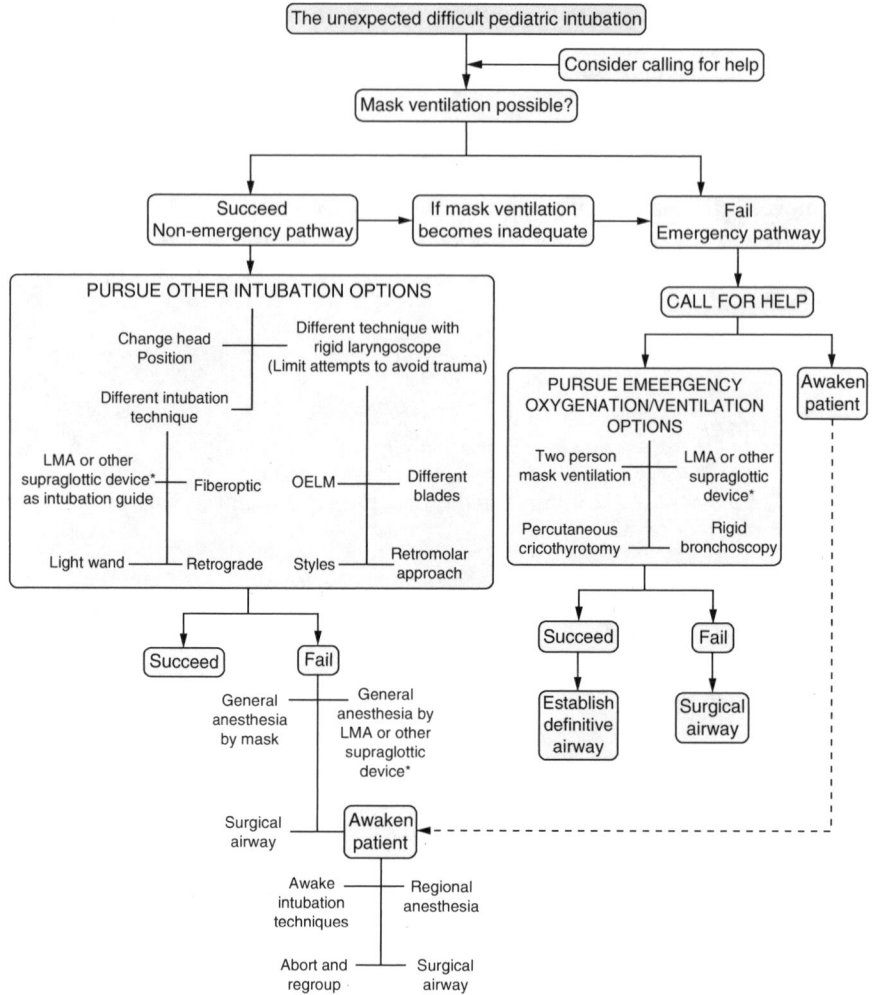

*Consider using PLMA if the child is at risk for aspiration or if high inflation pressures are needed

Fig. 52.1 A proposed algorithm for the management of the unexpected difficult pediatric airway. *LMA* laryngeal mask airway, *OELM* optimal external laryngeal manipulation, *PLMA* pro Seal LMA (with permission from Elsevier, from Wheeler, M, Cote CJ, Todres ID. The pediatric airway. In: Cote CJ, Lerman J, Todres ID, editors. A practice of anesthesia for infants and children. 4th ed. Saunders Elsevier; 2009. p. 264)

Accurate assessment and replacement of blood loss in cranial vault repair is difficult, but most blood loss will occur during elevation of the vascular periosteum and then continue slowly throughout the procedure after the osteotomy has been performed. Blood loss will depend not only on the type of craniosynostosis but also

Fig. 52.2 Maximal allowable blood loss (MABL)

$$MABL = EBV\frac{(Ho - Hl)}{Ho}$$

EBV = Estimated blood volume

Ho = Baseline (preoperative) Hematocrit (%)

Hl = Lowest acceptable Hematocrit (%)

on the surgical technique, with procedures associated with more bony dissections, such as cranial vault remodeling, often resulting in higher blood loss. To minimize the risk of transfusion-related morbidity (post-transfusion hepatitis, acquired immunodeficiency, hemolytic transfusion reactions and allergic reactions, transfusion-related lung injury, and leukocyte-platelet allogenic immunization), use all appropriate strategies to decrease the need for homologous transfusion.

Prevention

The surgical technique will define the range of expected blood loss. The anesthesiologist must prepare before surgery to manage blood loss:

- Evaluate preoperative hematocrit, platelet count, and coagulation studies
- Type and cross for packed red blood cells and use

  - Leukocyte-depleted components
  - Cytomegalovirus seronegative products for children younger than 1 year
  - Red blood cells stored < 2 or 3 weeks

- Insert two large-bore intravenous catheters (22–20 gauge catheters for infants less than 6 months are adequate)
- Place an arterial line
- Consider monitoring central venous pressure, especially if large blood loss is anticipated
- Estimate the maximal allowable blood loss (MABL) before surgery (Fig. 52.2).

The following techniques may help to prevent blood transfusion:

- Preoperative treatment with recombinant human erythropoietin (300 U/kg erythropoietin every other day for 3 weeks with additional elemental iron μ [2 mg/kg TID])
- Perioperative blood salvage (Cell Saver)
- Acute normovolemic hemodilution, especially in older children.

Crisis Management

Signs of significant blood loss include:

- Tachycardia
- Low blood pressure
- Low CO_2 can be an indicator for diminished cardiac output
- Respiratory variation in arterial line pressure wave

Transfusion guidelines:

- As a rule of thumb: *Red blood cell transfusion* is rarely indicated when the hemoglobin concentration is >10 g/dL and is almost always indicated when the hemoglobin concentration is <6 g/dL. Sometimes, red blood cells must be given before the MABL is reached, e.g., with rapid blood loss or when hemodynamic instability occurs despite adequate volume replacement. Be aware that rapid blood transfusion in an infant can cause hyperkalemia and cardiac arrest, primarily because of the high concentration of potassium in stored blood.
- *Platelet transfusion* is usually required if the platelet count is $<50 \times 10^9$/L. The therapeutic dose is one platelet concentrate per 10 kg body weight or 5–10 mL/kg body weight.
- *FFP* is indicated to correct microvascular bleeding when prothrombin and partial thromboplastin times are >1.5 times normal or in the setting of massive transfusion when coagulation tests cannot be obtained in a timely manner. To achieve an increase in plasma factor concentration of 30%, 10–15 mL/kg FFP should be given.
- *Cryoprecipitate* must be considered when microvascular bleeding is present and fibrinogen levels are <80–100 mg/dL. One unit of cryoprecipitate per 10 kg body weight will normally raise the plasma fibrinogen concentration by approximately 50 mg/dL.
- *Calcium gluconate* (30–45 mg/kg) or calcium chloride (10–20 mg/kg via central venous line) may be indicated to stabilize myocardial function and to treat hypocalcemia, which occurs in cases requiring larger volumes of citrate-containing blood products.

Key Points

- Blood loss during craniosynostosis repair is very common, and blood transfusion is often necessary.
- Preparing for anticipated blood loss and using strategies to decrease homologous transfusion will contribute to an excellent patient outcome.

Venous Air Embolism

Overview

Venous air embolism has been reported in up to 83% of craniosynostosis repairs, most of them without hemodynamic consequences. Positioning the head above the heart and exposing open noncollapsible veins to air after opening the skull together with a decreased central venous pressure during rapid blood loss can result in a pressure gradient that favors venous air entry. And, moreover, the persistence of a patent foramen ovale in 50% of children younger than 5 years increases the potential for a paradoxical air embolism and may result in a coronary or cerebral embolism.

Prevention

- Avoid positioning the head above the heart as surgical indications allow.
- Avoid nitrous oxide due to its low blood/gas partition coefficient and its ability to increase the size of any air embolus that occurs.
- Use a precordial Doppler ultrasonic probe to detect venous air embolism early.
- Maintain adequate intravascular volume status, and avoid a sudden decrease in the central venous pressure.
- Control ventilation and prevent negative intrathoracic pressure.

Crisis Management

- Ventilate patient with 100% oxygen.
- Communicate with the surgeon immediately to treat early (flood the surgical field) and minimize further air entrainment.
- If central venous access is in place, try to aspirate air from the central venous pressure line.
- Consider compressing the jugular veins until the surgeon has occluded air entry.
- In the case of severe venous air embolism, consider lowering the head to decrease the rate of air entrainment.
- Do not use PEEP. This may cause a paradoxical air embolism by increasing right atrial pressures and opening a patent foramen ovale.

Key Points

- Venous air embolism is common in craniosynostosis repair, but usually asymptomatic.
- A precordial Doppler ultrasonic probe will detect venous air embolism immediately and, therefore, will allow early treatment.
- Communication with the surgeon is a key to early treatment.

Increased Intracranial Pressure

Overview

About 30–40% of patients with syndromes and complex craniosynostosis have intracranial hypertension, while 15–20% of patients with single suture craniosynostosis have increased ICP. Restricted skull volumes are responsible for this increase in pressure as well as anomalous intracranial venous drainage, hydrocephalus, and upper airway obstruction, especially in patients with craniofacial syndromes.

Prevention

Each patient should be assessed preoperatively for any signs or symptoms of increased ICP. In addition, preoperative studies such as CT scans or MRIs should be reviewed for signs of increased ICP. To prevent further increases in ICP

- Establish and secure the airway meticulously and control ventilation to minimize the risk of hypoxia and hypercapnia
- Avoid arterial hypertension
- Consider corticosteroids
- Position the head carefully, avoid Trendelenburg position if possible.

Crisis Management

- Check oxygenation and ventilation of the patient.
- Assess level of sedation, and increase anesthesia, if appropriate.
- Check head positioning to rule out venous outflow obstruction.
- Consider corticosteroids if not administered earlier.
- Consider moderate hyperventilation and maintain a normal arterial pressure.
- Consider mannitol and/or furosemide.

Key Points

- A significant number of patients for craniosynostosis repair may present with increased ICP.
- An established well-secured airway is the key to avoid hypoxia and hypercapnia and, therefore, to prevent a further increase in ICP.
- Moderate hyperventilation, corticosteroids, mannitol, and furosemide as well as positioning are important treatment options.

Suggested Reading

Difficult Airway

Butler MG, Hayes BG, Hathaway MM, et al. Specific genetic diseases at risk for sedation/anesthesia complications. Anesth Analg. 2000;91:837–55.
Wheeler M. Management strategies for the difficult pediatric airway. Anesthesiol Clin. 1998;16:743–56.

Blood Loss and Blood Transfusion

British Committee for Standards in Hematology Transfusion. Transfusion guidelines for neonates and older children. Br J Haematol. 2004;124:433–53.
Koh JL, Gries H. Perioperative management of pediatric patients with craniosynostosis. Anesth Clin. 2007;25:465–81.

Venous Air Embolism

Faberowski LW, Black S, Mickle JP. Incidence of venous air embolism during craniectomy for craniosynostosis repair. Anesthesiology. 2000;92:20–3.

Increased Intracranial Pressure

Tamburrini G, Caldarelli M, Massimi L, et al. Intracranial pressure monitoring in children with single suture and complex craniosynostosis: a review. Childs Nerv Syst. 2005;21:913–21.

Chapter 53
Challenges During Tumor Surgery in Children and Infants

Christopher Karsanac and Jayant Deshpande

Intracranial tumor resection in pediatrics represents a broad spectrum of surgeries. The surgical approach depends largely on tumor location. Specific complications accompany each surgery depending on that location. However, some complications are common regardless of neurosurgical approach. This section focuses on the more common possible complications associated with intracranial tumor resection: (1) neuromonitoring failure, (2) massive hemorrhage, (3) syndrome of inappropriate antidiuretic hormone secretion (SIADH), and (4) diabetes insipidus.

This is not an exhaustive list, as there are other complications that are associated with tumor surgery. These topics are discussed elsewhere (Chaps. 17, 36, and 42).

Neuromonitoring Failure

Overview

Evoked potentials increasingly are used in neurosurgery to monitor the integrity of specific sensory or motor pathways. Specific pathways that are monitored depend on the location of the tumor. Sensory evoked potentials (SEPs) can monitor somatosensory (SSEPs), brainstem auditory (BAEP), or visual (VEP) pathways. Motor evoked potentials (MEPs) can monitor the dorsolateral and ventral spinal cord or can be used to monitor cranial nerves.

C. Karsanac, MD (✉)
Department of Anesthesiology, Vanderbilt University Medical Center, Nashville, TN, USA
e-mail: christopher.j.karsanac@Vanderbilt.Edu

J. Deshpande, MD, MPH
Departments of Pediatrics and Anesthesiology, Arkansas Children's Hospital, University of Arkansas for Medical Sciences, Little Rock, AR, USA

A.M. Brambrink and J.R. Kirsch (eds.), *Essentials of Neurosurgical Anesthesia & Critical Care*, DOI 10.1007/978-0-387-09562-2_53,
© Springer Science+Business Media, LLC 2012

After an applied electrical stimulus, appropriately placed electrodes detect the transient potential differences along the neural pathway. Latency and amplitude of the potential differences are compared to values at baseline obtained before the initial incision is made. Significant increases in latency and/or decreases in amplitude may indicate compromise of the monitored neural pathway.

Prevention

Anesthetic, physiologic, and environmental factors are all capable of producing changes in evoked potentials that mimic pathway compromise. Communicating changes in both anesthetic dosing and monitored vital signs with the neuro-monitoring team is crucial to avoid confounding values.

All anesthetics that have been studied influence evoked potentials to some extent. Volatile agents have the most profound effect and, therefore, are often avoided all together in favor of a total intravenous anesthesia (TIVA) technique. A significant change in dosing regimen of an IV agent (e.g., boluses) will affect the neuromonitoring. Thus, any changes to anesthetic dosing must be communicated to the monitoring team.

Significant changes in most physiologic factors, such as temperature, blood pressure, PaO_2, and $PaCO_2$, can also alter signals from baseline. Much like anesthetic use, maintaining steady levels of these parameters are imperative to avoiding large changes in signal latency and amplitude.

Crisis Management

Significant changes in monitored evoked potentials should be immediately communicated by the neuromonitoring team to the surgeon and anesthesiologist. Concurrently, the anesthesia team should evaluate possible contributing factors, including (a) anesthetic changes (i.e., volatiles turned on, bolus agents given, paralytic agents given, etc.) or (b) significant decrease in cerebral/spinal cord oxygen delivery (e.g., hypotension, hypoxia). If using deliberate hypotension, discuss with the surgeon the possibility of returning blood pressure to baseline.

Key Points

- Evoked potential monitoring can guide the neurosurgeon and help to maintain cortical and spinal pathway integrity.
- The latency and amplitude of potentials are recorded to monitor any pathway compromise.
- Changes in anesthetics and physiological parameters can cause evoked potential changes that mimic pathway compromise.
- Maintaining systemic perfusion and oxygen delivery during any episode of possible pathway compromise is essential.

Massive Hemorrhage

Overview

The child has a smaller total circulating blood volume compare with an adult (Table 53.1). Blood loss that is inconsequential to adults may lead to circulatory collapse in children.

Close monitoring of blood loss is important and consists of evaluating not only blood in the suction canister but also that in the drapes and on surgical sponges. Large amount of blood loss may go undetected or may be difficult to control because of the constraints of the operative field or the inaccessibility of the offending vessels.

Prevention

Prevention revolves around making the operating field as accessible as possible for the neurosurgeon. The better the visualization, the easier it may be to avoid vessels and, if necessary, to respond to any hemorrhaging that does occur. Maintaining a low-normal $PaCO_2$ (35–40 mmHg) decreases cerebral blood volume and provides better surgical access. Deliberate hypotension may also be requested to reduce surgical bleeding.

Adequate IV access is important. At a minimum, the patient for intracranial tumor resection should have two large bore IVs that allow for rapid administration of fluids and resuscitation drugs.

Crisis Management

Large amounts of blood loss will result in hypovolemia as well as cerebral and systemic hypoperfusion. Acutely, blood pressure will decrease and heart rate will increase. If evoked potentials are being monitored, they will show increased latency and decreased amplitude as cerebral or spinal perfusion decreases. Maintaining oxygen delivery to vital organ systems is the goal of therapy.

- Oxygen delivery may be improved by increasing FiO_2 to 100%.
- Isotonic crystalloids (0.9% normal saline) or colloids can be given as a bolus (10–20 mL/kg).

Table 53.1 Total circulating blood volume (child)

Age	Total blood volume (mL/kg)
Newborn	80–85
6 Weeks to 2 years	75
2 Years to puberty	72

- Warmed packed red blood cells (PRBCs) should be transfused if the patient becomes hemodynamically compromised (start with 10 mL/kg).
- Coagulation studies and hematocrit levels should be obtained to help guide the use of PRBCs and other blood components (e.g., FFP or platelets); consider checking serum calcium levels after the use of blood products.

Key Points

- Massive hemorrhage may occur at any point during tumor resection.
- Adequate IV access and blood product availability is essential to treatment.
- In the unstable patient, blood loss should be replaced with a blood transfusion.
- Serial lab studies will help to guide further treatment after the acute hemorrhage has resolved.

SIADH

Overview

Antidiuretic hormone (ADH) is produced by the posterior pituitary gland. It promotes the resorption of free water in the collecting tubules of the kidneys. This causes a decrease in serum osmolality and subsequent increase in circulating blood volume. ADH release is regulated by numerous stimuli. The two main stimuli are changes in osmolality sensed in the hypothalamus and activation of stretch receptors located in the left atrium.

The SIADH occurs when there is excessive ADH present. SIADH results in an abnormal decrease in serum osmolality (<280 mOsm/kg), hypervolemia and urine output that is low volume and highly concentrated (>300–400 mOsm/kg and urine sodium >30 mEq/L). SIADH appears to be more common in children with tumors in the cerebral hemispheres or posterior fossa.

Prevention

While prevention might not be possible, early recognition is key in avoiding the complications secondary to the hyponatremia associated with SIADH. Hyponatremia can cause altered levels of consciousness, brain swelling, coma, and seizures. Hypotonic IV solutions must be avoided to minimize the incidence of these symptoms.

Crisis Management

Hyponatremia is treated according to etiology, the rapidity of onset, level of serum osmolality, and estimation of total body sodium (TBS). Since TBS is typically normal in SIADH, excess total body water should be calculated:

TBW (liters) = 0.611 (weight kg) + 0.251
Normal TBW = TBW × (serum sodium/140)
Excess TBW = TBW − normal TBW.

Severity of symptoms of hyponatremia relate to the rapidity of the drop in serum sodium levels. Symptoms usually begin to manifest postoperatively as serum sodium levels decrease. In the OR, symptoms may be masked by the anesthetic agents used. Treatment is guided by sodium levels and serum osmolality. Discontinuing hypotonic IV solutions in mild cases of hyponatremia may be all that is needed. Serum sodium levels <115–120 mEq/L require more aggressive therapy:

- Hypertonic 3% saline may be administered at a rate of 1–2 mL/kg/h to raise plasma sodium levels by 1–2 mEq/L/h but not >10 mEq/L/day.
- Normal 0.9% saline along with 0.5–1 mg/kg of IV furosemide may be used as an alternative.
- For persistent SIADH in children >8 years old, postoperative treatment with demeclocycline 6–12 mg/kg/day PO divided into two to four doses may be necessary.

Rapid correction may cause permanent neurologic sequelae secondary to osmotic pontine demyelination syndrome. Risk factors for osmotic demyelination syndrome include rapidity of correction and also duration of hyponatremia, the patient's nutritional status, and other underlying pathologies

Key Points

- SIADH results in a eunatremic, hypervolemic hyponatremia.
- SIADH is a diagnosis of exclusion that presents with decreased urine output, urine sodium >30 mEq/L, urine osmolality >300–400 mOsm/kg, and serum osmolality <285 mOsm/kg.
- Symptoms are related to the rapidity of onset and chronicity of the hyponatremia.
- Mild hyponatremia treatment consists of avoidance of free water and hypotonic fluids and fluid restriction.
- Severe hyponatremia should be corrected cautiously with frequent evaluation to avoid osmotic demyelination.

Central Diabetes Insipidus

Overview

Diabetes insipidus (DI) results from inadequate secretion of ADH or the inability of ADH to act on the kidneys. This results in polydipsia, hypernatremia, and large amounts of very dilute urine. Hypernatremia produces worsening neurological symptoms (mental status changes, coma, and seizures) and can cause renal insufficiency which may progress to renal failure. Reduction in brain volume may damage delicate vessels leading to subdural, subarachnoid, or even subcortical hemorrhage.

Patients with sellar and suprasellar tumors are more likely to have DI. Intracranial neurosurgical procedures, alone, may also cause DI. The clinical course varies and depends on the location and type of tumor and the amount of cerebral manipulation. Polyuria may be present for only a few days after surgery, be permanent, or may present in a triphasic sequence with return of function followed by recurrent DI.

Prevention

Similar to SIADH, prevention of DI may not be possible. However, the consequences of electrolyte derangement can be prevented. The most feared complication of acute hypernatremia is central pontine myelinolysis (CPM). CPM is nerve damage caused by the destruction of the myelin sheath covering nerve cells in the brainstem. In a patient with polyuria undergoing neurosurgical intervention, frequent electrolyte monitoring is needed to detect episodes of hypernatremia.

Patients already diagnosed with DI are often on DDAVP (desmopressin). It is a synthetic analog of ADH that can be given by a variety of routes. When given intranasally, it has prolonged antidiuretic activity (12–24 h) and is associated with a low incidence of pressor effects.

Crisis Management

The clinical signs of severe hypernatremia and hypovolemia associated with DI are largely masked by general anesthesia. However, polyuria in the face of rising serum sodium should raise suspicion. Typically, urine sodium is <10–15 mEq/L and urine osmolality is <400 mOsm/kg. Decreased blood pressure and tachycardia due to hypovolemia can also be seen, if DI has been allowed to progress. Total body water deficit (TBWD) can be calculated to help aide in fluid management: $TBWD = TBW \times [([Na] - 140)/140]$.

- Fluid replacement with isotonic IV solutions.
- DDAVP 0.3 mcg/kg IV as a slow push is useful as replacement therapy. Postoperatively, DDAVP can be administered intranasally.
- If the patient is on an intranasal dose of DDAVP, 1/10 of the nasal dose may be given IV.
- Serum electrolytes should be checked frequently to ensure that the decrease in plasma sodium is no faster than 1–2 mEq/L/h.

Hypotonic solutions are rarely needed. However, if the patient is actively seizing or is having severe neurologic symptoms, hypotonic solutions can be used cautiously. Overly aggressive correction may result in acute brain swelling.

Key Points

- Central DI results in the underproduction of ADH by the posterior pituitary.
- Diagnosis is made in the presence of polyuria with urine sodium <10–15 mEq/L, urine osmolality <400 mOsm/kg, and serum sodium >150 mEq/L.
- Symptoms are related to hypernatremia (changes in mental status, coma, and seizures) and hypovolemia (low blood pressure, tachycardia, and organ underperfusion).
- Treatment involves correction of hypovolemia (with isotonic IV solutions) and correction of hypernatremia (with DDAVP).
- Frequent electrolyte monitoring is recommended to avoid a too rapid correction of hypernatremia.

Suggested Reading

Barash, PF, Cullen BF, Stoelting RK. Clinical anesthesia. 5th ed. Philadelphia: Lippincott Williams & Wilkins; 2006. p. 760–3, 1149–50.

Cote CJ, Lerman J, Todres ID. A practice of anesthesia for infants and children. 4th ed. Philadelphia: Saunders Elsevier; 2008.

Jaffe RA, Samuels SI. Anesthesiologist's manual of surgical procedures. 3rd ed. Philadelphia: Lippincott Williams & Wilkins; 2004.

Matta BF, Menon DK, Turner JM. Textbook of neuroanesthesia and critical care. 1st ed. London: Greenwich Medical Media; 2000.

Steward DJ, Lerman J. Manual of pediatric anesthesia. 5th ed. Philadelphia: Churchill Livingstone; 2001. p. 29–30, 207.

Chapter 54
Challenges During Surgery for Vascular Anomalies in Pediatrics

Edward R. Smith, Craig D. McClain, and Sulpicio G. Soriano

Overview

Cerebrovascular disease (CVD) is rare in pediatric patients and commonly manifests its presence as hemorrhagic or ischemic stroke. Underlying vascular anomalies that can result in stroke can be categorized as follows:

1. Structural changes in preexisting blood vessels (aneurysms or arterial dissections)
2. Pathologic vascular structures [arteriovenous malformations (AVMs), vein of Galen malformations (VOGMs), arteriovenous fistulas (AVFs), and cavernous malformations (CMs)]
3. Progressive arteriopathies (moyamoya syndrome or heritable arteriopathies)

Prevention

The perioperative management of pediatric patients with vascular anomalies should focus on optimizing cerebral perfusion. Operative management is commonly associated with massive blood loss and these patients require several IV access sites and invasive hemodynamic monitoring. Hemodynamic stability during intracranial surgery requires careful maintenance of intravascular volume. Massive blood loss should be anticipated and treated with blood replacement therapy. Hypotension can transiently be treated with

E.R. Smith, MD
Department of Neurosurgery, Children's Hospital Boston, Harvard Medical School,
Boston, MA, USA

C.D. McClain, MD, MPH (✉) • S.G. Soriano, MD, FAAP
Department of Anesthesiology, Perioperative and Pain Medicine,
Children's Hospital Boston, Boston, MA, USA
e-mail: Craig.McClain@childrens.harvard.edu

A.M. Brambrink and J.R. Kirsch (eds.), *Essentials of Neurosurgical Anesthesia & Critical Care*, DOI 10.1007/978-0-387-09562-2_54,
© Springer Science+Business Media, LLC 2012

Table 54.1 Vascular anomalies in children

Aneurysms	Prevent hypertension preclip with vasodilators (labetalol and nitroprusside)
	Anticipate temporary clipping events with planned hypertension after clip
AVM/VOGM	Preoperative staggered embolization (interventional radiology)
	Postresection hypertension may result in hyperemic cerebral edema (consider antihypertensives)
Moyamoya	Maintain normocapnia and normovolemia

vasopressor infusion (e.g., dopamine, epinephrine, norepinephrine) during fluid resuscitation. Ischemia can result from blood loss or inadvertent occlusion of parent arteries by the surgeon. In both cases, avoidance of hypotension is critical to maintain collateral perfusion to compromised neural tissue. Table 54.1 lists management techniques for specific lesions.

Crisis Management

Pathophysiology and Clinical Presentation

Aneurysms

The pathogenesis of pediatric aneurysms includes trauma, infection, and predisposing genetic disorders. These manifest clinically as a subarachnoid hemorrhage (SAH), rapidly increasing intracranial pressure (ICP), and/or direct mass effect.

Postoperative complications

- Hydrocephalus – can result from subarachnoid blood; treat initially with external drain to lower CSF volume and monitor ICP. Approximately one-third of all SAH patients will ultimately require ventricular shunt.
- Vasospasm – Extremely rare in children, but has been reported. Occurs usually posthemorrhage day 4–14. Can be identified with transcranial Doppler (TCD) and angiography. Need to treat to prevent stroke. Treatment includes nimodipine, "triple-H" therapy (hydration, hemodilution, and hypertension), and angioplasty/intra-arterial vasodilators (suggestions are extrapolated from evidence in the adult; however, no clinical studies have proven these treatment options effective in children).
- Hyponatremia – can result from cerebral salt wasting (hypovolemic hyponatremia – treated with replacement) or SIADH (hypervolemic hyponatremia – treated with water restriction); accurate differential diagnosis based on laboratory results is of high importance to avoid further deterioration, particularly in the context of cerebral vasospasm.
- Rehemorrhage or stroke – can occur from faulty clip placement (very rare). Treat with evacuation of clot (if needed) and/or repositioning of clip.

AVM

AVMs consist of direct arterial-to-venous connections without intervening capillaries. They can occur in the cerebral hemispheres, brainstem, and spinal cord. Functional neural tissue does not reside within the lesion. Pathologically 80–85% of all pediatric AVMs present with hemorrhage. Clinically AVMs may present as seizures, headache, or focal neurologic deficits. Hemorrhagic AVMs have been associated with a 25% mortality rate. Rebleeding rates are approximately 6% for the first 6 months, then 3% per year afterwards. This lesion produces neurological deficits through mass effect or from cerebral ischemia that is due to diversion of blood to the AVM from the normal cerebral circulation ("steal").

Perioperative complications

- Hydrocephalus (see above).
- Rehemorrhage or stroke – can occur from faulty clip placement or residual AVM. Evaluate for residual lesion with vascular imaging if possible. Treat as above.
- Normal perfusion pressure breakthrough (NPPB) – a small number of patients with high-flow AVMs will experience postoperative parenchyma hemorrhage and cerebral edema resulting from markedly increased blood flow in cerebral vessels after in-toto embolization or surgical resection of the AVM. This NPPB phenomenon should be anticipated after treatment of high-flow lesions and can sometimes be avoided through staged embolization prior to surgical resection and maintenance of normal to slightly low blood pressure postoperatively.

Arteriovenous Fistulas/Vein of Galen Malformations

AVFs and VOGMs are direct connections between cerebral arteries and existing veins. Unlike AVMs, they do not usually have a nidus, and in some cases of AVFs, may exist as a single pathologic connection between an artery and vein. In VOGMs, single or multiple small arterial vessels directly drain into the vein of Galen. The result of this type of direct connection is markedly increased cerebral venous pressure; leading to an increased ICP and potential hemorrhage or even venous stroke. In some VOGMs, the connections have such rapid flow rates that children develop high-output cardiac failure. Carotid-cavernous fistulas (CCFs), a subtype of AVF, manifest as a pathologic connection between the carotid artery and cavernous sinus. They can result from trauma, infection, or iatrogenically. Patients present with proptosis, chemosis, pain, and visual problems (loss of acuity and ophthalmoplegia). In general, AVFs are either congenital or they are acquired: they may occur after trauma or in settings of venous stasis as is seen in transverse sinus thrombosis after severe mastoiditis; presumably by the connection of dural arteries in the wall of the sinus into the partially recanalized lumen of the dural sinus.

Perioperative complications: same as AVM. Additionally, patients with large VOGMs may have concomitant high output heart failure. This may require the use of inotropic cardiac support. Pharmacologic support may be weaned as tolerated immediately following embolization.

Moyamoya

Moyamoya is an arteriopathy characterized by chronic progressive stenosis to occlusion at the apices of the intracranial internal carotid arteries including the proximal anterior cerebral arteries and middle cerebral arteries resulting in ischemic stroke. Moyamoya *disease* is the idiopathic form of moyamoya, while moyamoya *syndrome* is defined as the arteriopathy found in association with another condition, such as prior radiotherapy to the head or neck for optic gliomas, craniopharyngiomas, and pituitary tumors; genetic disorders such as Down syndrome, neurofibromatosis type I (NF1) (with or without hypothalamic-optic pathway tumors), large facial hemangiomas, sickle cell anemia, and other hemoglobinopathies; autoimmune disorders such as Graves' disease, congenital cardiac disease or renal artery stenosis.

Perioperative complications

• Stroke and transient ischemic attacks (TIAs)

Patient Assessment

Many patients with intracranial vascular anomalies will have no antecedent history or findings on exam. However, clinicians should be attentive to specific "red flags" in the history or exam that may herald an emergency related to CVD (Table 54.2).

Review of Systems

Look for

• Headaches, seizures, focal neurological deficits (weakness, numbness, visual field problems), or cognitive.
• Previous TIAs or strokes.
• Systemic illnesses such as lupus erythematosus (SLE), congenital cardiac disease, or high-output cardiac failure and illicit drug use, such as cocaine.

Examination

• Typical patient may not have any obvious findings on general physical exam.
• Focal weakness or numbness in a cortical distribution, visual field deficits.
• Presence of a systolic bruit over the eye, head, or neck; present in 15–40% of patients with AVMs or carotid dissections.
• Intracranial arteriovenous shunts may be associated with tachycardia, cardiomegaly, and cardiac failure; especially in infants, consider VOGM.

Table 54.2 "Red flags" on examination or history

Bradycardia, hypertension, decreased respirations (Cushing response)
Dilated pupil, hemiparesis (Uncal herniation)
Fixed downward gaze (Parinaud's syndrome)
Lethargy, tense open anterior fontanel in infants
Ataxia with nausea and vomiting
Sudden onset of a third nerve palsy, including involvement of the pupil: would appear dilated
Sudden onset of severe headache

Radiographic Evaluation

- *Intracranial ultrasonography. Indications:* Infants with open fontanel as initial, nonurgent screening test; can detect hemorrhage, hydrocephalus, large infarcts, or lesions (AVM, VOGM).
- *Duplex ultrasonography* may be useful in children of any age if the diagnosis of an extracranial carotid dissection is being considered.
- *Computerized tomography (CT)/computerized tomography angiography (CTA). Indications:* CT is often the initial study for hemorrhage, delayed stroke, or larger vascular lesions. CTA is excellent for emergent evaluation of AVM, aneurysm: may help with identifying a dissection.
- *Magnetic resonance imaging (MRI) and magnetic resonance angiography (MRA). Indications:* Evaluation of urgent stroke with diffusion-weighted images – DWI, CMs (susceptibility imaging), and nearly all vascular lesions. Consider obtaining frameless stereotaxic sequences if desired in surgery.
- *Digital subtraction catheter angiography (DSA). Indications:* Gold standard for all vascular lesions *except* CMs.

Intervention/Treatment

The surgical treatment for aneurysms, AVMs, and AVF aims toward eliminating the malformation from the cerebral circulation in order to prevent intracranial hemorrhage. This requires clipping or coiling (aneurysm) or embolization and/or resection (AVM/AVF). Alternatively, AVM/AVFs are treated by Gamma-Knife over several months if the location precludes an operative approach.

Aneurysms

- *Diagnosis (CT/CTA)*: angiogram after patient stabilized. Lumbar puncture should be considered only if question of diagnosis from history with negative CT: remember to use small bore needle and limit CSF removal; xanthochromia useful in positive diagnosis for SAH.

- Blood pressure control (labetalol, nicardipine, or nipride) – (nimodipine to prevent vasospasm is controversial in children).
- ICP control – external ventricular drain (EVD) if hydrocephalus (avoid overdrainage of CSF to prevent rerupture; often no more than 5 ml at a time). Elevate the head of the bed.
- Consider antiepileptic medication (phenytoin, levetiracetam).

AVM/VOGM

- Most VOGMs and AVFs are treated endovascularly. Postocclusion hypertension and cerebral hyperemia should be treated aggressively with antihypertensives, e.g., vasodilators. Most high-flow lesions can be treated with staged embolization, reducing the risk of this complication.
- Hydrocephalus – High venous pressures from the fistula can impair CSF drainage, resulting in hydrocephalus. This hydrocephalus usually resolves following treatment of the lesion and often will not require shunting. There is a risk of hemorrhage from passing a ventricular catheter through a swollen brain with high venous pressures. As such, temporizing measures (such as head elevation and medical management) are useful while treating the primary cause of the problem – the fistula.

Moyamoya

The surgical treatment in patients with symptomatic Moyamoya disease or syndrome aims at improving cerebral perfusion distal to the lesions in order to prevent cerebral infarction. This requires the creation of one or more cerebrovascular bypass.

Preoperative

- As discussed in the preoperative section, careful management of moyamoya patients before they arrive in the OR can have a significant influence on complication avoidance; patients ideally should be neurologically stable prior to surgery, and at least 1 month should have passed after the last significant ischemic stroke. Patients must be medically optimized for surgery, including intravenous prehydration the night prior to surgery. Preoperative imaging is critical to planning vessel selection (the parietal branch of the superficial temporal artery (STA) may be small or absent, necessitating utilization of a frontal or retroauricular branch for the bypass). Preservation of spontaneous collateral vessels (as identified by the preoperative angiogram) from the external carotid system should be maintained during the craniotomy.

Intraoperative

- Avoid hyperventilation and hypotension at all times. Tight control of blood pressure and ventilatory parameters is crucial. The goal should be normotension and normocapnia based on preoperative values.

- Meticulous hemostasis.
- EEG is employed during surgery to identify focal slowing, indicative of compromised cerebral blood flow, so that immediate compensatory measures can be instituted by the operative team. EEG technicians must communicate changes in the EEG to allow the team to respond immediately, with appropriate changes in blood pressure, pCO2 and anesthetic agents.

Postoperative

- Continued IV fluids at 1.5× maintenance for 48–72 h until taking oral liquids.
- Frequent and detailed neurologic examinations to identify ischemia early.
- Aggressive pain control to minimize BP fluctuations and hyperventilation.

Key Points

- Intracranial vascular anomalies may be clinically silent prior to a catastrophic presentation – clinicians should be attuned to "red flags" on evaluation (Table 54.2).
- Preoperative imaging is critical to proper diagnosis, operative planning, and safe treatment.
- Key aspects of anesthetic management center on reliable IV access, careful hemodynamic monitoring, and anticipation of blood loss. The primary goal of perioperative management is maintenance of cerebral perfusion pressure.

Suggested Reading

Awad IA, Robinson Jr JR, et al. Neurosurgery. 1993;33(2):179–88. discussion 188.
Friedlander RM. N Engl J Med. 2007;356(26):2704–12.
Millar C, Bissonnette B, et al. Can J Anesth. 1994;41(4):321–31.
Sato K, Shirane R, et al. J Neurosurg Anesthesiol. 1999;11(1):25–30.
Smith ER, Scott RM. Skull Base Surg. 2005;15(1):15–26.
Soriano SG, Sethna NF, Scott RM. Anesth Analg. 1993;77(5):1066–70.

Chapter 55
Challenges During Epilepsy Surgery in Pediatric Patients

Abraham Rosenbaum and Zeev N. Kain

Overview

At least 1.5 million people in the USA have epilepsy – 0.5–1% of the population. Most often epilepsy presents during the first decade of life, with up to 50% of the cases occurring before the age of 5 years. Of these, 60% have focal epilepsy, and approximately 20% become drug resistant or refractory. Early onset of intractable seizures, particularly in children less than 3 years old, has a very poor prognosis. Epilepsy is considered refractory if seizures continue after 2 years of pharmacological treatment with 2–3 appropriately selected drugs with good patient compliance. Typically, the frequency or severity of seizures in this situation prevents normal function and/or development. Moreover, patients with refractory epilepsy commonly suffer from the side effects and complications of high-dose anti-epileptic drugs. Indeed, even in the therapeutic range, antiepileptic medications can significantly influence the developing brain. In addition to the risk of cognitive dysfunction, physical issues are also associated with medically intractable seizures. These patients have higher rates of accidental death or sudden death, ranging from 2 to 18%, as compared to cause of death in all people with epilepsy. Only half of the patients with medically intractable seizures or refractory epilepsy are able to become self-supporting on reaching adulthood. Therefore, early surgical intervention increases the chances of significantly reducing or eliminating seizures, improving quality of life, reducing the risk of cognitive, behavioral and motor developmental damage and decreasing the risk for permanent brain injury in infants and young children. Common causes of pediatric refractory epilepsy that are amenable to surgery include tumors, cortical malformations, vascular abnormalities, and certain epileptic syndromes. Consequently, approximately one-third of children with

A. Rosenbaum, MD (✉) • Z.N. Kain, MD
Department of Anesthesiology and Perioperative Care, University of California,
Irvine Medical Center, Orange, CA, USA
e-mail: arosenba@uci.edu

A.M. Brambrink and J.R. Kirsch (eds.), *Essentials of Neurosurgical Anesthesia & Critical Care*, DOI 10.1007/978-0-387-09562-2_55,
© Springer Science+Business Media, LLC 2012

refractory epilepsy are candidates for surgery. Of those, children with refractory *unifocal* epilepsy are the best candidates for surgical interventions.

Although freedom from seizures is important in defining surgical success in the pediatric population, preventing cognitive and developmental decline or stagnation may be an equally, if not more, important measure.

Implications for the Neurosurgical Patient

Surgical therapy for medically intractable epilepsy has traditionally been viewed as an extreme measure, reserved as a last resort when the disease becomes a life-threatening condition or a progressive neurologic disorder. However, recent publications have shown a favorable outcome following surgery in young children with catastrophic epilepsy. For these patients, *when* to have the surgery is a critical factor in the decision to have the surgery. Some argue that the young brain demonstrates high neuroplasticity, allowing for better behavioral and cognitive development following trauma or surgery, and, thus, surgery is appropriate for this age group.

In order to determine who will benefit most from surgery, four questions need to be answered: (1) Are the seizures truly epileptic? (2) Is there a focal origin? (3) Are there more than one foci? (4) Is this an excisable lesion? General contraindications such as acute psychiatric disorder, neurodegenerative disorder, and medical contraindication need to be established as well. The initial epilepsy evaluations should include characterization of the seizures and optimizations of the medical therapy. A detailed history should include previous central nervous system infection, trauma, family history, range of previous drugs used and patient compliance. Neuropsychological assessment is necessary to lateralize brain dominance and speech and memory areas for future follow-up. Further evaluation should include localization of the seizure focus zone. During the last decade, multiple diagnostic modalities, such as multichannel EEG and video monitoring, high resolution magnetic resonance imagining (MRI), proton emission tomography (PET), and single proton emission computed tomography (SPECT), have been developed to allow for noninvasive evaluation of patients. Certain invasive techniques, including depth and surface electrodes, have also been shown to be safe and, indeed, more efficacious under certain circumstances.

Radiological evaluation is classically defined as structural and functional; for example, MRI supplemented by CT or cerebral angiography can detect structural pathologies. On the other hand, functional MRI (fMRI) can elucidate active areas of the functioning cortex during simple tasks. PET can show focal inter-ictal reduction in metabolism, and SPECT can show focal increase in blood flow. Scalp EEG can exclude the possibility of a focal locus by demonstrating multifocal seizure activity. In cases where there is inconclusive data from noninvasive techniques, invasive extradural/subdural or parenchymal electrodes placed surgically can be used both for electro-corticography and cortical stimulation during the operation. Other diagnostic techniques worth mentioning are experimental Magneto-encephalography,

Fig. 55.1 Summary of the most common surgical interventions for intractable seizure disorder (partially adopted from Elger CE, Schmidt D. Modern management of epilepsy: A practical approach. Epilepsy Behav. 2008;12: 501–39)

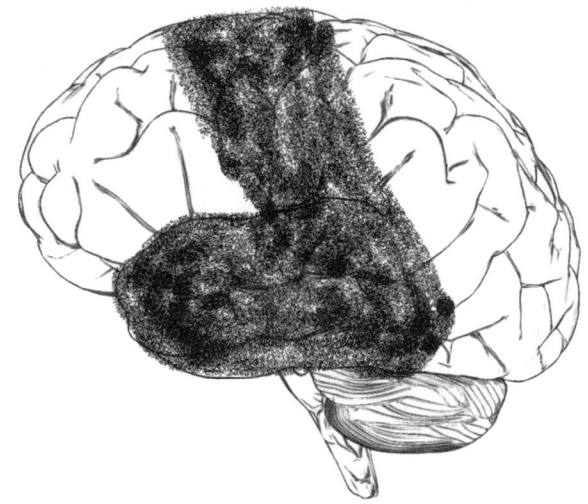

which records the electronic field of epileptic locus, and the WADA test, in which half of the brain is "anesthetized" by injecting amobarbital through one of the internal carotid arteries. While the brain is partially anesthetized, speech and memory are tested to verify that these critical cognitive functions will be maintained after surgery.

Surgical Techniques (Fig. 55.1)

Surgical techniques can be classified into removal of the epileptic lesion, isolation of the focus, and functional operations (neurostimulation). Hemispherectomy is the most invasive form of surgery, while vagus nerve stimulation (VNS) is the least invasive.

Temporal Lobectomy

Temporal lobe epilepsy is not the most common etiology of childhood seizures. Nonetheless, this syndrome is usually focal and easily accessible and so has become the most common surgically treated type of epilepsy. Indeed, 56% of all of pediatric epilepsy surgeries are temporal lobe resections. Temporal lobe surgery has been modified over the last 30 years as our understanding of the etiologies and treatments of epilepsy has progressed. The standard operation for temporal lobe epilepsy is anterior medial temporal resection (*temporal lobectomy*). This surgery involves the removal of a significant portion of the brain. There are, however, two techniques that, although technically challenging, reduce the impact on the cortex (i.e., nonselective amygdalohippocampectomy and selective amygdalohippocampectomy, using the transsylvian route).

Surgeries for extratemporal (topectomy) foci have been less successful compared to other epilepsy surgeries, particularly in the absence of defined structural lesion. Extratemporal epilepsy has a more diffuse epileptogenic zone, as well as invasion of these zones to deeper structures. Therefore, extratemporal surgeries are almost always preceded by invasive monitoring. An awake craniotomy is a common technique many surgeons choose when operating on this type of pathology.

Hemispherectomy/Hemispherotomy

The most invasive and radical surgical technique for intractable epilepsy is *hemispherectomy*. Typically, children with extensive hemispheric damage, such as seen in Sturge–Weber syndrome, are candidates for hemispherectomy. However, this surgical technique has evolved toward a less-invasive approach to avoid fatal long-term complications; *hemispherotomy*, the disconnection of the epileptogenic hemisphere from the subcortical centers and from the other hemisphere, has fewer complications as compared to hemispherectomy. Approximately 80% of children who undergo this surgery become seizure free while another 15% show improvement.

Corpus callosotomy is performed in patients without identifiable epileptogenic foci. The purpose of this type of surgery is to disrupt the propagation of seizure discharge from one hemisphere to the other, although the indication for this surgery might be broadened to many intractable epilepsy situations. However, the high complication rate and the degree of invasiveness reduced its acceptance. Reduction of generalized seizures with this type of surgery ranges from 56 to 100%, and 30% of the patients become seizure free after this operation.

Multiple subpial transections (MSTs) is a surgical technique where a well-identified epileptogenic locus exists in a cortical area that cannot be sacrificed. After identifying the epileptogenic locus, multiple cuts are made in the carefully marked cortex zone. This procedure isolates small cortical sections from each other while still allowing other useful outflow to persist. This technique is very time consuming.

Gamma knife surgery (stereotactic radiosurgery) is a technique that uses a high-energy photon beam directed at a single point in the brain. The tissue in the epileptogenic area becomes necrotic or neurologically altered without harming the surrounding tissue. Generally, there is a lag time of 12–36 months between the treatment and a seizure-free state.

VNS is the least invasive technique for the control of intractable epilepsy. This technique is efficacious as a neurophysiological treatment for patients with refractory epilepsy who are unsuitable for resective and potentially curative surgery. VNS is usually done under general anesthesia although some centers use local anesthesia. The VNS mechanism of action is far from understood although the pathway, via the nucleus of the solitary tract, has been demonstrated. Experience with VNS in children is less extensive as compared to adults; however, two studies have demonstrated a reduction in seizure activity of 60% in 80% of the cases and of 50% in 38% of the children. The patient can be also provided with a magnet, which, by passing the magnet over the generator for 1–2 s, increases stimulation in the case of an aura or a seizure. The magnet can also inhibit stimulation by keeping it over the generator. Currently FDA indication for VNS covers patients 12 years and older, although studies have shown clinical efficacy in younger pediatric patients as well.

Concerns and Risks

Surgical risk must be taken into consideration during preoperative patient counseling, given that, in at least two studies, the overall complication rate was around 3%. Surgical risk can be further divided into transient (infection, hematoma, DVT, hydrocephalus, CSF leakage) and permanent complications (hemiparesis, hemianopia, cranial nerve injury, and dysphasia).

Temporal Lobectomy

This procedure has an infrequent morbidity with 0% mortality. The risk of temporal lobe resection is related to the proximity of the Sylvian vessels as well as to the vessels and optical tract in the ambient cistern. The most common neurological side effect is homonymous superior quadrantanopsia resulting from interruption of the optic tract. Language and verbal deficits occur when these particular areas in the dominant hemisphere are resected, although this is usually transient and often not a problem in children younger than 9 years. Other neurological deficits may occur as a result of Sylvian vessels vasospasm, infection of bone flap, wound infection, transient cranial nerve palsies, postoperative psychosis and postoperative depression. One study found a 5.1% mortality rate, attributable primarily to continuation of seizures after the surgery. Accidents and suicide were also among the causes of mortality.

Hemispherectomy

Blood loss and requirement of blood transfusion are a major concern following this surgery and is most common in patients with malformation of cortical development, Rasmussen's encephalitis and Sturge–Weber syndrome. Consequently, strategies such as autologous blood transfusion and staging of the hemispheric surgery in very young patients may be necessary. Other reported complications include hydrocephalus, recurrent seizures that required re-operation (usually because of incomplete disconnection) and syndrome of inappropriate ADH secretion (SIADH). There is an expected motor impairment and worsening of preoperative hemiplegia. Homonomous hemianopia is another expected complication, as is loss of useful hand function.

Postoperative severe headache and chronic intracranial hypertension have been reported, as well as new onset of migraine. Poor postoperative cognitive and maladaptive functions have a direct relationship with the duration of the seizure activity, possibly by affecting the nonoperated hemisphere. Thus, as suggested by some authors, early surgical intervention should be high priority, and a young age at surgery is an important factor for favorable outcome. Postsurgical linguistic outcome is related to the side of the damage and resection, age at the time of surgery, seizure control, and etiology. Most patients show only moderate change in cognitive performance, with variable changes in intelligence quotient.

Corpus Callosotomy

Reported acute complications were wound infection and CSF leak, hydrocephalus requiring shunt, and chemical meningitis/ventriculitis. Hemispheric edema may occur due to prolonged and vigorous retraction of the hemisphere. Corpus callosotomy is known for *acute postoperative neurological syndrome* that includes mutism, nondominant arm and leg apraxia, bilateral Babinski signs and urinary incontinence. These complications are almost always transient, with mutism usually resolving within several weeks. More long-term complications are corpus callosotomy with forniceal injury, possibly resulting in memory disturbances. Damage to the corona radiata may lead to motor weakness. Injury to the pericallosal arteries of vasospasm from excessive manipulation can result in lower-extremity weakness secondary to ischemia. Permanent side effects of callosotomy are relatively uncommon, with weakness or apraxia and language/behavior impairment occurring 8–12% of the cases. Dysphasia and dysgraphia were observed in patients with mixed or crossed cerebral dominance. Some patients have difficulty learning new bimanual tasks, but previously acquired bimanual tasks remain intact. Most of the persisting deficits following corpus callosotomy involve the incomplete integration of information processing across the hemispheres, often referred as *disconnection syndrome*. These changes are subtle and require neuropsychological testing to be detected. Recognition of this phenomenon led to a two-stage procedure, initiated by partial callosotomy and followed by a period of 6–12 months to evaluate the need for total callosotomy.

Vagus Nerve Stimulator

VNS is a relatively safe, well-tolerated procedure with low rate of complications. The most common side effects were noted during stimulation of the vagus nerve consisting of hoarseness, voice alteration, coughing, discomfort, dyspnea, vomiting and local neck/throat paraesthesias, all of which subside in time. Surgical complications include device failure, left vocal cord paralysis, lower facial muscle paresis, and fluid accumulation around the generator and infection around the device. Erosion of the generator through the chest wall is a rare complication and of more concern in small children with little subcutaneous fat. There is a rare reporting of transient bradycardia and asystole during intraoperative testing of the device. No long-term cardiovascular effects were reported.

Intracranial Electrodes

Complication rate of intracranial electrode placement as part of intractable epilepsy workup and diagnosis is as low as 3%, and these mainly include intracranial hemorrhage, infection (meningitis), status epilepticus, aseptic meningitis, and transient neurological deficit. Age, gender, number of electrodes and number of days with the electrodes does not influence the complication rate.

Key Points

- Up to one-third of children with epilepsy are refractory to medical therapy.
- Far beyond mere seizure control, enhancing development and cognitive potential, treating psychological and behavior problems and avoidance/reduction of brain damage are goals for treatment in children with intractable seizure disorders.
- Additional complicating factors must be considered, such as the cause of epilepsy, the effect of drugs on the developing brain and brain plasticity, when determining the course of treatment.
- Epilepsy surgery is now widely accepted and has a high success rate.
- Temporal lobectomy is the most common epilepsy procedure in children, followed by extratemporal lesion resection, callosotomy, multiple lobar transections, hemispherectomy/hemispherotomy, and MSTs.
- Complication rate of epilepsy surgery is low and can be divided into transient (infection, hematoma, DVT, hydrocephalus, CSF leakage), and permanent complications (hemiparesis, hemianopia, cranial nerve injury, and dysphasia).
- Vagus nerve stimulator has been proven to be an efficient, noninvasive modality of seizure suppression and control, both in adults and children.

Suggested Reading

Albright AL, Pollack IF, Adelson PD. Principles and practice of pediatric neurosurgery. New York: Thieme; 2008. p. 1056–68, 1078–86, 1115–8.
Basheer SN et al. Hemispheric surgery in children with refractory epilepsy: seizure outcome, complications, and adaptive function. Epilepsia. 2007;1:133–40.

Boon P et al. Vagus nerve stimulation for refractory epilepsy. Seizure. 2001;10:448–55.

Gonzalez-Martinez JA et al. Hemispherectomy for catastrophic epilepsy in infants. Epilepsia. 2005;9:1518–25.

Jea A et al. Corpus callosotomy in children with intractable epilepsy using frameless stereotactic neuronavigation: 12-year experience at the Hospital for Sick Children in Totronto. Neurosurg Focus. 2008;3:E7.

Kemeny AA. Surgery for epilepsy. Seizure. 2001;10:461–5.

Chapter 56
Challenges During Pediatric Endoscopic Neurosurgery

Nina Deutsch

Overview

Endoscopic neurosurgery has become an important modality in the treatment of several pediatric neurologic conditions. With improvements in imaging, fiberoptic technology, and equipment, minimally invasive techniques have allowed for safe visualization and manipulation of areas that were previously difficult to access through conventional neurosurgical procedures. Table 56.1 summarizes some of the more common pediatric conditions treated with endoscopic neurosurgery and the preferred noninvasive interventions.

For the procedure, the endoscope is introduced through a burr hole and placed through the frontal cortex into the ventricle. To visualize the structures, the surgeon uses continuous irrigation with warmed saline or lactated Ringers solution through the scope, with drainage of cerebrospinal fluid through the scope or burr hole. Significant complications occur very rarely, with varying incidence depending on the procedure performed and the patient's condition and anatomy.

Endoscopic neurosurgery has been shown to improve patient safety and allow for shorter hospital stays with virtually no mortality (0–1%) when compared to conventional open procedures. The incidence of intraoperative and postoperative complications varies widely from 5 to 30%, based on published patient series from several centers. In noncommunicating hydrocephalus, endoscopic third ventriculostomy has become the standard surgical treatment (success rate of 60–90%) and has allowed patients to live without indwelling shunts in the majority of cases, thereby, reducing overall morbidity (endoscopic surgical risk of 5%) in this patient population. The more commonly associated complications of endoscopic neurosurgery are summarized in Table 56.2.

N. Deutsch, MD (✉)
Department of Anesthesiology and Pain Medicine, Children's National Medical Center, Washington, DC, USA

A.M. Brambrink and J.R. Kirsch (eds.), *Essentials of Neurosurgical Anesthesia & Critical Care*, DOI 10.1007/978-0-387-09562-2_56,
© Springer Science+Business Media, LLC 2012

Table 56.1 Pediatric indications for endoscopic neurosurgery

Diagnosis	Intervention
• Hydrocephalus	• Third ventriculostomy for aqueductal stenosis, for fourth ventricular outlet obstruction, for septostomy
• Arachnoid cysts	• Fenestration
• Colloid cysts	• Endoscopic removal
• Periventricular tumor	• Biopsy
• Pituitary tumor	• Endoscopic transnasal hypophysectomy
• Cranial synostosis	• Endoscopic strip craniectomy
• Hematoma or brain abscess	• Endoscopic drainage

Table 56.2 Complications of endoscopic neurosurgery

Complications
- Cardiovascular
  - Arrhythmia
  - Hypertension
- Neurologic
  - Increased intracranial pressure
  - Delayed emergence
  - Nerve palsy
  - Venous/arterial hemorrhage
  - CSF leakage
- Diabetes insipidus or SIADH
- Disturbances in temperature regulation
- Electrolyte disturbances

Prevention

The likelihood of successful outcomes increases greatly with appropriate patient selection (anatomy conducive to the procedure) combined with a neurosurgeon experienced with these techniques. By tailoring the anesthetic to the anticipated procedure, the anesthesiologist can also help to decrease the probability of complications. The following points need to be considered.

Anesthetic Technique

- Despite the less-invasive aspect of endoscopic neurosurgery, anesthetic considerations do not differ greatly from conventional neurosurgical procedures.
- Preoperatively, patients may present with symptoms of increased intracranial pressure (ICP) such as vomiting, headache, confusion, or altered mental status. A full neurologic exam should be documented. Preoperative anxiolytics may need to be used sparingly, if at all, due to both the preoperative neurologic status, as well as the desire to prevent delayed emergence after the procedure.

- Intraoperatively, general anesthesia is the preferred method to ensure immobility throughout the procedure. Arrhythmias or hemodynamic instability can occur without warning, necessitating constant vigilance on the part of the anesthesiologist who should intervene when appropriate and modulate systemic hemodynamics to allow for optimal surgical conditions. ICP can also rise during the procedure, often necessitating treatment, including hyperventilation and blood pressure management to maintain cerebral perfusion pressure. Drainage of CSF may also be performed by the surgeons. Nitrous oxide should be avoided as it can cause expansion of ventricular air bubbles that are introduced by the endoscope. Use of shorter-acting opioids will allow for rapid emergence and early neurologic examination.
- Postoperatively, continued neurologic examination and monitoring of serum electrolytes is important for early detection of postoperative bleeding, increased ICP, diabetes insipidus or hypothalamic dysfunction.

Communication

- The importance of communication between the anesthesiologist and the surgical team cannot be underestimated and should be ongoing. Some examples specific to endoscopic procedures are as follows:
  - The incidence of cardiovascular instability is more likely to occur during third ventriculostomy when the surgeon is stimulating the floor of the third ventricle with the tip of the endoscope. Notifying the anesthesiologist of this event helps him/her to prepare for and more quickly treat such an occurrence. Likewise, communication to the surgeon of arrhythmias can allow for him/her to pull back the endoscope, which is often the only treatment necessary.
  - The occurrence of bleeding should always be communicated to allow for blood pressure control and transfusion when appropriate.
  - The need to convert to an open procedure or to abort the current procedure should be part of the ongoing dialogue between teams.

Crisis Management

Cardiovascular Instability

Cardiovascular instability (reported in 28–32% of patients) most often manifests as arrhythmias (bradycardia most commonly) and hypertension. Ventricular irritability and sudden cardiac arrest, though rare, have also been reported. Table 56.3 summarizes the more common cardiovascular findings.

Table 56.3 Cardiovascular instability

Pathophysiology and presentation	Patient assessment	Treatment/intervention
• Arrhythmias secondary to increased pressure in the ventricular system (related to increased irrigation and CSF drainage) and direct stimulation of the floor of the third ventricle with the endoscope • Most commonly seen bradycardia • Hypertension secondary to increased ICP	• Is there evidence of raised ICP? • Is it associated with painful stimuli? • Is there adequate analgesia? • What are the pulse, rhythm, and BP? • Is there hypoxia?	• Have surgeon pull the scope away from floor of third ventricle • Check that there is appropriate drainage of fluid through the endoscope • May need pharmacologic treatment (atropine for unresolving bradycardia, antihypertensives, or analgesics) • Treat ICP

Venous/Arterial Hemorrhage

Several neurologic complications can develop during and after endoscopic neurosurgery, including increased ICP, delayed emergence, nerve palsy, and CSF leakage. Part of the management of these patients is to be aware of these complications and tailor the anesthetic to allow for rapid emergence and full neurologic examination as soon as possible. One of the most severe complications, however, is the development of hemorrhage, which is summarized in Table 56.4.

Diabetes Insipidus or SIADH

Diabetes insipidus (DI) or syndrome of inappropriate secretion of ADH (SIADH) can develop either intraoperatively or postoperatively. Each is thought to be due to hypothalamic dysfunction from injury caused by the endoscope or higher pressures generated by the irrigation fluid. Diabetes insipidus is typically self-limited. The presentation, patient assessment, and treatment of each are summarized in Table 56.5.

Electrolyte Disturbances

Postoperative electrolyte imbalances often occur in patients undergoing endoscopic neurosurgery. While disturbances in sodium can be attributed to DI or SIADH with hypothalamic injury, one often sees hyperkalemia in the postoperative period. Table 56.6 summarizes the findings with electrolyte disturbances.

Table 56.4 Venous/arterial hemorrhage

Pathophysiology and presentation	Patient assessment	Treatment/intervention
• Basilar artery disruption is most significant but rare • Venous bleeding from disruption of subependymal vessels or the choroid plexus by the endoscope • Hemorrhage at the insertion site or the burr hole • Bleeding can prevent further visualization through the scope and surgeon may need to abandon endoscopic procedure and convert to open procedure	• Is bleeding visualized in the scope's field of vision? • What are the pulse, rhythm and BP (signs of increased ICP)? • Is there delayed emergence? • Is there a progressive change in the neurologic exam postoperatively?	• Supportive care in arterial bleeding including transfusion and control of BP • Continuous irrigation of venous bleeding by surgeon can be enough to stop it • Be prepared to rapidly convert to open procedure for uncontrolled bleeds • Treat ICP • Postoperative EVD may be necessary

Table 56.5 Diabetes insipidus and SIADH

Pathophysiology and presentation	Patient assessment	Treatment/intervention

• Diabetes insipidus:
  – Increased dilute urine output developing either during or after the procedure associated with hypernatremia
  – Can lead to dehydration and hypotension if not recognized and treated
• SIADH:
  – See hyponatremia, concentrated urine and water retention w/o hypertension
  – Can develop postoperative headache, nausea, vomiting, confusion, or seizures
	• What are the serum electrolytes?
	• What is the concentration of the urine?
	• What are the pulse and BP?
	• Is there delayed emergence?
	• Is there a progressive change in the neurologic exam?
		• Diabetes insipidus:
		  – Continued hydration with balanced electrolyte solution and continued monitoring of electrolytes
		  – Often self-limited; may need short course of desmopressin
		• SIADH:
		  – Follow serum sodium levels; replace as needed; fluid restriction
		  – Monitor for seizures

Table 56.6 Electrolyte disturbances

Pathophysiology and presentation	Patient assessment	Treatment/intervention
• Hyperkalemia appears to increase with use of lactated Ringer's solution for irrigation of surgical field • Normal saline irrigation produces a relative hypokalemia, though not usually clinically significant • Disturbances in sodium discussed above	• What are the pulse and rhythm? • What are the postoperative serum electrolytes? • Is there delayed emergence? • Is there a progressive change in the neurologic exam?	• Close monitoring of serum electrolytes • Treat potassium if cardiac rhythm disturbances appear • Lactated Ringer's irrigation closer physiologically to CSF but can increase potassium levels • Normal saline may have less effect on potassium

Table 56.7 Delayed emergence

Pathophysiology and presentation	Patient assessment	Treatment/intervention
• Residual anesthetic, including inhalational agents, opioids, paralytic agent, or premedication • Neurologic causes, including intraventricular bleed, edema, increased ICP, structural damage to the brain, ischemia • Electrolyte abnormalities • Hypoglycemia • Hypoxia • Hypotension/arrhythmia • Can see focal deficits or generalized obtundation	• What are the SpO2 and EtCO2? • What are the pulse, rhythm, and BP? • What are the serum electrolytes/glucose? • Were there signs of bleeding during the procedure or high irrigation pressures? • Is there a focal neurologic deficit on the exam or signs of high ICP? • Have paralytics been reversed? Is there residual inhalation agent present? Could this be residual opioid or premed?	• Close monitoring of vital signs and treatment of hypotension, hypertension, hypoxia • Correct electrolyte abnormalities and glucose • Reversal of all anesthetic agents • Imaging studies to evaluate neurologic causes (bleeding, ischemia) • ICP monitoring?

Delayed Emergence

Delayed emergence can be related to the surgical procedure or the anesthetic management of the patient and warrants immediate investigation into the cause to allow for immediate management. Table 56.7 summarizes the salient features of delayed emergence.

Key Points

- Endoscopic neurosurgery allows for less-invasive and safe treatment of several neurologic conditions in the pediatric population.
- Complete preoperative assessment, including full history, physical, neurologic exam, and laboratory evaluation should be well documented and help guide the anesthetic management of the patient.
- Good communication with the surgeon and constant vigilance on the part of the anesthesiologist are invaluable to help ensure the safety of the patient.
- Know what the most common complications of endoscopic neurosurgery are and how to treat them.
- Always be prepared to convert to an open procedure in case of emergency.
- Continued evaluation of the patient in the postoperative period can help to prevent catastrophic complications from going unnoticed.

Suggested Reading

Baykan N, Isbir O, Gercek A, et al. Ten years experience with pediatric neuroendoscopic third ventriculostomy. J Neurosurg Anesthesiol. 2005;17:33–7.

El-Dawlatly AA. Endoscopic third ventriculostomy: anesthetic implications. Minim Invasive Neurosurg. 2004;47:151–3.

El-Dawlatly AA, Elgamal E, Murshid W, et al. Anesthesia for third ventriculostomy. A report of 128 cases. Middle East J Anesthesiol. 2008;19:847–57.

Johnson JO. Anesthesia for minimally invasive neurosurgery. Anesthesiol Clin North America. 2002;20:361–75.

Schubert A, Deogaonkar A, Lotto M, et al. Anesthesia for minimally invasive cranial and spinal surgery. J Neurosurg Anesthesiol. 2006;18:47–56.

Part X
Postoperative Concerns in Neuroanesthesia for Children and Infants

Chapter 57
Emergence from Anesthesia Following Pediatric Neurosurgery

Kirk Lalwani

Overview

Emergence from general anesthesia and tracheal extubation may be associated with tremendous physiologic and metabolic stress in patients. These stress-induced alterations in physiologic parameters may be harmful to patients as they can exacerbate preexisting disease or produce medical or surgical complications in the recovery period. It is important therefore, to implement measures that minimize these stress-induced changes during emergence from anesthesia, particularly in patients at higher risk or after procedures where complications may result in significant morbidity or even mortality.

Implications for the Neurosurgical Patient

Pediatric Considerations

Neonatal blood pressure range for cerebral autoregulation has been estimated to be similar to that in adults, with no age-related differences in autoregulatory capacity. The steep slopes at either end of this range predispose the neonate to cerebral ischemia or intraventricular hemorrhage in the event of hypotension or hypertension, respectively. Intracranial compliance in infants is generally higher in the presence of gradually increasing ICP as a result of open fontanelles and cranial sutures. Children, on the other hand, have decreased intracranial compliance compared to adults as a result of higher brain water content, less CSF volume, and a higher ratio of brain content to intracranial capacity. Therefore, children may be at higher risk

K. Lalwani, MD, FRCA, MCR (✉)
Department of Anesthesiology and Perioperative Medicine,
Oregon Health & Science University, Portland, OR, USA

A.M. Brambrink and J.R. Kirsch (eds.), *Essentials of Neurosurgical Anesthesia & Critical Care*, DOI 10.1007/978-0-387-09562-2_57,
© Springer Science+Business Media, LLC 2012

for ischemia and herniation in the event of similar relative increases in ICP when compared to adults as a result of lower intracranial compliance. Much of the work on emergence from anesthesia following craniotomy has not been performed in children; therefore, studies on adults will also be discussed in this chapter in the interest of understanding concepts and applying techniques that in all probability fulfill the same goals in both children and adults.

Metabolic Changes

Recovery from general anesthesia is associated with sympathetic stimulation, increased catecholamine secretion, increased oxygen consumption (VO_2), tachycardia, and systemic hypertension, which in turn may lead to intracranial hypertension. It has been demonstrated that independent of whether propofol or isoflurane is used, cerebral blood flow velocity increases by 60% above the awake value at extubation and is significant for at least 30 min following extubation. Interestingly, this increase did not correlate with MAP or $PaCO_2$ at any time, likely as a result of central adrenergic stimulation during emergence from anesthesia. Multiple additional sources of stress such as stimulation by the endotracheal tube, coughing, suctioning of the oropharynx or trachea, awareness of surroundings, auditory stimulation, shivering, emergence agitation, and pain related to surgery may greatly magnify the hemodynamic response to emergence (Fig. 57.1).

Early Versus Delayed Emergence

Early Emergence

Patients undergoing neurosurgical procedures that involve intracranial structures are particularly prone to the devastating effects of surgical hemorrhage or brain edema postoperatively, mostly as a result of pressure effects on the brain within the confines of the rigid cranium. Early detection is therefore critical in order to avoid permanent morbidity or death. This is typically accomplished by early and frequent neurological examination following surgery to determine the presence of any neurologic deficits. In high-risk cases, this may be supplemented by early CT imaging of the brain, often prior to, or immediately after emergence from anesthesia and tracheal extubation.

It seems intuitive, therefore, that rapid emergence and early awakening following craniotomy is a prerequisite for early neurological examination. In practice, however, achieving rapid emergence and awakening is often accompanied by profound alterations in physiologic parameters related to the stress of emergence and extubation, unless the anesthetic technique is tailored to specifically prevent these changes. Paradoxically, the techniques that attenuate these hemodynamic changes may

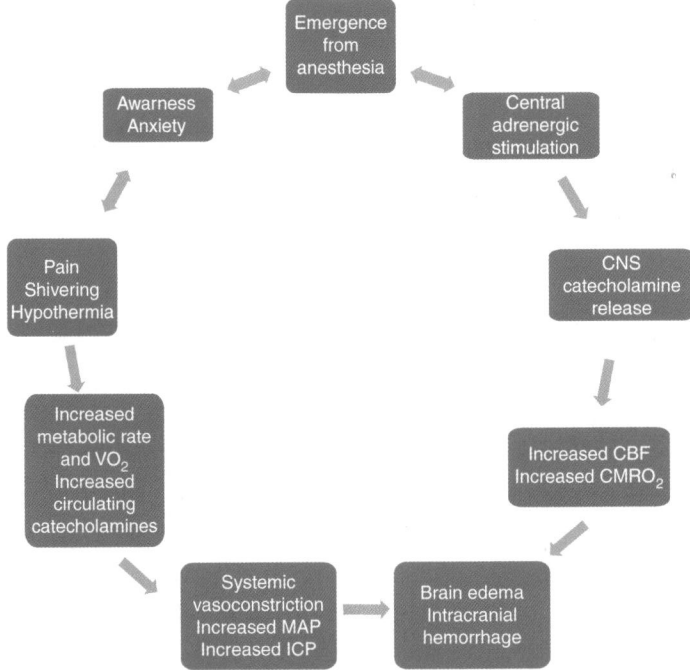

Fig. 57.1 Stress-induced changes during emergence from anesthesia

adversely affect early awakening and return to consciousness. Therefore, careful planning is required to balance the dual requirements of early awakening versus meticulous hemodynamic control following craniotomy.

Delayed Emergence

There exists a subgroup of patients in whom early awakening and emergence entails significant risk, and postoperative ventilation is desirable. These high-risk patients must be identified as early as possible in the perioperative period in order to optimize intraoperative anesthetic care as well as postoperative requirements for imaging, continued ventilation, sedation, correction of acid-base, electrolyte, temperature, and coagulation parameters prior to extubation on the ICU.

It is important to realize that the effect of delayed extubation (2 h of propofol sedation after surgery) exacerbates the production of markers of stress when compared to early (immediate) extubation following surgery, and therefore cannot be recommended for this purpose alone. However, likely candidates for delayed extubation are patients with altered consciousness preoperatively, lengthy surgery (>6 h), large tumor resection with preoperative midline shift, injury to cranial nerves (especially IX, X, XI), complications during surgery, intraoperative brain swelling, hypothermia, coagulopathy, and significant acid-base or electrolyte abnormalities.

To facilitate early diagnosis of intracranial complications in patients for whom delayed extubation is planned, many surgeons routinely request a CT scan en route from the operating room to the ICU, or soon after arrival on the ICU as a substitute for early awakening and neurological examination.

Concerns and Risks

Neurological Complications

In a prospective study of 162 adult patients, the incidence of complications following craniotomy in the first 6 h postoperatively was reported to be as high as 57%, of which 3% were neurological complications such as seizures, neurologic deficits, and delayed awakening. Of the patients who experienced complications, 45% had more than one complication. In a retrospective study of perioperative complications after pediatric craniotomies, von Lehe et al. noted that the incidence of new neurologic deficits was higher in posterior fossa craniotomies when compared to supratentorial (23.6% vs. 6.7%, respectively); the incidence of postoperative bleeding requiring reoperation was 1.7%, and the incidence of other severe systemic complications (sepsis, pneumonia, etc.) was 3.8%.

Intracranial hemorrhage has been linked to intraoperative hypertension; patients with postoperative intracranial hypertension were 3.6 times more likely to be hypertensive than matched controls. There was also a strong association between intracranial hemorrhage and patients who were normotensive during surgery, but hypertensive in the postoperative period, presumably as a result of inadequate hemostasis at a lower range of blood pressures. Intracranial hypertension is common after craniotomy (12–18%), and was associated with clinical deterioration in 52% of adult patients, and CT findings of cerebral edema and cerebral hemorrhage. Intracranial hypertension in premature infants or newborns can result in intraventricular hemorrhage as a result of impaired autoregulatory ability coupled with rapid alterations in cerebral blood flow and pressure. In addition, children may be at increased risk of herniation compared with adults as a result of low intracranial compliance. Neonates and infants, on the other hand, are able to tolerate fluctuations in intracranial pressure and volume better than older children as a result of open fontanelles and sutures.

Shivering

Hypothermia after surgery is more common in infants and children as a result of several factors. Neonates have a skin-surface area to body mass ratio of ~1, whereas in adults this ratio is about 0.4. Neonates also lose heat easily via thermal conduction as a result of a thin layer of subcutaneous fat; in addition, the ambient temperature limit of thermoregulation for neonates is 22°C compared to 0°C in adults. This propensity to lose heat more rapidly coupled with the decreased ability to regulate body temperature requires careful attention during surgery in order to prevent hypothermia. Shivering related to hypothermia or volatile anesthetic agents can increase VO_2 by 200–400% and MAP by approximately 35% or more. Patients who develop mild hypothermia during surgery experience a much greater increase in norepinephrine concentration, more significant vasoconstriction, and increased systemic blood pressure in the early postoperative period compared to normothermic patients. Even in the presence of mild hypothermia, forced air warming decreases the incidence and intensity of shivering. It is useful to remember that though shivering may occur in neonates following emergence from anesthesia, it is unimportant as a method of thermogenesis in this age group, and tends to occur more commonly in children over 6 years of age.

Pain

Pain is a significant stress factor that increases VO_2 and induces catecholamine release in the postoperative period, and the use of intraoperative analgesia attenuates these metabolic changes in the postoperative period. One study demonstrated that the use of morphine analgesia reduced VO_2 in critically ill patients by 20%, but the effect of analgesics on VO_2 in restless patients may be even greater as a result of the additional sedative benefits conferred by opioid analgesics. Peripheral nerve blocks of the scalp are effective in decreasing postoperative pain following craniotomy, and the effect may persist for as long as 48 h after surgery, even if the block is performed at the end of surgery. Scalp nerve blocks may also decrease postoperative opioid consumption and reduce postoperative nausea and vomiting (PONV). Wound infiltration with local anesthetic has also been shown to result in decreased pain scores for up to an hour after arrival in the PACU.

In children, pain must be distinguished from separation anxiety, hunger, disorientation to surroundings, a full bladder, and emergence delirium. Simple comfort measures are often all that is required to placate a child following surgery; if pain is the likely diagnosis, opioids should be titrated to effect. Acetaminophen is useful rectally or orally, but ketorolac is usually avoided in the immediate postoperative period for fear of altered platelet function that could exacerbate bleeding.

Emergence Agitation

Agitation on emergence may occur in children or adults as a result of pain, bladder distention, hypoxia, airway obstruction, unfamiliar surroundings, disorientation, hunger, electrolyte imbalance, and paradoxical reactions to drugs such as midazolam or diphenhydramine, or true emergence delirium that occurs more often in children following the use of volatile anesthetic agents, particularly sevoflurane. It is important to exclude and treat remediable causes such as pain, avoid agents that may precipitate the condition in patients with the history of a previous episode following anesthesia, and employ strategies to decrease the incidence in susceptible patients by the use of prophylactic opioids, propofol, clonidine, or dexmedetomidine. If suspected, propofol in a dose of 0.5–1 mg/kg terminates the episode rapidly without the potential hazard of excessive opioid use, and may decrease the likelihood of morbidity related to intracranial complications, loss of surgical drains, surgical site bleeding, and injury to patients and providers.

Anesthetic Techniques and Drugs

Stress Response

Techniques

A prospective randomized trial by Bhagat et al. of three different anesthetic techniques for reduction of stress related to early emergence from anesthesia and for up to 1 h following extubation concluded that a low-dose fentanyl infusion (1.5 mcg/kg/h) was superior to a propofol infusion (3 mg/kg/h) or to low-dose isoflurane inhalation (end-tidal concentration of 0.2%) in allowing early awakening, and limiting emergence hypertension when each regimen was administered from the start of dural closure until the start of skin closure. In addition, patients in the propofol group had a significantly higher incidence of hypotension at the time of dural closure; there were no statistically significant differences in the incidence of PONV, return to full Glasgow Coma Scale, postoperative complications, or length of stay in the ICU. One significant predictor of emergence hypertension in this study was a preoperative midline shift of >5 mm on cerebral imaging scans. In children, titration of intravenous fentanyl is usually adequate to ensure smooth extubation with minimal coughing following emergence. This can be supplemented with intravenous lidocaine (1 mg/kg) if necessary. Following neurovascular surgery, "deep" extubation may be the best way to avoid coughing; however, if there is any suspicion of respiratory or airway compromise, the patient should be left intubated and transferred to ICU with additional sedation to minimize intracranial hypertension.

Drugs

Beta blockers such as labetalol and esmolol can be effective in preventing the stress response to emergence and extubation in neurosurgical patients, though their effect may be unpredictable, or associated with bradycardia and conduction delays, respectively. Calcium channel antagonists such as nicardipine, while effective, cause dose-dependent cerebral vasodilatation, inhibition of autoregulation, and frequent hypotension. Dexmedetomidine, an alpha-2 agonist is gaining popularity in this area as a result of its sedative, sympatholytic, and analgesic effects. In a double-blind, prospective, randomized, placebo-controlled trial comparing a supplemental dexmedetomidine infusion to placebo for craniotomy patients undergoing anesthesia with sevoflurane, opioids, and antihypertensive medications at the discretion of the blinded neuroanesthesiologists, patients in the dexmedetomidine group had improved hemodynamic stability without episodes of hypotension or bradycardia despite the best efforts of the anesthesiologists. Fewer patients in the treatment group required antihypertensive medications (42% vs. 86%), and patients in this group were discharged from the PACU earlier (91 min vs. 130 min). Despite numerous reports of the widespread use of Dexmedetomidine in children, it has not been approved for use in this age group, and no data exists for its use in this scenario in children.

Respiratory Complications

Techniques to minimize coughing and tracheal stimulation can effectively blunt the large increases in ICP that may result during emergence and extubation. Intravenous or intratracheal lidocaine with or without short-acting opioids such as alfentanil or remifentanil decrease coughing, agitation, cardiovascular stimulation, and emergence hypertension. In addition, care should be taken to ensure adequate preoxygenation prior to extubation, full reversal of neuromuscular block, and a patent, unobstructed airway following extubation to minimize hypoxia and/or hypercarbia. Specifically, measures to prevent and treat airway or soft tissue edema, laryngospasm, stridor, postobstructive pulmonary edema, pulmonary aspiration, and bronchospasm are fundamental in this regard. Clinical evaluation should always precede extubation to ensure optimal conditions for safe extubation. It is imperative to monitor children for respiratory obstruction following extubation, particularly in infants and younger children, or in the presence of significant facial edema. Vocal cord paralysis as a result of cranial nerve dysfunction following removal of posterior fossa tumors is an important cause of postoperative respiratory obstruction that usually requires immediate reintubation.

Postoperative Nausea and Vomiting

The incidence of PONV in children and adults following craniotomy is reported to be as high as 50–60%. PONV is unpleasant, can raise blood pressure and intracranial pressure and may cause dehydration and alkalosis, all of which may lead to morbidity following intracranial surgery. Prevention of PONV following craniotomy with the use of one or more prophylactic antiemetic drugs should be a part of routine management of these patients. A meta-analysis looking at the use of 5-HT$_3$ receptor antagonists in 448 patients showed a significant reduction in the risk of emesis at 24 (relative risk = 0.50, 95% C.I. 0.38–0.66) and 48 h (relative risk = 0.52, 95% C.I. 0.36–0.75) following craniotomy, but had no effect on nausea. Interestingly, the use of prophylactic ondansetron alone has not been shown to be effective in preventing postoperative vomiting in children following craniotomy when compared to placebo. It is likely that the use of other agents such as dexamethasone, low-dose droperidol, and propofol can lower the incidence of PONV in this age group. School-age children (4–12 years of age) are more likely to vomit in the first 24 h following surgery compared to adolescents.

Key Points

- Emergence from anesthesia and tracheal extubation are associated with tremendous physiological stress that result in hypertension, increased oxygen consumption, and central and peripheral adrenergic stimulation.
- The metabolic stress response may cause devastating complications such as intracranial bleeding and/or dangerously elevated intracranial pressure. Premature infants have a high risk of intraventricular hemorrhage as a result of impaired autoregulatory capacity.
- The anesthesiologist should decide early on whether the child is suitable for early emergence and extubation, or would benefit from a period of postoperative ventilation; anesthetic management should be tailored to best achieve this outcome while taking steps to minimize the metabolic stress response during emergence and following extubation.
- In children, prevention or attenuation of hypothermia, shivering, anxiety, pain, coughing, airway obstruction, emergence agitation, and PONV will reduce but not eliminate the stress response to emergence and extubation.
- Peripheral nerve blocks of the scalp, intravenous lidocaine at extubation, and low-dose fentanyl during wound closure are useful in attenuating the stress response to emergence and extubation in children.
- Prophylaxis of PONV with 5-HT$_3$ receptor antagonists is ineffective in children, therefore alternative agents should be considered for prophylaxis of PONV.

Suggested Reading

Basali A, Mascha EJ, Kalfas I, Schubert A. Relation between perioperative hypertension and intracranial hemorrhage after craniotomy. Anesthesiology. 2000;93(1):48–54.
Bekker A, Sturaitis M, Bloom M, et al. The effect of dexmedetomidine on perioperative hemodynamics in patients undergoing craniotomy. Anesth Analg. 2008;107(4):1340–7.

Bhagat H, Dash HH, Bithal PK, Chouhan RS, Pandia MP. Planning for early emergence in neurosurgical patients: A randomized prospective trial of low-dose anesthetics. Anesth Analg. 2008;107(4):1348–55.

Bruder NJ. Awakening management after neurosurgery for intracranial tumours. Curr Opin Anaesthesiol. 2002;15(5):477–82.

Bruder N, Ravussin P. Recovery from anesthesia and postoperative extubation of neurosurgical patients: A review. J Neurosurg Anesthesiol. 1999;11(4):282–93.

Eldredge EA, Soriano SG, Rockoff MA. Pediatric neurosurgical anesthesia. In: Cote CJ, Todres DI, Ryan JF, Goudsouzian NG, editors. A practice of anesthesia for infants and children. 3rd ed. Philadelphia, PA: W. B. Saunders; 2001. p. 493–521.

Magni G, La Rosa I, Gimignani S, Melillo G, Imperiale C, Rosa G. Early postoperative complications after intracranial surgery: Comparison between total intravenous and balanced anesthesia. J Neurosurg Anesthesiol. 2007;19(4):229–34.

Udomphorn Y, Armstead WM, Vavilala MS. Cerebral blood flow and autoregulation after pediatric traumatic brain injury. Pediatr Neurol. 2008;38(4):225–34.

Vlajkovic GP, Sindjelic RP. Emergence delirium in children: Many questions, few answers. Anesth Analg. 2007;104(1):84–91.

Chapter 58
Postanesthesia Care Unit Risks Following Pediatric Neurosurgery

Sally E. Rampersad and Lynn D. Martin

Overview

In this chapter, we will review the issues that are of importance in the initial postoperative recovery of the pediatric neurosurgical patient. The pediatric anesthesiologist is able to control many factors that influence cerebral blood flow (CBF), cerebral metabolic rate for oxygen ($CMRO_2$), and intracranial pressure (ICP). When there are immediate post-surgical concerns, failure to awaken or new neurological signs, the actions of the anesthesiologist may be instrumental in determining the outcome. The advantages and disadvantages of obtaining a CT or MRI scan prior to emergence from anesthesia versus a delayed or "as-needed" scan will be discussed. Emergence from anesthesia, management of the airway and postoperative delirium are discussed in Chap. 57.

The goal of the pediatric neuroanesthesiologist is to provide stability of hemodynamics, respiratory parameters, temperature control, and of metabolic and endocrine factors. This stability must continue into the postoperative period to insure an optimal neurological outcome.

Implications for the Neurosurgical Patient

Blood Pressure Control

A normal newborn autoregulates intracerebral blood flow at mean blood pressures between 20 and 60 mmHg, with a steep rise and fall at either end of the autoregulatory curve. The brain of an infant or child receives a relatively larger percentage of the

S.E. Rampersad, MB, FRCA (✉) • L.D. Martin, MD, FAAP, FCCM
Department of Anesthesiology and Pain Medicine, Seattle Children's Hospital,
University of Washington, Seattle, WA, USA

A.M. Brambrink and J.R. Kirsch (eds.), *Essentials of Neurosurgical Anesthesia & Critical Care*, DOI 10.1007/978-0-387-09562-2_58, © Springer Science+Business Media, LLC 2012

cardiac output as compared to adults. After traumatic brain injury, young age (less than 4 years) has been shown to be an independent risk factor for impaired cerebral autoregulation. These factors place pediatric neurosurgical patients at particular risk for ischemia at low blood pressures and for hemorrhage at high blood pressures. Short-acting vasoactive agents such as intravenous esmolol or labetalol may be needed in PACU for acute control of hypertension and adequate fluid and blood replacement must be given to avoid hypotension.

Pain Management

Adequate analgesia is essential, so that the hyperventilation that may occur with crying can be avoided. Short-acting intravenous opioids such as fentanyl or remifentanil may be used intraoperatively, but there is then a need to titrate in a longer-acting intravenous agent during emergence. If remifentanil has been used, there is the possibility of acute tolerance with an unexpectedly high opioid requirement in PACU; although studies have not universally confirmed this finding. An age-appropriate pain scale must be used accurately to determine the level of pain, so that it may be adequately controlled. Some scales to consider include the modified infant pain scale (MIPS); the FLACC behavioral scale; the Wong–Baker FACES scale and the Oucher. Older children may be asked to report using the familiar 0–10 visual analogue scale (VAS). If opioids are needed, a patient-controlled analgesia (PCA) system may be a good option for delivery, so that the older child can titrate to an adequate level of analgesia but can also avoid sedation that may occur if opioids are given by continuous infusion or by RN-administered bolus doses. Excessive treatment of pain may result in sedation of the patient, making neurological assessment difficult. In addition, there may be respiratory depression leading to elevated arterial levels of carbon dioxide (CO_2) which may in turn cause somnolence. Patients who have had surgery close to the brain stem, such as a Chiari decompression, may be especially sensitive to even a mildly elevated level of CO_2 Hence there is a need to balance treatment of pain versus the risk of somnolence and impaired neurological assessment. Administration of intravenous naloxone to relieve narcotic-induced somnolence or respiratory depression can cause significant hypertension, so opioids must be titrated with care to avoid the need for reversal of their effects.

Temperature Management

Shivering significantly raises oxygen consumption and so efforts should be made to maintain normothermia and to treat shivering promptly with warming blankets or with low-dose meperidine if it occurs. Hyperthermia may occur with either an infectious or noninfectious etiology and should be treated, no matter what the cause. Combination therapy (acetaminophen, ibuprofen, and physical cooling) may be needed effectively to maintain normothermia.

Postoperative Nausea and Vomiting

Postoperative nausea and vomiting (PONV) should be treated to avoid the potentially deleterious effects of a Valsalva maneuver during vomiting which may transiently raise ICP or increase the risk for intracranial hemorrhage. Fortunately, the 5-HT$_3$-receptor antagonists, such as ondansetron, can provide a useful anti-emetic effect without the problematic sedative side effects that occurred with some older agents such as droperidol and promethazine.

Endocrine Issues

A few patients who have had surgery in or close to the pituitary fossa, will need close monitoring for early signs of the development of diabetes insipidus, manifested by abnormally high volumes of dilute urine. Other endocrine derangements such as hyperglycemia or hypoglycemia are also possible. One study demonstrated a poor outcome following brain injuries in children when blood glucose levels were elevated (above 250 mg/100 ml).

Respiratory Management

Neurogenic pulmonary edema (NPE) is a complication unique to neurosurgical patients who have had intracranial surgery or injury. It can be life-threatening and the exact etiology and pathophysiology are incompletely understood. The neuroanesthesiologist must be ready to provide respiratory support, including reintubation and ventilation, if this complication develops in order to maintain oxygenation and normocarbia.

Concerns and Risks

Elevated ICP

Neurosurgical patients experience cerebral hyperemia during emergence from general anesthesia, independent of the anesthesia technique used. Delay of extubation does not attenuate the increase in heart rate, mean arterial pressure and oxygen consumption and catecholamine surge that occur at extubation. For patients whose raised ICP has not been alleviated by surgery, who had surgery of long duration, had major blood loss, or may have cranial nerve damage that impairs airway-protective reflexes, controlled ventilation with adequate sedation may be necessary after surgery. When the time comes to extubate such patients, one should remember that raised ICP has an association with delayed gastric emptying, so suction must be available and the patient should be fully awake and optimally positioned to reduce the possibility of aspiration.

Seizures

Seizures significantly raise the cerebral metabolic rate for oxygen. Early postoperative seizures are defined as those occurring within the first week after surgery. They occur in 15–20% of patients who have had a supratentorial tumor resection. Close monitoring for postoperative seizures is necessary. Prophylaxis for seizures is generally left to the neurosurgeon's preference as prospective trials are lacking. Phenytoin is commonly given in the perioperative period.

Postoperative Neuroimaging

Timing of postoperative CT or MRI scans is controversial. At our institution, it is common practice to get an immediate postoperative CT scan and then to extubate the patient in PACU, if postoperative ventilation was not planned. This practice is not universal; some institutions scan on an as-needed basis only (change in neurological status or seizures being indications to scan) while other institutions scan routinely on postoperative day 1. There is a strong argument for rapid awakening of these patients to allow early neurological assessment and early diagnosis of adverse postoperative neurological outcomes. The anesthesiologist in PACU must be able to respond in a timely manner to adverse hemodynamic and respiratory events. Delayed response to these hemodynamic and respiratory changes can theoretically result in cerebral ischemia, raised ICP, altered consciousness level, and long-term adverse outcomes.

Failure to Awaken

The following goals are desirable clinical targets in the pediatric neurosurgical patient. One or more of these factors may need to be corrected for the patient who fails to awaken at the end of surgery (Table 58.1).

If all of the above parameters have been considered and corrected if necessary, emergent imaging and neurosurgical consultation may be needed to rule out postoperative hemorrhage or edema for any patient who fails to awaken.

New Neurological Signs

A concerning development in PACU is the occurrence of new neurological signs and symptoms. These must be assessed promptly by both neurosurgeon and anesthesiologist (Fig. 58.1).

Table 58.1 Failure to awaken

Normothermia (>36°C, avoid hyperthermia)

Normoglycemia (glucose > 60 mg/100 ml and <200 mg/100 ml)

Spontaneous ventilation without hypercapnia (<50 mmHg) or hypoxemia (SaO_2 >94%)

Normal osmolality (>275 mOsm kg^{-1} and <300 mOsm kg^{-1})

Normal circulating blood volume and pressure

Adequate reversal of muscle relaxants

No significant brain edema

No ongoing seizure activity

Hematocrit, coagulation within acceptable limits

Intact cranial nerves for airway protection

Normal, or near-normal preoperative neurological state

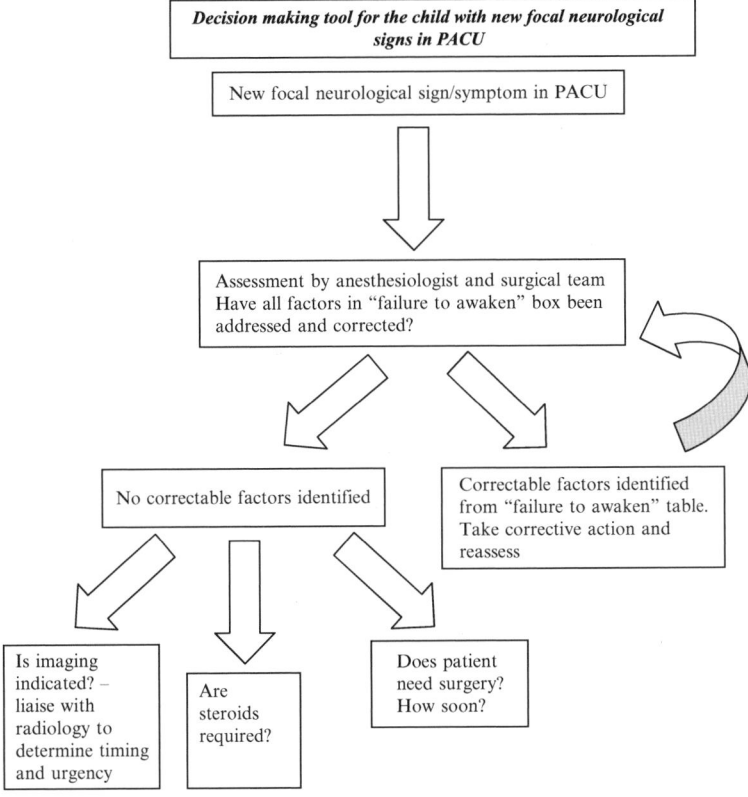

Fig. 58.1 Decision making tool for the child with new focal neurological signs in PACU

Key Points

- The major concern when caring for a pediatric neurosurgical patient in the PACU is finding the balance between adequate analgesia while providing an alert, interactive patient for confirmation that no new neurological deficits have occurred.
- The effect of any intervention (or lack of intervention) on ICP, the threshold for seizure activity or altering level of consciousness must always be considered as etiologies for postoperative neurologic dysfunction.
- Meticulous attention to pain control, control of PONV, careful management of fluid status to achieve euvolemia and maintenance of normothermia, normal osmolality, and normoglycemia are essential.
- In pediatric neurosurgical patients it is particularly important to avoid hypoxemia, hypercarbia, and hyper/hypotension, since derangements in arterial blood gases or in blood pressure can have profound effects on the cerebral vasculature, resulting in intracranial hemorrhage, raised ICP or in vasospasm, causing new neurological deficits.

Suggested Reading

Brown JM, Udomphorn Y, Suz P, Vavilala M. Antipyretic treatment of noninfectious fever in children with severe traumatic brain injury. Childs Nerv Syst. 2008;24:477–83.

Bruder N, Stordeur J-M, Ravussin P, et al. Metabolic and hemodynamic changes during recovery and tracheal extubation in neurosurgical patients: Immediate versus delayed recovery. Anesth Analg. 1999;89:674–8.

Bruder N, Pellissier D, Grillot P, Gouin F. Cerebral hyperemia during recovery from general anesthesia in neurosurgical patients. Anesth Analg. 2002;94:650–4.

Fàbregas N, Bruder N. Recovery and neurological evaluation. Best Pract Res Clin Anaesthesiol. 2007;21(4):431–47.

Freeman SS, Udomphorn Y, Armstead WM, et al. Young age as a risk factor for impaired cerebral autoregulation after moderate to severe pediatric traumatic brain injury. Anesthesiology. 2008;108(4):588–95.

Michaud LJ, Rivara FP, Longstreth Jr WT, et al. Elevated initial blood glucose levels and poor outcome following brain injuries in children. J Trauma. 1999;31:1356–62.

Pryds O. Control of cerebral circulation in the high-risk neonate. Ann Neurol. 1991;30:321–9.

Šedý J, Zicha J, Kunes J, et al. Mechanisms of neurogenic pulmonary edema development. Physiol Res. 2008;57:499–506.

Sulpicio GS, Eldredge EA, Rockoff MA. Pediatric neuroanesthesia. Anesthesiol Clin North America. 2002;20:389–404.

Chapter 59
Intensive Care Risks of Pediatric Neurosurgery

Craig D. McClain and Michael L. McManus

Introduction

Pediatric patients who have undergone intracranial neurosurgical procedures are generally best managed in a critical care setting. These patients may experience hemodynamic, respiratory, and neurologic fluctuations postoperatively and will therefore need frequent assessment to ensure a stable recovery. In centers with high-volume, specialized neurocritical care teams have been demonstrated to improve patient outcomes for both adult and pediatric populations. The transition from operating suite to ICU should begin with clear communication of the patient's history, intraoperative course (including relevant events such as airway issues, bleeding, and brain edema), and anticipated postoperative course including potential concerning focal neurologic deficits.

All new admission to the ICU will require a thorough physiologic and neurologic assessment. These assessments should be repeated frequently, as changes in the neurologic exam will be sensitive indicators of potential postoperative complications.

Respiratory Support

- While it is desirable, not all patients meet extubation criteria prior to admission to the ICU.
- Postoperative mechanical ventilation aims to support gas exchange while permitting ongoing neurological assessment.

C.D. McClain, MD, MPH (✉)
Department of Anesthesiology, Perioperative and Pain Medicine, Children's Hospital Boston, Boston, MA, USA
e-mail: Craig.McClain@childrens.harvard.edu

M.L. McManus, MD, MPH
Department of Anesthesiology, Perioperative and Pain Medicine, Children's Hospital Boston, Harvard Medical School, Boston, MA, USA

A.M. Brambrink and J.R. Kirsch (eds.), *Essentials of Neurosurgical Anesthesia & Critical Care*, DOI 10.1007/978-0-387-09562-2_59, © Springer Science+Business Media, LLC 2012

- Triggered modes (i.e., pressure support) offer a method for providing support without losing respiratory drive as a marker of neurologic function and minimize respiratory muscle deconditioning.
- PEEP should be used with caution as even small amounts may impair venous return and decrease cerebral compliance.
- In infants with open fontanelles, there is no association between mean airway and intracranial pressures (ICPs).

Hemodynamic Support

Overview

- Goals – avoid hypotension and maintain adequate cerebral perfusion pressure (CPP).
- In sick neonates, intermittent pressure passivity of the cerebral circulation is present and can predispose to intracranial hemorrhage.
- Even in very low-birth-weight infants, both dopamine and epinephrine are effective in supporting systemic pressure and restoring cerebral blood flow.

Implications for the Neurosurgical Patient

- When increased ICP is present, critical CPP for preschool children (2–6 years) is approximately 50 mmHg, rising to 55–60 mmHg in older children.
- The lower limit of pressure autoregulation in infants and prematures is approximately 30 mmHg.

Fluid Management

Overview

Meticulous fluid management is critical in the care of neurosurgical patients. Small size, immature renal function, and variable intake make fluid and electrolyte imbalances common in pediatrics. These dispositions are further magnified in neurosurgical patients by the disruption of normal homeostatic controls.

- Overall, more than 10% of all children experience postoperative hyponatremia and this percentage is likely higher after neurosurgery.

- Elevated ADH levels can result from a variety of stimuli ranging from surgical manipulation, to postoperative pain and nausea to fluid shifts and intravascular hypovolemia.
- Since sudden, unrecognized falls in serum sodium can provoke seizures, it is prudent to follow electrolytes closely throughout the perioperative period.

Concerns and Risks

- Nonosmotic secretion of ADH makes hyponatremia common after neurosurgery, despite intraoperative fluids that are high in sodium and isotonic – or slightly hypertonic – to plasma (lactated Ringer's, 272 mOsm/L; normal saline, 308 mOsm/L).
- When significant hyponatremia occurs, treatment may include hypertonic saline with free water excesses addressed through fluid restriction and administration of diuretics.
- Small premature infants, with limited reserves of glycogen and limited gluconeogenesis; require continuous infusions of glucose at 5–6 mg/kg/min in order to maintain serum levels.
- The stress of critical illness and resulting insulin resistance can produce hyperglycemia that, in turn, is associated with neurologic injury, infection, and poor outcomes in adults.

    - Tight glycemic control has been widely recommended.
    - In pediatrics, hyperglycemia has been linked to poor outcome but it remains unclear that tight glycemic control offers significant benefits to children.
    - Limited evidence now suggests that tight control may carry undue risk of hypoglycemia.
    - A conservative approach that maintains random serum glucose levels below 180 mg/dL may be utilized.

Key Points

- Avoid hypotonic solutions altogether in the perioperative period.
- Infants are at particular risk for hypoglycemia. Monitoring of serum glucose is crucial during the perioperative period in these patients.

Fluid and Electrolyte Abnormalities in the ICU

Syndrome of CSW

- Common in children, can be seen following head trauma and many neurosurgical procedures.
- Has been diagnosed with increasing frequency and reported in association with

  - Meningitis
  - Calvarial remodeling
  - Tumor resection
  - Hydrocephalus

- Incidence is approximately 11.3/1,000 procedures with mean duration of symptoms of 6 days, with a range of one to five.
- Marked by polyuria and natriuresis leading to hyponatremia and hypovolemia.
- Result of excessively high atrial or brain natriuretic peptide levels, which also block steroidogenesis – cerebral salt wasting (CSW) is typically accompanied by mineralocorticoid deficiency.
- Classic treatment involves saline administration; more rapid resolution has been achieved with fludocortisone.

Diabetes Insipidus

- Complication of procedures involving the pituitary and hypothalamus.
- Most frequently seen in association with craniopharyngioma, where it can be a presenting symptom in 40% of the cases.
- Noted by an elevated serum sodium (>150 mg/dL) and polyuria (>4 mL/kg/h).
- Severe dehydration and hypovolemia may result.
- A standardized protocol is helpful when postoperative care is multidisciplinary.

  - Unconscious patients, those unable to take oral fluids, or those in whom normal thirst mechanisms are impaired, are best managed using a continuous infusion of vasopressin titrated to minimize urine output (1–0.5 mL/kg/min) – other clinical markers of volume status must be followed.
  - Awake and thirsty patients may be transitioned to oral fluids and DDAVP.

Sedation

Overview

Pain control and sedation present unique challenges in the pediatric intensive care unit. Ideally, postoperative neurosurgical patients are comfortable, awake, and cooperative with their care. In pediatrics, some level of sedation is often necessary to insure a safe recovery. While the ideal sedation regime would include short-acting or reversible agents that can be withdrawn intermittently to permit neurologic assessment, a single agent suitable for children has yet to be developed.

Implications for the Neurosurgical Patient

Propofol

- Propofol is a potent, ultra-short-acting, sedative-hypnotic that is extremely useful in adult neurocritical care with limited utility in pediatrics because of its association with a fatal syndrome of bradycardia, rhabdomyolysis, metabolic acidosis, and multiple organ failure when used over extended periods in small children.
- The mechanism of this remains unclear; it appears related to both the duration of therapy and the cumulative dose. These difficulties are much less common in adults.
- If propofol is utilized, continuous infusions of limited duration are recommended.

Opioids/Benzodiazepines

- The mainstay of sedation in the pediatric intensive care unit remains a combination of narcotic and benzodiazepine administered via continuous infusion.
- Titration to a validated sedation score is advised and regular "drug holidays" help insure that excessive sedation is avoided.
- Infants and children receiving opioid and/or benzodiazepine infusions for more than 3–5 days are subject to tolerance and experience symptoms of withdrawal when infusions are discontinued.

Dexmedetomidine

- An ultra-short-acting single-agent sedative to be used in the postoperative period but apnea is not a problem with spontaneous breathing easily maintained.
- Pediatric studies are limited but the drug appears to be safe and effective when used for periods of 24 h or less.

- Pharmacokinetics of dexmedetomidine in pediatric patients are similar to published adult values.
- Opioid cross-tolerance makes it a useful agent for treatment of fentanyl or morphine withdrawal.
- Transient increases in blood pressure can be seen with boluses followed by hypotension and bradycardia as sedation deepens. In our experience, both hypo- and hypertension can occasionally be observed with long-term infusions and a withdrawal syndrome results when extended infusions are discontinued.

Seizures

Overview

Seizures are a common manifestation of neurological illness in pediatrics. In the child with unexplained, altered mental status, nonconvulsive status epilepticus is also an important consideration. Prophylaxis in the perioperative period and aggressive treatment of new seizure activity are well-recognized mainstays of care.

Agents

- While phenytoin is the agent used most commonly for prophylaxis, maintaining therapeutic serum levels can be a challenge.
- Alternative agents include phenobarbital, carbamazepine, and valproic acid.
- Though potentially compounding respiratory depression, Phenobarbital 20 mg/kg is also an effective first-line antiepileptic drug.
- For status epilepticus, lorazepam 0.1 mg/kg IV or diazepam 0.5 mg/kg PR are effective.
- Lorezepam may be repeated after 10 min and accompanied by fosphenytoin 20 mg/kg IV or IM if initial doses are ineffective.
- Increasingly, levetiracetam is being used for seizure prophylaxis and treatment. Purported benefits over phenytoin include the following:

  - No need to follow drug levels
  - Lack of significant drug interactions
  - Similar bioavailability between oral and intravenous forms
  - Broad spectrum of antiepileptic activity

Status Epilepticus

- Refractory status epilepticus continues to present a significant challenge.
- Chemically induced coma remains the mainstay of care with AEDs titrated to EEG burst suppression.

- Pentobarbital, midazolam, or phenobarbital may be employed in bolus-infusion regimes with adjustments directed by continuous EEG.
- Mechanical ventilation and invasive monitoring are necessary since therapy often results in hypotension and myocardial depression. In addition, barbiturates have been associated with depression of immune function and increased rate of nosocomial infection.
- Propofol is also effective in quenching seizures and inducing coma, but the propofol infusion syndrome limits its use in pediatrics.

Seizure Prophylaxis for Head Trauma

- The utility of seizure prophylaxis after pediatric head trauma continues to be controversial.
- Although some data suggest that children may benefit more than adults from routine prophylaxis, the overall risk of seizures is low after blunt injury.

Intracranial Pressure

Overview

- ICP monitoring is desirable in trauma and in neurosurgical patients at risk for brain swelling or sudden expansion of a mass lesion.
- Symptoms are nonspecific in children and intermittent apnea may be its first sign in infancy.
- Low thresholds are kept for invasive monitoring of unconscious patients since physiologic parameters are less sensitive than mental status changes.
- In babies, split sutures and bulging fontanelles provide clinical evidence of increasing ICP, but noninvasive quantitative measures are not reliable.
- The treatment of increased ICP in infants and children is still largely informed by adult data.

  – A notable exception to this, as discussed above, is that target thresholds for mean arterial pressure and CPP vary with age.

- Osmotherapy with 3% (hypertonic) saline is widely used in boluses or infusion to control ICP; it may more rapidly lead to severe hypernatremia in small children than in adults.
- Other elements of management extrapolated from adult data include avoidance of steroids, the preference of crystalloid over colloid resuscitation fluids, and the reluctance to employ hyperventilation.

- Regarding the latter, it is particularly important to recognize that small children are subject to inadvertent overventilation and that hyperventilation-associated cerebral ischemia can occur. Careful monitoring of blood gasses, minute ventilation, and end-tidal carbon dioxide tensions are therefore recommended.

- When CPP is low and ICP remains high despite medical management, decompressive craniectomy may have a better outcome in children than adults.

Brain Death

Overview

- Determination of brain death in older children is similar to adults but the diagnosis is difficult in infancy.
- Uniform Determination of Death Act defines death as "irreversible cessation of circulatory and respiratory function or irreversible cessation of all functions of the entire brain, including the brainstem."
- Diagnosis requires

  - Normothermia
  - Normotension
  - Normal systemic oxygenation
  - Absence of confounding toxins or medications

- An apnea test (documenting the absence of respiratory effort despite $pCO_2 > 60$ torr) is conducted last since elevated pCO_2 may exacerbate neurologic injury.
- To establish irreversibility, age-related observation periods are necessary:

  - For premature newborns and infants under 7 days of age, no such period has been established.
  - For infants 1–8 weeks of age, our institution utilizes two exams and two iso-electric electroencephalograms 48 h apart.
  - Infants 2–12 months of age require two clinical exams separated by 24 h.
  - Patients older than 1 year require exams 6–12 h apart, or 24 h if the proximate cause of death is hypoxia-ischemia.

- The exam seeks to establish the complete absence of cortical and brainstem function.
- Cerebral ^{99}Tc-ECD single photon emission computed tomography (SPECT) scanning is used to document the absence of cerebral perfusion when confounders complicate the clinical diagnosis.

Key Points

- Extubation and initial neurological assessment are ideally accomplished in the operating room.
- Postoperative mechanical ventilation aims to support gas exchange while permitting ongoing neurological assessment.
- Hemodynamic goals are to avoid hypotension and maintain adequate CPP.
- Sudden, unrecognized falls in serum sodium can provoke seizures, and can be life threatening.
- Avoid hypotonic solutions altogether in the perioperative period.
- Ideally, postoperative neurosurgical patients are comfortable, awake, and cooperative with their care.
- Seizure prophylaxis in the perioperative period and aggressive treatment are well-recognized mainstays of care.
- ICP monitoring is desirable in trauma and in neurosurgical patients at risk for brain swelling or sudden expansion of a mass lesion.
- In babies, split sutures and bulging fontanelles provide clinical evidence of increasing ICP, but noninvasive quantitative measures are not reliable.
- Uniform Determination of Death Act defines death as "irreversible cessation of circulatory and respiratory function or irreversible cessation of all functions of the entire brain, including the brainstem."

Suggested Reading

Abend NS, Dlugos DJ. Nonconvulsive status epilepticus in a pediatric intensive care unit. Pediatr Neurol. 2007;37:165–70.

Bell MJ, Carpenter J, Au AK, et al. Development of a pediatric neurocritical care service. Neurocrit Care. 2009;10(1):4–10.

Caricato A, Conti G, Della Corte F, et al. Effects of PEEP on the intracranial system of patients with head injury and subarachnoid hemorrhage: the role of respiratory system compliance. J Trauma. 2005;58:571–6.

Huang SJ, Hong WC, Han YY, et al. Clinical outcome of severe head injury using three different ICP and CPP protocol-driven therapies. J Clin Neurosci. 2006;13:818–22.

Mathur M, Petersen L, Stadtler M, Rose C, et al. Variability in pediatric brain death determination and documentation in southern California. Pediatrics. 2008;121(5):988–93.

Skippen P, Seear M, Poskitt K, et al. Effect of hyperventilation on regional cerebral blood flow in head-injured children. Crit Care Med. 1997;25:1402–9.

Wise-Faberowski L, Soriano SG, Ferrari L, et al. Perioperative management of diabetes insipidus in children [corrected]. J Neurosurg Anesthesiol. 2004;16:14–9.

Part XI
Fundamentals of Interventional Neuroradiology

Chapter 60
Radiation Safety in Interventional Neuroradiology

Justin P. Dodge, Neil E. Roundy, and Kenneth C. Liu

Overview

Information obtained using radiation is clinically valuable and often could not be obtained by any other reasonable means. Thus the radiation exposure of the patient is warranted as the clinical benefit typically exceeds the potential risk. In contrast, the health-care provider receives no benefit from the radiation; therefore, the radiation exposure should be kept as low as possible. The most common exposure of health-care personnel to medical X-rays comes from the use of fluoroscopy units. It should be noted that there are many other sources of naturally occurring and other man-made sources of radiation (including other sources of medical radiation). *The essence of radiation safety in relation to medical X-rays involves three basic principles – time, distance, and shielding.* The information within this chapter should be regarded as a minimalist approach in understanding the basics of limiting radiation exposure. A good radiation safety program will utilize a Health Physics office or equivalent. The Health Physics office has many important roles, including safety information, equipment inspections, and the management of the radiation exposure monitoring (dosimetry).

J.P. Dodge, MD (✉)
Department of Radiology, Landstuhl Regional Medical Center, Landstuhl, RP, Germeny
e-mail: justin.dodge.md@gmail.com

N.E. Roundy, MD
Department of Neurological Surgery, Oregon Health & Science University, Portland, OR, USA

K.C. Liu, MD
Departments of Neurological Surgery and Radiology, University of Virginia Health System, Charlottesville, VA, USA

A.M. Brambrink and J.R. Kirsch (eds.), *Essentials of Neurosurgical Anesthesia & Critical Care*, DOI 10.1007/978-0-387-09562-2_60, © Springer Science+Business Media, LLC 2012

Background

Many scientific units are used to measure radiation. The units that are most important to the health-care worker are the rad (*r*adiation *a*bsorbed *d*ose) and the rem (*r*adiation *e*quivalent [dose in] *m*an). System International (SI) unit conversions are 100 rad = 1 Gray (Gy), and 100 rem = 1 Sievert (Sv). These units and conversions are provided for familiarity purposes.

Fluroscopy

A fluoroscopy unit or C-arm is the most commonly encountered X-ray-generating device in the operating room or angiographic suite. Several specific concepts are import when using or being exposed to the X-rays produced by a fluoroscopy unit. The radiation effect most important in increasing the health-care worker's exposure is through scattered radiation which is ideally approximately 0.1% of the radiation exposure of the patient at 1 m. A key element in reducing scatter includes keeping the Image Intensifier (X-ray detector) as close to the patient as possible.

Time

Time is the easiest principle to understand. *The actual time the fluoroscopy unit is generating X-rays is directly related to exposure.* That is to say if the X-ray generator is active for twice as long, radiation exposure cumulatively increases by twice as much. Keeping this principle in mind during a procedure means being aware of the amount of time the X-ray unit is on, limiting the time the unit is on to the minimum amount to effectively care for the patient, and learning to be as efficient with radiation utilization as possible.

Distance

Distance from the radiation source is an important principle, and most important for the personnel not actively involved in patient care. *The distance from the radiation source correlates to exposure by the inverse square law.* This means that doubling the distance from the X-ray source, radiation exposure is reduced by a factor of four. Furthermore, tripling (or quadrupling) the distance from the X-ray source, radiation exposure is reduced by a factor of 9 (or 16). Keeping this principle in mind during a procedure simply means spending most of your time as far from the X-ray source as possible while still being able to effectively care for the patient. Particularly critical is keeping your body outside of the direct beam unless absolutely necessary.

Shielding

Shielding personnel from radiation exposure is the principle that the health-care provider has the most direct control over. Shielding is a material that effectively "absorbs" the energy of the radiation and thus protects the health-care worker. The effectiveness of shielding is a much more complex calculation and not practical for the scope of this chapter.

Shielding is present in many forms from the design of the room and equipment to barrier devices. Most of the personnel reading this chapter will not have control over the design of the room or equipment. *The critical portion of this principle is that the safety devices that are not used will offer no protection.* Commonly used safety equipment utilized includes lead aprons, thyroid shields, and lead glasses. Specialized devices are also available for additional body parts that are routinely exposed to the X-ray beam by the nature of the procedure. These devices effectively absorb between 90 and 99.5% of the radiation depending on several variables such as the thickness and design of the shielding device and the energy of the X-ray being generated. "Leaded glass," commonly made of special plastic, is also available and can be placed between the health-care worker and the X-ray source in addition to worn safety devices.

Implications for the Patient

During fluoroscopy, the patient is directly in the X-ray beam. In other words, the patient is receiving approximately 1,000 times or more the radiation exposure as the health-care worker. Due to the nature of the procedure and the design of the equipment several items should be reviewed in regards to patient safety.

In regards to time, the longer the fluoroscopy unit is on the more radiation exposure the patient receives. Using effective collimation (narrowing of the X-ray beam), keeping the tube current as low as possible to obtain a diagnostic image, and using the last image hold feature (if available) are all easy steps that can greatly reduce radiation exposure. Using "pulsed" instead of continuous fluoroscopy imaging can significantly reduce the time factor.

Distance from the X-ray generator to the patient (source object distance) is fixed in many systems, but again, the furthest distance from the patient decreases the radiation exposure. When using a C-arm this concept becomes particularly important as the distance from the X-ray generator to the image intensifier is fixed. *It is desirable to keep the image detector as close to the patient as possible, therefore making the X-ray generator as far as possible from the patient* (Fig. 60.1). This is a win–win scenario where the patient radiation exposure is decreased (the distance component) and the health-care radiation exposure is decreased (the scatter effect).

The last of the principles is again shielding. Shielding the patient can usually be done only for body parts outside the region of treatment interest. Commonly used patient shield devices include breast, gonad, and thyroid shields which are designed to protect the most radio-sensitive organs.

Fig. 60.1 Illustration demonstrating the ideal configuration of the C-arm with the image intensifier placed close to the patient and the X-ray generator far from the patient

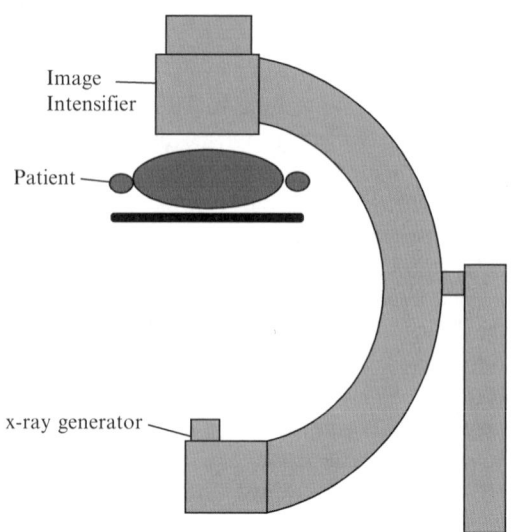

Concerns and Risks

The radiation used in medical imaging is ionizing radiation. This means that the radiation can cause biologic damage on the molecular level. There are four main negative effects (risks) of radiation exposure, including tissue damage, radiation-induced cancers, genetic effects, and fetal exposure. As a general rule, a rapidly dividing cell type is more sensitive to the effects of radiation.

In the practical use of medical X-rays, hair loss, skin erythema, and desquamation are the most commonly encountered tissue damage and typically occur on the order of 3 weeks after the exposure. These effects occur in a threshold model. This means that a certain level of radiation exposure must be reached before the effect occurs.

The carcinogenic effects of radiation are not completely understood but several general statements can be made. The higher the radiation exposure(s) are, the higher the risk becomes. There is typically a one to several decade delay between the radiation exposure and the development of cancer. Children are at the highest risk of radiation induced cancer. The most common radiation induced cancers are breast, thyroid, lung, leukemia, and GI cancers. Genetic effects of radiation are not typically encountered at the doses used in medical imaging and are felt to occur at a much lower rate than the carcinogenic effects.

The rapidly growing fetus is extremely sensitive to radiation exposure; therefore, limiting exposure to pregnant patients or health-care workers is highly desirable. Fetal gestation is divided into three major components: preimplantation, organogenesis, and fetal growth. During the preimplantation stage, the fetus is particularly sensitive, and excessive radiation exposure typically results in fetal demise. Radiation exposure during organogenesis has a higher likelihood of causing organ malformations. The fetal growth phase radiation exposure most commonly results in neurologic and sense organ anomalies and childhood cancers.

Dosimetry

Monitoring the exposure of radiation health-care workers is important for safety and in many places for legal purposes. A Health Physics office typically monitors this program and assesses the individuals' appropriate monitoring requirements based on their exposure to medical radiation. Special requirements are utilized for pregnant personnel. Monitoring devices most commonly used are film badges and less commonly dosimeters. These devices allow the health-care worker to monitor their radiation exposure and to compare their exposure rates to established limits. *The most important principle in dosimetry is that the required monitoring devices are worn appropriately*. Dosimeters are typically worn *outside* of lead shielding on the front of the body. Special care should be taken to store the dosimetry units in a location that is reasonably excluded from radiation exposure.

Key Points

While using or being exposed to medical radiation, the health-care worker should understand the basic principles of radiation safety. Most health-care workers should also be familiar with the *ALARA* concept which means keeping the radiation exposure *as low as reasonably achievable*.

- Keep the time of the procedure and the radiation exposure as short as reasonable possible from the X-ray source.
- Increase the distance of the health-care worker as far as reasonably possible from the X-ray source.
- Utilize safety devices and shielding whenever possible.
- Be familiar with the appropriate use of fluoroscopy and the specific techniques to reduce radiation exposure for both the health-care workers and the patient.

Suggested Reading

Bushberg JT et al. The essential physics of medical imaging. 2nd ed. Philadelphia: Lippincott Williams & Wilkins; 2002.

Chapter 61
Understanding Basic Techniques and Procedures in Interventional Neuroradiology

Kenneth C. Liu, Lori E. Guidone, and Stanley L. Barnwell

Overview

Interventional neuroradiology (or endovascular neurosurgery) is a fairly nascent and rapidly evolving field specializing in minimally invasive, image-based technologies/procedures used in the diagnosis and treatment of diseases of the head, neck, and spine. While the majority of the procedures are endovascular and target vascular pathology, interventional neuroradiologists also specialize in the percutaneous treatment of spinal disorders that do not use the circulatory system as the conduit for therapy (e.g., vertebroplasty, kyphoplasty, facet arthrodesis). Interventional neuroradiology is a unique subspecialty in that it represents a veritable melting pot of specialists, including radiologists, neurosurgeons, neurologists, and cardiologists. Because the nomenclature can be confusing, the term "surgeon" is used here to refer to the physician performing the procedure. In the future, these specialists will refer to themselves as neurointerventional surgeons.

K.C. Liu, MD (✉)
Departments of Neurological Surgery and Radiology, University of Virginia Health System, Charlottesville, VA, USA
e-mail: KCL3J@hscmail.mcc.virginia.edu

L.E. Guidone, PA-C
Department of Neurological Surgical, Oregon Health & Science University, Portland, OR, USA

S.L. Barnwell, MD, PhD
Department of Neurological Surgery and Dotter Interventional Institute, Oregon Health & Science University, Portland, OR, USA

A.M. Brambrink and J.R. Kirsch (eds.), *Essentials of Neurosurgical Anesthesia & Critical Care*, DOI 10.1007/978-0-387-09562-2_61,
© Springer Science+Business Media, LLC 2012

Implications for the Neurosurgical Patient

The workhorse of the neuroangiography suite is the biplane fluoroscopy unit, which uses two C-arm X-ray heads to image the patient in two planes, usually orthogonal to each other. These imaging heads are fairly bulky and because the majority of interventional neuroradiology procedures treat pathology in the cranium, the heads are typically centered around the patient's head. As the imaging heads each rotate in two axes, there needs to be sufficient room around the patient's head to accommodate not only the image intensifiers, but the anesthesia machines and associated equipment as well. Three-dimensional imaging is also being used more frequently as the technology becomes more widely available. Acquisition of three-dimensional imaging involves one of the C-arm heads spinning rapidly around the area of interest, typically the head. To avoid inadvertent collision of equipment and traction on tubing, careful planning by both anesthesia, surgical, and radiology technician staff is required to arrange the equipment in a manner that allows for both the anesthesiologist and surgeon to work unencumbered. Careful spacing of IV poles and making sure IV and endotracheal tubing is long enough are ways to do this.

Because the procedures are image-based, live image processing by workstations occurs. This often consists of overlaying digitally processed images over live images. Any patient motion degrades the quality and utility of these overlays and because of this, the surgeons will often request that neuromuscular blockade be used to ensure that patients remain motionless. Oftentimes, when images are being acquired, the surgical team will ask for temporary apnea so that ventilatory chest motion does not degrade the quality study.

Interventional neuroradiologists typically target diseases of the blood vessels in the head and neck. This comprises intracranial aneurysms, arteriovenous malformations (AVMs) of brain, dura, and face, uncontrolled epistaxis, carotid stenosis, and acute ischemic stroke. Treatment of the disease states that can lead to hemorrhages (aneurysms, AVMs) typically involves using an embolic agent to exclude the pathology from normal circulation. These agents can be solid (platinum coils) or liquid (glue polymer). Balloons and stents are used to assist in coil embolization of aneurysms or for revascularization in the carotid or intracranial circulation (i.e., stenosis, vasospasm). Stents are associated with thromboembolic complications if patients are not adequately pre-treated with anti-platelet agents (e.g., aspirin, clopidogrel, ticlodipine). Intravenous heparinization is also used at the time of the intervention to control embolic complications from catheter movement within the arteries.

Common spinal procedures performed in the angiography suite are vertebroplasty and kyphoplasty. These are most commonly used to treat vertebral compression fractures of the thoracic and lumbar spine. Under fluoroscopic guidance, a needle is introduced percutaneously from a posterior approach transpedicular into the vertebral body where cement is then injected. This stabilizes the fracture and typically brings significant pain relief to the patient. Kyphoplasty involves using a balloon to create a cavity prior to cement injection. Because a foreign material is injected, the patient must have received pre-operative antibiotics prior to the case, unlike intracranial interventional procedures where antibiotics are usually not needed.

Concerns and Risks

The majority of neurointerventional procedures are directed towards intracranial vascular pathology, including cerebral aneurysms (ruptured and unruptured), AVMs and fistulas, and diseases of the dural sinuses (thrombosis, stenosis). The procedures often involve the manipulation of micro-guidewires and the navigation of microcatheters through the intracranial circulation. This presents risk to the patient of guidewire perforation or vessel rupture. Unlike open procedures where the vessel is directly visualized, periprocedural hemorrhage or other untoward events can occasionally go unnoticed and may be manifested only by changes in the patient's vital signs. Following an intracranial bleed these can be as subtle as a very transient bradycardic episode or as evident as a brisk Cushing's response. Also, it can be difficult to control unexpected intracranial bleeding in the neuroangiography suite. Sometimes, balloons are used to occlude the point of hemorrhage. Blood pressure should be lowered during periods of acute intracranial hemorrhage. Acute ruptures are also managed by placing an external ventricular drain at the bedside to relieve intracranial pressures. Rarely, extracranial vessel injury may result and manifest as, e.g., retroperitoneal hematoma, which frequently goes undetected until significant compromise of the systemic circulation is encountered.

Even though most of these intracranial interventional procedures are performed with the patient under general anesthesia, the movement of guidewires, catheters, and balloons in the intracranial vessels is very stimulating, as these arteries are highly innervated. Changes in the blood pressure and heart rate are often seen and can be variable from patient to patient. Traction on intracranial arteries often induces a transient bradycardia. Likewise, balloon angioplasty for carotid stenting places pressure on the carotid bulb disrupting vagal tone to the cardiovascular system. The surgeon will often ask for the anesthesiologist to administer an anticholenergic agent (e.g., atropine) prior to dilating the carotid bulb. Even so, carotid angioplasty can cause a severe enough hypotensive state that vasopressor support is needed. These patients will often have atherosclerotic disease in their coronary circulation and need pressor support to avoid cardiac ischemia.

Anesthesia providers are typically located near the patient's airway and need to be cognizant of their proximity to the X-ray tubes. Proper shielding should be worn at all times and distance should be maximized as much as is safely possible without compromising the patient's care.

Key Points

- Patient motion can severely degrade imaging quality and compromise the surgeons' ability to deliver optimal care; the use of neuromuscular blockade should be discussed with the surgeons preoperatively
- Neurovascular structures are exquisitely sensitive to the intraluminal movement of wires and catheters as well as extraluminal traction; unexpected changes in heart rate and blood pressure can occur during manipulation and should be anticipated
- Because direct visualization of vascular structures is impossible, subtle changes in the patient's vital signs can signify the presence of a wire perforation or hemorrhage
- Maintain adequate lead shielding and follow radiation safety guidelines at all times

Suggested Reading

Hurst RW, Rosenwasser RH, editors. Interventional neuroradiology. New York: Informa Healthcare; 2008.
Osborn AG, editor. Diagnostic cerebral angiography. 2nd ed. Philadelphia: Lippincott Williams & Wilkins; 1999.

Chapter 62
Basics of Image Interpretation in Interventional Neuroradiology

Wibke Müller-Forell

Overview

The majority of patients with cerebral vascular diseases, demanding neuroradiological interventions are those, who present with potential life-threatening spontaneous intracranial/intracerebral haemorrhages due to cerebral aneurysms or/and arteriovenous malformations (AVMs) or with cerebral infarction due to intra-arterial thrombi in cerebral arteries. Neuroradiological procedures (interventional neuroradiology) (IN), always, performed in general anaesthesia can be divided into occluding and opening interventions.

Examples of occluding interventions include endovascular occlusion of cerebral aneurysms (with platin-coils, sometimes in a combination with endovascular stent application), AVMs and dural fistula (often performed with a combination of coils and glue administration). The most frequently used glues are *N*-butyl cyanoacrylate (Histoacryl®) or ethylene-vinyl-alcohol combined with dimethyl sulfoxide (DMSO) and tantalum (Onyx®). These procedures should be performed only by experienced neuroradiologists, as they carry the risk for severe complications as for instance intracerebral haemorrhage or ischemic stroke (Table 62.1).

Examples of opening interventions include revascularization by local medical lysis/direct, mechanical removal (aspiration) of embolic thrombi from main cerebral vessels (i.e. endovascular treatment of ischemic stroke) or arterial application of vasodilators in cerebral vessels affected by vasospasm following aneurysmal subarachnoid haemorrhage (SAH).

W. Müller-Forell, MD, PhD (✉)
Institute for Neuroradiology, University Medical Center Johannes Gutenberg University,
Mainz, Germany
e-mail: mueller-forell@neuroradio.klinik.uni-mainz.de

A.M. Brambrink and J.R. Kirsch (eds.), *Essentials of Neurosurgical Anesthesia & Critical Care*, DOI 10.1007/978-0-387-09562-2_62,
© Springer Science+Business Media, LLC 2012

Table 62.1 Overview of diagnostic procedures, therapy (alternative therapy), and complication of neuroradiological interventions (1–3 demand occluding, 4 and 5 opening procedures)

Disease	Diagnostic imaging	Therapy	Complications of NR interventions

1. Cerebral aneurysm	1. CT/CTA
	2. DSA
		Interventional:
		  1. Coiling
			Acute : arterial rupture
			Follow-up: vasos-
			  pasm → interventional
			  procedure (see below)

		2. Coiling + stent Neurosurgical: clipping	
Iatrogenic aneurysm		Interventional: stent	Vessel occlusion

2. AVM	1. MRI/MRA	Interventional:
		  glue/(coils)
			Rupture with intracere-
			  bral haemorrhage and/

	2. DSA	Neurosurgical: extirpation	or CSF disturbance
	3. (CT/CTA)	(Radiation)	

3. Dural fistula	1. CT/CTA
	2. MRI/MRA
		Interventional: glue/
		  coils (venous >
		  arterial approach)
			Rupture
			Intracerebral
			  haemorrhage

	3. *DSA*		CSF disturbance

4. Arterial thrombi/ stenosis	1. CT/CTA	Interventional: local
		  lysis, aspiration
		  of the thrombus,
		  stent (balloon
		  dilatation)
			Failure of recanalization,
			  arterial emboli in
			  distant territory,
			  arterial rupture

	2. DSA	(Conservative: systemic lysis)	

5. Vasospasm	CT/CTA,
	  perfusion map
		Local lysis (papaverine,
		  nimodipine)
		Balloon dilatation
			Arterial rupture

Implications for Neurosurgical Patients

The imaging method of choice in emergency cases is computed tomography (CT). In combination with CT angiography (CTA; CT plus iodinated contrast injection followed by 3D reconstruction to identify vascular pathology or cerebral tumours), computer tomography today allows a quick and exact structural overview, and also helps to diagnose site and size of an aneurysm, presence of space occupying intracerebral haemorrhage, acute CSF disturbance, and existence/extend of perfusion deficits.

The main diagnostic tool for interventional neuroradiological procedures, and still the gold standard in patients with cerebrovascular vascular diseases, is the digital subtraction angiography (DSA). In combination with 3D angiography, DSA allows to determine the exact size, width, and configuration of the neck and dome of cerebral aneurysms.

Table 62.2 Characteristic findings of CT/CTA

	Native CT	CTA	Additional findings
SAH	Hyperdensity of the basal cisterns	Site/width/configuration of the aneurysm	Hydrocephalus caused by CSF disturbance
AVM	– Intracerebral haemorrhage – Density disturbances (caused by combination of enlarged vessels, parenchymal defects)	– Width of the nidus – Enlarged feeding arteries – Enlarged draining veins	Hydrocephalus due to intraventricular haemorrhage
Dural fistula	– Intracerebral haemorrhage – General brain oedema – Uncommon vessels	Uncommon, enlarged (mainly) extracerebral vessels	Hydrocephalus due to venous congestion
Arterial thrombi	Hyperdense vessel sign (basilar, middle cerebral artery)	Vessel occlusion at the site of the thrombus	Malignant brain oedema
Vasospasm	Hypodense territories (infarction)	Narrowed vessels	Perfusion deficit

Magnetic resonance imaging (MRI)/MR angiography is less important in the early phase of emergency care for these patients, but plays an important role in pre-therapeutic imaging of AVMs or in the follow-up of coiled aneurysms.

Independent of the imaging technique used, timely image interpretation by a specialized neuro radiologist is essential to assure the best possible and most immediate therapeutic intervention.

Cerebral Aneurysms

The underlying pathology of spontaneous, non-traumatic SAH is the rupture of a cerebral artery aneurysm. The most common location for a cerebral aneurysm (due to hemodynamic factors) is at the level of Willis. Therefore, with aneurysm rupture, blood commonly collects in basal cisterns. Neuroradiological intervention with the application of multiple individual platinum coils inside the aneurysm is an alternative therapy to neurosurgical clipping (Table 62.2).

On CT acute haemorrhage presents with hyperdensity, in case of SAH in the basal cisterns. Distribution and amount of the SAH may suggest approximate

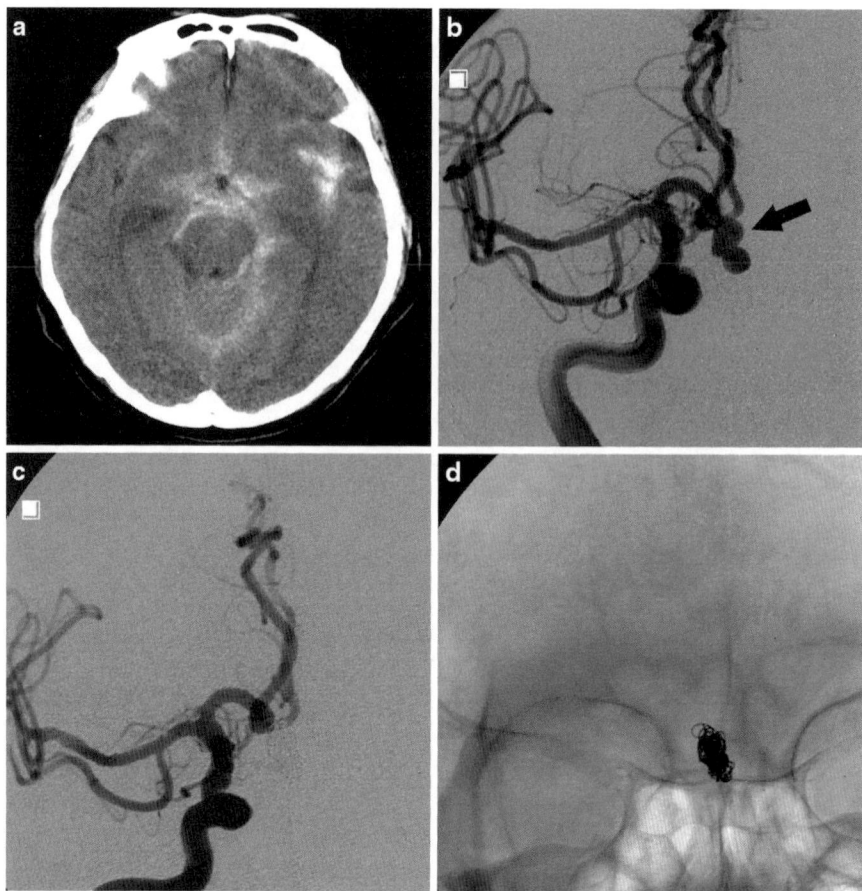

Fig. 62.1 Subarachnoid haemorrhage (SAH). 43-Year-old man with acute headache, meningism, and progressing vigilance deficits. (**a**) Native CT, demonstrating the hyperdensity of the basal cistern, due to acute subarachnoid haemorrhage. (**b**) DSA of the right internal carotid artery in frontal view, demonstrating an aneurysm of the anterior communicating artery (*arrow*). (**c**) Corresponding view after coiling of the aneurysm. (**d**) Corresponding unsubtracted view, showing the coil package

location of the aneurysm, while CTA and DSA (including 3D rotational angiography) confirm the exact size, width, and configuration of the aneurysm neck and dome. This information is critical to allow the clinician to make therapeutic decisions regarding the best approach (i.e. surgery or IN). In the event that the treatment team recommends IN, CTA and DSA are also critical in helping the team determine if a stent should be placed to guarantee the stable delivery and safe placement of the coils inside the aneurysm (Fig. 62.1).

In case of iatrogenic aneurysms, that, although rare, occur as a complication of neurosurgical or ENT operations, occlusion of the leak is usually achieved with covered stents (Fig. 62.2).

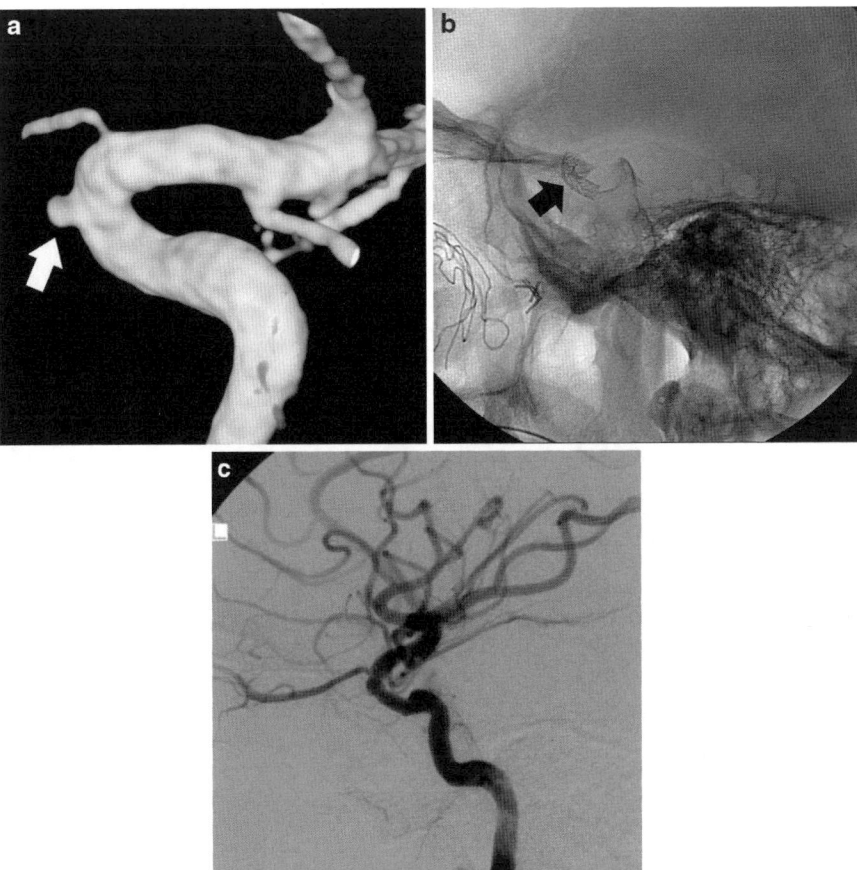

Fig. 62.2 Iatrogenic aneurysm. 24-Year-old woman, who presented with arterial bleeding in the course of an ENT operation (nasal polyposis). (**a**) 3D angiography of the right internal carotid artery. The *arrow* marks the aneurysm at the carotid syphon, due to a fracture of the sphenoid sinus wall. (**b**) Unsubtracted lateral view, demonstrating the stent (*arrow*). (**c**) Corresponding lateral view of the post-interventional DSA showing a nearly normal carotid syphon

Cerebrovascular Vasospasm

Vasospasm, associated with delayed cerebral ischemia, represents a severe (but common) complication in the early (first 2 weeks) postoperative course after aneurismal SAH, and remains a major cause of morbidity and mortality in this patient population. Repeated neurologic examination and monitoring with transcranial Doppler ultrasound, CT perfusion measurements, and CTA are helpful in these patients to guide the need for DSA and intervention. The focus for IN treatment is improvement in cerebral perfusion (as evidenced by vasodilation on angiography, reduction of Doppler blood flow velocities, and improved clinical exam) either by

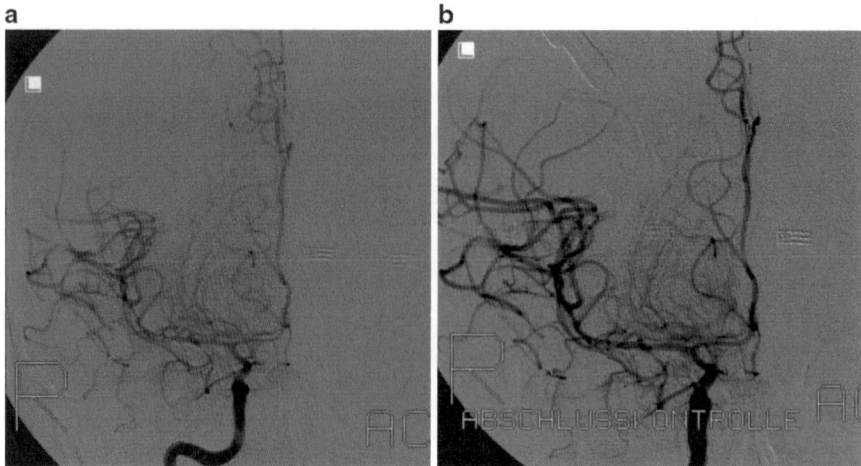

Fig. 62.3 Vasospasm. 56-Year-old woman with bilateral flow acceleration in transcranial Doppler measurements, 5 days after clipping of an ACM aneurysm of the right side. (**a**) DSA of the right ICA, frontal view, demonstrating the marked narrowing of the M1- and A1 segment. (**b**) Corresponding post-interventional view (intra-arterial application of nimodipine plus balloon dilatation), demonstrating the normalization of the calibres of ACM and ACA not only at the main trunks but in the periphery as well

intra-arterial drug administration (e.g. papaverine, verapamil, and nimodipine) or local vessel (balloon) dilatation (Fig. 62.3).

Arteriovenous Malformation

The majority of cerebral AVM are believed to be a congenital disorder, they mainly present with haemorrhage, seizure, chronic headache, or focal neurological deficits. The pathological substrate is the lack of capillaries, leading to a compact or diffuse network of channels interposed between feeding arteries and draining veins, the so-called nidus, the target of the occlusion with glue, which is frequently followed by surgical resection. On MRI, the nidus presents as an area of intraparenchymal pathological vessels; on DSA as a convolution of enlarged arteries and draining veins (Fig. 62.4). Especially in complex AVMs, neuroradiological interventions mainly are preoperative procedures to minimize the size of the AVM nidus by intra-arterial embolization with glue.

Dural arteriovenous fistula (DAVF) (syn. dural arteriovenous malformation [DAVM]) are rare lesions, are characterized by abnormal connections (shunts) between arterial and venous intradural vessels, mainly located in the skull base. Their clinical presentation depends on the venous drainage pattern. Especially in the more benign types of DAVM, where non-invasive imaging (CT, MRI, and MRA) may not have adequate diagnostic sensitivity, the gold standard of identification,

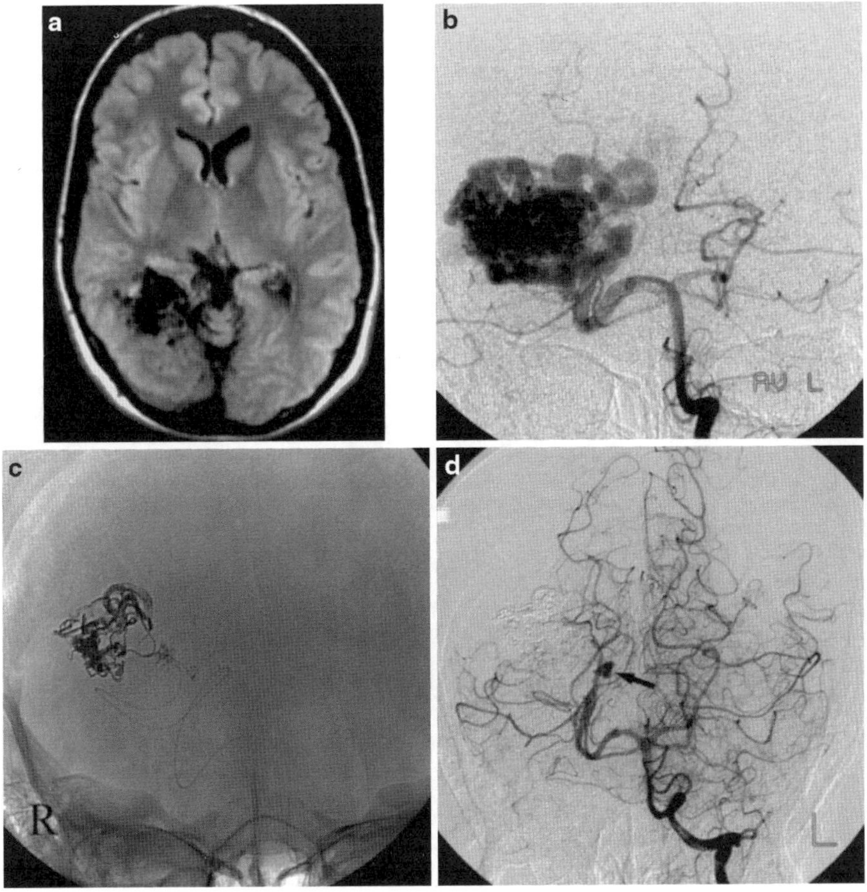

Fig. 62.4 Arteriovenous malformation (AVM). 30-Year-old woman with acute homonymous hemianopia to the left. (**a**) T2-weighted (T2w) axial MRI showing the nidus of the AVM in the right occipital lobe. (**b**) DSA of the left vertebral artery in frontal view. Note the enlarged diameter of the right posterior cerebral artery in comparison to the left, due to high arteriovenous shunt volume. (**c**) Corresponding unsubtracted view, where the way of the microcatheter to the nidus is apparent. Note the (radiologically marked) glue in the nidus. (**d**) Corresponding frontal view after neurointervention (transarterial glue application) demonstrating a small, flow-related aneurysm (*arrow*) of the distal perimesencephalic segment (P3) of the posterior cerebral artery (PCA), as the only pathological remnant

analysis, and classification of the lesion is DSA. Indication for IN treatment (Fig. 62.5), with the target of occlusion of the shunt area(s), performed either by transvenous application of coils into the affected sinus or transarterial application of glue, depends on the prognosis of the disease. The main indication for interventional therapy is a venous drainage into superficial cerebral veins, as this finding harbours the risk of intracerebral haemorrhage, due to venous congestion.

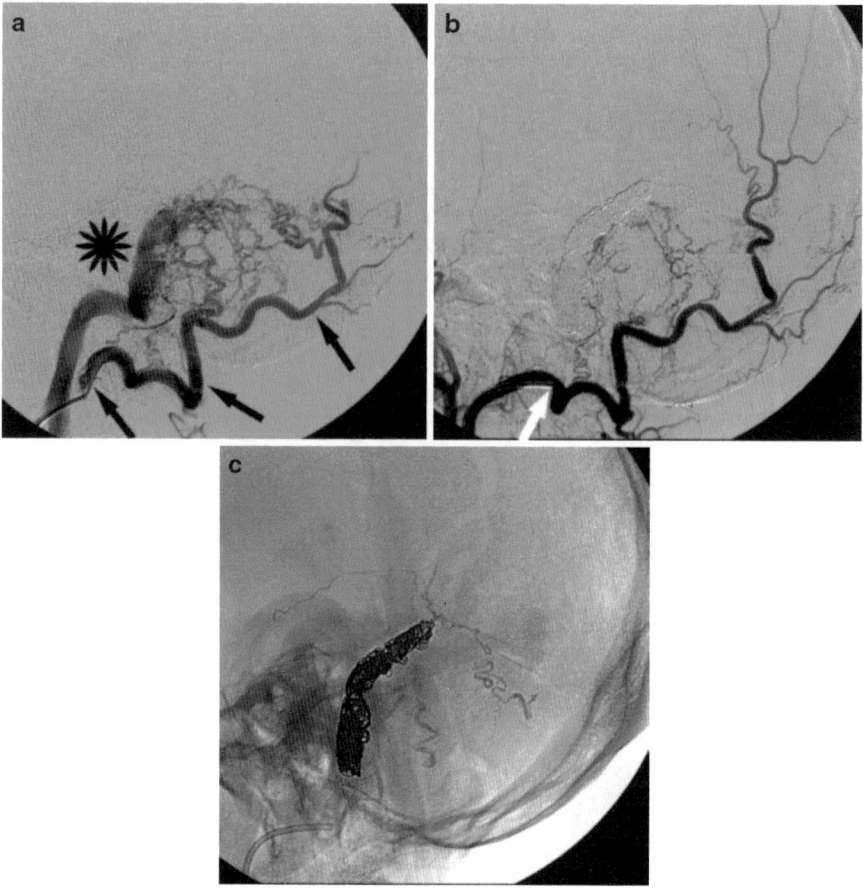

Fig. 62.5 Dural fistula. DSA of a 64-year-old man with pulsatile tinnitus of the left side. (**a**) Lateral view of the left occipital artery (*arrows*), showing the extent of the involved part of the sigmoid sinus with intradural arteries, shunting the ipsilateral sigmoid sinus (*star*), and the jugular bulb. (**b**) Post-interventional corresponding view (transvenous coiling of the sigmoid sinus plus intra-arterial glue). No av shunts are seen, although some enlarged collaterals are still apparent (the *white arrow* marks the end of the catheter in the occipital artery). (**c**) Corresponding unsubtracted view, demonstrating the coils in the entire sigmoid sinus and glue in some feeding arteries

Arterial Thrombosis (Ischemic Stroke)

Depending on the size of intra-arterial thrombi, a main trunk of cerebral vessels may be occluded, leading to an infarction of the cerebral territory. On CT, the thrombus may be apparent due to its hyperdensity (positive vessel sign) (Fig. 62.6), sometimes with additional slight hypodensity of the affected vessel territory.

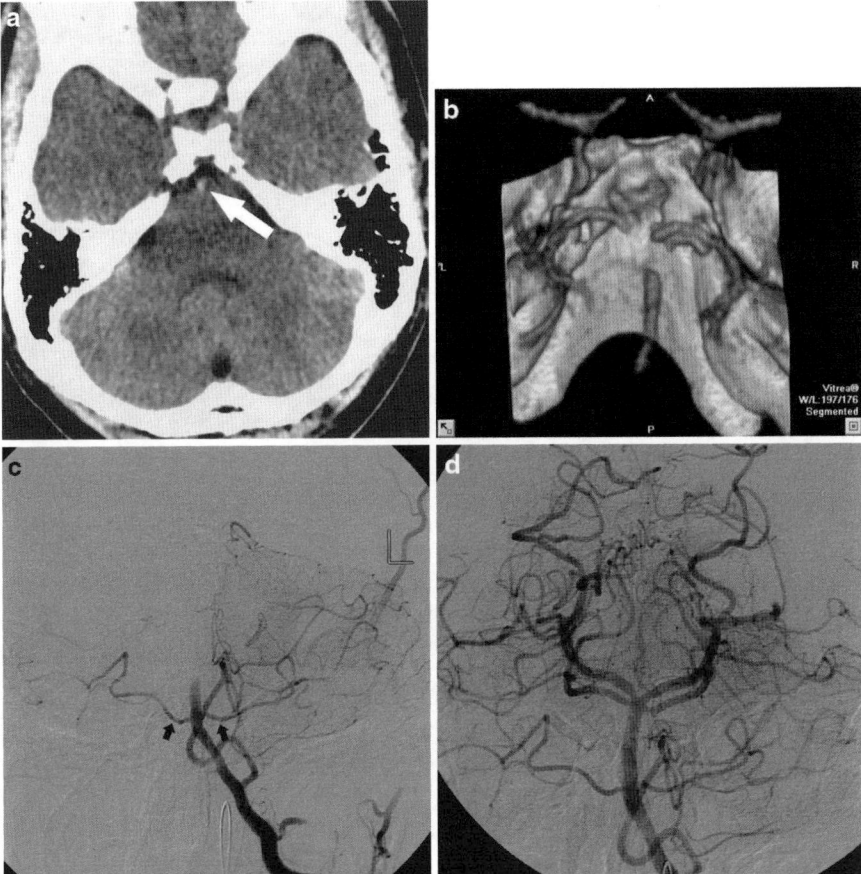

Fig. 62.6 Thrombosis of the basilar artery. 36-Year-old man with acute vigilance deficit, and horizontal nystagmus. (**a**) Native axial CT. The hyperdensity (*arrow*) is due to the thrombus in the basilar artery (*positive vessel sign*). (**b**) 3D-CTA (pa view) demonstrating the closed distal part of the basilar artery. (**c**) DSA of the left vertebral artery with KM-stop of the basilar artery distal to the branching of both inferior cerebellar arteries (AICA) (*small arrows*). (**d**) Corresponding post-interventional view (aspiration of the thrombus) with complete filling of the arteries of the basilar territory (both superior cerebellar and posterior cerebral arteries)

The consequence of untreated basilar thrombosis is severe morbidity, or even death of the patient. This is known too in the course of a thrombotic occlusion of the main trunk of the middle cerebral artery (MCA), as the natural history of brain swelling leads to brain herniation and death (so-called malignant infarction). The target of IN intervention is the recanalization performed either with intra-arterial application of thrombolytic agents or direct aspiration of the thrombus (Fig. 62.7).

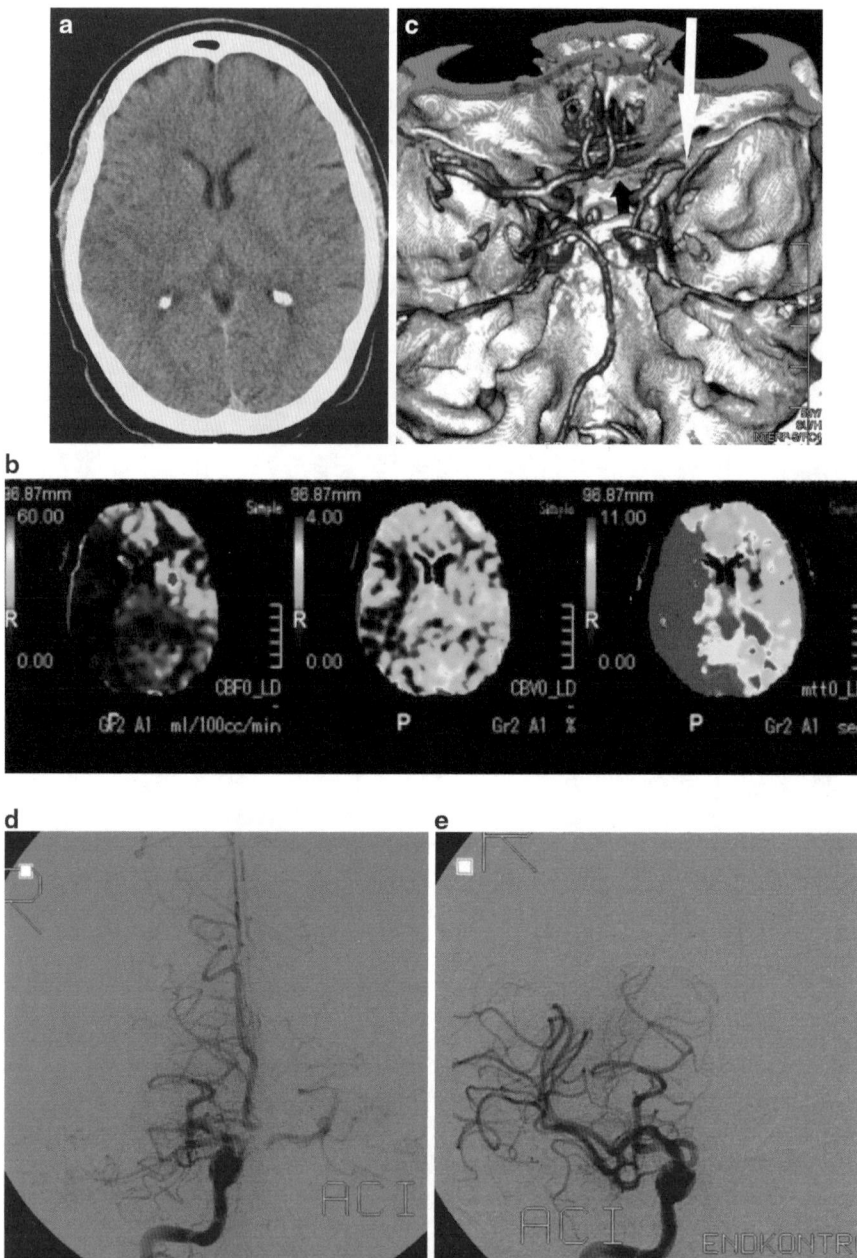

Fig. 62.7 Thrombosis of the MCA. 60-Year-old man with acute hemiplegia of the left side (time window: 1.5 h). (**a**) Native CT with slight hypodensity of the right territory of the medial cerebral artery (MCA): Note the effacement of the grey and white matter distinction of the insular, basal ganglia, and fronto-temporal region with slight narrowing of the cortical sulci, compared with the left hemisphere, as early signs of infarction. (**b**) CT-perfusion map, demonstrating the different

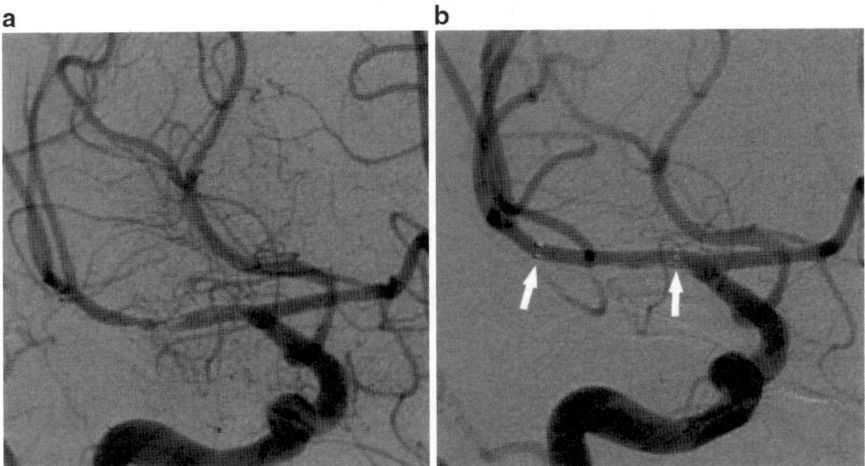

Fig. 62.8 Atherosclerotic stenosis of the MCA. DSA of an 81-year-old woman with recurrent embolic infarction of the MCA territory, suggested to arise from an M1 stenosis, seen on MR angiography (not shown). (**a**) Frontal view with narrowing of the distal M1 segment of the right MCA. (**b**) Corresponding view after placement of the stent (*white arrows*)

An increasing indication for IN intervention is stenting of intracerebral stenosis mainly of the basilar or medial cerebral artery (Fig. 62.8), to avoid total occlusion with subsequent fatal course of territorial infarction.

Concerns and Risks

As a substantial part of neuroradiological interventions concern life-threatening diseases and are frequently emergency procedures (especially in patients with cerebral artery thrombosis or symptomatic vasospasm, which need immediate endovascular intervention), timely IN is mandatory in every case. Although IN may provide life-saving treatment, many of these procedures are associated with significant risk of complications, including rupture of a main artery and embolism from glue, particles, and coils.

Fig. 62.7 (continued) areas of perfusion parameters with a related mismatch: elongated mean transit time (MTT) (*right*), reduced cerebral blood flow (CBF) (*left*), but relatively small reduction of cerebral blood volume (CBV) (*middle*). (**c**) 3D-CTA with complete occlusion of the left (MCA) (*white arrow*). Note the hyoplasia of the left anterior cerebral artery (ACA) (*small black arrow*). (**d**) DSA of the right ICA (ap view) with complete loss of vascularization of the media territory, but filling of the small, hyoplastic ACA, and ipsilateral posterior cerebral artery (PCA) via posterior communicating artery (Pcom). (**e**) Corresponding post-interventional DSA (intra-arterial application of r-tPA and aspiration of the thrombus) with recanalization of the media territory, but (due to normalization of the intravascular pressure) lack of contrast in the ACA, which was seen in the filling of the contralateral ICA (not shown)

Key Points

- Neuroradiological interventions concern life-threatening diseases and are frequently emergency procedures.
- Amendable to neuroradiologic intervention are patients with cerebrovascular aneurysms (coiling/stenting), arteriovenous malformations (gluing/coiling), cerebral artery thrombosis (clot removal), vascular stenosis (angioplasty, stenting), and cerebral vasospasm (intra-arterial vasodilators).
- While often life-saving many procedures are associated with significant risk of complications, including intracranial haemorrhage due to vascular injury and ischemic stroke secondary to embolism from dislodged coils or glue.
- Neurointerventional procedures basically can be divided into occluding (coiling and glue) and opening interventions (thrombus aspiration, intra-arterial vasodilators).
- Although CT/CTA and MRI/MRA plus computerized 3D reconstruction are emerging techniques, DSA remains the main diagnostic tool and gold standard in cerebrovascular diseases.
- Timely image interpretation by a specialized neuroradiologist is essential to assure the best possible and most immediate therapeutic intervention.

Suggested Reading

Cognard C, Spelle L, Pierot L. Pial arteriovenous malformations. In: Forsting M, editor. Intracranial malformations and aneurysms. From diagnostic work-up to endovascular therapy. New York: Springer; 2004. p. 39–100.

Gnanalingham KK, Apostolopoulos V, Barazi S, O'Neill K. The impact of the international subarachnoid aneurysm trial (ISAT) on the management of aneurismal subarachnoid hemorrhage in a neurosurgical unit in the UK. Clin Neurol Neurosurg. 2006;108:117–23.

Molyneux A, Kerr R, Stratton I, Sandercock P, Clarke M, Shrimpton J, et al. International Subarachnoid Aneurysm Trial (ISAT) of neurosurgical clipping versus endovascular coiling of 2143 patients with ruptured intracranial aneurysms: a randomised trial. Lancet. 2002;360: 1267–74.

Müller Forell W, Engelhard K. Neuroimaging for the anaesthesiologist. Anesthesiol Clin. 2007;25: 413–39.

Sayama CM, Liu JK, Couldwell WT. Update on endovascular therapy for cerebral vasospasm induced by aneurismal subarachnoid hemorrhage. Neurosurg Focus. 2006;21:E12.

Szikora I. Dural Arteriovenous malformations. In: Forsting M, editor. Intracranial malformations and aneurysms. From diagnostic work-up to endovascular therapy. New York: Springer; 2004. p. 101–42.

Wanke I, Dörfler A, Forsting M. Intracranial aneurysms. In: Forsting M, editor. Intracranial malformations and aneurysms. From diagnostic work-up to endovascular therapy. New York: Springer; 2004. p. 143–247.

Part XII
Specific Concerns Regarding Anesthesia for Interventional Neuroradiology

Chapter 63
Procedural Challenges in Interventional Neuroradiology

William L. Young

Preventing and responding to procedural complications are perhaps the greatest contribution an anesthesiologist can provide to the care of the patient undergoing interventional neuroradiologic procedures. Below we discuss two of the most important occurrences requiring expert input from the anesthetist (see Table 63.1).

Acute Occlusive Ischemia

Overview

During acute arterial occlusion, usually the only immediate way to improve perfusion of territories distal to the occluded site is by increasing collateral blood flow. This must be done by overcoming collateral cerebrovascular resistance. Although theoretically possible by selective vasodilation of collateral resistance vessels, practically the only choice currently available is to drive collateral perfusion pressure by increasing the systemic arterial blood pressure.

There are two primary sources of collateral pathways in the cerebral circulation. The Circle of Willis is a primary collateral pathway, composed of the large interlocking vessels at the base of the brain. However, in as many as 21% of otherwise normal subjects, the circle may not be complete. There are also secondary collateral channels that bridge adjacent major vascular territories, e.g., pial vessels at the border zones of the territories subserved by the long circumferential arteries that supply the hemispheric convexities. These pathways are known as the pial-to-pial or leptomeningeal collateral pathways.

W.L. Young, MD (✉)
Departments of Anesthesia and Perioperative Care, Neurological Surgery and Neurology, University of California, San Francisco, CA, USA
e-mail: YoungW@Anesthesia.ucsf.edu

A.M. Brambrink and J.R. Kirsch (eds.), *Essentials of Neurosurgical Anesthesia & Critical Care*, DOI 10.1007/978-0-387-09562-2_63, © Springer Science+Business Media, LLC 2012

Table 63.1 Management of intracranial catastrophes[a]

Initial resuscitation:
Communicate with endovascular therapy team
Assess need for assistance; call for assistance
Secure airway ventilate with 100% O_2
Determine if problem is hemorrhagic or occlusive
Hemorrhagic: immediate heparin reversal (1 mg protamine for each 100 units of heparin given) and low normal mean arterial pressure
Occlusive: deliberate hypertension, titrated to neurologic exam, angiography or physiologic imaging studies; or to clinical context
Further resuscitation:
Head up 15° in neutral position, if possible[b]
$PaCO_2$ manipulation consistent with clinical setting, otherwise normocapnia
Mannitol 0.5 g/kg, rapid i.v. infusion
Titrate i.v. induction agent (thiopental or propofol) to EEG burst suppression
Passive cooling to 33–34°C
Consider ventriculostomy for treatment or monitoring of increased ICP
Consider anticonvulsants, e.g., phenytoin or phenobarbital

[a]These are only general recommendations and drug doses which must be adapted to specific clinical situations and in accordance with a patient's preexisting medical condition. In some cases of asymptomatic or minor vessel puncture or occlusion, less aggressive management may be appropriate

[b]This maneuver is a standard one; however, a corresponding decrease in cerebral perfusion pressure results from placing the head in an elevated position above the right atrium

Partial arterial occlusion is usual seen in the case of symptomatic vasospasm after aneurysmal subarachnoid hemorrhage. In addition to the collateral pathways described above, there is also the residual lumen of the spastic vessel, which usually remains patent to a variable degree. Therefore, increasing proximal arterial pressure will also serve to minimize the pressure drop across the stenotic vessel segment. Direct intra-arterial vasodilators are commonly used to treat vasospasm, as well as balloon angioplasty. In the pretreatment phase, induced hypertension may be the only temporizing method available to improve tissue perfusion.

Prevention

Other than careful control of anticoagulation, a shared responsibility (see below), prevention of acute occlusive ischemia per se is generally not under the anesthetist's control. Rather, it is tied to the interventionalist's technique and a patient's particular anatomical and physiological circumstances. However, the potential harm caused by any instance of ischemia might be mitigated with certain preparatory considerations or maneuvers on the part of the anesthetist.

To effectively augment blood pressure, one must have a clear sense of what a particular patient's normal baseline blood pressure is. A sense of both the normal average blood pressures at which a patient functions, as well as the range of blood pressures that are tolerated, are useful benchmarks.

For procedures involving the blood supply to the CNS, beat-to-beat blood pressure monitoring is necessary, considering the rapid-time constants in this setting for changes in systemic or cerebral hemodynamics. In those cases, where intra-arterial catheters are used, the concordance between blood pressure cuff and intra-arterial readings needs to be considered; preoperative blood pressure range is likely only to be known through blood pressure cuff values. One may over- or underestimate the true normal for a given patient if only intra-arterial measurements are used without consideration of cuff pressures.

Relative normocapnia or mild hypocapnia (33–35 mmHg) consistent with the safe conduct of positive pressure ventilation should be maintained during procedures involving the cerebrovascular tree. Although there are theoretical reasons why hypocapnia might be useful in augmenting collateral perfusion pressure, it is unpredictable (hypocapnia induces "inverse steal phenomena," decreasing blood flow to normal tissue, while accentuating blood flow to abnormal tissue). If a patient has increased intracranial pressure, prophylactic moderate hypocapnia may be indicated.

There is no clear superiority of one modern anesthetic over another in terms of pharmacological protection against ischemic injury. The specific choice of anesthesia may be guided primarily by other cardio- and cerebrovascular considerations, not the least of which is the facility with which one can effectively maintain arterial blood pressure. An argument could be made for avoiding N_2O because of the possibility of introducing air emboli into the cerebral circulation during endovascular procedures, and also because of reports that it worsens outcome after experimental brain injury.

Crisis Management

In the setting of vascular occlusion, the goal is to increase distal perfusion by blood pressure augmentation. Blood pressure augmentation is a *temporizing measure*. Definitive treatment requires removal of the obstructing clot or hardware, thrombolysis, intra-arterial vasodilators, and/or balloon angioplasty.

The extent to which the blood pressure has to be raised depends on the condition of the patient and the nature of the disease. The endpoints would be classed generally as (1) empiric, (2) cerebrovascular, and (3) cardiac.

In most settings, deliberate hypertension entails increasing systemic blood pressure, which is raised by 30–40% above the baseline. In the absence of other endpoints, such an increase would be an empiric target.

Positive cerebrovascular endpoints would include findings such as resolution of ischemic symptoms in an awake patient or imaging evidence of improved perfusion.

Improved perfusion is unlikely to be measured directly, as this would require being in a tomographic imaging device such as a CT, MR or PET scanner, or possibly in one of few centers that utilize 2-D isotope methods to measure CBF, e.g., 133-Xe. Angiography is unreliable in determining tissue perfusion. Although not sensitive to changes in perfusion, gross absence of opacification after adequate contract injection is a specific indicator of inadequate flow. Negative endpoints would be worsening symptoms or perfusion, consistent with acute hemorrhage or brain swelling.

Cardiac endpoints are negative ones and represent adverse events. Most typically, the EKG and ST segment monitor should be carefully inspected for signs of myocardial ischemia. Other adverse endpoints would be the appearance of arrhythmias, e.g., ectopy, escape beats, or bradycardia. The level of blood pressure augmentation can be titrated against cerebral and cardiac endpoints.

Increasing systemic vascular resistance is the most rapid and effective way to augment blood pressure. It is, however, predicated on adequate preload. Therefore, euvolemia is essential for the conduct of induced hypertension. Phenylephrine is usually the first-line agent for deliberate hypertension and is titrated to achieve the desired level of blood pressure. However, in patients with low baseline heart rates, other sympathomimetic agents may be used. If myocardial dysfunction is present, an inotrope may be appropriate. This may be particularly important in patients with a recent SAH and the attendant neurocardiac injury. Improving cardiac output per se does not improve cerebral perfusion unless a low output state causes arterial hypotension, venous hypertension, or sympathetic constriction of large conductance vessels supplying the brain.

In most patients, in most settings, the amount of time needed to definitively treat the vascular occlusion should be minutes to hours, such that the adverse effects of central and peripheral vasoconstriction should not adversely affect other organ systems. In addition to cardiac monitoring, careful monitoring of renal function during periods of vasoconstrictor therapy would seem prudent.

The risk of causing hemorrhage into an ischemic area must be weighed against the benefits of improving perfusion, but augmentation of blood pressure in the face of acute cerebral ischemia is probably protective or therapeutic in most settings. How long does it take for the blood brain barrier to become disrupted after an acute ischemic event? This is difficult to predict clinically, but in the face of ongoing ischemia, the benefit of preventing an infraction most probably outweighs the risk of promoting vasogenic edema or causing hemorrhage in the acute setting.

There is also a risk of rupturing an aneurysm or AVM with induction of hypertension. There are no data that speak to this directly. For intracranial aneurysms, older case series report rupture during anesthetic induction in the range of about 1%, presumably due to acute hypertension. For AVMs, cautious extrapolation of observations for head-frame application suggests the rarity of AVM rupture from acute blood pressure increases.

Key Points

- In symptomatic patients, it is common to induce generous increases above baseline MAP in the range of 30–50%.
- Specific endpoints would be an improvement in neurological status in an awake patient, or some imaging evidence of improved perfusion.
- The EKG should be monitored carefully for signs of myocardial ischemia.
- If the patient has an unsecured intracranial aneurysm that has recently ruptured or has another form of intracranial, this target may be tempered.
- Phenylephrine is the most widely used and versatile agent, but other agents may be chosen given mitigating circumstances, e.g., low-resting heart rate.
- If myocardial dysfunction is present from neurogenic injury, addition of an inotrope may be appropriate.

Cerebral Hemorrhage

Overview

Intracranial hemorrhage (ICH) is an ever-present complication of interventional imaging or manipulation of the cerebral circulation. This may derive from a technical complication, a delayed response to an ischemic injury or a part of the natural history of the type of cerebrovascular disease being evaluated and treated, e.g., vascular malformations such as intracranial aneurysms or arteriovenous malformations. The anesthesiologist should be prepared for vascular malformation rupture at all times. The morbidity and mortality of intra-procedural rupture is high.

Cerebral hemorrhages in the interventional suite can be classified as: (a) natural history bleeds from disease, i.e., vascular malformations, which are unrelated to the procedure; (b) anatomic trespass, i.e., the rupture of a blood vessel or malformation; (c) post-reperfusion hemorrhage. The acute management is similar for all types in terms of initial resuscitation.

Regarding the first two types of bleeds, whether an instance of ICH is due to a natural history event or some technical misadventure is not always knowable. The third type of bleeding – post-reperfusion – can come from reperfusing an area distal to an acute or chronic occlusion. It may also occur after closure of a significant arteriovenous shunt, such as after the treatment of an arteriovenous malformation, dural a-v fistula, or carotid cavernous fistula.

In acute occlusive stroke, it is possible to recanalize the occluded vessel by superselective intra-arterial thrombolytic therapy. Thrombolytic agents can be delivered in high concentration by a microcatheter navigated close to the clot. Neurological deficits may be reversed without additional risk of secondary hemorrhage if treatment is completed within several hours from the onset of carotid territory ischemia, and somewhat longer in vertebrobasilar territory. Intra-arterial thrombolysis is currently an "off label" use. Despite an increased frequency of early symptomatic hemorrhagic complications, treatment with intra-arterial pro-urokinase within 6 h of the onset of acute ischemic stroke with MCA occlusion significantly improved clinical outcome at 90 days.

A newer and promising approach is the use of mechanical retrieval devices to physically remove the offending thromboembolic material from the intracranial vessel. Such devices appear to be efficacious in recanalizing occluded vessels, and early restoration of flow appears to reduce the volume of infracted brain.

Both t-PA and mechanical retrieval have an inherent risk of promoting hemorrhagic transformation, just as in the case of intravenous thrombolysis. This is an important area for investigation because hemorrhagic transformation, or its threat, has great impact on clinical practice. t-PA promotes expression and activity of matrix metalloproteinase-9 (MMP-9), a key protease for tissue remodeling involved in various kinds of vascular injury that can damage the neurovascular unit and promote hemorrhage. t-PA can increase MMP-9 expression in the brain endothelium, acting through the low-density lipoprotein receptor-related protein (LRP), and promotes upregulation after focal cerebral ischemia. Patient MMP-9 plasma levels are also increased after treatment.

Prevention

Anticoagulation is used prophylactically for acute management during cases of intracranial catheter navigation to minimize thromboembolic complications. Anticoagulation is also an important component of the management of various forms of cerebrovascular disease. Understanding the approaches to anticoagulation is important to rationally manage its emergent reversal.

Heparin is routinely used for procedural anticoagulation. Generally, after a baseline-activated clotting time (ACT) is obtained, intravenous heparin (70 U/kg) is given to a target prolongation of 2–3 times of baseline. Then heparin is given continuously or as an intermittent bolus with hourly monitoring of ACT.

Heparin-induced thrombocytopenia (HIT) is a rare but important adverse event for heparin anticoagulation. Development of heparin-dependent antibodies after initial exposure leads to a prothrombotic syndrome. In high-risk patients, direct thrombin inhibitors can be used. Direct thrombin inhibitors inhibit free and clot-bound thrombin, and their effect can be monitored by either aPTT or ACT. Lepirudin and bivalirudin, a synthetic derivative, have half-lives of 40–120 min and about 25 min, respectively. Because these drugs undergo renal elimination, dose adjustments may be needed in patients with renal dysfunction. Argatroban is an alternative agent that undergoes primarily hepatic metabolism.

Antiplatelet agents (aspirin, the glycoprotein IIb/IIIa receptor antagonists, and the thienopyridine derivatives) are increasingly being used for cerebrovascular disease management. Although still controversial, they may be of use for acute treatment of thromboembolic complications. Abciximab ReoPro has been used to treat thromboembolic complications. Abciximab, eptifibatide, and tirofiban are glycoprotein IIb/IIIa receptor antagonists. Activation of the platelet membrane glycoprotein (GP) IIb/IIIa leads to fibrinogen binding and is a final common pathway for platelet aggregation.

The long duration and potent effect of Abciximab also increase the likelihood of major bleeding. The smaller molecule agents, eptifibatide and tirofiban, are competitive blockers and have a shorter half-life of about 2 h. Thienopyridine derivatives (ticlopidine and clopidogrel) bind to the platelet's ADP receptors and permanently alter the receptor; therefore, the duration of action is the life span of the platelet. The addition of clopidogrel to the antiplatelet regimen is commonly used for procedures that require placement of hardware (e.g., stents, coiling, or stent-assisted coiling) primarily in patients who have not had an acute event, such as unruptured aneurysms.

Crisis Management

In conscious patients, bleeding catastrophes are usually heralded by headache, nausea, vomiting, and vascular pain related to the area of perforation. Sudden loss of consciousness is not always due to ICH. Seizures, as a result of contrast reaction or transient ischemia, and the resulting post-ictal state, can also result in an obtunded patient. In the anesthetized or comatose patient, the sudden onset of bradycardia and hypertension (Cushing response) or the endovascular therapist's diagnosis of extravasation of contrast may be the only clues to a developing hemorrhage.

If an ICH occurs, anticoagulation must be immediately reversed. Heparin may be reversed with protamine. Since there is no specific antidote for the direct thrombin inhibitors or the antiplatelet agents, platelet transfusion is a nonspecific therapy, should reversal be indicated. There is no currently available accurate test to measure platelet function in patients taking the newer antiplatelet drugs. Desmopressin (DDAVP) has been reported to shorten the prolonged bleeding time of individuals taking antiplatelet agents such as aspirin and ticlopidine. There are also increasing recent reports on using specific clotting factors, including recombinant factor VIIa and factor IX complex, to rescue severe life-threatening bleeding, including ICH uncontrolled by standard transfusion therapy. The safety and efficacy of these coagulation factors remain to be investigated. Prothrombotic effects of factor VIIa is of particular concern.

In a significant bleeding event, the airway must be secured and ventilation controlled using 100% O_2 and mild hyperventilation until the extent of the mass effect is clear. A Cushing response (hypertension and bradycardia) may develop. CPP should be maintained at adequate levels.

Most cases of vascular rupture can be managed in the angiography suite. Most vascular perforations do require interventional treatment, although occasionally glues or coils will be used to seal off the rupture site. The procedure can be aborted or brought to a stable intermediate point along the spectrum of treatment. If needed, a ventriculostomy catheter may be placed emergently in the angiography suite. Some authors even suggest that ventriculostomy catheters should be placed prior to the procedure in selected high-risk patients, i.e., those with ventriculomegaly. Postprocedure, patients with suspected rupture will require a CT scan, but emergent craniotomy is usually not indicated.

All types of reperfusion settings probably result in some degree of cerebral hyperemia, for both ischemic stroke treatment and vascular malformation obliteration. This hyperemia is probably exacerbated by uncontrolled increases in systemic arterial blood pressure. In the absence of collateral perfusion pressure inadequacy, fastidious attention to preventing hypertension is warranted. Complicated cases may go first to CT or some other kind of tomographic imaging; critical care management may need to be extended during transport and imaging. Symptomatic hyperemic complications are more uncommon than "silent" hyperemic states; with the use of more sensitive MR imaging, ischemic events are probably more common than previously suspected.

Key Points

- ICH is an ever-present complication of interventional imaging or manipulation of the cerebral circulation.
- ICH may derive from a technical complication, a delayed response to an ischemic injury or as part of the natural history of the type of cerebrovascular disease being evaluated and treated. The acute management is similar for all types in terms of initial resuscitation.
- Bleeding catastrophes are usually heralded by headache, nausea, vomiting, and vascular pain related to the area of perforation. In the anesthetized or comatose patient, the sudden onset of bradycardia and hypertension (Cushing response) or the endovascular therapist's diagnosis of extravasation of contrast may be the only clues to a developing hemorrhage.
- If an ICH occurs, anticoagulation must be immediately reversed. Protamine can be used for heparin, but since there is no specific antidote for the direct thrombin inhibitors or the antiplatelet agents, platelet transfusion is a nonspecific therapy, should reversal be indicated.
- Most cases of vascular rupture can be managed in the angiography suite. The INR team can attempt to seal the rupture site endovascularly and abort the procedure; a ventriculostomy catheter may be placed emergently in the angiography suite.
- All types of reperfusion settings probably result in some degree of cerebral hyperemia, for both ischemic stroke treatment and vascular malformation obliteration. This hyperemia is probably exacerbated by uncontrolled increases in systemic arterial blood pressure. In the absence of collateral perfusion pressure inadequacy, fastidious attention to preventing hypertension is warranted.

Acknowledgments   The authors would like to thank the members of the UCSF Brain AVM Study Project and the Center for Cerebrovascular Research (http://www.avm.ucsf.edu) for the opportunities to learn more about cerebrovascular disease and anesthetic management; John Pile-Spellman, Lotfi Hacein-Bey, Lawrence Litt, Tomoki Hashimoto, Chanhung Z. Lee, Michael T. Lawton, Randall T. Higashida, and Van Halbach for their insights and collaboration on efforts to advance knowledge in this area.

Suggested Reading

Connolly Jr ES, Lavine SD, Meyers PM, Palistrandt D, Parra A, Mayer SA. Intensive care unit management of interventional neuroradiology patients. Neurosurg Clin N Am. 2005;16: 541–5, vi.

Drummond JC, Patel PM. Neurological anesthesia. In: Miller RD, Eriksson LI, Fleisher LA, Wiener-Kronish JP, Young WL, editors. Miller's Anesthesia, vol. 2, chapter 63. 7th ed. Philadelphia: Churchill Livingstone, 2009. p. 2045–87.

See JJ, Manninen PH. Anesthesia for neuroradiology. Curr Opin Anaesthesiol. 2005;18:437–41.

Tsuji K, Aoki T, Tejima E, Arai K, Lee SR, Atochin DN, et al. Tissue plasminogen activator promotes matrix metalloproteinase-9 upregulation after focal cerebral ischemia. Stroke. 2005;36:1954–9.

Young WL. Anesthesia for endovascular neurosurgery and interventional neuroradiology. Anesthesiol Clin. 2007;25:391–412.

Young WL, Pile-Spellman J. Anesthetic considerations for interventional neuroradiology. Anesthesiology. 1994;80:427–56.

Young WL, Dowd CF. Interventional neuroradiology: anesthetic management. In: Cottrell JE, Young WL, editors. Cottrell and Young's Neuroanesthesia, chapter 14. 5th ed. Philadelphia: Mosby Elsevier, 2010. p. 247–63.

Chapter 64
Anesthesiological Challenges During Neuroradiological Interventions

Michael Aziz and Ansgar M. Brambrink

Anesthesiologists are asked with increasing frequency to assist with cases involving interventional neuroradiology (INR). The anesthesia team should be aware of potential complications. Rarely, problems such as stroke from coil dislodgement, glue embolization, cranial vessel dissection, acute hemorrhage from occult large vessel dissection, undiagnosed coagulopathy, groin hematoma, and reperfusion edema may occur. This section will focus on three more common complications associated with neuroradiologic procedures: (1) acute reactions to contrast medium, (2) contrast-induced nephropathy, and (3) periprocedural arterial hypertension.

Contrast Reactions

Overview

Intravascular contrast medium facilitates visualization of neurovascular structures. Administration of contrast agents can cause severe complications. For all settings the estimated incidence of adverse reactions is 5–8%. The incidence of life-threatening reactions is 1 in 1,000–2,000 examinations, and fatal reactions have been reported.

M. Aziz, MD (✉)
Department of Anesthesiology and Perioperative Medicine,
Oregon Health & Science University, Portland, OR, USA
e-mail: azizm@ohsu.edu

A.M. Brambrink, MD, PhD
Departments of Anesthesiology and Perioperative Medicine, Neurology and Neurologic Surgery,
Oregon Health & Science University, Portland, OR, USA

A.M. Brambrink and J.R. Kirsch (eds.), *Essentials of Neurosurgical Anesthesia & Critical Care*, DOI 10.1007/978-0-387-09562-2_64,
© Springer Science+Business Media, LLC 2012

Reactions to contrast media are classified as anaphylactoid or chemotoxic. Anaphylactoid reactions occur at certain threshold levels and are not dose-dependent. Contrast can cause direct release of histamine from mast cells or can activate complement, but the exact mechanism of reaction is poorly understood. Anaphylactoid reactions present as nausea, urticaria, bronchospasm, angioedema, laryngospasm, hypotension, or seizures. Patients at higher risk for anaphylactoid reactions are those with a history of multiple allergies, asthma, or previous reaction to contrast media.

Chemotoxic reactions result from chemical effects of the agent on the vessel or organ perfused. These reactions are dose-dependent (i.e., increased dose; repeated administration = increased likelihood). Types of chemotoxic reactions include fluid shifts due to the hyperosmolar nature of media and renal toxic effects (discussed further below). Patients at risk for these chemotoxic reactions are those with significant medical comorbidities. Patients with renal and cardiovascular disease are at particular risk due to the effects of fluid shifting and nephropathy.

Prevention

Preparation is paramount to prevention and appropriate treatment of contrast reactions. Administer contrast to patients only in settings equipped for cardiopulmonary resuscitation with skilled providers who know the patient's medical history.

Patients at risk for anaphylactoid reactions should be pretreated with adequate hydration, corticosteroids, and histamine-blocking agents.

Patients at risk for chemotoxic reactions should be adequately hydrated throughout and particularly after administration of contrast. When possible, use lower osmolality, nonionic contrast media. The minimum amount of contrast medium necessary should be administered. Patients at risk for renal complications are discussed below.

Crisis Management

Table 64.1 summarizes the key treatment strategies for contrast reactions.

Table 64.1 Key treatment strategies for contrast reactions

Reaction	Treatment	Potential adverse effects
Nausea/vomiting	Ondansetron or other 5HT3 agent	Migraine headache
Urticaria	Diphenhydramine	Drowsiness
	Cimetidine or ranitidine	
Bronchospasm – mild	Supplemental oxygen	
	Albuterol	
	Subcutaneous epinephrine	Tachycardia, hypertension, cardiac dysrhythmias
Bronchospasm – severe	Supplemental oxygen	
	Corticosteroid	
	Albuterol or terbutaline	Tachycardia
	IV epinephrine	Tachycardia, hypertension, potentially malignant cardiac dysrhythmia
Angioedema	Secure airway	Tachycardia, hypertension, potentially malignant cardiac dysrhythmia
	Corticosteroid	
	Epinephrine	
Laryngospasm	Positive pressure ventilation	
	Succinylcholine	Paralysis may require endotracheal intubation (provider skilled in airway management should be readily available)
Vagal Reaction	IV fluids	Fluid overload
	Elevate patient's legs/ Trendelenburg	
	Atropine	Tachycardia, dysrhythmias
Hypotension – mild	IV fluids	Fluid overload
Hypotension – severe	IV fluids	Fluid overload
	Epinephrine	Tachycardia, hypertension, cardiac dysrhythmia
Seizures	Diazepam or other benzodiazepine	Respiratory depression, sedation

Key Points

- Contrast reactions can be classified as anaphylactoid or chemotoxic.
- Patients at risk for anaphylactoid reactions include those with multiple allergies, asthma, or previous reaction to contrast media; patients with medical comorbidities are at risk for chemotoxic reactions.
- In preparation, carefully evaluate the patient and ensure that the facility is equipped for resuscitation and that skilled providers are readily available.
- Reactions can manifest as nausea, bronchospasm, hypotension, or seizures or as large fluid shifts (anaphylactic), and renal toxic effects (chemotoxic).
- Severe reactions should be treated quickly and aggressively according to the manifesting symptoms as some reactions can be fatal.

Contrast-Induced Nephropathy

Overview

Contrast-induced nephropathy is one of the most common causes of renal failure in hospitalized patients. This nephropathy increases morbidity and mortality of the primary disease, prolongs hospitalizations, increases costs, and may lead to long-term hemodialysis requirement. It occurs in 1–15% of all patients undergoing invasive angiography procedures and in as many as 50% of patients with preexisting renal dysfunction or diabetes mellitus. Definition of nephropathy is often a measured serum creatinine ≥25% above baseline or ≥0.5 mg/dL above baseline.

Contrast agents produce renal dysfunction by several mechanisms. Contrast causes an initial dilation of renal vasculature followed by prolonged renal vasoconstriction, which reduces renal blood flow. Reductions in blood flow, as well as direct osmotic toxicity, can cause necrosis of medullary epithelial cells. Subsequent oxidative radical formation injures the renal tubules. Additional mechanisms for nephropathy are thrombo-embolic events during arterial cannulation and catheter manipulation.

Patients at particular risk for contrast-induced nephropathy are summarized in Table 64.2.

Prevention

Multiple interventions have been employed to prevent contrast-induced nephropathy both in patients at risk and as global prophylaxis. While many agents have

Table 64.2 Patients at particular risk for contrast-induced nephropathy

Patient risk factors	• Chronic kidney disease
	• Left ventricular pressure ejection fraction <40%
	• Urgent procedure
	• Congestive heart failure
	• Advanced age
	• Arterial hypertension
	• Low hematocrit
	• Diabetes mellitus
	• Hypovolemia
History of exposure to particular drugs	• Nonsteroidal anti-inflammatory drugs
	• ACE inhibitors/angiotensin receptor blockers
	• Aminoglycoside antibiotics
Contrast-related factors	• Contrast volume
	• Ionic contrast
	• Viscosity
	• Contrast osmolarity

shown some benefit in various experimental models, few agents are proven to have benefits based on human randomized controlled trials. The best prevention likely comes from adequate periprocedure hydration. Table 64.3 summarizes reported interventions, their mechanism, potential side effects and results from related human trials to date.

Crisis Management

The serum creatinine of patients at risk for contrast-induced nephropathy should be followed 24–48 h after the procedure. Those at low risk may be followed for symptoms of renal dysfunction and evaluated subsequently for problems. Any dysrhythmia, difficulty in breathing, change in neurologic status, weight gain, or other sign of fluid overload should be promptly evaluated. A small rise in serum creatinine may be followed by prolonged hospitalization and repeat creatinine measurements. A significant rise in serum creatinine warrants immediate evaluation by a nephrologist as well as strict monitoring of acid/base status, serum electrolytes, and volume status. Treatment should focus on electrolyte and fluid derangements but may also involve some duration of hemodialysis or necessitate even renal transplantation surgery in some cases.

Table 64.3 Reported interventions, mechanisms, effects, clinical investigations

Intervention	Mechanism	Potential adverse effects	Results of clinical investigations
Hydration	Increases renal blood flow	Volume overload	Study results *strongly support* this intervention
N-Acetylcysteine (150 mEq in 850 mL D5. Infuse at 3 mL/kg/h for 1 h, then 1 mL/kg/h for 6 h)	Scavenging oxygen-free radicals	Flushing, itching, rash, congestive heart failure, GI side effects	Mostly supportive. May be more protective when given IV
Sodium bicarbonate (600 mg IV BID for 3 doses)	Limits the production of oxygen-free radicals	Metabolic alkalosis	Mostly supportive
Calcium channel blockers	Increases renal blood flow	Excessive vasodilation	Mixed results, but benefits may outweigh risks
Theophylline	Increases renal blood flow	Arrhythmia, GI side effects, headache, tremor, restlessness, seizure	Mixed results
Fenoldopam	Increases renal blood flow	Headache, dizziness, hypotension, flushing, tachycardia	Study results *do not support* this intervention
Dopamine	Increases renal blood flow	Tachycardia, hypertension	Not supportive
Atrial natriuretic peptide	Increases renal blood flow	Volume overload	Not supportive
Allopurinol	Reduces effects of oxygen-free radicals	Skin rash, GI side effects, fatigue	Not supportive
Periprocedural hemodialysis	Removal of contrast media	Hypotension, electrolyte disturbance, bleeding	Mixed results
Furosemide	Diuresis	Hypotension, hypokalemia	Not supportive
Prostaglandin E1	Increases renal blood flow	Flushing, peripheral edema, hypotension	Not supportive

Key Points

- Patients at risk for renal disease must be identified, and prophylaxis prior to contrast administration should be strongly considered.
- When possible, low volume, nonionic, low osmolality contrast should be used.
- The most effective prophylactic strategy remains adequate IV hydration prior to contrast exposure. Patients at higher risk likely also benefit from preemptive intravenous application of N-acetylcysteine and sodium bicarbonate (see doses in Table 64.3).
- Other prophylactic measures have not produced consistent results or were harmful in human randomized controlled trials or meta-analysis.
- Treatment should focus on monitoring and treatment of fluid, electrolyte, and acid/base disorders and may require hemodialysis.

Arterial Hypertension

Overview

Elevated arterial blood pressure is problematic in INR. An acute rise in blood pressure can precipitate rupture of an aneurysm and cerebral edema. In contrast, an acute increase in arterial blood pressure at any time during the procedure may, among other things, indicate an acutely elevated ICP and requires immediate attention. The key to successful anesthetic management is a balance between adequate cerebral blood flow and prevention of aneurysm rupture or the precipitation of hypertensive encephalopathy/brain edema formation. A patient with an unsecured aneurysm requires precise blood pressure control to avoid rises that could precipitate rupture. Conversely, if an aneurysm rupture is suspected and the patient has a declining neurologic status, mean arterial pressure may need to be elevated to overcome a high intracranial pressure.

Prevention

Preparation begins with detailed patient history and preoperative evaluation. Because cerebral vessels are manipulated and blood pressure can change acutely, most providers advocate the use of invasive arterial monitoring. Since the neuroradiologist places an arterial catheter for access, a separate arterial catheter is not used by some. However, a preoperative arterial line facilitates a hemodynamically stable anesthetic induction as well as constant monitoring during periods when the femoral arterial pressure is not transduced.

Table 64.4 Events/problems requiring manipulation of hemodynamics

Events/problems	Patient presentation indication	Therapeutic intervention/diagnostic intervention
Laryngoscopy/ endotracheal intubation	Tachycardia and hypertension	Treatment with esmolol, lidocaine, opioid, IV antihypertensive agent, or deepened anesthesia
Cannulation of the femoral artery	Brief stimulating response	Opioid or short-acting antihypertensive
Carotid occlusion trial	To confirm cerebrovascular reserve in patients undergoing carotid occlusion	Induced hypotension may be necessary
Coil placement in wide-necked aneurysms	Repeated failed attempts	Deliberate hypotension or brief cardiac standstill (adenosine) to facilitate placement are options
Embolization of brain arteriovenous malformations	To prevent embolization or acute hemorrhage from glue dislodging into a draining vein	Deliberate hypotension may facilitate glue placement
Acute rise in intracranial pressure	May present as hypertension and bradycardia (potential causes include aneurysmal rupture, brain edema, intraparenchymal hemorrhage)	Relieve elevated ICP via acute hyperventilation, osmotherapy, ventriculostom, or emergent surgical intervention. Maintain high MAP to allow adequate CBF – cerebral perfusion pressure-guided
Aneurysmal rupture	May manifest as an acute rise in arterial blood pressure	Evaluate for extravasation of contrast medium. Reverse anticoagulant. Consider emergency surgery
Cerebral edema	Signs of intracranial hypertension	Consider ICP measurement to guide therapy. Osmodiuretics, deepen anesthesia, maintain adequate perfusion pressure
Cerebral vasospasm	Declining neurologic status days after subarachnoid hemorrhage	Medically induced hypertension, hypervolemia, hemodilution. Continue calcium channel blockers; statins. Consider balloon angioplasty and intra-arterial application of vasodilatory drugs

Crisis Management

The evidence to support a specific antihypertensive regimen is weak. Calcium channel blockers may be preferred in patients with aneurysmal subarachnoid hemorrhage as these drugs have been shown to improve long-term outcomes secondary to positive effects on cerebral vasospasm. Otherwise, blood pressure can be controlled with various antihypertensive agents and/or inhalation or intravenous anesthetics. Table 64.4 summarizes several events or problems that may require immediate intervention to manipulate hemodynamics accordingly.

Key Points

- Precise control of blood pressure is crucial to prevent rupture of an aneurysm and cerebral edema.
- Invasive arterial monitoring facilitates precise control.
- For ruptured aneurysms or brain edema, MAP needs to be elevated in order to allow for adequate CBF; consider ICP monitoring for CPP-driven therapy.
- To control hypertensive responses, multiple antihypertensive or anesthetic agents can be used.

Suggested Reading

Contrast Reaction

Bush WH, Swanson DP. Acute reactions to intravascular contrast media: Types, risk factors, recognition, and specific treatment. AJR Am J Roentgenol. 1991;157:1153–61.

Contrast-Induced Nephropathy

Merten GJ, Burgess WP, Gray LV, Holleman JH, Roush TS, Kowalchuk GJ, et al. Prevention of contrast-induced nephropathy with sodium bicarbonate: A randomized controlled trial. JAMA. 2004;291:2328–34.

Pannu N, Wiebe N, Tonelli M, Alberta Kidney Disease Network. Prophylaxis strategies for contrast-induced nephropathy. JAMA. 2006;295:2765–79.

Stenstrom DA, Muldoon LL, Armijo-Medina H, Watnick S, Doolittle ND, Kaufman JA, et al. N-acetylcysteine use to prevent contrast medium-induced nephropathy: Premature phase III trials. J Vasc Interv Radiol. 2008;19:309–18.

Tepel M, van der Giet M, Schwarzfeld C, Laufer U, Liermann D, Zidek W. Prevention of radiographic-contrast-agent-induced reductions in renal function by acetylcysteine. N Engl J Med. 2000;343:180–4.

Arterial Hypertension

Osborn IP. Anesthetic considerations for interventional neuroradiology. Int Anesthesiol Clin. 2003;41:69–77.

Young WL. Anesthesia for endovascular neurosurgery and interventional neuroradiology. Anesthesiol Clin. 2007;25:391–412, vii.

Chapter 65
Specific Challenges During Neuroradiological Interventions in Pediatric Patients

Tariq Parray and Timothy W. Martin

Overview

Interventional radiology procedures performed on the brain and spinal cord of children may be diagnostic, therapeutic, or palliative, and may be performed on either a "stand alone" basis or combined with an open surgical procedure. Most procedures are performed with high speed fluoroscopy and digital subtraction angiography for imaging, and the use of microcatheters that permit superselective catheterization of blood vessels.

While either transarterial or transvenous routes can be used, including the umbilical vessels in neonates, the transfemoral arterial approach is selected most commonly. In children, these procedures are typically done under general anesthesia requiring endotracheal intubation, as cases may be long and require a motionless state. With endotracheal intubation, the airway and ventilation can be controlled to optimize cerebral perfusion and deal with possible periprocedural complications. Laryngeal mask airways are appropriate in some cases. Table 65.1 lists common neuroradiologic diagnostic and therapeutic procedures in children, while Table 65.2 lists possible complications that can occur during or following these procedures.

The listed anesthetic complications of loss of airway or intravenous access, while not specific to neuroradiologic procedures, may be more likely to occur during these cases due to frequent movement of the patient or radiologic equipment and the typical

T. Parray, MD (✉)
Department of Anesthesiology Arkansas Children's Hospital, University of Arkansas for Medical Sciences, Little Rock, Arkansas, USA

T.W. Martin, MD, MBA
Department of Anesthesiology, Arkansas Children's Hospital, UAMS College of Medicine, Little Rock, AR, USA

A.M. Brambrink and J.R. Kirsch (eds.), *Essentials of Neurosurgical Anesthesia & Critical Care*, DOI 10.1007/978-0-387-09562-2_65,
© Springer Science+Business Media, LLC 2012

Table 65.1 Common neuroradiological procedures in children

Diagnostic procedures	
Cerebral angiography	Catheter-based cerebral angiography useful in defining both intra and extracranial vascular anatomy and pathology
Lumbar puncture (LP)	Guided LP for failed lumbar puncture in patients with spinal deformities or anomalies
Myelography	Evaluation of congenital spinal anomalies, disc disease, and radiculopathy
Image-guided biopsies or aspirations	Biopsies or aspirations of intracranial masses
Therapeutic procedures	
Vascular embolization	Intracranial aneurysm, cerebral arteriovenous malformation, spinal arterioveno fistula, and malformations
Tumor embolization	Meningiomas, glomus tumor, and nasopharyngeal angiofibroma
Thrombolysis	Local intra-arterial lysis treatment for stroke

Table 65.2 Potential complications of pediatric patients during interventional neuroradiology procedures

Procedural complications
- Intracranial hemorrhage
- Occlusive complications/thromboembolic stroke
- Contrast reactions
- Contrast nephropathy
- Hematoma and hemorrhage from the vessel puncture site

Anesthetic complications
- Hypothermia
- Loss or disruption of airway or breathing circuit integrity
- Loss of intravenous access
- Protamine allergy
- Heparin overdose

increased distance of the anesthesia provider from the patient. These complications are not discussed separately in this chapter, but are included in Table 65.2 in the interest of creating awareness and completeness.

Prevention

Most of the complications that may occur in pediatric interventional neuroradiologic procedures can be prevented by thoroughly evaluating the patient's coexisting disease (with particular attention to cardiac, pulmonary, and renal function) and allergy status, having a clear understanding of the planned procedure and anticipated movement of the patient and imaging equipment, and meticulous preparation of all medications (anesthetic and procedure related). Specific preventive measures will be described in the discussion of each potential complication.

Crisis Management: Intracranial Hemorrhage

Intracranial hemorrhage from aneurysm or arteriovenous malformation rupture may occur as a result of pathology of the vessels themselves, acute rise of blood pressure, or intracranial vessel injury, perforation or dissection directly by vascular manipulation during the procedure. This may result in permanent neurological disability or death (Tables 65.3 and 65.4).

Table 65.3 Signs and symptoms of intracranial hemorrhage

- Awake patients may complain of sudden headache, nausea, vomiting, progressive neurologic deficit, confusion, seizure, or loss of consciousness
- Patients under anesthesia may have a seizure, bradycardia, abrupt rise in mean arterial blood pressure
- Extravascular extravasation of contrast agent seen during the procedure

Table 65.4 Management of intracranial hemorrhage

- Communicate with the interventional radiologist; call for help
- Secure the airway if patient is not intubated for the procedure
- Hyperventilate with 100% oxygen to bring $PaCO_2$ between 26 and 30 mmHg. This will induce cerebral vasoconstriction and reduce the bleeding
- Immediately stop heparin infusion
- Immediate reversal of the heparin with protamine. Typically, 1 mg of protamine is administered for every 100 units of heparin. This may be done after checking the activated clotting time (ACT). Treat severe hypertension with caution to avoid lowering cerebral perfusion below a safe value
- Initiate measures to lower ICP including optimizing head position, diuresis, and ventricular drainage
- Consider antiseizure medications
- Order cross matching of blood for possible blood transfusion
- Aneurysm perforation may be treated by endovascular placement of coils by the interventional radiologist or emergency craniotomy with clipping of the aneurysm, though outcomes are usually poor

Key Points

- Intracranial hemorrhage can be life threatening or result in devastating neurological compromise.
- Ventilate with 100% O_2 and keep pCO_2 26–30 mmHg to induce cerebral vasoconstriction.
- Reverse any active heparin with protamine.
- Lower the systemic arterial pressure while maintaining the cerebral perfusion.
- Blood should be available for possible transfusion.
- Utilize measures to lower ICP (e.g., mannitol; ventriculostomy).
- Avoid anesthetic agents that may raise ICP.

Crisis Management: Occlusive Complications

Occlusive complications can result from embolic material being dislodged from a thrombosed aneurysm site, intraprocedural thrombosis, accidental embolization of occlusive material to an unintended target site, or vasospasm induced by the vascular manipulation. These events can occur during or following the procedure and may compromise cerebral perfusion leading to cerebral ischemic injury and infarction, and the development of new neurological deficits.

Cyanoacrylate adhesives are embolic agents used in treating arteriovenous malformations that can cause arterial ischemia and microcatheter "gluing," with compromise of the blood supply. Cyanoacrylate can also result in asymptomatic and symptomatic pulmonary emboli and possible respiratory failure.

Most of these complications are diagnosed when the patient recovers from the anesthetic (Table 65.5).

Diagnosis

An occlusive site can be seen and confirmed by an angiogram (Table 65.6).

Table 65.5 Signs and symptoms of occlusive crisis

- Change in the mental status in a awake patient preoperatively or postoperatively
- Development of new neurologic deficits
- Possible respiratory compromise or failure

Table 65.6 Management of occlusive crisis

- Communicate with the interventional radiologist to determine the extent of occlusion; call for help as necessary
- Secure the airway to maintain oxygenation and ventilation
- Ventilate with 100% oxygen
- Decrease the anesthetic depth
- Maintain normocarbia to hypercarbia, to increase the cerebral blood flow
- Induced hypertension to increase the cerebral blood flow, increase the MAP 30–40% above baseline to drive adequate flow through collaterals
- Malpositioned embolic material compromising the cerebral perfusion may be possibly retrieved by interventional radiologist
- Failure to retrieve may require craniotomy by the neurosurgeon
- Microcatheter imbedded in glue may be removed by snare or surgically
- Thrombus revealed on angiogram may be treated by intra-arterial tissue plasmogen activator

> **Key Points**
>
> - Patient should be ventilated with 100% oxygen
> - Increase the arterial blood pressure to increase collateral blood flow
> - Continuous infusion of heparinised saline should be used during the procedure to prevent thrombosis and maintain catheter patency
> - Removal of malpositioned embolic material may be attempted by the radiologist or may require surgical intervention

Crisis Management: Contrast Reactions

Contrast agents improve the visualization of anatomical structures which are not easily seen normally. They can be administered by intravenous, intra-arterial or intrathecal routes. The most commonly used intravenous contrast agents are iodinated ionic and nonionic compounds.

Pediatric contrast reactions are usually anaphylactoid, with rates of 0.18–3% for low osmolality contrast media and 3–13% for high osmolality contrast media. Most contrast reactions occur within 3–5 min of injection. Severe hypersensitivity reactions are likely to occur in patients with a history of allergy, atopy, or asthma. Patients with a previous reaction have increased chances of recurrence on reexposure (Tables 65.7–65.9).

Table 65.7 Types of contrast reaction

Type of reaction	Mechanism	Remarks
Anaphylactic	IgE mediated	Rare, but life threatening
Anaphylactoid/ idiosyncratic	Non-IgE-mediated histamine and serotonin release/activation of the complement system	Reactions can be mild to severe
Nonanaphylactoid/ physiochemotoxic/ nonidiosyncratic	Nonimmunological; dependent upon ionicity and osmolality, volume and route of administration	Reactions are usually mild to moderate

Table 65.8 Clinical manifestations of contrast reactions

Pruritis, flushing, erythema, urticaria, angioedema, nausea, vomiting, abdominal pain, laryngeal edema, hoarseness, chest tightness, cough, dyspnea, wheezing, light headedness, syncope, tachycardia, dysrhythmias, and hypotension

Table 65.9 Signs of severe reactions under general anesthesia	Cutaneous	Flushing
		Urticaria
		Erythema
		Angioedema
	Respiratory	Wheezing
		Cyanosis
		Increase in peak airway pressure
	Cardiovascular	Tachycardia
		Hypotension
		Dysrhythmias
		Cardiovascular collapse

Prevention of Contrast Reactions

Pretreatment of these patients with antihistamines and corticosteroids is not effective in preventing anaphylactic reactions, but can be helpful in patients with previous nonimmunologic mediated radiocontrast reactions. These patients are usually pretreated with antihistamines (H1 and H2 antagonists) and corticosteroids.

Management of Contrast Reaction

The reactions can range from mild to life-threatening events and could be either anaphylactic or anaphylactoid reactions, which may not be clinically distinguished.

A mild reaction of short duration may be treated with antihistamine and intravenous fluid while life-threatening reactions should be treated aggressively and immediately (Tables 65.10 and 65.11).

Key Points

- Contrast reactions can be anaphylactic, anaphylactoid, or chemotoxic, and usually cannot be distinguished clinically
- Life-threatening reactions can occur; as such all equipment, drugs, and staff should be available to aggressively treat the patient
- Airway should be secured immediately, before angioedema develops
- Epinephrine should be used to treat severe hypotension
- Antihistamines and steroids are used to prevent histamine, serotonin, complement release

Table 65.10 Treatment of mild contrast reaction

* Stop the administration of contrast agent
* Maintain adequate oxygenation and ventilation
* IV fluids for volume expansion to treat hypotension
* Antihistamines (diphenhydramine 0.5–1 mg/kg) to treat pruritis, flushing, erythema, urticaria
* Bronchospasm may be treated with albuterol or terbutaline, and if refractory, with epinephrine
* Epinephrine may be used to treat hypotension not responding to volume expansion
* Hydrocortisone 1–2 mg/kg body weight, then repeated after 4–6 h

Table 65.11 Treatment of acute anaphylactic reaction

* Stop the administration of contrast agent
* Secure the airway and ventilate with 100% oxygen
* Discontinue all anesthetic agents, since they are cardiovascular depressants
* Epinephrine should be 10 mcg/kg body weight IV, if patient has cardiovascular collapse. The dose may be repeated as needed. If patient is hypotensive, epinephrine 1–2 mcg/kg may be given and gradually increased every 30–60 s until blood pressure improves
* Insert large bore IV
* Rapid intravenous fluids expansion
* CPR if needed
* Diphenhydramine 0.5–1 mg/kg IV body weight
* Hydrocortisone 1–2 mg/kg body weight then repeated after 4–6 h
* For persistent hypotension start epinephrine 0.05–0.1 mcg/kg/min norepinephrine or dopamine infusion may be used if the clinical condition demands
* Invasive arterial line and venous catheter for monitoring and infusion of vasoactive drugs
* For persistent hypotension, consider vasopressin
* Arrange for PICU monitoring for 24 h
* Evaluate the airway for edema before extubation

Crisis Management: Contrast Nephropathy

Contrast nephropathy is the impairment of renal function occurring within 3 days following the administration of intravascular contrast agent. Creatinine increases 25% or 0.5 mg/dl from the baseline within 72 h after the contrast is given. In most cases the disorder is self-limited; however, the nephropathy can persist for weeks in some patients, leading to renal failure requiring dialysis.

The commonly used contrast media are either ionic or nonionic. Ionic contrast agents have high osmolality (1,400–2,400 $Osm/kg/H_2O$). Nonionic contrast agents have a lower osmolality (411–796 $mOsm/kg/H_2O$). These agents are generally safer, have less toxicity and a lower incidence of adverse events, and are generally better tolerated.

Table 65.12 Prevention of contrast nephropathy

- Use low osmolality contrast agent media
- Use lowest possible dose of contrast agent
- Contrast studies should be spaced more than 3 days apart whenever feasible
- Discontinue nephrotoxic drugs if possible before the procedure
- Hypovolemia should be corrected before the procedure, and the intravascular volume status of the patient should be optimized perioperatively
- Consider using N-acetylcysteine or intravenous hydration with sodium bicarbonate as prophylaxis for contrast nephropathy

Table 65.13 Management and treatment of contrast nephropathy

- Patients at risk for the development of nephropathy should be monitored by measuring serum creatinine levels before the procedure and once daily for 5 days post procedure
- Any nephrotoxic drugs should be avoided and further contrast studies avoided in this period
- The volume status of patients should be optimized, with careful monitoring of fluid input–output and weight gain
- Patient needs to be hospitalized with monitoring of serum electrolytes, acid base balance, and volume status
- Once the diagnosis of contrast nephropathy is established, the management is the same of renal failure
- Some of the patients will need hemodiaylsis

The pathogenesis is probably related to intrarenal endothelin and adenosine-induced vasoconstriction, leading to reduction in glomerular filtration rate (GFR) and renal ischemia, impaired nitric oxide production, direct cellular toxicity and oxygen-free radical formation. Patients at risk of developing nephropathy include those with preexisting renal disease, diabetes mellitus, heart failure, volume depletion, use of a high dose of contrast agent, use of high osmolality ionic contrast agent, and use of other nephrotoxic drugs (Tables 65.12 and 65.13).

Key Points

- Patients at risk for contrast nephropathy should be identified
- Preexisting renal dysfunction should be corrected if possible
- Nephrotoxic drugs should be avoided or stopped
- Dehydration or hypovolemia should be corrected
- Low osmolality contrast agent media should be used
- Contrast studies should be spaced with a 3-day interval, whenever possible
- Patients developing renal dysfunction need to be carefully monitored and treated

Crisis Management: Hemorrhage/Hematoma at Vessel Puncture Site

Bleeding may occur around the catheter site at the time of placement, during the procedure or after decannulation. Even small amounts of blood loss may be significant in infants (Tables 65.14 and 65.15).

Table 65.14 Prevention of hemorrhage/hematoma at vessel puncture site

- Avoid multiple attempts at catheter placement
- Catheter site should be checked perioperatively and postperatively for any bleeding
- Tubing should have tight connections, and preferably luer-locking connections should be used
- Emergence of the patient should be smooth; coughing, straining, or emergence agitation should be avoided

Table 65.15 Management of hemorrhage/hematoma at vessel puncture site

- Application of direct pressure for 10–15 min and temporary pressure dressing at the site after catheter removal will limit the hematoma formation
- Narcotics or propofol may be given to ensure smooth emergence
- Antiemetic should be given to avoid nausea and vomiting on emergence
- Residual heparin effect should be ruled out

Key Points

- Multiple attempts for catheter placement should be avoided
- Catheter site must be regularly inspected
- After catheter removal application of manual pressure for 10–15 min followed by pressure dressing

Crisis Management: Hypothermia During Neuroradiologic Interventions

Hypothermia is defined as core body temperature of less than 35°C. General anesthesia inhibits thermoregulation, and the cold temperature in the procedure room causes further heat loss. Heat is lost to the environment by conduction, convection, evaporation, and radiation, besides the depression of metabolic heat production during anesthesia (Tables 65.16–65.19).

Table 65.16 Etiology of hypothermia in children

- Larger surface area to body mass ratio compared to adults results in more heat loss
- Higher conductivity than adults, less subcutaneous fat
- Evaporation is higher due to lower keratin content in skin
- Reduced capacity for heat production
- Significant heat loss from head, which forms nearly 20% of body surface area in neonates and infants. The head may remain exposed during the procedure
- IR procedures may be of prolonged duration
- Cool interventional radiology rooms
- Use of room temperature fluids

Table 65.17 Diagnosis of hypothermia

- Body temperature lower than normal, either in perioperative or postoperative period
- Shivering may be present in older children although in infants it will be absent
- Cutaneous vasoconstriction, piloerection
- Delayed awakening, decreased level of consciousness

Table 65.18 Clinical implications of hypothermia

- Increased blood viscosity, impaired platelet function, platelet sequestration in portal circulation, abnormal blood coagulation cascade, and increased blood loss
- Left shift of oxy-hemoglobin dissociation curve, increase in pulmonary vascular resistance, decrease oxygen consumption and decreased CO_2 production, VQ mismatch
- Arrhythmias, bradycardia, prolonged PR interval, widened QRS interval, prolonged QT interval, ventricular fibrillation, asystole when core body temperature is less than 30°C
- Delayed postanesthetic recovery

Table 65.19 Management of hypothermia

- Increase the room temperature to reduce radiant heat loss
- Use forced air warming blanket
- Cover exposed portions of patient whenever possible; the head may be covered with a clear plastic bag
- Use warm intravenous fluids
- Use low flow of inhaled gases and humidifier
- In postoperative period warming lights may be used for neonates and infants

> **Key Points**
>
> - Infants and particularly neonates are prone to hypothermia during neuroradiologic interventions
> - Mild hypothermia may not impair post anesthesia recovery if the procedure is short
> - Moderate hypothermia causes prolonged drug effects, impaired coagulation, and hemodynamic effects
> - Hypothermia can be prevented or minimized by increasing temperature in the procedure room, use of warming devices, and intravenous fluid warming

Crisis Management: Heparin Overdosage

Flush solutions containing heparin are used to maintain the patency of catheters during the procedure and to prevent thromboembolic complications. This is accomplished by using a pressurized infusion bag or syringe pump. The concentration of heparin is usually 10 units/ml for infants less than 10 kg weight and 100 units/ml for patients over 10 kg. Massive doses of heparin can be given because an incorrect amount of concentrated heparin is used to prepare the flush solution. It is important to regulate the volume of flush solution to prevent fluid overload and provide an accurate dose of heparin.

The newborn has increased clearance of heparin because of increased volume of distribution and accelerated metabolism. The half-life of unfractionated heparin is 25 min at term compared to 70 min in adults (Tables 65.20 and 65.21).

Table 65.20 Prevention of heparin overdosage

- Recheck the concentration of the heparin vial before using it
- Use a syringe infusion pump to regulate the volume infused
- Record the total dose of heparin
- Check baseline-activated clotting time (ACT) and check ACT every hour for long procedures

Table 65.21 Management of heparin overdosage

- If wrong concentration of heparin infusion is suspected or there is an unexpected hemorrhagic complication, heparin should be immediately stopped
- ACT should be checked and heparin can be reversed with protamine
- If bleeding has occurred, blood transfusion and supportive measures may be needed

> **Key Points**
>
> - Term neonates have increased heparin requirements while preterm neonates have reduced heparin requirements
> - The concentration of heparin must be rechecked before infusion
> - The infusion must be through syringe pump to regulate the volume and accurate dose of heparin
> - Heparin may be reversed with protamine depending on activated clotting time (ACT)

Crisis Management: Protamine Reaction

Protamine is a specific heparin antagonist used to neutralize the effects of heparin at the end of a procedure or during the procedure in the event of unanticipated intracranial hemorrhage. The heparin–protamine complex does not have any anticoagulant activity. One hundred units of heparin are antagonized by 1 mg of protamine. Complications are rarely seen in interventional neuroradiology because the doses of heparin are small and rarely need to be neutralized. The common complication seen is hypotension, while pulmonary hypertension and anaphylaxis are rare (Tables 65.22 and 65.23).

Table 65.22 Clinical presentation of protamine reaction

- *Hypotension*: This usually occurs with rapid administration and is associated with tachycardia and flushing. This results from histamine release and release of nitric oxide-related substances. This can be avoided by slow IV injection
- *Pulmonary hypertension*: Protamine reaction with heparin can result in complement activation and thromboxane release resulting in pulmonary vasoconstriction, pulmonary hypertension, right heart failure, and systemic hypotension
- *Allergic reactions*: The allergic reactions may range from anaphylactic reactions to anaphylactoid reactions. True anaphylactic reaction occurs as a result of specific antiprotamine IgE antibody seen in patients who use protamine zinc insulin or who have been previously exposed to protamine. Anaphylactoid reactions are the result of the heparin–protamine complex

Table 65.23 Management and treatment of protamine reaction

- Protamine should be given by slow intravenous injection
- Hypotension can be treated with increased IV fluid volume, ephedrine, phenylephrine, and antihistamines
- In case of severe reaction or cardiovascular collapse, protamine administration should be stopped, and the patient treated as for a severe anaphylactic reaction

Key Points

- Protamine is given at end of procedure to reverse the effect of heparin
- Protamine reaction can cause mild hypotension to severe cardiovascular collapse
- It should be given slowly IV
- The most common reaction is hypotension which can be treated with fluid volume, ephedrine, phenylephrine, and antihistamines

Suggested Reading

Bochner BS, Lichtenstein LM. Anaphylaxis. N Eng J Med. 1991;324:1785.

Dillman R, Strouse PJ, Ellis JH, et al. Incidence and severity of acute allergic-like reactions to IV nonionic iodinated contrast material in children. AJR Am J Roentgenol. 2007;188:1643–7.

Levy JH. Anaphylactic and anaphylactoid reactions. Emilo B Lobato, Nikolaus Gravenstein, Robert R Kirby (eds.) In: Complications in anesthesiology. Philadelphia: Lippincott Williams & Wilkins; 2008. p. 701–11.

Singh J, Daftary A. Iodinated contrast media and their adverse reactions. J Nucl Med Technol. 2008;36(2):69–74.

Varma MK, Price K, Jayakrishnan V, et al. Anaesthetic considerations for interventional radiology. Br J Anaesth. 2007;99(10):75–85.

Part XIII
Challenges During Postoperative Anesthesia Care After Neurosurgery

Chapter 66
Surgical Emergencies After Neurosurgery

R. Alexander Schlichter

Care of the neurosurgical patient by the anesthesiologist extends beyond the operating suite. Complications can occur in the postanesthesia care unit (PACU) that require intervention by the anesthesiologist. Common postoperative emergencies in the neurosurgical patient include depression of airway reflexes, hemodynamic instability, increased intracranial pressure (ICP), and bleeding complications. This section will focus on etiology, prevention, and treatment of three common postsurgical complications: (1) hemorrhage from the surgical site, (2) coagulopathy, and (3) hematoma formation.

Hemorrhage

Overview

Despite apparent hemostasis at the end of a neurosurgical procedure, postoperative hemorrhage can occur, leading to serious and sometimes fatal complications of neurosurgery. Given that the cranial vault is a rigid structure with a fixed total volume, bleeding after an intracranial procedure can lead to an increased ICP. The elevation of the ICP can lead to not only changes in mental status, but hematoma in extreme situations. In addition, heme can irritate brain parenchyma leading to seizure and vasospasm. Although a majority of cases occur at the primary surgical site, there are case reports of remote cerebellar hemorrhage (RCH) after supratentorial surgery, usually associated with loss of cerebrospinal fluid (CSF) during the procedure.

R.A. Schlichter, MD (✉)
Department of Anesthesiology and Critical Care,
University of Pennsylvania School of Medicine, Philadelphia, PA, USA
e-mail: Rolf.Schlichter@uphs.upenn.edu

A.M. Brambrink and J.R. Kirsch (eds.), *Essentials of Neurosurgical Anesthesia & Critical Care*, DOI 10.1007/978-0-387-09562-2_66,
© Springer Science+Business Media, LLC 2012

Table 66.1 Causes of postoperative hemorrhage

Inadequate surgical hemostasis	Bucking/coughing at extubation
Coagulopathy	Emesis/retching
Uncontrolled hypertension	Trauma to head when moving patient

Table 66.2 Risk factors for postoperative hemorrhage

Bleeding disorders (hemophilia)	Cirrhosis
Antiplatelet therapy (aspirin, clopidogrel)	History of motion sickness
DVT prophylaxis/treatment (heparin, LMWH, and argatroban)	History of PONV
Chronic hypertension	Alcohol use
Respiratory disease (coughing)	Tobacco use
Vascular disease	Illicit drug use (cocaine, PCP, and opioids)

Bleeding related to neurosurgical procedures remote from the cranium involve a unique set of complications. Hemorrhage after carotid endarterectomy (CEA) can lead to hematoma formation, compromising the airway and cerebral blood flow. Bleeding after spinal surgery can lead to significant blood loss, pressure on the spine, and spinal ischemia. The multiple etiologies of postoperative hemorrhage are summarized in Table 66.1.

Prevention

A thorough preoperative assessment of the patient can reveal potential risk factors to postoperative hemorrhage (Table 66.2). Perioperative preparation also plays an important role: smooth emergence and extubation should be achieved by optimization of equipment and intraoperative medications, stable blood pressure (intra-arterial blood pressure monitoring and antihypertensives), and aggressive antiemesis. If intraoperative hypothermia was employed during aneurysm clipping, the patient needs to be rewarmed, as hypothermia can worsen coagulopathies. After multiple blood transfusions, plasma and platelet administrations should be addressed to prevent a dilutional coagulopathy (see below). Careful positioning and transferring the patient from OR bed to stretcher will prevent trauma or stress on the surgical site.

Crisis Management

Crisis management strategies for addressing possible causes of postoperative hemorrhage are listed in Table 66.3.

Table 66.3 Crisis management for hemorrhage

Risk factor	Treatment	Potential adverse effects
Hypertension	Opioids	Over sedation
	Labetalol	Bradycardia/hypotension
	Esmolol	Bradycardia
	Nicardipine	Hypotension
Emesis/Retching	Ondansetron	Migraines
	Droperidol	Oversedation
	Compazine	Extrapyramidal side effects
	Promethazine	Sedation
	Propofol	Sedation/loss of airway
Mental status changes	Reverse sedation	Pain/delirium
	Full neurological exam	
	CT scan	
	Surgical reexploration	Risks of surgery and anesthesia
Hypothermia	Warming blankets	Low risk for burns
	Warm IV fluids	Hypervolemia
	Hot lights	
Coagulopathy	See Table 66.4	
Hematoma formation	See Table 66.4	

If the patient has a suspected postoperative hemorrhage after a neurosurgical procedure, a full neurological exam should be performed at bedside and the neurosurgical team should be immediately notified. The intervention performed depends on the severity of the exam. If a patient has a change in neurological exam, but is still arousable and can move appropriate extremities, a conservative "watch and see" approach is appropriate. Any further changes in mental status or neurological exam warrant imaging, usually a CT scan. If major hemorrhage is suspected (loss of consciousness, obtundation, loss of extremity function), immediate surgical reexploration of the wound is required.

Key Points

- Postoperative hemorrhage is a serious and sometimes fatal complication of neurosurgery.
- Although the majority of cases occur at the primary surgical site, RCH has been reported after supratentorial surgery.
- Patients should be carefully evaluated for possible risk factors that can lead to postoperative hemorrhage.
- Proper equipment and medications should be available to treat hypertension, prevent coughing, insure a smooth extubation, warm the patient, treat coagulopathy, and prevent and treat PONV.
- Frequent and thorough neurological exams of the patient in the PACU can detect changes that might indicate a possible hemorrhage. Communication with the neurosurgical team is important to determine if the patient needs further evaluation or reexploration of the surgical site.

Coagulopathy

Overview

Coagulopathy is a serious postoperative complication that can lead to hemorrhage and hematoma formation. Despite adequate intraoperative hemostasis, a coagulopathy may be present. If unrecognized intraoperatively, the coagulopathy may lead to intracranial hemorrhage, further complicating a patient already experienced with acute brain injury. Coagulopathy can be caused by low plasma levels of clotting factors or platelets, by a breakdown in the enzymatic systems that insure proper coagulation and platelet function, or by hyperfibrinolysis. Risk factors are summarized in Table 66.4.

Prevention

A proper history, physical, and laboratory tests are essential in preventing post operative coagulopathy. The patient needs to be asked about bleeding disorders, easy bruising, petechiae, medications (clopidogrel, aspirin, Warfarin, and LMWH), nutrition (vitamin K deficiency), and alcohol use. Appropriate preoperative laboratory tests for coagulopathy include a platelet count, a prothrombin time (PT), and a partial thromboplastin time (PTT). Bleeding time, activated clotting time (ACT), fibrinogen level, and thromboelastogram are not necessary, but may be useful to follow the patient's coagulation profile intra- and postoperatively. If the patient is at an elevated risk for intra- or postoperative-coagulopathy (including acute brain injury), adequate large bore venous access must be obtained, including possible central venous access. Intra-arterial monitoring can be useful if large amounts of colloid are going to be transfused or frequent laboratory tests are needed to follow the patient's coagulation profile. Type and Cross is necessary to insure appropriate amounts of packed red blood cells, fresh frozen plasma, platelets, and other clotting factors are available for the surgical procedure.

Table 66.4 Common risk factors for postoperative coagulopathy

Hereditary (hemophilia, Von-Willebrand's)	Dilutional (massive transfusion)
Vitamin K deficiency (malnutrition)	Hypothermia
Antiplatelet therapy	Consumptive (ITP)
Heparin therapy	Cirrhosis
Warfarin therapy	Nitroprusside
Disseminated intravascular coagulopathy	Hetastarch
Acute head injury	Hyperfibrinolysis

Crisis Management

Postoperative coagulopathy requires immediate intervention in the PACU. Treatment is focused on using the appropriate blood factors to reverse the coagulopathy. If the patient has a high PT/INR, vitamin K 10 mg subcutaneously or intramuscularly should be administered. If the patient is hypothermic, warming should be implemented with a warm air blanket, hot lights, and fluids and blood products should be warmed before being administered ("blood warmer"; water bath temperature set to 42°C). If large volumes of blood products are given, the patient's fluid status needs to be monitored to prevent fluid overload and pulmonary edema. Appropriate diuretics should be used to prevent fluid overload.

If plasma transfusion does not correct the coagulopathy, cryoprecipitate may provide clotting factors not concentrated in FFP. Recently, recombinant Factor VII 20 mcg/kg has been found to be successful in patients with acute brain injury not responding to FFP or cryoprecipate. If platelet dysfunction is suspected, desmopressin 0.3 mcg/kg can be administered. The role of antifibrinolytics has been studied in prevention of rebleeding, but not in active treatment of coagulopathy. The treatments are summarized below in Table 66.5.

Table 66.5 Blood products and clotting factors

Blood product	Clotting factors present	Clinical use
Fresh frozen plasma	II, V, VII, IX, X, XI, antithrombin III, Proteins C + S Inadequate fibrinogen, VWF	Treating coagulopathy with elevated PT, PTT DIC Reversing heparin Replacing deficient clotting factors except Fibrinogen and VWF
Cryoprecipitate	VIII, XIII, VWF, fibrinogen	Replacement of these factors DIC Use if FFP is not reversing coagulopathy
Platelets	Platelets	Thrombocytopenia Platelet dysfunction ITP, TTP Reverse antiplatelet drugs
Recombinant factor VII	Factor VII	DIC Hemorrhage in acute brain injury Use when FFP, cryo not reversing coagulopathy

Key Points

- Coagulopathy can be caused by low plasma levels of clotting factors or platelets, by a breakdown in the enzymatic systems that insure proper coagulation and platelet function, or by hyperfibrinolysis.
- Bleeding disorders, easy bruising, petechiae, medications (clopidogrel, aspirin, Warfarin, and LMWH), nutrition (vitamin K deficiency), and alcohol use should be assessed. Appropriate preoperative laboratory tests for coagulopathy include a platelet count, a prothrombin time (PT), and a PTT.
- Bleeding time, ACT, fibrinogen level, and thromboelastography are not necessary, but may be useful to follow the patient's coagulation profile intra- and postoperatively.
- The appropriate blood components need to be given based on laboratory data, medication history, and clinical exam.
- Hypothermia should be reversed and fluid status should be monitored if large amounts of colloid are transfused.

Hematoma

Overview

The combination of coagulopathy and hemorrhage can lead to hematoma formation. Subdural hematomas occur between the brain and the dura and are generally caused by rupture of a sinus or bridging vein. By expanding against other parts of the brain, a subdural hematoma can increase ICP and cause ischemia. Increased pressure on the brain can lead to changes in mental status, hypertension, and bradycardia. Epidural hematomas are caused by rupture of meningeal arteries and place pressure on the adjacent spinal cord (or brain if intracranial) causing a change in neurological exam or spinal ischemia. Hematomas from neurosurgical procedures not involving the CNS may also lead to postoperative complications. Airway compromise can occur from direct pressure on the trachea or compression of the recurrent laryngeal nerve. A decrease in cerebral blood flow can result from a regional hematoma following a CEA. The patient presents with neck swelling accompanied by change in voice, difficulty swallowing, or changes in mental status.

Prevention

The prevention of hematoma formation depends on preventing possible sources of bleeding. Strategies include the above for treating hemorrhage (Table 66.3) and coagulopathy (Table 66.5).

Table 66.6 Crisis management in hematoma formation

Hematoma location	Diagnosis	Treatment
Intracranial	Neurological exam	Observation
	Neuroimaging	Surgical evacuation
Carotid	Neurological exam	Secure airway
	Physical exam	Surgical reexploration and evacuation
	Airway exam	
Epidural	Neurological exam	Observation
	Neuroimaging	Surgical evacuation

Crisis Management (Table 66.6)

All hematomas should be treated as serious emergencies. If a hematoma formation is suspected, a quick but thorough neurological exam should be performed immediately. The neurosurgical team should be informed and an operating room is made available for possible surgical exploration. If the patient's neurological exam is stable, the neurosurgical team might initially obtain a CT scan.

Key Points

- All hematomas should be treated as serious emergencies.
- The combination of coagulopathy and hemorrhage can lead to hematoma formation.
- Hematomas following CEA can compromise the airway and cerebral blood flow.
- If a hematoma formation is suspected, a quick but thorough neurological exam needs to be performed. The neurosurgical team should be immediately informed and an operating room is made available for possible surgical exploration.

Suggested Reading

Hemorrhage

Friedman M, Piepgras PG, Duke DA, et al. Remote cerebellar hemorrhage after supratentorial surgery. Neurosurgery. 2001;49:1327–40.
Manninen PH et al. Early postoperative complications following neurosurgical procedures. Can J Anaesth. 1999;46(1):7–14.

Coagulopathy

Roitberg B et al. Human recombinant factor VII for emergency reversal of coagulopathy in neuro-surgical patients: A retrospective comparative study. Neurosurgery. 2005;57(5):832–6.

Hematoma

Hou J et al. Risk factors for spinal epidural hematoma after spinal surgery. Spine. 2002;27(15): 1670–3.

Palmer JD et al. Postoperative hematoma: a 5 year survey and identification of avoidable risk factors. Neurosurgery. 1994;35(6):1061–5.

Self D et al. Risk factors for post-carotid endarterectomy hematoma formation. Can J Anaesth. 1999;46(7):635–40.

Chapter 67
Airway Emergencies After Neurosurgery

Yulia Ivashkov and Karen B. Domino

Postoperative respiratory complications contribute to length of hospital stay, morbidity, and mortality. Hypoxemia and hypercapnia in neurosurgical patients have particularly grave consequences, such as cerebral vasodilatation, increases in ICP, and hypoxic brain damage.

This chapter gives an overview of postoperative respiratory complications according to the traditional pathophysiological classification by hypercarbic hypoxia and hypoxic normocarbia. However, the classification is schematic, and in reality each disorder usually falls under two or more pathophysiologic criteria. The pathophysiologic mechanisms and causes of arterial hypoxemia are summarized in Table 67.1.

Upper Airway Obstruction

Overview

Upper airway obstruction is the most common early respiratory complication that leads to hypoxemia and hypercarbia after neurosurgical procedures. The major risk factors for its development are sleep apnea, residual anesthetic agents, and trauma of the upper airway. Laryngospasm may be triggered by extubation during light anesthesia, accumulated secretions, and inadequate pain control. The etiologic factors include supraglottic, glottic, or subglottic causes, and are shown in Table 67.2.

Y. Ivashkov, MD
Department of Anesthesiology and Pain Medicine, University of Washington, Seattle, WA, USA

K.B. Domino, MD, MPH (✉)
Department of Anesthesiology and Pain Medicine, University of Washington School
of Medicine, Seattle, WA, USA
e-mail: kdomino@u.washington.edu

A.M. Brambrink and J.R. Kirsch (eds.), *Essentials of Neurosurgical Anesthesia & Critical Care*, DOI 10.1007/978-0-387-09562-2_67,
© Springer Science+Business Media, LLC 2012

Table 67.1 Pathophysiologic mechanisms of arterial hypoxemia

Arterial hypoxemia

Decreased P$_I$O$_2$	Alveolar hypoventilation	Impaired alveolar-capillary diffusion	Ventilation–perfusion mismatch	Pulmonary shunt
Unlikely in monitored environment	See Table 67.2	Very rare within clinically significant limits, mostly accompanies restrictive lung disease	See Table 67.3	An extreme example of ventilation–perfusion mismatch

Prevention

The best prevention of postoperative airway obstruction is a thorough assessment prior to extubation. An awake and alert patient with no signs of respiratory depression or excessive swelling of the airway has a low chance for airway obstruction. A "leak" test should be performed prior to extubation in prone cases and in those who have received a significant amount of crystalloid solutions. Discussion with the surgeon regarding possible upper airway compromise is particularly important in prone cervical spine and posterior fossa cases.

Crisis Management

Pathophysiology and Clinical Presentation

Obstruction to air flow develops when oropharyngeal tissues lose their baseline tone, swell, or confine the airway by active contraction. Mucus, blood, vomitus, or foreign body (e.g., tooth or throat pack) can also block the airway. Complete obstruction not only causes hypoventilation and arterial desaturation, but the forceful respiratory attempts against a closed glottis may result in the rapid development of negative-pressure or postobstructive pulmonary edema.

The clinical picture of an upper airway obstruction is usually very obvious, unless the initial presentation was missed and respiratory distress progressed to apnea. Snoring, gurgling, and high-pitched stridorous sounds accompany the labored breathing. Nasal flaring and sternal or intercostal muscle retractions represent the use of the accessory muscles. In the case of complete obstruction, no noise may be present since the effective respiration has ceased. Forced expiration efforts using accessory muscles may also be present. If conscious, the patient may appear diaphoretic and agitated. With the ongoing hypoxemia, agitation may progress to stupor. Hypoxemia and hypercarbia result in profound autonomic discharge leading to tachycardia and hypertension; severe hypoxemia ultimately causes myocardial failure and circulatory arrest.

Table 67.2 Causes for alveolar hypoventilation

Mechanisms of alveolar hypoventilation

Obstructive mechanisms			Impaired regulatory mechanisms	Restrictive mechanisms
Supraglottic	Glottic	Subglottic		
(a) Tongue/soft tissue obstruction	(a) Laryngospasm	(a) Bronchospasm	(a) Trauma, swelling, and excessive pressure involving regulatory centers	(a) Involving lung tissue (these disorders often are accompanied by right-to-left shunting)
				– Pneumonia
				– Acute lung injury (ARDS)
				– Interstitial lung diseases (pulmonary fibrosis – not a common reason for postoperative respiratory insufficiency)
(b) Foreign bodies (blood, secretions, etc.)	(b) Vocal cord paralysis	(b) Exacerbation of COPD	(b) CNS depression by chemicals (opiates, residual anesthetics)	(b) Involving pleural space
				– Pleural effusion
				– Pneumothorax
(c) Tissue swelling and edema (anaphylaxis, trauma, impaired venous drainage)	(c) Trauma	(c) Foreign bodies		(c) Involving respiratory muscles
				– High spinal cord injury
				– Residual neuromuscular blockade
	(d) Swelling			(d) Involving thoracic cage
				– Obesity
				– Chest trauma (flail chest)

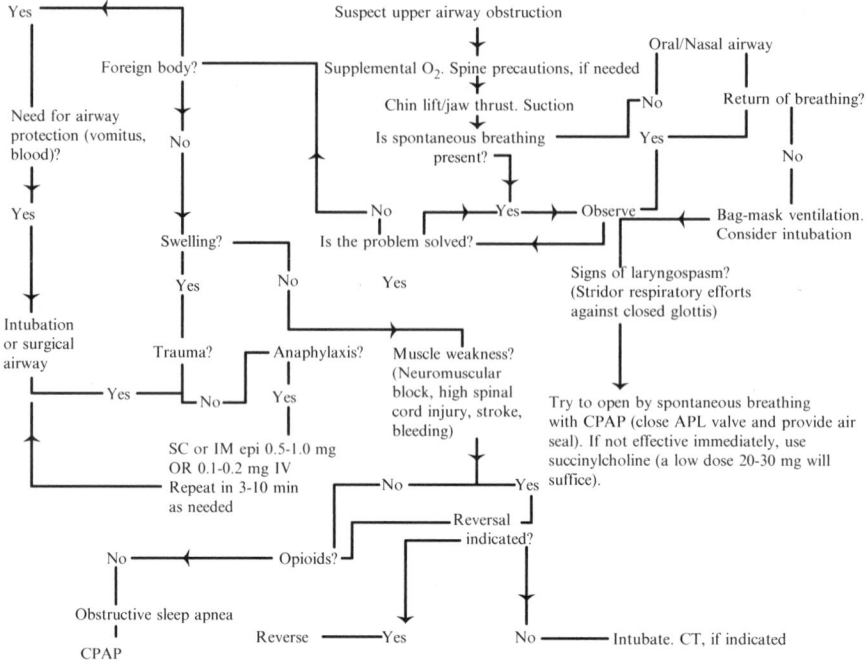

Fig. 67.1 Algorithm of action for possible upper airway obstruction

Patient Assessment

If upper airway obstruction is present, start with oxygen treatment prior to any other intervention, and establish monitoring if not already present. Monitoring oxygen saturation, respiratory rate, and end-tidal CO_2 during the event is crucial. For differential diagnosis of airway obstruction refer to Table 67.2 and Fig. 67.1. An arterial blood gas measurement is useful when the obstruction persists and reintubation is considered. If the cause of upper airway obstruction cannot be easily found, fiberoptic laryngoscopy may be indicated to rule out vocal cord paralysis or the presence of a foreign body.

Intervention/Treatment

Treatment options depend upon the cause of airway obstruction and are shown in Fig. 67.1.

> **Key Points**
> - Plan for extubation ahead of time.
> - Extubate the patient only if all of standard extubation criteria are met, including a "leak" test if indicated.
> - Airway obstruction may lead to rapid deterioration. Give oxygen immediately and restore assisted ventilation as soon as possible. If the obstruction was not relieved by the therapeutic maneuvers such as chin lift, jaw thrust, or supraglottic airway, do not hesitate to insert an LMA or reintubate. You can always remove the endotracheal tube later.

Obstructive and Restrictive Pulmonary Disorders

Overview

Obstructive pulmonary diseases include asthma, emphysema, chronic bronchitis, and bronchiectasis. Restrictive pulmonary diseases include interstitial pulmonary disease, diseases of the chest wall, and neuromuscular disorders. Etiology, pathophysiology, and clinical presentation of these disorders are shown in Table 67.3.

Exacerbation of chronic obstructive lung disease, particularly chronic bronchitis, increases the risk of pulmonary infection. Obstructive severe restrictive lung disease can lead to prolonged ventilator support, also increasing the possibility of ventilator-associated pneumonia.

Prevention

Preexisting pulmonary disease, emergent procedures, and prolonged surgery are the major independent risk factors for postoperative pulmonary complications. Thus, preoperative medical management of chronic medical conditions as well as minimizing the surgical and anesthesia time are important. Postoperative antibiotics do not decrease the incidence of pulmonary infections in patients undergoing major head and neck surgery. Only the prevention and aggressive treatment of postoperative atelectasis significantly reduces the infection risk.

Administration of albuterol preoperatively and prior to extubation helps reduce bronchospasm associated with endotracheal intubation. Inhaled ipratropium bromide may be added as well. Consider oral prednisone in patients with poorly controlled asthma or COPD. After initial brief course of 40 mg, prednisone is tapered rapidly (e.g., 40, 40, 40, then 20, 10, off). If *preventive* corticosteroids were not

Table 67.3 Causes for ventilation–perfusion $(\dot{V_A}/\dot{Q})$ mismatch

Ventilation–perfusion ratio imbalance	
Relative or absolute increase in dead space ventilation	Relative or absolute increase in perfusion of poorly ventilated alveoli
Hypovolemia (blood loss, diuresis)	Hypocapnia • Mechanical hyperventilation (to treat increased ICP) • Spontaneous as a response to pain or as a sign of respiratory distress

Decreased cardiac output
 (CHF, pharmacological vasodilatation)
	Loss of alveolar space
	• Pulmonary edema
	  – Postobstructive (negative pressure)
	  – Neurogenic
	  – Cardiogenic
	  – Transfusion-related acute lung injury (TRALI)
	• Acute lung injury/acute respiratory distress syndrome (ARDS)
	• Aspiration pneumonitis
	• Pneumonia
	• Atelectasis
	• Pneumothorax
	• Modest decrease of hypoxic pulmonary vasoconstriction by volatile agents with increase of intrapulmonary shunt fraction

Pharmacological influence on the airways (atropine)	
Pulmonary vasoconstriction (pulmonary embolism)	
Supine position	
Abdominal obesity	

effective, then steroid *treatment* is indicated. Start hydrocortisone intravenously, bolus of 300 mg followed by 200 mg intravenously every 4 h thereafter until the patient is better; continue oral prednisone or methylprednisolone.

Crisis Management

Pathophysiology and Clinical Presentation

Hypoventilation with the increase in arterial and alveolar CO_2 initially leads to hypoxia due to decrease of P_AO_2, and later hypoxia may worsen due to increased $\dot{V_A}/\dot{Q}$ mismatch. Clinical presentation may give important cues for diagnosis; nevertheless, dyspnea and wheezing may accompany many clinical conditions, so additional tests such as chest X-ray and arterial blood gases are often needed.

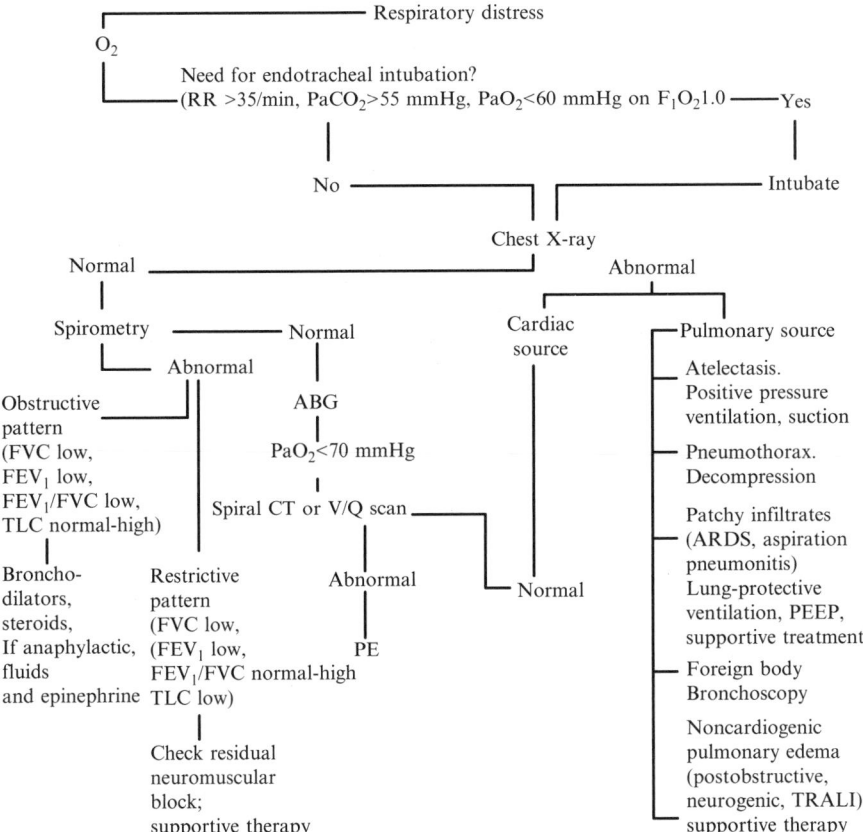

Fig. 67.2 Algorithm of diagnostic and therapeutic approach to respiratory distress

Patient Assessment

Assessment and management strategies for disorders associated with dyspnea are represented in Fig. 67.2.

Intervention/Treatment

For management of disorders associated with alveolar hypoventilation please refer to Figs. 67.1 and 67.2

Key Points

- Assess pulmonary function prior to the surgery, primarily based upon history and physical examination.
- Chest x-rays, spirometry, and arterial blood gases are not routinely recommended for the preoperative evaluation.
- Chronic lung disease, particularly chronic bronchitis, poses a significant risk factor for postoperative infection. Preexisting restrictive lung disease combined with postoperative respiratory depression by opioids and anesthetics may lead to severe hypercapnia and respiratory failure.
- Prophylactic administration of albuterol and possibly ipratropium bromide helps reduce reflex-induced bronchospasm associated with endotracheal intubation.

Ventilation–Perfusion Ratio ($\dot{V}_A/\dot{Q}$) Mismatch and Right-to-Left Shunt

Overview

Any condition that leads to anatomical or functional exclusion of a number of the lung units from the gas exchange creates a predisposition to $\dot{V}_A/\dot{Q}$ mismatch. The etiologic factors are presented in the Table 67.4. The predisposing factors are case-specific. Atelectasis may be caused by the low-volume ventilation, obesity, endobronchial intubation, and administration of 100% oxygen. Aspiration may follow stomach distention and regurgitation or vomiting. Intracranial hypertension is a risk factor for development of neurogenic pulmonary edema.

Prevention

Prevention mostly consists of maintaining both optimal ventilation and perfusion. Maintaining euvolemia, treating hypotension, and deep venous thrombosis/pulmonary embolism prophylaxis will help to avoid hypoperfusion. Postoperative lung expansion with incentive spirometry, chest physical therapy, postural drainage, and continuous positive-airway pressure are useful for prevention of the uneven ventilation. $\dot{V}_A/\dot{Q}$ matching is improved in the prone position compared to the supine position.

Table 67.4 Obstructive versus restrictive lung disease

	Obstructive lung disease	Restrictive lung disease
Risk, incidence, epidemiology	Risk increases with preexisting lung disease and prolonged surgery	Risk increases with obesity, high spinal cord injury, chest wall deformities, intrinsic restrictive lung disease, and long surgery, residual neuromuscular blockade
Etiology, pathophysiology	Increase of airway resistance due to (a) narrowing of the airways with inflammation, secretions, compression or contraction of the smooth muscles, and (b) dynamic compression of the airways with the forceful expiration, when pleural pressure exceeds airway pressure	Decrease of lung expansion and increase of work of breathing due to (a) intrinsic increase of elastic lung recoil, or (b) extrinsic obstacle to chest expansion (pleural effusion, obesity, chest wall deformity, muscle weakness)
Clinical presentation	Dyspnea, cough, wheezing, prolonged exhalation, distress	Rapid shallow respirations, respiratory distress, dry cough, muscle weakness in cases of neuromuscular disorders

Crisis Management

Pathophysiology and Clinical Presentation

The clinical presentation depends on the primary pathology, though hypoxia is the universal feature. Aspiration may present with cough and wheezing. Pulmonary edema will manifest itself with bronchospasm, respiratory distress, cyanosis, tachypnea, copious frothy secretions, or hemoptysis.

Patient Assessment

The severity of $\dot{V}_A / \dot{Q}$ mismatch may be established based on the response to O_2 treatment (Fig. 67.2). In the case of $\dot{V}_A / \dot{Q}$ mismatch, PaO_2 will increase with oxygen treatment. However, in the extreme of $\dot{V}_A / \dot{Q}$ mismatch, when some areas of the lung receive zero ventilation (true shunt), oxygen will not have much effect on PaO_2. The higher is the shunt fraction, the less the response to oxygen will be.

To find the alveolar to arterial O_2 tension difference [P(A–a)O_2], an arterial blood sample should be obtained. To calculate the alveolar gas equation, $[P_AO_2 = FiO_2 \times (P_B - P_{H_2O}) - P_ACO_2]$ is used.

The shunt magnitude is estimated by the shunt equation:

$$\dot{Q}s/\dot{Q}t = (Cc'O_2 - CaO_2)/(Cc'O_2 - C\overline{v}O_2),$$

where $\dot{Q}s/\dot{Q}t$ is a shunt fracture in %, $Cc'O_2$ is the end-capillary blood and ideally equals P_AO_2, and CaO_2 is the arterial oxygen content and is calculated as:

$$CaO_2 = Hb\,(g/dL) \times 1.34\,ml\,O_2/gHb \times SaO_2 + PaO_2 \times (0.003ml\,O_2/mmHg/dL).$$

$C\bar{v}O_2$ represents the mixed venous oxygen content and is calculated accordingly as:

$$C\bar{v}O_2 = Hb\,(g/dL) \times 1.34ml\,O_2/gHb \times S\bar{v}O_2 + P\bar{v}O_2 \times (0.003ml\,O_2/mmHg/dL).$$

$P\bar{v}O_2$ could be measured in the blood aspirated through the distal port of pulmonary artery catheter.

Intervention/Treatment

Start treatment with oxygen administration. A shunt of 15–30% requires various levels of oxygen support, and shunt over 30% causes profound hypoxemia that usually requires mechanical ventilation and positive end-expiratory pressure. If atelectasis is present, chest physiotherapy should be the first line of treatment (e.g., incentive spirometry, chest percussion), and if that does not help, consider the noninvasive positive pressure ventilation (NPPV), namely continuous positive-airway pressure (CPAP) and bi-level positive-airway pressure (BiPAP). The advantages of NPPV over traditional ventilation through endotracheal tube include elimination of intubation-related stress and trauma, decreased incidence of ventilator-associated pneumonia, shorter hospital stay and lesser expenditures. NPPV is more effective in a relaxed and cooperative patient. It is contraindicated, when respiratory arrest, hemodynamic instability, increased aspiration risk, facial fractures, severe hypoxemia, or impaired mental status is present. If NPPV trial failed, or could not be employed, proceed to intubation and invasive positive pressure ventilation. Think of fiberoptic bronchoscopy if a thick mucus plug or foreign body is present.

Key Points

- $\dot{V}_A/\dot{Q}$ mismatch and shunt are the most common reasons for decreased PaO_2.
- Decreased PaO_2 will improve with oxygen treatment in the case of $\dot{V}_A/\dot{Q}$ mismatch, but will not improve with true shunt.
- Atelectasis is one of the major factors that lead to postoperative shunting and hypoxia.

Suggested Reading

Ahrens T, Rutherford K. Essentials of oxygenation: implications for clinical practice. Boston: Jones & Bartlett; 1993.

Gravenstein N, Lobato EB, Kirby RR. Complications in anesthesiology. 3rd ed. Philadelphia: Lippincott Williams & Wilkins; 2007.

Luce JM, Tyler ML, Pierson DJ. Intensive respiratory care. Philadelphia: Saunders; 1984.

Newfield P, Cottrell JE. Handbook of neuroanesthesia. 4th ed. Philadelphia: Lippincott Williams & Wilkins; 2007.

Rozet I, Domino KB. Respiratory care. Best Pract Res Clin Anaesthesiol. 2007;21(4):465–82.

Stockley RA, Rennard S, Rabe K, Celli B. Chronic obstructive pulmonary disease: a practical guide to management. Malden, MA, Oxford: Blackwell Publishing; 2007.

Weinberger SE, Cockrill BA, Mandel J. Principles of pulmonary medicine. 5th ed. Philadelphia: Saunders/Elsevier; 2008.

Chapter 68
Neurologic Emergencies After Neurosurgery

Doortje C. Engel and Andrew Maas

Overview

Care during the postoperative phase is critical and fundamental to the success of neurosurgical operations to the brain and spinal cord.

The result of a complex but technically perfect operation can be ruined by inadequate postoperative care. Conversely, a complicated operative procedure will necessitate expert care to optimize conditions for preserving and restoring brain function. Assessment and reassessment, as well as careful clinical and neurological monitoring, are required. Complications, such as a postoperative hematoma with rapid neurological deterioration, require prompt intervention. In some centers, all patients are admitted directly to the ICU following intracranial surgery. In other centers, patients are observed in the PACU for 24 h. In yet other centers, the PACU is utilized as an intermediate intensive care, providing advanced monitoring facilities for critical patients, awaiting transfer to the ICU. Thus, within the PACU environment, a wide spectrum of neurosurgical pathology and disease severity is treated.

The aim of this chapter is to review general and disease-specific complications after neurosurgical procedures and to summarize the essential aspects of care for the neurosurgical patient in the PACU environment, as seen from the neurosurgical perspective.

D.C. Engel, MD, PhD, MBA (✉)
Department of Neurosurgery, Cantonal Hospital St. Gallen, St Galle, Switzerland
e-mail: doortje.engel@kssg.ch

A. Maas, MD
Department of Neurosurgery, University Hospital Antwerp,
Edegem, Belgium

A.M. Brambrink and J.R. Kirsch (eds.), *Essentials of Neurosurgical
Anesthesia & Critical Care*, DOI 10.1007/978-0-387-09562-2_68,
© Springer Science+Business Media, LLC 2012

Table 68.1 CNS complications according to localization of surgery/disease

CNS complications	Consequences
Supratentorial surgery	
– Hematoma (subgaleal, epi- or subdural, intracerebral)	– Brain compression, raised ICP, herniation
– Swelling/edema	– Raised ICP, herniation
– Seizures	– Massive vasodilatation, swelling
– Infection: meningitis/ventriculitis; abscess/empyema; bone flap infection	– Toxic effects on CNS tissue
Infratentorial surgery	
– Hematoma	– Brain stem compression/inverse cerebellar herniation
	– Disturbed gag reflex, aspiration, hypoxia
– Cranial nerve palsy	– Hydrocephalus
	– Circulatory collapse
– CSF obstruction	– Raised ICP
– Air embolism (sitting position/opening of large cerebral veins during surgery)	– Slit ventricles
– Cerebellar mutism	– Ventriculitis
– Aseptic meningitis	
Shunt surgery	
– Dysfunction (obstruction, dislocation)	– Peritoneal shunt: dysfunction due to adhesions of the omentum
– Overdrainage	Peritonitis/intraperitoneal abscess
– Infection; proximal	– Cardiac shunt: bacteremia/sepsis
– Infection; distal	Risk of late glomerulonephritis
Spine surgery	
– Postoperative hematoma	– Compression of spinal cord/cauda equina with development of neurological deficits
– Spinal instability	– Spinal cord/cauda equina damage
Brain and spinal surgery	
– CSF leakage	– Increased risk of meningitis
	– Intracranial hypotension syndrome
	– Chronic, low-grade infection
	– Meningitis, empyema
– Infection of implanted foreign material; for example, in spinal instrumentation, cranioplasty	– Wound dehiscence
	– Spinal column instability

General Complications

A technically excellent and flawless procedure with rapid recovery is what every patient and doctor wishes. Reality is, however, sometimes different because of surgical problems and/or postoperative complications. Knowledge of details of surgery and anesthesia is essential for anticipating possible problems. Complications after surgery may be neurosurgical or systemic (Tables 68.1 and 68.2).

Table 68.2 Systemic complications

Systemic complications	Consequences
– Hypovolemia (insufficient pre- and perioperative hydration, blood loss)	– Hypoperfusion, ischemia
– Coagulation disorders (blood loss, imbalance coagulation factors (i.e., AT3. factor XIII))	– Increased risk of postoperative hemorrhage
– Pulmonary (atelectasis, pneumothorax)	– Hypoxemia→ischemia – Hypercapnia→ cerebral vasodilatation
– Thromboembolic (DVT, pulmonary embolism, myocardial infarction)	– Ischemia, hypoxemia
– Infection (pneumonia, urinary tract infection, catheter sepsis)	– Ischemia, increased risk of hemorrhage

Table 68.3 "Red alert": signs that should trigger immediate response

- Decreasing level of consciousness
- Development of pupillary abnormalities
- Development of focal deficits
- Increasing ICP
- Extreme agitation and repeated vomiting

CNS complications after surgery result, in principle, from only a few causes whether surgery is performed supra-/infratentorial or spinal: hemorrhage, ischemia, raised intracranial pressure (ICP), dysfunctional CSF circulation, damage to CNS tissue and infection. All of these may coincide and initiate or aggravate each other.

Systemic complications, even when relatively minor from the systemic perspective, may cause substantial secondary damage to the CNS tissue, rendered more vulnerable following the surgical procedure.

Postoperative hematomas following cranial surgery may be subgaleal, epidural, subdural, or intraparenchymal. Subgaleal hematomas occur in up to 11% of procedures, but generally are of little consequence. Intracranial hemorrhages are more serious and may be life threatening. Approximately one-half of these are intraparenchymal, one-third epidural and 5–7% in the subdural space. These hematomas may be life threatening, due to raised ICP. Raised ICP is one of the most feared complications after cranial surgery and may further result from swelling/edema, vasodilatation or dysfunctional CSF circulation. Raised ICP has two profound and potentially fatal consequences:

(1) Herniation, consequently brain stem compression.
(2) Decrease in cerebral perfusion pressure, resulting in insufficient cerebral blood flow and ischemia.

Clinical signs of raised ICP and impending herniation include decreasing level of consciousness and the development of pupillary abnormalities. These signs should trigger immediate response (Table 68.3).

Table 68.4 Seizures in the direct postoperative phase

Cause	Prophylaxis
On anticonvulsants	– Balance between benefit/risk
– Low plasma levels due to:	
(a) Blood loss	High-risk indications:
(b) Hemodilution	– Arteriovenous malformation
(c) Did not receive normal dose	– Convexity/parasagital meningeoma
of anticonvulsive medication	– Subdural empyema/cerebral abscess
on the morning of surgery	– Penetrating head injury
	– Compound depressed skull fracture
No anticonvulsants:	
– Cortical irritation	

Seizures in the direct postoperative phase constitute a serious complication, due to the associated vasodilatation and subsequent brain swelling. Seizures also increase the risk for a postoperative hematoma. Every attempt should therefore be made to prevent the occurrence of seizures (Table 68.4) and – when occurring – immediate treatment may be life saving (see *Crisis Management*). When considering antiseizure prophylaxis, a balance should be sought between the risk for seizures developing and the possible risk of adverse events of anti/epileptic therapy.

Disease-Specific Complications

Although the general complications, listed in Table 68.1, may occur in any disease entity (e.g., oncologic, vascular, or trauma surgery), certain complications are more disease specific.

Aneurysm Treatment

The main complications in cerebrovascular surgery for an aneurysm are rebleed, acute or delayed ischemia and hydrocephalus, due to decreased CSF resorption or obstruction of CSF flow and vasospasm. Acute hydrocephalus (within the first 24 h) occurs in 20% of patients with an aneurysmal subarachnoid hemorrhage and is treated by external CSF drainage. Special vigilance is required on the patency of the drainage system. Complications of aneurysm treatment, their cause and treatment, differentiated per treatment modality, are summarized in Table 68.5.

Traumatic Brain Injury

Traumatic brain injury is a heterogeneous disease, in which raised ICP and ischemia are the most common problems. The cause and treatment of complications following TBI is summarized in Table 68.6.

Table 68.5 Complications of aneurysm treatment

Complications	Cause	Treatment
Surgical clipping		
– Postoperative hematoma	– Insufficient hemostasis – Surge in blood pressure	– Reoperation
– Rebleed		
	– Incomplete clipping	– Reoperation
	– Migration of clip	– Endovascular treatment
– Ischemia	– Low blood pressure	– Volume administration/ vasopressors
	– Vessel (partially) obstructed, intraoperative temporary clipping – Thrombosis	– Triple H therapy, calcium channel blockers
	– Vasospasm	– Consider thrombolysis – Triple H therapy[a], calcium channel blockers
	– Kinking of artery due to clip	– Consider reoperation
Coiling		
– Rupture of aneurysm during procedure	– Coil, stent manipulation, catheter manipulation	– Consider temporary balloon occlusion; complete procedure
– Arterial dissection	– Catheter manipulation	– Endovascular stenting
	– Catheter manipulation	
– Ischemia	– Low blood pressure	– Volume administration/ vasopressors
	– (Partial) migration of coils	
– Embolus	– Vasospasm	– Embolectomy/anticoagulants, stent/anticoagulants, reposition/ anticoagulants, volume administration/vasopressors, Triple H therapy, calcium channel blockers
Medical management		
HHH therapy		
– Heart failure	– Excessive volume load	– Diuretics, limit volume load
– Electrolyte disorders	– Iatrogenic/disease related	– Correction with IV fluids
– Bowel ischemia	– Excessive dose vasopressors	– Reduce dose vasopressors; bowel resection
– Calcium channel blocker	– Hypotension	– Reduce dose; administer vasopressors if necessary

[a] Triple H therapy: hypervolemia, hypertension, hemodilution

Table 68.6 Traumatic brain injury

Complications	Cause	Treatment
Raised ICP	– Hematoma	– Surgery
	– Edema	– ↓ICP/↑CPP therapy, decompressive craniectomy
	– Vasodilatation	– Hyperventilation/barbiturates
	– CSF flow disturbance	– CSF drainage
Ischemia	– Hypoxia/hypotension	– Medical management as appropriate
	– Vasospasm, microcirculatory disturbance	– Hemodilution/CPP therapy
	– Mitochondrial dysfunction	– Adequate sedation
CSF leak	– Skull (base) fracture	– External CSF drainage
		– Skull (base) reconstruction
Infection/meningitis	– CSF leak/air sinus wound	– Antibiotics/repair leak
Cerebral abscess	– Penetration foreign body	– Surgical debridement; antibiotics

Spinal Cord Surgery

In spinal cord surgery, prevention of ischemia and maintenance of adequate perfusion is just as important as in surgery to the brain. Careful observation of the neurological function is required following any type of spinal operation with specific attention for motor and sensory function as well as bowel/bladder function. The occurrence of increased or new deficits is suspect for compression of the spinal cord or cauda equina due to a postoperative hematoma or instability. In patients with spinal cord damage, specific and life-threatening or potentially debilitating complications include

- Urinary tract infection/pyelonephritis
- DVT and pulmonary embolism
- Pressure sores due to immobility and autonomic dysregulation
- Low blood pressure due to autonomic disturbance

Evaluation, Assessment, and Treatment in the Direct Postoperative Phase

Intake and Assessment

Following admission to the PACU, the first priority is to establish adequate monitoring; second, to gain an orientation on the patients history with a focus on the preoperative situation, intraoperative details (anesthesia and surgical) and postoperative instructions followed by a full evaluation (including focused physical examination). Relevant aspects for the postoperative intake are summarized in Table 68.7.

Table 68.7 Postoperative intake after neurosurgical operations

Preoperative situation	• Neurological deficit, e.g.: – Level of consciousness – Focal paresis – Sensory loss – Cranial nerve lesions – Hormonal deficits • Preexisting disease (especially pulmonary and cardiac) • Preoperative medication • History of seizures • Allergy
Intraoperative details (anesthesia)	• Narcotic agents and antagonists • Blood loss and substitution • Intraoperative laboratory values • Intraoperative secondary insults, diabetes insipidus, etc.
Intraoperative course (surgical)	• Indication, approach, and duration of surgery • Immobilization/positioning of patient • Surgical difficulties and complications, e.g.: – Brain swelling – Difficult hemostasis – Temporary or definite vascular occlusions – Opening of air sinus – Dura opening/closure – Intraoperative extraventricular drainage
Postoperative instructions	• Time of extubation • Instructions for postoperative care and monitoring • Instructions for removal of drainage, tubes, and stitches • Preferred duration of postoperative artificial ventilation • Instructions for follow-up CT/early postoperative MRI (if indicated) • Postoperative medication (including duration), e.g., – Anticonvulsants – Antibiotics – Steroids – Mannitol – Antithrombosis prophylaxis

A full assessment of the patient's neurological status is often impossible shortly after surgery if the patient arrives in the PACU still intubated and sedated. Yet, the clinical neurologic exam is the most sensitive monitor to detect structural lesions and the onset of postoperative complications. At arrival, the assessment of the pupillary reactivity and size is frequently the only reliable parameter. Every attempt should, however, be made to obtain some indication of the level of consciousness and of possible focal deficits as early as possible.

Assessment and reassessment are the keywords for monitoring a patient in the direct postoperative phase. The relevant parameters and their significance are summarized in Table 68.8. In this table, symptoms which should trigger immediate diagnostic or therapeutic interventions (see also Table 68.3) are highlighted.

Table 68.8 Assessment and reassessment

Parameter	Symptom	Significance
Level of consciousness	– Decreasing – Depressed	– ALARM – Anesthetic effect?
Pupillary reactivity	– Asymmetry/unreactive	– ALARM
Focal deficits	– Paresis/paralysis, cranial nerve palsy	– Deteriorating: ALARM
		– Stable: may indicate operative damage
Wound drainage	– Excessive	– Inadequate hemostasis? – Coagulopathy?
		May indicate:
Blood pressure	– High	– Raised ICP or – Inadequate analgesia
		Higher risk of bleeding!
	– Low	– Hypovolemia? – Sedative effect?
Volume status/ electrolytes	– Disorders may cause secondary damage	– Require correction
Blood gases	– Hypoxia*	– Aggravates ischemic damage
	– Hypocapnia	– Aggravates ischemic damage by vasoconstriction
	– Hypercapnia	– Increasing cerebral blood volume and ↑ICP by vasodilatation
CSF drainage	– No drainage/absent pulsations	– Catheter blocked, dislocated? – Accidentally removed
(ICP)	– Increasing ICP	– ALARM
	– Increased ICP > 20 mmHg	– Raised blood pressure/stress? – Postoperative intracranial hematoma? – Brain swelling/edema? – Extracranial cause?

*In addition to atelectasis and pneumonia as common causes of hypoxia, decreased oxygenation may indicate neurogenic pulmonary edema, impending cardiac or respiratory failure because of prolonged effects of anesthesia

Routine blood tests are indicated at time of admission to PACU/ICU and should include at least:

- Sodium
- Potassium
- Hemoglobin
- Glucose
- Blood gas analysis (pO2, pCO2, base excess, pH)
- Coagulation status (INR, PTT)

Table 68.9 Extubating the
neurosurgical patient

- Avoid coughing/straining
- Assess:
  - Adequate respiration?
    (a) Normal oxygenation
    (b) CPAP for at least 10 min
    (c) No apnea periods
  - Able to swallow?
  - Ability to communicate/obey commands
  - Pupillary reactivity
  → When all "yes" → proceed to extubate

Extubation

In most cases after elective surgery, the anesthesiologist and neurosurgeon will order often an early extubation, particularly in order to allow evaluation of the postoperative neurologic status. Criteria for extubation are summarized in Table 68.9.

If the patient does not fulfill these criteria or extubation cannot be performed "quietly," it may be preferable to prolong sedation with a bolus of a short-acting anesthetic agent, such as propofol or dexmeditomidine. During extubation it is essential to prevent coughing and straining, as this may provoke bleeding in the surgical field early after surgery. Extubation of the trachea should only occur when a health-care provider is present who is able to reintubate the airway in the event that the patient develops respiratory distress following extubation. Following emergency surgery, after complex procedures or when operative complications occurred, it may be preferable to prolong sedation and keep the patient intubated and ventilated in the immediate postoperative period. The appropriate anesthetic and sedative agents should then be instituted (e.g., midazolam/fentanyl).

Raised ICP

In more severe patients, in whom early extubation is not considered appropriate, and observation of the neurological status is therefore not possible, monitoring of ICP may be performed. If ICP increased to values above 20 mmHg, ICP-directed therapy is indicated (see Table 68.10), particularly in the setting of reduced cerebral perfusion. First, however, remediable extracranial causes should be excluded (Table 68.11).

ICP-directed therapy is, however, not without risk or complications (Table 68.12).

Care should therefore be taken not to treat ICP unnecessarily or to "over treat" patients.

Table 68.10 Remediable extracranial causes of intracranial hypertension

Calibration errors	Wrongly connected, not calibrated, unknown
Airway obstruction	Kinked endotracheal tube, tongue, sputum retention, pneumothorax
Hypoxia	FIO2, lung disease/collapse
Hypercapnia	Hypoventilation
Hypertension	Pain, sedation, coughing, straining
Hypotension	Hypovolemia, sedation, cardiac
Posture	Trendelenburg position, neck rotation
Hyperpyrexia	Infection, autonomous
Seizures	See Table 68.4
Hypo-osmolality	Sodium, protein

Table 68.11 Complications of ICP-directed therapy

Treatment modality	Problem		Result	Prevention
Hypocapnia	–	Excessive vasoconstriction	– Ischemia/infarction	Always maintain PaCO2 ≥ 30 mmHg (4 kPa) unless additional monitoring of CBF and oxygenation implemented
Mannitol	–	Hyperosmolarity	– Kidney damage	Maintain serum osmolarity (<315 mmol/l)
	–	Rebound phenomenon	– Increased ICP	If prolonged treatment required, dose at least 6×day
Hypertonic saline	–	Hypernatremia	– Decreased level of consciousness – Seizures	Maintain serum sodium (<150 mmol/l)
Barbiturates	–	Hypotension	– Ischemia	Maintain systolic BP>100 mmHg or MAP>60
CPP therapy	–	Volume overload	– Aggravate brain edema – May cause ARDS – Protracted course of raised ICP	Systemic monitoring
Sedation	–	Propofol syndrome	– Multiple organ failure	1 mg/kg/h, max 5 mg/kg/h no longer than 7 days continuously

Table 68.12 Response to alarm signs

Immediate treatment to lower ICP	Acute management of seizures:
– CSF drainage (only if ventricular catheter present)	– Immediate antiepileptic medication by IV route, e.g.:
– Hyperosmolar agents; choice between mannitol dose: 1 g/kg body weight IV hypertonic saline dose	– Diazepam 10 mg i.v. – Depakine 500–1,000 mg i.v. – Lorazepam 4 mg i.v.
– (Mild) hyperventilation; keep PaCO2 ≥ 30 mmHg (4 kPa)	– Phenytoin 15 mg/kg i.v. (to be administered over at least 2 h because of the risk of cardiac arrhythmias)
– Give vasopressors to maintain CPP if necessary	Further management:
• Contact neurosurgeon	*On anticonvulsants*:
• Initiate diagnostic tests (CT) and implement causal therapy	– Check plasma levels – Administer additional dose
	No anticonvulsants: – Initiate antiseizure medication

Patients can deteriorate quickly within hours to days after the operation, therefore reassess frequently!

Crisis Management

Crisis management is indicated when signs indicating critically raised ICP and impending herniation are noted or when seizures occur. In crisis management following intracranial surgery, the immediate priority is symptomatic treatment. Approaches are summarized in Table 68.10. The second priority is to contact the neurosurgeon and to initiate diagnostic tests (CT) and implement causal therapy.

> **Key Points**
>
> The status/condition of a patient in the direct postoperative phase can change rapidly within minutes to hours. Continued vigilance assessment and reassessment and necessary appropriate action remains indicated throughout the direct postoperative period.
>
> Overtreatment or inappropriate treatment can be just as dangerous or risky as undertreatment. Reassessment and a high level of awareness for possible complications can, however, never be exceeded.
>
> - Assess and reassess the patient.
> - Communication and documentation: get full postoperative intake.
> - Involve the neurosurgeon in case of any suspicion of problems or complications.
> - Awareness of possible complications.
> - Immediate response to alarm signs or seizures.
> - Do not be reluctant to initiate further diagnostic tests (e.g., CT scan).
> - Call for help early. Consulting with another provider is a sign of strength, not weakness.

Suggested Reading

Brain Trauma Foundation. Guidelines for the management of severe traumatic brain injury, 3rd edition. J Neurotrauma. 2007;24 Suppl 1:S1–106.

Constantini S, Cotev S, Rappaport ZH, Pomeranz S, Shalit MN. Intracranial pressure monitoring after elective intracranial surgery: a retrospective study of 514 consecutive patients. J Neurosurg. 1988;69:540–4.

Lee KH, Lukovits T, Friedman JA. "Triple-H" therapy for cerebral vasospasm following subarachnoid hemorrhage. Neurocrit Care. 2006;4(1):68–76.

Chapter 69
Hemodynamic Complications After Neurosurgery

Jeffrey Yoder and Rene Tempelhoff

Postoperative cardio-pulmonary complications may present following neurologic surgery and include hyper- or hypotension, bradycardia, myocardial ischemia, and hypoxemia. These physiologic disturbances may result secondary to the effects of surgical stress on preexisting medical comorbidities such as essential hypertension, coronary artery disease, or cardiomyopathy. Emergence hypertension, pain, and agitation can produce tachycardia and increase myocardial oxygen demand resulting in ischemia in susceptible patients. Electrolyte disturbances and intravascular volume shifts secondary to hyperosmotic therapy can precipitate arrhythmias, hypotension, or cardiac failure. Fluid loading and vasopressor administration such as for hypertensive, hypervolemic (triple H) therapy during treatment for cerebral vasospasm can precipitate pulmonary edema and heart failure.

Cardio-pulmonary complications may also occur as a result of interactions between the central nervous system and the cardiac and/or autonomic systems. While some of these effects have been recognized for nearly a century, most remain incompletely understood. Neurogenic pulmonary edema (NPE) may complicate traumatic brain injury, subarachnoid hemorrhage (SAH), or herniation syndromes. Electrocardiographic disturbances, myocardial injury, and heart failure may develop following SAH. Cushing's triad occurs in association with increased intracranial pressure and is comprised of bradycardia, hypertension, and respiratory failure.

J. Yoder, MD (✉)
Saint Anthony's Hospital, Denver, CO, USA
e-mail: jyoder8@gmail.com

R. Tempelhoff, MD
Department of Anesthesiology, Washington University School of Medicine, St. Louis, MO, USA

A.M. Brambrink and J.R. Kirsch (eds.), *Essentials of Neurosurgical
Anesthesia & Critical Care*, DOI 10.1007/978-0-387-09562-2_69,
© Springer Science+Business Media, LLC 2012

Neurogenic Pulmonary Edema

Overview

Neurogenic pulmonary edema (NPE) may result following multiple different types of neurologic injury and results in significant morbidity and mortality in affected patients. Insults such as traumatic brain or spinal cord injury, intracranial hemorrhage, intracranial hypertension, epileptic seizure, and SAH are all associated with the development of NPE. Tachypnea, tachycardia, hypoxemia, and diffuse bilateral pulmonary infiltrates are typical findings. Pulmonary vascular congestion, accumulation of protein-rich alveolar fluid, and intra-alveolar hemorrhage often result in significant hypoxemia. Treatment is primarily supportive.

Multiple pathophysiologic mechanisms have been proposed, although this process is not completely understood. Trigger zones consisting of specific vasomotor centers have been identified in the brainstem and hypothalamus. Injury to these regions and/or increased ICP are thought to elicit NPE through destabilization of pulmonary autonomics, massive catecholamine surge, and release of other vasoactive substances. Rapid sympathetic activation, as well as increased pulmonary capillary permeability, results in intra-alveolar exudates. Neurogenic stunned myocardium and cardiac failure may also contribute to the formation of pulmonary edema in some patients.

Prevention

There are no proven prophylactic measures to prevent NPE in man. In laboratory animals, lesions which produce NPE are much less likely to do so when the animal is concurrently anesthetized with high concentrations of volatile anesthetics. It is possible that tight hemodynamic control and blunting of the response to catecholamines may limit the generation of NPE. Treatment of the underlying condition (such as surgical clipping of an aneurysm) may also improve NPE outcome.

Crisis Management (Table 69.1)

Key Points

- NPE may be elicited by multiple different injuries to the CNS.
- Significant hypoxemia may develop, and morbidity is high.
- Treatment is supportive.

Table 69.1 Presentation/assessment/intervention

Presentation	Assessment	Intervention
• Tachycardia	• Check vital signs	• Treatment is supportive
• Tachypnea/dyspnea	• Arterial blood gas – hypoxemia is the most common finding	• Supplemental oxygen and mechanical ventilation if required
• Hypoxemia	• Chest X-ray – typically diffuse bilateral infiltrates	• Hemodynamic support as necessary
• Respiratory failure	• Differentiate from other causes of pulmonary edema. Consider TTE to assess cardiac function	• Expect clearance within 24–48 h (= additional diagnostic evidence)
	• Assess need for mechanical ventilation	

Pulmonary Embolism

Overview

Patients for craniotomy or major spine surgery are at increased risk for the development of deep venous thrombosis (DVT) and venous thromboembolism (VTE). Specific risk factors include immobility secondary to neurologic deficit and/or prolonged surgery, malignancy, advanced age, venous stasis, and avoidance of pharmacologic DVT-prophylaxis due to concern of increased risk of bleeding. A state of relative hypercoagulability has been described following many neurologic events.

The reported incidence of lower extremity DVT and VTE varies based on patient population, risk factors, type of screening, and presence and type of prophylaxis. DVT is unfortunately quite common in the neurosurgical patient population with a reported incidence as high as 20–40% during hospital stay. Clinically significant VTE is more rare, with a reported incidence of <5% in most studies, although it is thought that the majority of VTE are "silent." Practices that support the routine use of PICC lines also observe an increased frequency of DVT and VTE in the upper extremity.

Prevention

Various prophylactic measures against DVT are employed in hospitalized patients. Commonly used techniques include elastic stockings, intermittent pneumatic compression devices (IPC), subcutaneous unfractionated heparin, and low-molecular weight heparin. Elastic stockings and IPCs are generally the only prophylactic measures taken during the perioperative period due to concerns that heparin could increase the risk of bleeding. In recent meta-analysis of mixed neurosurgical patients, IPCs appear of similar efficacy to low-molecular weight heparin in prevention of VTE during the immediate perioperative period. However, it is likely that patients with multiple risk factors might benefit from a combined regimen. During surgery, patients should be positioned such that venous return is not impeded (avoidance of excessive flexion of the hips/knees in prone patients). Postoperatively medical prophylaxis should be resumed as soon as it is deemed safe to do so by the surgical team. Concerns about the appropriate timing of pharmacologic thrombophrophylaxis remain particularly high for patients after intracranial hemorrhage due to their high risk for both rebleeding as well as thrombus formation. Currently, clinical practice of DVT-prophylaxis in this patient population is guided by personal experience rather than by scientific evidence, secondary to a paucity of reliable data. The avoidance of PICC lines in the absence of pharmacologic prophylaxis may be an important consideration to reduce the incidence of upper extremity DVT.

Crisis Management (Table 69.2)

Table 69.2 Presentation/assessment/intervention

Presentation	Assessment	Intervention
• Tachycardia	• Check vital signs	• Supportive care
• Tachypnea/dyspnea	• Assess oxygenation and ventilation, check for change in $ETCO_2$ in intubated patients	• Supplemental oxygen and/or mechanical ventilation as necessary
• Hypoxemia	• ABG – typically shows hypoxemia. $PaCO_2$ may be significantly higher than $EtCO_2$	• Hemodynamic support if required
• Increased gradient between $EtCO_2$ and $PaCO_2$	• Differentiate from other causes of hypoxemia including pulmonary edema, atelectasis, etc.	• Consider IVC filter placement (particularly if LE venous Doppler studies demonstrate clot)
• Anxiety	• Chest X-ray – often negative in PE	• Consider anticoagulation (heparinization) depending upon type and duration out from surgical procedure
• Hemodynamic instability	• PE protocol CT (or V/Q scan in patients with significant renal impairment) • Consider lower extremity Doppler's (may influence decision for early IVC filter if positive)	• Consider intravascular clot retrieval by skilled interventional radiologist

Key Points

- Neurosurgical patients are at high risk for DVT.
- IPC and/or compression stockings are the most commonly employed prophylaxis during the perioperative period.
- Clinically significant VTE present with hypoxemia and tachycardia.
- IVC filter placement should be considered in patients with VTE and DVT, given bleeding risk from early anticoagulation.

Blood Pressure Dysregulation

Overview

Blood pressure lability is common in postoperative neurosurgical patients and may result from a variety of neurogenic, cardiogenic, or systemic causes. Emergence hypertension, pain, and agitation are common. The Cushing's response to raised ICP, or cerebral ischemia can result in significant increases in blood pressure. Patients with spinal cord lesions whether acute (spinal shock) or chronic (autonomic hyperreflexia) may develop blood pressure instability in the perioperative period. Seizures may result in labile blood pressures. Following carotid endarterectomy many patients experience blood pressure dysregulation, most commonly hypertension, as a result of baroreceptor dysfunction.

Systemic causes of hemodynamic instability are numerous and include hypovolemia, anemia, and pulmonary embolism. Myocardial infarction, arrhythmias, and cardiac failure can also present with significant hemodynamic instability.

Careful attention to blood pressure must always be paid in order to ensure adequate perfusion pressure to critical organs such as the brain and myocardium, but hypertension cannot be allowed to go unchecked. Emergence from anesthesia is frequently accompanied by postoperative hypertension and cerebral hyperemia. There is a significant association between postoperative hypertension and intracranial hemorrhage, thus this response should be controlled by beta-blockers and other antihypertensives.

Prevention

Postoperative blood pressure lability may be limited by careful intraoperative management of blood pressure, volume status, and hematocrit. Significant emergence hypertension should prompt early treatment with beta-blockers (which have the advantage of not effecting ICP) and other antihypertensives, as well as effective treatment of pain and agitation. Dexmedetomidine has shown promise in preliminary studies in reducing hypertensive events in the perioperative period in patients undergoing craniotomy.

Crisis Management (Table 69.3)

Table 69.3 Cause/assessment/intervention

Cause	Assessment	Intervention
• Pain	• Check vital signs, neurologic assessment, and pain score	• Supportive care for patient
• Agitation	• Assessment of volume status, recent drugs administered, hematocrit	• Identify and treat underlying cause (if possible)
• Emergence hypertension	• Consider underlying etiology – neurogenic, cardiogenic, metabolic	• Antihypertensive therapies
• Elevated ICP		– β blockade (i.v. esmolol 10–50 mg, metoprolol 1–5 mg, labetolol 5–20 mg)
• Cerebral ischemia		– Hydralazine (5–15 mg i.v.)
• Seizure		– Nicardipine (0.25–2 mcg/kg/min i.v. infusion)
• Spinal cord injury		• Antihypotensive therapies
• Baroreceptor dysfunction		– Treat significant bradycardia with anticholinergics
• Essential hypertension		– Ephedrine (5–10 mg i.v.)
• Drug effect		– Phenylephrine (0.25–2 mcg/kg/min i.v. infusion) Caution in the context of bradycardia
• Hypovolemia/Anemia		– Norepinephrine (0.02–0.2 mcg/kg/min iv infusion)
• Myocardial infarction/Cardiac failure		
• Arrhythmia		
• Pulmonary embolism		

Key Points

- Postoperative blood pressure instability can present secondary to multiple neurogenic or cardiac causes.
- Blood pressure should be carefully regulated in the postoperative period to ensure effective perfusion to organs and reduce the risk of hemorrhage.

Bradycardia

Overview

Bradycardia is frequently noted in neurosurgical patients during the perioperative period. Identification of cause is important for effective therapy. This response may be elicited by multiple neurogenic, cardiac, or metabolic factors.

Cushing's triad of bradycardia, hypertension, and apnea in response to elevated ICP may occur in patients with mass effect from tumor, edema, intracranial hemorrhage, or acute hydrocephalus. Bradycardia may also occur in association with spinal cord injury (SCI), such as acute spinal shock secondary to transection of sympathetic pathways or autonomic dysreflexia in chronic SCI patients. Bradycardia may also be seen with seizures and can be triggered via reflex pathways such as the baroreceptor or trigeminal-cardiac reflex.

Cardiac etiologies of bradycardia may include nodal or conduction deficits, as well as other arrhythmias. Myocardial ischemia and cardiac failure can also precipitate bradycardia. Metabolic causes are numerous. Many drugs may produce bradycardia through direct or indirect effects. Electrolyte disturbances may be precipitated by diuretics or hyperosmolar therapy. Endocrine disorders such as hypothyroidism may also contribute to bradycardia.

Prevention

As significant bradycardias are not infrequent in neurosurgical patients, resuscitative drugs, particularly atropine should always be readily available. Patients at high risk for such complications include those after surgeries on/and around the brain stem or the cerebral-pontine angle, and those after endovascular carotid stenting. In high-risk cases or when bradycardias are frequently noted, prophylactic administration of anticholinergics such as glycopyrrolate may be beneficial.

Crisis Management (Table 69.4)

Key Points

- Bradycardia is frequent and has multiple potential etiologies in neurosurgical patients.
- Bradycardia may be a sign of impeding clinical deterioration of the patient.
- Treatment involves identifying cause, anticholinergics, and pacing in refractory cases.

Table 69.4 Cause/assessment/intervention

Cause	Assessment	Intervention

• Increased ICP
  – Edema
  – Hemorrhage
  – Hydrocephalus
  – Pneumocephalus
    (tension)
	• Check vital signs, including BP and oxygenation, and neurologic assessment
	
	• Check rhythm strip (p wave, narrow/wide complex)
		• Anticholinergics (e.g., glycopyrolate 0.2–1.0 mg; atropine 1 mg i.v. for significant bradycardia) – avoid lower doses in adult patients due to risk of paradoxical bradycardia

• Vagal	• Evaluate for cause	• Support hemodynamics and oxygenation
• Spinal cord injury	– Drug administration	• Identify/treat underlying cause (if possible)
• Cardiac, nodal/ Conduction deficits	– Reflex	• Consider temporary pacing (transvenous) in refractory cases
• Drug effect	– Cardiac	
• Metabolic	– Increased ICP	
	• Consider imaging (head CT)	

Myocardial Infarction

Overview

Postoperative myocardial infarction (MI) is fortunately a rare event. Often affected patients have preexisting medical comorbidities such as coronary artery disease, or its risk factors such as smoking, diabetes, or others. Coronary insufficiency can lead to infarction when stress of surgery is superimposed. Independent of surgery, severe brain injury states may also cause significant elevations in catecholamines which can precipitate ischemia and infarction. EKG changes suggestive of myocardial injury occur in up to 80% of patients following subarachnoid hemorrhage. While these patients often exhibit elevation of cardiac enzymes and regional wall motion abnormalities, this form of myocardial injury is more commonly neurogenic stress cardiomyopathy than traditional myocardial infarction.

In patients with risk factors or known coronary artery disease, preoperative optimization is often limited to medical therapies. Invasive coronary interventions typically require anticoagulation and wait times for stent stabilization. Given the often urgent nature of neurosurgery and the risk of significant complications with surgical bleeding, coronary intervention may not be feasible or able to effectively reduce risk. These limitations can also complicate management of active myocardial ischemia in the patient immediately postop from brain or spine surgery. Furthermore in patients with preexisting coronary stents, perioperative discontinuation of aspirin and/or clopidogrel may precipitate acute coronary syndromes from in-stent thrombosis.

Prevention

Guidelines for preoperative cardiac evaluation are published by the American Heart Association and frequently updated. Currently, diagnostic testing (such as stress testing) is recommended only in high-risk patients, and only if results will significantly affect the surgical decision or perioperative management. Urgent surgeries generally should be delayed for medical optimization in patients with active cardiac conditions such as myocardial ischemia, decompensated heart failure, or significant arrhythmias. Patients with a history of coronary artery disease should be evaluated to ensure that they are medically optimized, such as effective beta-blockade and heart rate control. Perioperatively, patients with significant risk of cardiac ischemia should be carefully monitored and their hemodynamics aggressively controlled. Prevention of tachycardia and maintenance of an effective blood pressure are the primary goals.

Crisis Management (Table 69.5)

Table 69.5 Presentation/assessment/intervention

Presentation	Assessment	Intervention
• Chest pain and/or dyspnea	• Check vital signs with attention toward HR, BP, and oxygenation	• Limit tachycardia – treat pain, β blockade as tolerated (i.v. metoprolol)
• ECG abnormalities (ST segment depression or elevation)	• Obtain 12 lead ecg	• Ensure adequate oxygenation
• Hemodynamic instability	• Obtain labs for serum troponin-I, Hgb/Hct, and electrolytes	• Ensure an adequate blood pressure (for coronary and cerebral perfusion)
• Arrhythmia or cardiac failure		• Consider nitrates (however, these may increase CBF and ICP in at risk patients)
		• Early cardiology consultation for discussion of anticoagulation and/or invasive intervention

Key Points

- In neurosurgical patients, preoperative cardiac optimization is predominantly medical.
- Avoidance of tachycardia and maintenance of adequate coronary perfusion pressure are primary goals to prevent myocardial ischemia.
- Beta-blockade and other supportive care is first line therapy.
- Treatment of MI in the early postoperative period with antiplatelet agents and heparinization is complicated by the increased risk of bleeding.

Suggested Reading

Agrawal A, Timothy J, Cincu R, Agarwal T, Waghmare LB. Bradycardia in neurosurgery. Clin Neurol Neurosurg. 2008;110:321–7.

Basali A, Mascha EJ, Kalfas I, Schubert A. Relation between perioperative hypertension and intracranial hemorrhage after craniotomy. Anesthesiology. 2000;93:48–54.

Bekker A, Sturaitis M, Bloom M, Moric M, Golfinos J, Parker E, et al. The effect of dexmedetomidine on perioperative hemodynamics in patients undergoing craniotomy. Anesth Analg. 2008;107:1340–7.

Chan AT, Atiemo A, Diran LL, Licholai GP, Black PM, Creager MA, et al. Venous thromboembolism occurs frequently in patients undergoing brain tumor surgery despite prophylaxis. J Thromb Thrombolysis. 1999;8:139–42.

Collen JF, Jackson JL, Shorr AF, Moores LK. Prevention of venous thromboembolism in neurosurgery. Chest. 2008;134:237–49.

Fleisher LA, Beckman JA, Brown KA, Calkins H, Chaikof E, Fleischmann KE, et al. ACC/AHA 2007 Guidelines on perioperative cardiovascular evaluation and care for noncardiac surgery: a report of the American College of Cardiology/American Heart Association task force on practice guidelines. Circulation. 2007;116:e418–99.

Hacke W (ed). Neurocritical care. Ch. 34: Acute autonomic instability. Springer;1994.

Schubert A. Cardiovascular therapy of neurosurgical patients. Best Pract Res Clin Anaesthesiol. 2007;21:483–96.

Sedy J, Zicha J, Kunes J, Jendelova P, Sykova E. Mechanisms of neurogenic pulmonary edema development. Physiol Res. 2008;57:499–506.

Stoneham MD, Thompson JP. Arterial pressure management and carotid endarterectomy. Br J Anaesth. 2009;102:453–62.

Chapter 70
Endocrinologic Emergencies After Neurosurgery

Ola Harrskog and Robert E. Shangraw

Overview

Severe and potentially life-threatening endocrine conditions in neurosurgical patients most often are secondary to dysfunction of the hypothalamus–pituitary–adrenal axis. The pituitary gland, frequently called the "master endocrine gland," is confined within a bony space – the sella turcica – and is subdivided, both anatomically and functionally, into anterior (anterior pituitary) and posterior (neurohypophysis) components. The anterior pituitary has a vulnerable portal blood supply. The posterior portion connects to the hypothalamus via long sensitive nerve endings. This arrangement makes the pituitary especially susceptible to traumatic brain injury, brain edema, space-occupying intracranial lesions, and surgery.

Hormones secreted by the pituitary regulate metabolic homeostasis, fluid and electrolyte balance, and circulatory stability. The anterior pituitary secretes six hormones: growth hormone, adrenocorticotropic hormone (ACTH), thyroid-stimulating hormone (TSH), follicle-stimulating hormone (FSH), lutenizing hormone, and luteotropic hormone. Control of the anterior pituitary comes from the hypothalamus, via releasing factors secreted into the hypothalamic-hypophyseal portal system. There is a negative feedback control system, by which end products of anterior pituitary activity inhibit corresponding stimulatory hormone secretion by anterior pituitary and the upstream releasing factor secretion by the hypothalamus, to maintain homeostasis. ACTH released from the anterior pituitary stimulates the adrenal cortex to release cortisol and to a much lesser extent mineral-corticosteroid (aldosterone) and androgen (DHEA). Circulating cortisol feeds back to both the pituitary and hypothalamus to reduce stimulatory activity. Cortisol is vital to cellular homeostasis and metabo-

O. Harrskog, MD, DEAA • R.E. Shangraw, MD, PhD (✉)
Department of Anesthesiology and Perioperative Medicine,
Oregon Health & Science University, Portland, OR, USA
e-mail:shangraw@ohsu.edu

A.M. Brambrink and J.R. Kirsch (eds.), *Essentials of Neurosurgical Anesthesia & Critical Care*, DOI 10.1007/978-0-387-09562-2_70, © Springer Science+Business Media, LLC 2012

lism and is needed for both catecholamine-mediated and angiotensin-mediated maintenance of vascular tone, which is essential for hemodynamic stability.

The posterior pituitary secretes antidiuretic hormone (ADH), also known as vasopressin, and oxytocin. Its function is more directly regulated by the hypothalamus through neural connections. Through ADH secretion, the posterior pituitary (neurohypophysis) regulates both intravascular volume and serum osmolarity. ADH is a nonapeptide which acts on aquaporin 2 in the renal collecting tubule to increase water permeability and, in turn, retain water from the urinary space (antidiuretic effect). Physiologic control of ADH secretion is maintained via osmoreceptors located in the hypothalamus that increase ADH secretion in response to hyperosmolarity (most often hypernatremia). ADH plays a vital role in maintaining salt and water balance. ADH also has direct vasoconstrictor activity and is used as an effective non-catecholamine pressor agent in pharmacological concentrations. Its role in maintaining normal vascular tone under physiological conditions is less clear.

Anterior Pituitary Insufficiency

Severe illness, trauma, or other insults trigger a metabolic "stress" response, mediated in large part by the neuro-endocrine system. Under some circumstances, the stress response can be maladaptive and may need to be inhibited. During anesthesia, the stress response may be altered if not prevented.

Adrenal insufficiency, the inability to mount an appropriate level of cortisol secretion, can be relative or absolute. An intact hypothalamic-pituitary-adrenal axis, with cortisol as the centerpiece, is essential to maintaining stable hemodynamics during stress. Patients who receive preexisting glucocorticoid treatment are at risk for developing an absolute adrenal insufficiency because the adrenal gland atrophies. If, as in most cases, the glucocorticoid dose is low, the adrenal gland cannot provide the higher glucocorticoid concentration needed during a stress state. Less common causes of absolute adrenal insufficiency are congenital adrenal hypoplasia or destruction of the adrenal gland secondary to infection (e.g., Addison's disease) or surgery. The common endpoint of these conditions is an inability to increase cortisol production in response to stress.

Relative adrenal insufficiency is associated with critical illness, especially sepsis, and with head trauma, systemic inflammatory response, advanced age, and certain drugs. Among drugs associated with relative adrenal insufficiency, the sedative-hypnotic etomidate deserves special mention. Since its US release in 1972, etomidate has been known to attenuate the hypercortisolemic response to surgery. Although it was initially thought to produce a "stress-free" surgery, etomidate directly inhibits cortisol synthesis by the adrenal gland. Etomidate infusion in the intensive care unit has been associated with increased mortality secondary to adrenal suppression, and even a single induction dose of etomidate can suppress cortisol secretion for 4–12 h. Etomidate exposure is an important risk factor for relative adrenal insufficiency in critically ill, septic patients and is associated with higher mortality in these patients unless supplemental steroids are administered. Physiological doses of glucocorticoids improve outcome in septic patients, but supraphysiological doses provide no definite advantage. For nonseptic high-risk patients, the value of physiologic or supraphysiologic glucocorticoid administration on outcome is less clear.

Incidence. Adrenal insufficiency, as indexed by cortisol response, has an incidence of 30–40% in the general critically ill population and about 25% after traumatic brain injury. The underlying medical condition and the magnitude of stress stimulus are important for defining relative risk.

Prevention

Patients with a history of current or recent (within 2 months) glucocorticoid therapy should be considered at risk for relative adrenal insufficiency, even if signs or symptoms are absent. A daily dose of prednisolone 7.5 mg, or its equivalent, for 2 weeks or longer is sufficient to suppress the adrenal stress response; and the hypo-responsiveness can persist for 2 months after steroid therapy has been discontinued. Depending on the anticipated stress event, one should consider supplemental prophylactic glucocorticoid administration ("stress steroids"). Reasonable choices before major surgery are hydrocortisone 100 mg q 8 h × 3 doses or dexamethasone 8–10 mg with the same dosing regime.

Crisis Management

Clinical presentation. An unstressed patient with an underlying adrenal insufficiency may be asymptomatic, with no revealing signs. Clinical signs, if present, are constitutional and vague: asthenia, muscle weakness, anorexia, abdominal pain, or other referred gastrointestinal complaints. More pronounced insufficiency can lead to hypoglycemia, hyponatremia, and/or hyperkalemia. The electrolyte abnormalities may induce severe muscle weakness.

Diagnosis of a relative adrenal insufficiency, where the signs and symptoms are vague, requires a high level of suspicion. Superimposition of physiological stress (e.g., trauma, infection, and surgery) or sudden cessation of chronic steroid intake can trigger an acute crisis. In an acute adrenal crisis, the patient often develops a profound and refractory hypotension in addition to muscle weakness and hypoglycemia. Hypotension in this setting is due to a confluence of impaired catecholamine synthesis, hypo-responsive beta-adrenoreceptors, and an inability of vascular smooth muscle to contract in response to either circulating catecholamines or angiotensin. Clinical presentation of refractory arterial hypotension without obvious cause should include suspicion of acute adrenocortical insufficiency in the differential diagnosis.

Patient assessment. A random cortisol level is the definitive diagnostic test. The serum specimen should be collected before empirical steroid therapy commences; otherwise, timing is not important. Critically ill patients do not exhibit predictable diurnal cycling of cortisol secretion. In general, a cortisol value >35 μg/dL is normal in the critically ill patient with normal adrenal function, whereas a value <15 μg/dL is consistent with adrenal insufficiency. Intermediate results may indicate further testing. If the results are borderline, the corticotrophin-stimulating test may help to identify patients who may benefit from chronic glucocorticoid supplements. Serial measurements of serum electrolytes are indicated to detect hyponatremia, hyperkalemia, and/or hypoglycemia. Urine electrolytes are also useful because high urine sodium excretion may occur despite functional hypovolemia. An arterial blood gas will reveal whether there is an accompanying metabolic or respiratory acidosis.

Treatment. Treatment of an acute Addisonian crisis is often empirical because the turnaround time for serum cortisol analysis is often on the order of 24 h. Hydrocortisone 100 mg IV q 8 h or dexamethasone 10 mg IV q 8 h are both good choices. Hemodynamic support, fluid administration, and vasopressors are given as necessary. Other causes for hypotension, such as myocardial dysfunction (ischemia or infarction) or sepsis, should be evaluated and ruled out. If hypotension is precipitated by adrenal insufficiency, the patient will become quickly responsive to inotropes such as ephedrine or epinephrine within an hour after steroid supplementation.

If it appears that a critically ill patient may have an adrenal insufficiency, treatment with stress doses of hydrocortisone should be given as above. Patients with suspected relative adrenal insufficiency should be treated with titrated doses, i.e., in most nonseptic patients, the equivalent of dexamethasone 2–10 mg should suffice. Because cortisol is much less potent as a mineralocorticoid than as a glucocorticoid, the volume deficit in patients with adrenal crisis is rarely more than 10% of the total body water. Normal saline is the usual fluid for volume expansion. Hypoglycemia, which is usually mild, is treated carefully with glucose 5% added to the normal saline.

Monitoring. Frequent electrolyte, glucose, and arterial blood gas measurements are important. Invasive hemodynamic monitoring via arterial line and central venous line will be necessary to guide treatment in unstable patients.

Posterior Pituitary (Neurohypophysis) Dysfunction

Posterior pituitary dysfunction most often presents as disorders of water and salt balance. These are common in patients with traumatic brain injury or disease in the area of the hypothalamus and the pituitary gland. Dysfunction of the neurohypophysis can result in either overproduction or underproduction of ADH. Some disease states, such as pulmonary diseases (e.g., oat cell carcinoma) or extra neural neoplasms, are associated with ectopic production of ADH. Three conditions have important implications for salt and water homeostasis in patients with cerebral disease processes: diabetes insipidus (DI), syndrome of inappropriate ADH secretion (SIADH), and cerebral salt-wasting syndrome (CSWS). It is extremely important to recognize these conditions and their pathophysiology early to maximize the potential for recovery.

Diabetes Insipidus

DI is a syndrome characterized by polyuria, polydipsia, and excessive thirst. Patients with DI experience excessive loss of free water into the urine causing increased concentration of solutes throughout the body, and hemodynamic instability secondary to hypovolemia. DI is divided into two subtypes: (1) nephrogenic and (2) central (or neurogenic).

Nephrogenic DI, due to the failure of the kidney to appropriately respond to physiological levels of circulating ADH, and involves dysfunction of aquaporin 2, the intrinsic receptor that increases renal collecting tubule permeability to water. Central DI, the more common subtype in the neurosurgical patient, results from insufficient ADH release into the circulation from the posterior pituitary.

Normally, up to 12% of glomerular filtrate is reabsorbed under the influence of ADH. Complete absence of ADH results in excessive loss of free water (20 L/24 h) into the urine, leading to polyuria of extremely low osmolarity. Frequently, the ADH deficiency is relative, and the volume of hypotonic urine is 5–10 L/24 h. DI is usually transient but can be permanent.

Incidence. Transient DI after traumatic brain injury occurs in up to 50% of patients and is permanent in up to 10% of cases. After transphenoidal hypophysectomy, 18% of patients are affected at least transiently, and 2% require long-term treatment. In general, any prolonged episode of increased intracranial pressure, such as intracranial hemorrhage or a tumor, can impair ADH secretion by the neurohypophysis, independent of etiology.

Crisis Management

Clinical presentation. Onset of polyuria is usually sudden after trauma, regional surgery, or sella radiotherapy. If the patient is awake and alert, this will manifest as polydipsia. If the patient is not fully conscious, however, inadequate fluid intake may result in hypovolemia and hypernatremia. Replacement of lost water with a balanced intravenous salt solution leads to apparent sodium accumulation, and serum hypernatremia worsens. Severe hypernatremia induces central nervous system dysfunction, presenting progressively as delirium, confusion, somnolence, and finally coma. The marked interindividual variability in CNS response to high sodium concentration precludes assigning trigger sodium concentrations at which symptoms will occur. Once systemic hypernatremia has occurred, rapid correction of hyperosmolality can produce brain edema.

Patient assessment. Fulminant DI causes a copius and very hypotonic (50–200 mOsm/kg) urine. Incomplete DI is still characterized by polyuria, but the urine sodium concentration can be higher (up to 700 mOsm/kg), especially if the patient is hypovolemic and/or if intravenous saline has been given. The most important finding is that urine osmolality is inappropriately low compared with plasma osmolality

Table 70.1 Summary of differences in volume status and laboratory tests in postoperative neurosurgical patients

Dysfunction	Body water (fluid status, CVP)	Urine output	serum-[Na⁺]	Urine-[Na⁺]	Serum-[ADH]
CSWS	↓	↑	↓	↑	↑ or →
SIADH	↑ or →	↓ or →	↓	↑	↑
DI-Central	↓	↑↑	↑	↓ or →	↓
DI-Nephrogenic	↓	↑↑	↑	↓ or →	↑ or →

CSWS, cerebral salt-wasting syndrome; SIADH, syndrome of inappropriate release of antidiuretic hormone; DI, diabetes insipidus; ↓, lower than normal; ↑, higher than normal; →, no difference from normal

(ratio less than 2). If plasma Na > 145 mmol/L and plasma osmolality > 300 mOsm/kg, in concert with diluted polyuria (> 3.5 L/24 h), the most likely diagnosis is DI. Free water deficit can be estimated by the equation: Water deficit (liters) = 0.6 × body weight (kg) × ((current [Na]/desired [Na]) − 1) where the desired [Na] is taken to be 140 mmol/L.

The definitive test to discern central DI from nephrogenic DI is to assay the serum ADH concentration. ADH is low in central DI but normal in nephrogenic DI (Table 70.1).

Treatment. The goals of interventions are to: (1) correct intravascular volume and total body water deficits, (2) replace ongoing water losses, (3) reduce ongoing water losses, and (4) prevent hyperosmolality. Given these guidelines, treatment is individualized based on the severity and anticipated duration of the dysfunction. In an awake patient with an intact thirst mechanism (with free access to water), observation and monitoring may suffice.

If the condition is prolonged or the diuresis exceeds practical oral water intake, modified ADH (desmopressin, DDAVP) is the agent of choice to restore more normal renal water reabsorption. DDAVP can be administered by oral, nasal, or intravenous route. For acutely ill patients, parenteral administration is preferred, and the recommended dose is 1–4 μg q 8–12 h. Alternatively, unmodified vasopressin may be used, to help retain free water, but its short half-life limits utility.

Intravenous fluid replacement should maximize free water and limit sodium concentration because the goal is to compensate for the loss of free water. Aqueous glucose (D5% W) is usually the first choice in patients who cannot take in adequate oral fluid to cover the losses and deficits. Careful serum glucose management is warranted in such cases to prevent hyperglycemia and possible consequent brain injury.

Syndrome of Inappropriate Antidiuretic Hormone Secretion

SIADH is a condition of excessive ADH secretion (Table 70.1). High circulating ADH concentration promotes a pathologically increased free water reabsorption by the kidney, leading in turn to hypervolemia and hyponatremia. Concomitant renal sodium excretion may be normal or increased. The neurohypophysis is the source of the excessive ADH secretion in disease states such as intracranial infection, trauma, bleeding, or infection. However, tumors of extraneural origin, such as oat cell lung carcinoma, can serve as a pathologic ectopic source of ADH.

Incidence. In patients suffering traumatic brain injury, the incidence of SIADH is reported to be 2.3–37%. Single case series place the incidence of SIADH at 12.8% after transsphenoidal hypophysectomy, and 6.9% after major spine surgery.

Crisis Management

Clinical presentation. CNS manifestations of SIADH are usually mild as long as the plasma Na^+ concentration >125 mmol/L. Once the Na^+ concentration drops to <120 mmol/L, pronounced CNS signs and symptoms become more likely. The mildest presentation is headache, which may progress to nausea, confusion, coma, and seizures. The sensitivity of patients to hyponatremia depends in large part to the speed with which it unfolds. Very rapid progression also raises the risk of cerebral edema and its consequent events. Some individuals may tolerate serum sodium levels of <115 mmol/L without clinical symptoms for a long period of time, if the onset is gradual, such as over months.

Patient assessment. Patients with SIADH have hypotonic hyponatremia with urine osmolality greater than plasma osmolality. Sodium excretion exceeds 20 mmol/L while the serum osmolality is <280 mOsm/kg. The patient is not likely to present with circulatory instability unless there is congestive heart failure, which could be exacerbated by the hypervolemia. Symptomatic hyponatremia is typically produced by the coincidence of overhydration (positive balance 6–8 L) and a sodium deficit of 200–400 mmol.

Treatment. The treatment strategy depends upon presence or absence of clinical manifestations. If the patient is asymptomatic, the condition is treated by fluid restriction and identification of precipitating factor(s). If CNS manifestations are present, the sodium concentration must be increased to approximately 130 mmol/L, at a rate not to exceed 1–2 mmol/L/h. Normal (0.9%) saline is usually administered to correct hyponatremia at a rate that does not exceed urinary losses. Too rapid a correction of hyponatremia is carries the risk of demyelinating the brain (central pontine myelinolysis). On the other hand, if the patient has seizures, it is important to treat not only the seizures but also to begin prompt treatment of cerebral edema and a more rapid initial correction of the hyponatremia. Mannitol (100 g) or low-dose hypertonic saline have both been proposed in the setting of seizures.

Cerebral Salt-Wasting Syndrome

CSWS has been proposed as an alternative cause of hyponatremia in patients suffering neurological disease. CSWS and SIADH have many similar laboratory characteristics (Table 70.1). They differ, however, in that patients with SIADH are normovolemic or slightly hypervolemic, whereas those with CSWS are hypovolemic. The molecular mechanism underlying the excessive urinary sodium loss of CSWS following intracranial disease processes is unclear. One hypothesis is that as-yet unidentified natriuretic factor(s) is/are released by the injured or dysfunctional brain. Candidates for the diuretic factor include atrial natriuretic peptide (ANP) and brain natriuretic peptide (BNP). Circulating ADH concentration is normal in patients with CSWS, in contrast to the elevated ADH concentration in patients with SIADH.

Incidence. The incidence of CSWS is unknown. Controversy in the literature today centers on (1) whether the CSWS syndrome actually exists and (2) whether a number of patients with the diagnosis of SIADH should instead have been diagnosed with CSWS.

Crisis Management

Clinical presentation. CSWS usually appears the first week after an insult to the brain, whether trauma, tumor, infection, or surgery. It usually persists for a few weeks and is self-limited. Clinical characteristics are polyuria, increased urinary sodium loss, hyponatremia, and hypovolemia.

Patient assessment. The main clinical challenge is to distinguish CSWS from SIADH. Plasma ADH in CSWS is either within normal limits or may be increased as part of the physiological response to hypovolemia.

Treatment. Once the diagnosis of CSWS is made, treatment goals are to maintain adequate fluid hydration plus replace sodium losses. This regimen contrasts with the treatment of SIADH, the other major cause of hyponatremia, which is to restrict fluids to normalize the serum sodium levels. Incorrectly limiting intravenous (or oral) fluids in a patient with CSWS brings the risk of hypoperfusing an already compromised brain, with consequent morbidity and mortality. Some clinical examples of settings where CSWS inappropriately treated by fluid restriction could exacerbate brain injury are cerebral vasospasm, ischemic cerebral infarction, or myocardial ischemia. Since the major endpoint of therapy is to preserve volume status, invasive hemodynamic monitoring including arterial and central venous pressure (CVP) monitoring may be indicated, even if the patient appears to be hemodynamically stable. In addition, the propensity to hyponatremia must be corrected, which sometimes requires a hypertonic saline (e.g., 3% NaCl) infusion. Alternatively, normal saline can be used, and all infusions should be guided by frequent measures of plasma electrolyte concentrations. Severe CSWS episodes require the addition of a mineral corticoid to the treatment plan.

Key Points

- The hypothalamic-pituitary-adrenal axis underlies most critical endocrine conditions in the neurosurgical patient.
- Stress increases the requirement for cortisol, and stressed patients at risk for insufficient cortisol response should receive glucocorticoid supplement.
- Short-term steroid treatment has few negative effects and may be life-saving in the neurosurgical population.
- The patient at risk for adrenal insufficiency with circulatory instability should be treated empirically with steroids.

Patients with intracranial injury should have serum electrolytes, urine electrolytes, plasma glucose, body weight, and water balance monitored frequently to detect postoperative endocrine problems early.

Suggested Reading

Agha A, Thornton E, et al. Posterior pituitary dysfunction after traumatic brain injury. J Clin Endocrinol Metab. 2004;89(12):5987–92.

Agha A, Sherlock M, et al. The natural history of post-traumatic neurohypophysial dysfunction. Eur J Endocrinol. 2005;152(3):371–7.

Bloomfield R, Noble DW. Etomidate, pharmacological adrenalectomy and the critically ill: a matter of vital importance. Crit Care. 2006;10(4):161.

Brimioulle S, Orellana-Jiminez C, et al. Hyponatremia in neurological patients: cerebral salt wasting versus inappropriate antidiuretic hormone secretion. Intensive Care Med. 2008;34(1):125–31.

Cardoso AP, Dragosavac D, et al. Syndromes related to sodium and arginine vasopressin alterations in post-operative neurosurgery. Arq Neuropsiquatr. 2007;65:745–51.

Clapper A, Nashelsky M, et al. Evaluation of serum cortisol in the postmortem diagnosis of acute adrenal insufficiency. Am J Forensic Med Pathol. 2008;29(2):181–4.

Cooper MS, Stewart PM. Corticosteroid insufficiency in acutely ill patients. N Engl J Med. 2003;348(8):727–34.

Cotton BA, Guillamondegui OD, et al. Increased risk of adrenal insufficiency following etomidate exposure in critically injured patients. Arch Surg. 2008;143(1):62–7. discussion 67.

Dumont AS, Nemergut 2nd EC, et al. Postoperative care following pituitary surgery. J Intensive Care Med. 2005;20(3):127–40.

Fleisher LA. Evidence-based practice of anesthesiology. Philadelphia: Saunders; 2004.

Gibson SC, Hartman DA, et al. The endocrine response to critical illness: update and implications for emergency medicine. Emerg Med Clin North Am. 2005;23(3):909–29, xi.

Jackson Jr WL. Should we use etomidate as an induction agent for endotracheal intubation in patients with septic shock?: a critical appraisal. Chest. 2005;127(3):1031–8.

Mohammad Z, Afessa B, et al. The incidence of relative adrenal insufficiency in patients with septic shock after the administration of etomidate. Crit Care. 2006;10(4):R105.

Nemergut EC, Dumont AS, et al. Perioperative management of patients undergoing transsphenoidal pituitary surgery. Anesth Analg. 2005;101(4):1170–81.

Nielsen S, Chou C-L, et al. Vasopressin increases water permeability of kidney collecting duct by inducing translocation of aquaporin-CD water channels to plasma membrane. Proc Natl Acad Sci USA. 1995;92(2):1013–7.

Powner DJ, Boccalandro C. Adrenal insufficiency following traumatic brain injury in adults. Curr Opin Crit Care. 2008;14(2):163–6.

Ullian ME. The role of corticosteroids in the regulation of vascular tone. Cardiovasc Res. 1999;41(1):55–64.

Venkataraman S, Munoz R, et al. The hypothalamic-pituitary-adrenal axis in critical illness. Rev Endocr Metab Disord. 2007;8(4):365–73.

Verbalis JG. Management of disorders of water metabolism in patients with pituitary tumors. Pituitary. 2002;5(2):119–32.

Zaloga GP, Marik P. Hypothalamic-pituitary-adrenal insufficiency. Crit Care Clin. 2001;17(1): 25–41.

Chapter 71
Postoperative Paralysis, Skin Lesions, and Corneal Abrasions After Neurosurgery

Martin H. Dauber and Steven Roth

Although many complications attributed to anesthesia occur during the intraoperative period, several manifest later. In the postanesthesia care unit (PACU) problems that are dreaded and some that are non-life-threatening may manifest. Postoperative paralysis is a serious complication of neurosurgery, whereas skin lesions and corneal abrasions can be bothersome, but are rarely considered major issues. This section focuses on these three problems for patients following brain and spine-related procedures.

Postoperative Paralysis

Overview

Paralysis is the loss of voluntary control of skeletal muscle function caused by failure of nerve conduction of electrical impulse. This can occur centrally or be a result of peripheral nerve problems, and the differential diagnosis is critical in the postoperative period. Paralysis following intracranial surgery may be anticipated as a result of resection of tumor in proximity to the motor cortex. Similarly, following peripheral nerve resection an element of local paralysis may manifest.

Preexisting paresis or paralysis pose the greatest risk factors for paralysis presenting in the PACU. Many of these patients will indeed be weak or paralyzed after the surgery. A preanesthetic history and physical should thoroughly document the degree of neurologic impairment of all patients. This is particularly so in neurosurgical spine and intracranial procedures where, due to their typical long duration, it is common for the anesthesia team present upon emergence to be different from the team which started the case.

M.H. Dauber, MD (✉) • S. Roth, MD
Department of Anesthesia and Critical Care, The University of Chicago Medical Center, Chicago, Illinois, USA
e-mail: MDauber@dacc.uchicago.edu

A.M. Brambrink and J.R. Kirsch (eds.), *Essentials of Neurosurgical Anesthesia & Critical Care*, DOI 10.1007/978-0-387-09562-2_71,
© Springer Science+Business Media, LLC 2012

It is rare to have any paralysis in the PACU patients, in general, and the incidence may be higher in patients following neurosurgery. This elevated risk is due to three primary factors:

1. Location and nature of surgical site
2. Patient position during surgery (full or partially prone, sitting, lateral, etc.)
3. Long duration.

The location of surgery may increase the risk for central paralysis, whereas the other factors may elevate risk for peripheral neuropathies. It is these peripheral neuropathies that are most under the control of the anesthesiologist.

Prevention

Surgical attention to the possibility of paralysis both in the head and in the spine is the key to preventing the paralysis seen in the PACU that is related to surgical site. Details of this are beyond the scope of anesthesia practice, except in the broadest sense. Peripheral neuropathies leading to paralysis, however, are very much the concern of anesthesiologists. Although studies have failed to confirm with scientific certainty the relationship of positioning to peripheral neuropathies, the American Society of Anesthesiologists issued a practice advisory for the prevention of perioperative neuropathies.

Crisis Management and Assessment

Immediate diagnosis of paralysis upon emergence is the shared responsibility of the nurses caring for the PACU patient as well as of the neurosurgical and anesthesia teams. Centrally related paralysis needs to be differentiated from peripherally caused problems. Timely diagnosis is critical in these cases as certain causes indicate immediate surgical intervention. As soon as the finding of paresis or paralysis is revealed, both the surgeons and anesthesiologists need to be aware; the surgeons so they can pursue diagnosis or reexploration and the anesthesiologists so they can facilitate the emergency anesthetic.

Peripheral neuropathies are less likely to be surgical emergencies, unless they are as a result of arterial embolic phenomenon. Accordingly, the affected extremity must be examined for pulses, pain, and pallor.

Hemodynamic stability and oxygenation status are always important in the PACU, and even more so in the patient who may be required to go back to the operating room. Raising systemic arterial blood pressures to the high end of normal may increase perfusion to neural cells at ischemic risk, thereby protecting them and minimizing permanent injury. In the setting of presumed spinal cord injury, as the cause of new paralysis/paresis, high-dose corticosteroids have been advocated by many,

Key Point

- Postoperative paralysis is a potentially devastating complication of neuro-surgical procedures that may first manifest in the PACU. Central or surgical field-related etiologies are the most likely, though peripheral neuropathies can cause more localized paralysis. Anesthesiologists must be aggressive in the maintenance of hemodynamics and oxygen carrying capacity to prevent further deterioration of paresis or paralysis. Operating room care and early PACU diagnosis in the event of problems can lead to improved outcomes.

though there is little evidence upon which to base this. Methylprednisolone 30 mg/kg intravenously bolused over 15 min followed by a 23 h infusion of 5.4 mg/kg/h is the recommended dose.

Anemia and electrolyte imbalance must be aggressively addressed to rule out these as causes or contributing factors. Aggressive transfusion of red blood cells should be performed to raise hemoglobin concentrations over 10 g/dL, although the critical hematocrit has not been determined for this patient population. Depending on neurosurgical impressions, emergency imaging, such as MRI, may be indicated, and this may require the presence of the anesthesiologist if the patient has not made adequate progress toward recovery.

Skin Lesions

Overview

Dermatologic complications following neurosurgical procedures seem to occur with higher frequency than following surgery to other systems. However, there is sparse literature to support this impression. Since skin lesions can be painful, alarming for patients and others to see and potential sources of infection they can be troublesome. Nonetheless, skin problems following these cases can be divided into three broad categories:

1. Minor abrasions
2. Deep dermal damage
3. Complete skin disruption.

Most of these injuries occur through excess pressure over long time periods. Iatrogenic skin disruption during removal of electrodes or tape may also occur. This section discusses these various types of injuries and their diagnosis and treatment.

Presentation and Treatment

In the PACU after the basic recovery issues are handled, the nurse who performs the complete secondary survey will identify any dermal lesions. Additionally patients may complain of pain or burning sensation at affected areas. Erythema, bleeding, and tenderness may be present. In cases of complete skin disruption due to the skin's adherence to tape or the like, immediate diagnosis is important, as salvage of autogenous skin is possible. If the removed skin can be located, it should rapidly cleaned and then replaced in situ and secured with staples and sutures. A loose Vaseline dressing can then be applied. Infection is extremely rare eliminating the need for prophylactic antibiotics.

Prevention

Neurosurgical procedures are often performed in positions that put patients at risk for dermal damage, and have a long duration, further exacerbating any problems. Intraoperative attention to positioning can be the most protective mechanism against perioperative skin changes. Soft surfaces should be provided in any area of contact with the patient and bed, supports or other equipment. Pressure at boney prominences should be minimized as much as possible. Many use gel-filled pads where contact pressure is high, such as under the iliac crests and knees in prone patients. There are many pillows and other devices to position the head for prone cases that are non-abrasive, in addition to the other purported benefits. The female breasts should be positioned midline toward the head to allow adequate perfusion which primarily comes from the internal thoracic and internal mammary arteries.

Anesthesiologists often use tape and adhesives that may cause complete skin disruption upon removal. Additionally, neurosurgical patients are often subject of peripheral neurological monitoring, and neurophysiologists need to be attentive to this risk. Some patients, such as the elderly or those with "fair skin" may be more susceptible.

Key Point

- Skin lesions can be a nuisance type complication following any surgery, and neurosurgical patients seem to be at higher risk. Proper equipment to aid positioning and meticulous attention to the comfort of the anesthetized patient as well as protection of the skin may decrease the incidence. Visible skin lesions never threaten life but can cause disfigurement that is permanently bothersome to the patient who suffers this problem.

Corneal Abrasions

Overview

A corneal abrasion is a painful scrape or scratch of the surface of the clear part of the eye known as the cornea. This transparent window covers the iris, the circular-colored portion of the eye. The cornea has many nerve endings just under the surface, so that any disruption of the surface may be painful. Anytime a foreign body contacts the eye an abrasion is a possibility, particularly under general anesthesia when the eye does not have its protective reflexes. Corneal abrasions may also occur during anesthesia when the eye is not taped closed properly and the cornea becomes dry because the patient will not blink during anesthesia. The true incidence of corneal abrasions is not well documented for neurosurgical patients, but due to the exposure of the face and eyes to potential contact, it is assumed to be higher than for non-neurosurgical patients. In addition, during craniotomy or during prone cases the anesthesiologist is unable to monitor the eyes during the case to make sure the eyes remain completely closed during the entire case. Some patients also experience an itching sensation in their eyes upon awakening. In an attempt to alleviate the discomfort the still drowsy patient may try rubbing the eyes, which can easily result in corneal damage. The neuroanesthesiologist should be aware of any preexisting vision-related problems.

Crisis Management

Presentation

Following a neurosurgical procedure a patient may complain of:

1. Sensation of a foreign body in the eye.
2. Tearing of the eyes
3. Blurred vision or distortion of vision
4. Photophobia, especially to bright lights
5. Spasm of the periocular muscles causing squinting.

Any or all of these findings should lead to consideration of the possibility of a corneal abrasion. Although many advocate for immediate ophthalmologic evaluation, this can be difficult in some settings especially later in the evening when many neurosurgical cases are arriving in PACU.

Assessment

There are two principal parts of the diagnosis of corneal abrasion:

1. Ruling out the presence of a foreign body
2. Fluorescein ophthalmoscopic examination of the cornea.

Patients with corneal abrasions will be in pain, and this may make a proper examination difficult. The clinician must be relentless in his pursuit of diagnosis, nonetheless. The use of topical 1% tetracaine to the eye prior to exam has been recommended, but has been associated with the potential for worse healing. The upper and lower eyelids must be inverted and the fossae inspected. Then with either a drop of ophthalmic fluorescein (0.25%) or a fluorescein strip applied to the eye, an examination of the cornea can be performed under cobalt-blue filtered light. An abrasion will show as a disruption of the regular smooth surface of the cornea.

Management

If a foreign body is present on the eye, removal by irrigation may be possible. If not readily performed, emergency ophthalmologic consultation should be sought. In the case of a corneal abrasion:

1. Antibiotic eyedrops or ointment (such as erythromycin, tobramycin, or ciprofloxacin) may be applied. Some ophthalmologists advocate the addition of steroids to reduce inflammation and to avoid potential scarring.
2. Eye should not be patched. Recent evidence shows that patching the eye does not help and may actually have a negative impact on the healing process.
3. Mydriatics are no longer indicated.
4. Analgesics appropriate to patient's overall postoperative condition.
5. Follow-up examination by ophthalmologist after 24 h to assess the degree of healing and prognosticate about potential long-term sequellae.

Prevention

It is probably more true of the prevention of corneal abrasions that of many other iatrogenic injuries, that concern for the potential is the cornerstone of prevention. Many techniques have been advocated over the years, yet none has proven itself. Taping of the eyes early in peri-induction period may decrease the eyes' exposure to foreign bodies such as ID tags, endotracheal tube pilot balloons or laryngoscopes.

For craniotomies many use lubricants (lanolin based) to protect the corneas as well as to dilute any surgical prep solution that may enter under the tape. For prone cases where large volume shifts may occur some use hypertonic 3% saline ointment (e.g., Muro 128). Transparent adhesive medical dressings (e.g., Tegaderms) are occasionally put over the eyes for their protection, but skin abrasions have been noted. There is no foolproof method for absolute prevention that is standard of care.

Key Points

- Corneal abrasions can be bothersome to patients emerging from neurosurgical procedures. Although the incidence is low, these patients may be at higher risk because of the non-face-up positions that they may be in. Most anesthesia-related corneal abrasions heal within 24 h, though rarely can persist ophthalmoscopically for 3–4 months. Attention to prevention and rapid treatment and analgesia can improve the care of these patients.
- Although many anesthesia-related complications are noted in the operating room during the administration of general anesthesia, some are not noted until later. During emergence from anesthesia in the PACU major complications such as paresis or paralysis and minor ones such as corneal abrasions and skin lesions may manifest. Rapid attention to these complications can prevent further deterioration and possibly good outcomes.

Suggested Reading

Cheney FW, Domino KB, Caplan RA, Posner KL. Nerve injury associated with anesthesia. Anesthesiology. 1999;90:1062–9.

Roth S, Thistead RA, Erickson JP, Black S, Schreider BD. Eye injuries after nonocular surgery; a study of 60,965 anesthetics from 1988–1992. Anesthesiology. 1996;85:1020–7.

Chapter 72
Post-operative Pain Management in Patients After Neurosurgical Operations

Mary Newton and Tacson Fernandez

Overview

The management of post-operative pain in neurosurgical patients can be challenging.

Many neurosurgical patients may be denied adequate analgesia because of the mistaken belief that opioids may mask neurological deterioration. Despite the diversity of neurosurgical procedures and the multiplicity of pain presentations in this population, effective and safe pain relief is possible for the vast majority of patients.

A sound knowledge of the pathophysiology underlying the neurosurgical condition and an understanding of the complications associated with it are essential for optimizing safe post-operative analgesia. Many neurosurgical conditions are highly dynamic. A decrease in the Glasgow Coma Scale (GCS) must be carefully investigated as many neurosurgical complications may require urgent surgical and/or therapeutic intervention (Table 72.1). A deterioration in GCS must not be attributed solely to a relative opioid 'overdose' until other causes have been excluded.

Analgesia for major spinal surgery may be especially challenging. Many of these patients suffer from chronic pain and may present with a combination of nociceptive and neuropathic pain. A significant number of these patients may be taking opioids pre-operatively. Acute on chronic pain is typically more difficult to manage than isolated acute pain.

M. Newton, MBBS, FRCA (✉)
The National Hospital for Neurology and Neurosurgery, London, UK
e-mail: mary.newton@uclh.nhs.uk

T. Fernandez, MBBS, FCARCSI, FIPP, DPM
Department of Anaesthetics and Pain Medicine, Imperial College Hospitals
Healthcare NHS Trust, London, UK

A.M. Brambrink and J.R. Kirsch (eds.), *Essentials of Neurosurgical Anesthesia & Critical Care*, DOI 10.1007/978-0-387-09562-2_72,
© Springer Science+Business Media, LLC 2012

Table 72.1 Common causes of post-operative/post-procedure decrease in GCS

Common neurosurgical conditions	Potential causes of decreasing Glasgow Coma Scale (GCS)
Sub-arachnoid haemorrhage (SAH) (post-clipping/post-coiling)	Re-bleed
	Acute hydrocephalus
	Cerebral vasospasm
	Seizure
Traumatic brain injury (TBI)	Re-accumulation of haematoma
	Haemorrhage into contusion
	Oedema
	Seizure
Craniotomy	Haematoma (sub-dural/intracerebral etc.)
	Oedema
	Seizure
	Air encephalocoele
	Infection – e.g. meningitis etc.

Neuraxial opioids, alone or in combination with local anaesthetics, can be very effective following spinal surgery. However, the approach requires careful considerations; Neuroaxial local anaesthetic/opioids may be contraindicated if there is significant risk of an intraoperative dural tear which could result in unpredictable amounts of local anaesthetic/opioids reaching the cerebrospinal fluid (CSF). In some centres, administration of opioids (particularly those that are long-acting and water soluble) into the CSF would commit the patient to care high dependency (HDU) care post-operatively. Additionally, local anaesthetic-induced motor block may mask neurological deterioration secondary to spinal cord compression by, for example, haematoma or tissue swelling. If this analgesic technique is used, it is imperative that the patient is monitored by nursing staff familiar with its use in this specialized population of patients. There must be a strict local protocol for the action to be taken in the event of onset of reduced limb power.

Increasing or uncontrolled pain post-operatively requires reassessment and consideration of alternative causes (Table 72.2), for example, a surgical complication or neuropathic pain.

Prevention

Pain is the fifth vital sign and requires regular evaluation in combination with appropriate intervention to maximize pain relief. Effective management of acute post-operative pain reduces the incidence of chronic pain; additionally, it aids early mobilization and may decrease factors associated with immobility (e.g. venous thrombosis and pulmonary atelectasis). Education of patients and clinical staff is vital to optimize acute post-operative pain management.

Table 72.2 Post-operative complications which may increase pain

Complication	Cause of pain
Sub-arachnoid haemorrhage (SAH) (post-clipping/post-coiling)	Re-bleed
	Hydrocephalus
	Infection
Traumatic brain injury (TBI)	Wound infection
	Re-accumulation of haematoma
Craniotomy	Haematoma (e.g. sub-dural/intracerebral)
	Air encephalocoele
	Low ICP headache/CSF leak
	Infection – e.g. meningitis
Spinal decompression/fusion	Nerve root compression by disc remnant/haematoma/oedema
	Neuropraxia (C2 root especially common)
	Infection
	Malpositioned instrumentation
	Muscle spasm
Intradural/intramedullary spinal cord surgery	Wound infection
	Haematoma formation
	Meningitis
	Low ICP headache/CSF leak

Pain Scores

Pain is a subjective experience and most measures of pain are based on self-report. Numerous pain scales exist. Descriptive scales, where pain is described as 'none, mild, moderate or severe' are easy to use. Numerical scores are less easy to use but are more accurate at assessing the response to an intervention. The most popular numerical scale is the visual analogue score (VAS); it consists of a 100 mm line where 0 mm correlates with no pain and 100 mm correlates with 'worst pain possible'. The patient is asked to mark the line to 'score' their pain. VAS ratings of >70 mm are indicative of 'severe pain'.

Education

Education of patients pre-operatively can help to reduce anxiety, post-operative pain, and other associated symptoms. Ideally, it should begin pre-operatively with information about the planned surgical procedure, expected pain relating to it, the hospital's pain-scoring system (see below) and the importance of effective analgesia to aid early mobilization to reduce the clinical risks associated with immobility. Patients should be aware of the analgesic modalities available to them; this information will need to be reinforced repeatedly in the early post-operative phase.

All clinicians involved in the post-operative care of neurosurgical patients need on-going education in acute pain management and the additional considerations for this specialist group of patients. Familiarity with the operative procedure and

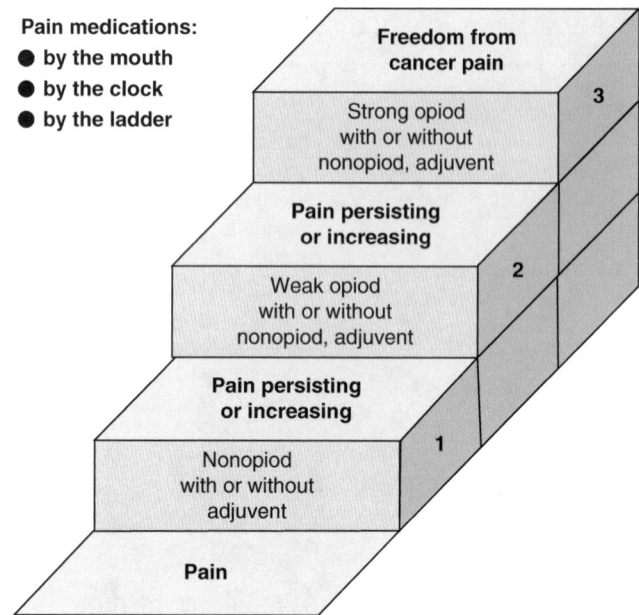

Fig. 72.1 WHO pain ladder

associated complications are particularly important. Clinical staff must be familiar with the hospital's pain-scoring system and the application of this to optimize analgesia. Standardized prescriptions for analgesia used in conjunction with frequent assessment of pain scores can improve post-operative pain management.

Recommended Analgesic Regimes

The World Health Organization (WHO) pain ladder (Fig. 72.1) describes a simplistic guide to the optimization of analgesia. Urgent action is required for patients in severe pain which frequently requires all three steps of the pain ladder to be initiated simultaneously, in combination with pharmacological adjuncts (Tables 72.4 and 72.5) and non-pharmacological adjuncts (e.g. reassurance, explanation of the cause of the pain and the intended management of it, careful positioning, cool/warm packs and eye shades). Prompt action in the provision of good pain relief reduces anxiety. Anxiety is known to exacerbate pain.

Table 72.3 is a guide to appropriate post-operative prescribing of multimodal analgesia in our unit where commonly performed neurosurgical procedures are categorized according to the *predicted* pain (VAS) in the post-operative period. Details of the timed introduction of multimodal analgesia for intra-cranial surgery are shown in Table 72.4 and for non-intracranial surgery in Table 72.5.

Table 72.3 Some common neurosurgical procedures are listed according to the *predicted* pain (VAS) in the post-operative period to guide appropriate post-operative prescribing of multimodal analgesia

Predicted pain scores without analgesia	Examples of surgical procedures in this category	Regular paracetamol (acetometophen)	Regular NSAID[a]	Regular oral or PCA morphine	'Rescue' opioid if required	Consider pharmaceutical adjunct (Table 72.5)
Minor pain (VAS 1–3)	Carpal tunnel	Yes	Yes	No	Yes	No
Intermediate pain (VAS 3–6)	Craniotomy/Lumbar microdiscectomy	Yes (i.v. first 24 h post-op)	≥6 h[a] post-op	Yes	Yes	No
Major pain (VAS 7–10)	Lumbar/cervical laminectomy	Yes (i.v. first 48 h post-op)	≥6 h[a] post-op	Yes (if no PCA consider slow release morphine preparation)	Yes (not with PCA)	No
Complex major pain (VAS 7–10)	Posterior spinal fusion thoracic discectomy	Yes (i.v. first 48 h post-op)	≥6 h[a] post-op	Yes (if no PCA consider slow release morphine preparation)	Yes (not with PCA)	Yes

[a]If no neurosurgical or medical contraindication

Table 72.4 Guidelines for multimodal analgesia following *intracranial surgery* – timing and analgesic considerations

Post-operative period	Recommended analgesia (aim for pain score ≤3)	Analgesic considerations	Evaluation of analgesia
Immediate (1–60 min)	Intravenous (i.v.) paracetamol +/– i.v. morphine Remember adjuncts (e.g. position, cool packs)	Severe pain post-craniotomy refractory to paracetamol and small amounts of i.v. morphine should prompt formal exclusion of complications	Frequent re-assessment of • Pain score • Response to intervention • Re-evaluate analgesic doses
Early (60 min–6 h)	Regular i.v. paracetamol 1 g 6-hourly Regular oral or PCA morphine Remember adjuncts (e.g. position, cool packs)	Paracetamol i.v. 6-hourly for first 48 h post-op for painful surgery Continuing severe pain – exclude complications	Frequent re-assessment of • Pain score • Response to intervention • Re-evaluate analgesic doses
Intermediate (>6–24 h)	Regular i.v. paracetamol 1 g 6-hourly Oral or PCA morphine Remember adjuncts (e.g. position, cool packs) *Consider regular*: oral/rectal/i.v. NSAIDs*	Paracetamol i.v. 6-hourly for first 48 h post-op for painful surgery *NSAIDs* see particular cautions relating to use in neurosurgical patients Continuing severe pain – exclude complications	Frequent re-assessment of • Pain score • Response to intervention • Re-evaluate analgesic doses
Late (>24 h)	Regular i.v. paracetamol 1 g 6-hourly Oral or PCA morphine Remember adjuncts (e.g. position, cool packs) *Consider regular*: oral/rectal/i.v. NSAIDs* +/– gabapentin	Paracetamol i.v. for first 48 h post-op for painful surgery *NSAIDs* see particular cautions relating to use in neurosurgical patients Continuing severe pain – exclude complications Consider introduction gabapentin 100 mg three times/day and titrate according to response	Frequent re-assessment of • Pain score • Response to intervention • Re-evaluate analgesic doses Reduce analgesia as pain improves (opioids first)

Table 72.5 Guidelines for multimodal analgesia following *non-intracranial surgery* – timing and analgesic considerations

Post-op period and recommended analgesia (aim for pain score ≤3)	Analgesic considerations	Evaluation of analgesia
Immediate (1–60 min) intravenous (i.v.) paracetamol +/– i.v. morphine *If severe pain persists consider:* Low-dose midazolam Clonidine Low-dose ketamine *For acute neuropathic pain consider:* Dexamethasone	*Midazolam* – useful post-spinal surgery if other analgesia unsuccessful. Use very low dose (0.5 mg) and be aware of intense synergism with opioids *Clonidine* – slow i.v. increments (15 µg) to maximum 150 µg. Monitor BP carefully *Ketamine* – dysphoria unlikely with very low bolus dose (0.1 mg/kg) *Dexamethasone* (4–8 mg) – may be helpful for acute neuropathic pain. Continue 4 mg four times daily for 48 h. Caution in diabetes	Frequent re-assessment of • Pain score • Response to intervention • Re-evaluate analgesic doses Severe pain? Consider post-op complications
Early (60 min – 6 h) As above but substitute i.v. morphine for regular oral *or* PCA morphine	As above *Paracetamol* i.v. 6 hourly for first 48 h post-op for painful surgery	As above
Intermediate (6–24 h) As above *Consider regular:* Oral/rectal/i.v. NSAIDs* *If severe pain persists consider:* Gabapentin Clonidine	As above **NSAIDs* see particular cautions relating to use in neurosurgical patients (above) *Gabapentin* – depending on age start at 100–200 mg three times daily and *clonidine* – start at 100 µg orally twice daily	As above
Late (24 h) As above If high opioid requirement consider switching to slow-release formulation *Consider regular:* Oral benzodiazepine for muscular wound pain	As above *Benzodiazepine* – low dose for 48–72 h, e.g. oral diazepam 2 mg three times daily	As above Severe pain? Consider post-op complications Consider reduction in analgesia as pain improves (opioids first)

Table 72.6 Preventive analgesic therapies that could be considered in expected 'Major' and 'Complex Major Pain' patient groups

Timing of adjunct	Dosage guidelines	Precautions
Pre-operative	*Gabapentin* 2 h pre-op (200–600 mg single dose, titrate dose according to age)	High-dose *gabapentin* may cause drowsiness. Dose reduction in renal failure
	Ketamine – not for intracranial surgery 5 min before skin incision – (0.1–0.5 mg/kg)	*Ketamine* – not for intracranial surgery Psychosis not usually a problem with low-dose ketamine
	Local anaesthetic block (LA)	LA – see notes in 'Overview'
Intraoperative	*ketamine* – not for intracranial surgery (0.1–0.25 mg/kg repeated at 1 h intervals)	*ketamine* – not for intracranial surgery Psychosis not usually a problem with low-dose ketamine
	Local anaesthetic block (LA)	LA – see notes in 'Overview'
Post-operative	*Gabapentin* (divided doses 200–1,800 mg/day titrate dose according to age. Caution in renal failure)	*Gabapentin* – dose reduction in renal failure. Continue for 1 month post-op. Wean off over 2 weeks
	Ketamine – not for intracranial surgery Avoid if possible in all patients post-op (10–50 mg orally three times daily)	*Ketamine* – not for intracranial surgery Psychosis not usually a problem with low doses

Preventive Analgesia

This describes a reduction in post-operative pain following the administration of a drug that has an effect longer than the expected duration of that agent. There is no evidence to support the best *timing* of this therapy in the perioperative period. The use of NMDA receptor antagonists has been advocated as preventive analgesic regime in the context of abdominal, gynaecological, orthopaedic and dental surgery. However, general concerns remain regarding the use of ketamine in neurosurgical patients because of its effect on intracranial pressure. Recent work has suggested a similar benefit following the use of gabapentin which would be more suitable in the context of neurosurgical interventions. Scalp blocks may provide effective and long-standing analgesia post-craniotomy; they are safe and simple to perform. As mentioned above, great care needs to be taken with the use of neuraxial opioids and local anaesthetic in spinal surgery. Potential preventive analgesic therapies that could be considered in expected 'Major' and 'Complex Major Pain' patient groups are shown in Table 72.6.

Relative Contraindications for Commonly Used Analgesics in the Neurosurgical Population

NSAIDs

The use of NSAIDs in neurosurgical patients is controversial. There are no published studies about their use in this population. Theoretically, they increase the risk of post-operative bleeding due to their inhibitory effect on platelet function, thus neurosurgeons have great concerns regarding their use, particular in the context of craniotomies and spinal surgery. Following elective supra-tentorial surgery it is highly unusual for patients to present with an intra-cranial haematoma if they have regained their pre-operative status by 6 h post-surgery. In our institution, we have applied this finding to our entire neurosurgical population and introduce NSAIDs after 6 h, if the post-operative course of any type of elective surgery has been uncomplicated and there is nothing to suggest a clotting disorder. Introduction of NSAIDs may be delayed in high-risk cases (e.g. spinal cord tumours, large meningioma resections, and 'deep brain' surgery).

Another concern with the use of NSAIDs is *possible* impairment of bone fusion (through interference with the complex regulatory system of bone formation that includes prostaglandins) which could be significant following spinal fusion. There is no evidence in humans to support this.

Opioids

If used in doses just sufficient to relieve pain, they will not significantly affect respiratory drive, thus avoiding an increase in $PaCO_2$ with consequent effects on increasing ICP.

Careful titration is the key to the safe use of opioids. Following craniotomy very small doses may be highly effective (e.g., 1–2 mg morphine repeated if necessary at 5 min intervals in the immediate post-operative phase followed by 5–10 mg orally at later stages). This is in contradistinction to patients in the 'Major' and 'Complex Major Pain' categories who invariably require much higher doses.

Patient-controlled analgesic (PCA) devices have been used successfully without complication following craniotomy and subarachnoid haemorrhage. For the use of morphine-PCA, some practitioners suggest low 4 h limits (e.g. 15 mg) and re-evaluate the patient before further dose increase. Patients after major spinal surgery frequently benefit from additional p.o. slow-release morphine preparations as supplementation of the PCA treatment due to more extensive pain levels; however, this requires a high level of patient supervision, such as an HDU environment. Endtidal CO_2-feedback-control PCA devices have been introduced in an attempt to improve patient safety when opioid self-administration is desired.

Crisis Management

Nociceptive Pain

Severe nociceptive pain is easier to treat than severe neuropathic pain. Whenever severe pain is present the cause of the pain should be actively sought. There should be a low threshold for further investigation, if it persists or is difficult to control. In the late post-operative phase, this may require admission to an HDU for rapid control of pain by intravenous boluses of opioids and other adjuncts.

Neuropathic Pain

Neuropathic pain is classically described as aching, burning, shooting, or stabbing. It may be paroxysmal or spontaneous with no precipitating cause and may be associated with hyperalgesia or allodynia. It may be a new phenomenon post-operatively or an exacerbation of pre-existing neuropathic pain. It can be very difficult to relieve. Although classically resistant to opioids these should be tried to assess whether they are of any benefit. Dexamethasone (4 mg four times daily for 48 h) can be very effective in the early post-operative phase, if oedema of nerve roots is thought a probable cause. There should be a low threshold to the introduction of gabapentin or amitriptyline if significant neuropathic pain persists. Carbamazepine is the most effective treatment for trigeminal neuralgia (sometimes exacerbated following microvascular decompression) but has a poor side-effect profile. There are successful reports of the use of intra-nasal sumatriptan in refractory cases of trigeminal neuralgia (caution should be exercised in patients with ischaemic heart disease).

Neuropathic pain following spinal cord injury and brachial plexus avulsion is common and can be severe. There is evidence to support benefit from opioids, ketamine infusion, and intravenous lidocaine. The latter two have to be administered in an HDU environment. Benzodiazepines may contribute to the management of refractory pain. Their use should be strictly short term and over-sedation and its attendant risks avoided.

Side Effects of Treatment

Constipation, nausea and so on are common post-operatively. They should be anticipated and active measures taken to prevent them. Several analgesic have sedative effects on the patients, particularly opioids. Awareness of the possible confounding effects of the analgesic treatment on mental status and neurologic presentation is of paramount importance in the perioperative management of neurosurgical patients. Overmedication with analgesics may result in differential diagnostic problems, which should trigger an immediate neurologic evaluation and frequently require emergency CT imaging of the cranium.

Key Points

- Acute pain management education of patients/clinical staff reduces the incidence of severe post-operative pain
- Post-operative pain management should be planned pre-operatively
- Consider the use of preventive analgesia in relevant patient groups
- Multimodal analgesia may improve the quality of analgesia and reduce the incidence of side effects
- PCA has a high patient satisfaction
- Be specific about site of pain and its potential causes
- Assess pain and the effect of interventions frequently
- Increasing or severe pain should prompt further investigation
- Monitoring in an HDU environment may be necessary for prompt and safe management of severe pain
- As pain improves focus should be provided to weaning analgesia to prevent dependence.

Suggested Reading

Acute Pain Management: Scientific Evidence – Australian and New Zealand College of Anaesthetists and Faculty of Pain Medicine. 2nd ed. 2005.

de Gray LC, Matta BF. Acute and chronic pain following craniotomy: a review. Anaesthesia. 2005;60:693–704.

Harmer M, Davies KA. The effect of education, assessment and a standardised prescription on postoperative pain management. Anaesthesia. 1998;53:424–30.

Kehlet H, Jensen TS, Woolf CJ. Persistent postsurgical pain: risk factors and prevention. Lancet. 2006;367:1618–25.

Pandey CK, Navkar DV, Giri PJ, et al. Evaluation of the optimal preemptive dose of gabapentin for postoperative pain relief after lumbar diskectomy: a randomized, double-blind, placebo-controlled study. J Neurosurg Anesthesiol. 2005;17:65–8.

Taylor WA, Thomas WM, Wellings JA, Bell BA. Timing of postoperative intracranial hematoma development and implications for the best use of neurosurgical intensive care. J Neurosurg. 1995;82:48–50.

Chapter 73
Management of Postoperative Nausea and Vomiting After Neurosurgery

Concezione Tommasino

Overview

Postoperative nausea and vomiting (PONV) constitutes a major unpleasant symptom after anesthesia and surgery. The current overall incidence of PONV for all surgeries is estimated to be 25–30%, whereas after craniotomies is more than 50%. In the absence of prophylactic antiemetics, in retrospective analysis, the incidence has been as high as 39% for emesis and 67% for nausea, while in prospective studies PONV incidence has been reported from 55 to 70%. The reasons for the high incidence of PONV in neurosurgical patients may relate to surgery being performed in close proximity to emetic centers of the brainstem, or on the structures integral to maintenance of equilibrium.

The exact etiology of PONV is unknown, but research suggests a multifactorial origin and risk factors are well established (Table 73.1). Other possible risk factors include history of migraine, better ASA physical status, anxiety, obesity, decreased perioperative fluids, general versus regional anesthesia or sedation, balanced versus total IV anesthesia, and use of longer-acting versus shorter-acting opioids.

Although PONV is almost always self-limiting and nonfatal, it can cause significant morbidity.

In addition to causing patient discomfort, protracted nausea and vomiting may cause dehydration, acid–base disturbances, and electrolyte imbalance. Despite the lack of documented cases of harm caused by postcraniotomy PONV, the physical act of vomiting may result in an increase in arterial, venous, and intracranial pressures, thereby potentially increasing the risk of intracranial hemorrhage and neurologic dysfunction. In patients with depressed airway reflexes during the early

C. Tommasino, MD (✉)
Department of Anesthesiology and Intensive Care, University of Milan,
H San Paolo Medical School, Milan, Italy
e-mail: concezione.tommasino@unimi.it

A.M. Brambrink and J.R. Kirsch (eds.), *Essentials of Neurosurgical Anesthesia & Critical Care*, DOI 10.1007/978-0-387-09562-2_73,
© Springer Science+Business Media, LLC 2012

Table 73.1 Risk factors for postoperative nausea and vomiting

Patient-specific risk factors	• Age
	• Female gender
	• Nonsmoking status
	• History of PONV/motion sickness
Anesthesia-related independent predictors	• Mask ventilation
	• Volatile anesthetics
	• Nitrous oxide
	• Intraoperative and postoperative opioids
	• Large-dose neostigmine
	• Long duration of anesthesia
	• Awake craniotomy *lower* risk than general anesthesia
Neurosurgical risk factors	• Infratentorial > supratentorial > transsphenoidal procedures
	• High risk in surgery near the area postrema at the floor of the forth ventricle (vomiting center located nearby)
	• Decompression of cranial nerves
	• Long duration of surgery
Emergence	• Rapid awakening
	• Movement
Other factors	• Hypotension
	• Pain

postoperative period, vomiting can cause pulmonary aspiration. The peak incidence of vomiting after neurosurgery is within the first few postoperative hours, rendering this complication one of the most frequent in the postanesthesia care unit (PACU) in this patient population, and each vomiting episode delays discharge from the recovery room by about 20 min.

Updated guidelines for managing PONV suggest that *prophylaxis* and *treatment* of nausea and vomiting improves patient comfort and satisfaction, reduces time to discharge, and should be done selectively.

No single drug or class of drug is fully effective in controlling PONV, presumably because none blocks all pathways to the vomiting center. However, because of the multi-receptor origin of PONV, combination therapy is being more widely employed.

The successful management of nausea and vomiting is a fundamental part of perioperative anesthesia treatment in neurosurgery and requires several steps:

1. recognition of patients at risk for PONV,
2. avoidance, when possibile, of factors precipitating PONV,
3. prophylaxis,
4. treatment.

Prevention

Identification of patients at moderate to severe risk for PONV enables targeting prophylaxis to those who will benefit most from it. Patient, anesthesia, and surgery-related risk factors have been identified (Table 73.1), and a number of PONV risk-scoring systems have been developed. Very simplified risk scores consider only few predictors and Tables 73.2 and 73.3 indicate the PONV incidence according to the presence of four or five of these predictors.

Both scores are very simple to use, and have demonstrated equivalent or superior discriminating power compared with more complex formulas. Koivuranta et al. simplified system (Table 73.3) has a statistically higher predictive value.

In children, risk of nausea and vomiting is highly associated with the type of surgery. Validated PONV-scoring systems are not available for children, but surgery lasting longer than 30 min, age of 3 years and older, a personal history and even a history of PONV in a close relative are all risk factors. The presence of all four factors increases the risk by 70%.

The simplified scoring systems obviate laborious calculations and may reduce the scope of required detailed history-taking. No risk model, however, can accurately predict the likelihood of an individual having PONV; risk models only allow clinicians to estimate the risk for PONV among patient groups.

The logical consequence of these risk scores is "the higher the risk, the more aggressive prevention should be," starting from strategies to reduce baseline risks (Table 73.4).

Table 73.2 Simplified risk score for PONV in adults based on four predictors: range of possibile score 0–4

Predictors (n=4)	Predictors	PONV risk by score (%)
• Female gender	0	10
• History of motion sickness or PONV	1	21
• Non-smoking status	2	39
• Postoperative opioids	3	61
	4	79

Table 73.3 Simplified risk score for PONV in adults based on five predictors: range of possibile score 0–5

Predictors (n=5)	Predictors	Risk of nausea by score (%)	Risk of vomiting by score (%)
• Female gender	0	17	7
• History of PONV	1	18	7
• History of motion sickness	2	42	17
• Nonsmoking status	3	54	25
• Duration of surgery > 60 min	4	47	38
	5	87	61

Table 73.4 Strategies to reduce baseline risk

Risk factors	Strategies
Anesthesia-related	• Awake craniotomy whenever applicable
	• Regional anesthesia whenever applicable
	• Propofol for induction and/or maintenance of anesthesia
	• Avoidance of high-dose volatile anesthetics[a]
	• Avoidance of nitrous oxide
	• Minimization of intraoperative and postoperative opioids[a]
	• Minimization of neostigmine (<2.5 mg)
	• Reduce duration of anesthesia
Surgery-related	• Reduce duration of surgery
Emergence-related	• Perform gastric aspiration/decompression
	• Plan a smooth awakening
	• Avoidance of sudden movements
Other factors	• Maintainance of hemodynamic stability
	• Adequate oxygenation
	• Adequate hydration
	• Adequate pain treatement

[a]Emetogenic effect of inhaled anesthetics and opioids appears to be dose-related

PONV is less common using propofol (induction and maintenance) and avoiding nitrous oxide. Hypotension causes brainstem hypoxia (vomiting center) and decreases blood flow to the chemoreceptor trigger zone (CTZ), both of which can induce nausea and vomiting. Keeping the patient well hydrated has been shown to reduce the incidence of PONV. Pain itself causes nausea and vomiting, and adequate control of pain is essential: the patient must not be deprived of analgesics under the false assumption that the medications are the only cause of PONV. It will be mandatory, however, to prevent opioid-induced emesis. Experienced PACU nurses are well aware that sudden changes of position and motion, including transportation by stretcher, may trigger vomiting. Upright positioning of a patient with hypotension, can also cause nausea. Controlling movement and surrounding activity, and decreasing noise and brightness will also reduce stimulation of the vestibular apparatus.

Nonpharmacologic Measures

Acupuncture, acupressure, and electrical stimulation of the P6 point have been shown to be effective in reducing nausea, at least in adults, which has been explained by endogenous β-endorphin release in the cerebrospinal fluid or a change in serotonin transmission, via the activation of serotonergic and noradrenergic fibers. It is unlikely that this approach will be the mainstay of reducing PONV, but it may have an effect when used as part of a multimodal approach.

Table 73.5 Receptor syte activity of antiemetic drugs and suggestions from the literature for their use in neurosurgery

Pharmacologic Group	Dopamine receptors	Muscarinic cholinergic receptors	Histamine receptors	Serotonin receptors	Literature suggestions
Butyrophenones					
Droperidol	++++	–	+	+	≤1.25 mg no sedative effects
Haloperidol	++++	–	+	–	
Phenothiazines					Not supported
Chlorpromazine	++++	++	++++	+	
Fluphenazine	++++	+	++	–	
Antihistamines					Not supported
Diphenhydramine	+	++	++++	–	
Promethazine	++	++	++++	–	
Anticholinergics					Not supported
Scopolamine	+	++++	+	–	
Benzamides					Supported
Metoclopramide	+++	–	+	++	≤10 mg no sedative effect
Antiserotonin					Supported
Ondansetron	–	–	–	++++	4 mg end of case
Granisetron	–	–	–	++++	1 mg end of case
Tropisetron	–	–	–	++++	2 mg end of case

The number of positive signs (+) indicates activity to the receptor type and negative sign (–) no activity

Pharmacologic Prophylaxis

Use of prophylactic antiemetics should be used only when the patient's individual risk is sufficiently high (Tables 73.2 and 73.3). This can be estimated by multiplying the expected incidence (baseline risk) by the relative risk reduction resulting from prophylaxis. As a rule of thumb, each effective antiemetic intervention will lead to a relative risk reduction of approximately 30%.

More aggressive prophylaxis is appropriate for patients in whom vomiting poses a particular medical risk, including those at risk for or with increased intracranial pressure, and when the anesthesia care provider determines the need or the patient has a strong preference to avoid PONV. Many patients are willing to pay out-of-pocket to avoid PONV, or would prefer to suffer pain over nausea and vomiting.

Available antiemetic agents work on different types of receptors involved in the etiology of PONV (Table 73.5). Clinicians, however, must carefully select an antiemetic for patients undergoing craniotomy. The need for ongoing neurocognitive monitoring makes the use of sedating antiemetics (such as anticholinergics, antihistamines, benzamides, and butyrophenones) undesirable (Table 73.5).

Table 73.6 Guidelines for identification and management of PONV

Risk	Management
Low (no risk factors)	Prophylaxis not recommended
Moderate (1–2 risk factors)	Use single agent prophylactic therapy such as dexamethasone, ondansetron, or droperidol
High (3–4 risk factors)	Treatment includes dexamethasone plus ondansetron or droperidol plus ondansetron
Very high (4 risk factors)	Treatment includes combination antiemetics plus total intravenous anesthesia with propofol

Because multiple receptor stimulation is usually involved, in patients at high risk several studies demonstrate better prophylaxis by the use of two or more antiemetics acting at different receptors compared with monotherapy. Combination therapy is recommended for both adults and children to prevent and manage PONV (Table 73.6).

In adults, 5-HT3-receptor antagonists, dexamethasone and droperidol, are equally effective; each reducing risk of nausea and vomiting by about 25%. In children, the 5-HT3-receptor antagonists are the drugs of choice (ondansetron: children < 40 kg = 0.1 mg/kg i.v.; >40 kg = 4 mg i.v.).

Dexamethasone, a corticosteroid, is an effective antiemetic drug. It reduces the incidence of PONV with delayed but prolonged efficacy. The antiemetic effect can be attributed to its strong anti-inflammatory action, which reduces the ascending impulses to the vomiting center. Other mechanisms discussed include decreased production of prostaglandins, blockade of the corticoreceptors in the nucleus tractus solitarius, release of endorphins, and reduction in the serotonin concentration in the brain and the gut. It should be administered before induction. Droperidol has been extensively used in neurosurgery. Nevertheless, in 2001, reports of cardiac rhythm changes after "large doses" droperidol, led the Food and Drug Administration to insert a black box warning in the package insert, although doses used for PONV management have never been associated with fatal cardiac arrhythmias.

The widespread use of drugs with pure 5-HT3 (serotonin) receptor antagonism in neurosurgical patients is based on their efficacy on vomiting and lack of side effects of sedation and extrapyramidal reactions. There is no evidence that any of the 5-HT3 antagonists are superior to or have less side effects than any other drug of that class. The evidence supports the administration of 5-HT3 antagonists at the end of surgery rather than prior to induction (Table 73.5).

Other antiemetics may be used, although the evidence supporting their use is less robust.

Multimodal Approach

A multimodal approach has been very effective in reducing early PONV in the highest risk group (PONV from 41% with no therapy to 2% with multimodal therapy).

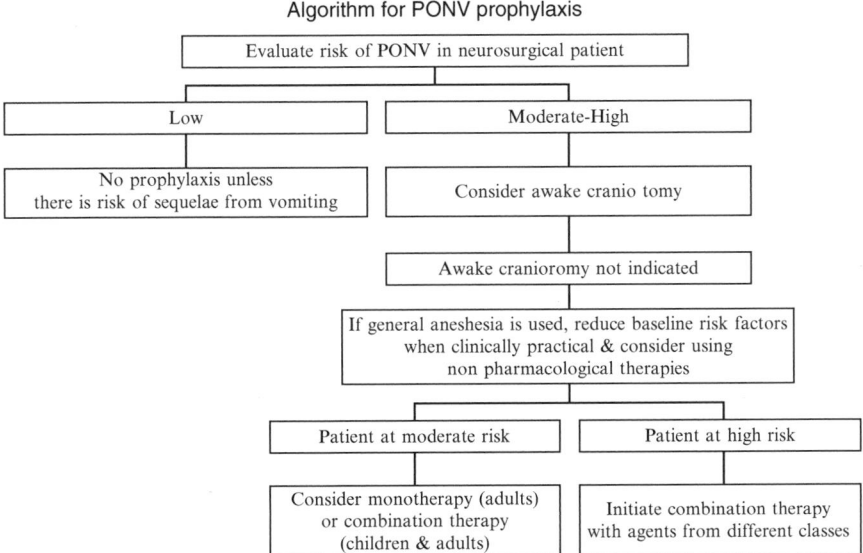

Fig. 73.1 Algorithm for PONV prophylaxis

This approach is based on avoiding *all* factors known to increase PONV and the combined administration of drugs known to reduce PONV (propofol, steroids, 5-HT3 antagonists, liberal intravenous fluids) (Tables 73.4 and 73.6). Figure 73.1 illustrates a suggested algorithm for PONV multimodal approach.

Crisis Management

Pathophysiology and Clinical Presentation

Nausea and vomiting are caused by the stimulation of neurologic mechanisms in the brain and the gastrointestinal tract (GIT). The complex act of vomiting involves coordination of the respiratory, gastrointestinal, and abdominal musculature. It is controlled by the vomiting center which is not a discrete anatomical site, but represents interrelated neuronal networks. The nucleus tractus solitarius, the dorsal motor nucleus of the vagus, and the nucleus ambiguous are the three nuclei that comprise the vomiting center. Inputs to the vomiting center include vagal sensory pathways from the GIT and neuronal pathways from the labyrinths, higher centers of the cortex, intracranial pressure receptors, and the CTZ, which is located in the area postrema, on the dorsal surface of the medulla oblongata at the caudal end of the fourth ventricle. The vomiting center is stimulated by histamine, dopamine, serotonin, and acetylcholine.

The vomiting reflex has two main detectors of the need to vomit: the GIT and the CTZ. The vagus is the major nerve involved in the detection of emetic stimuli from the GIT and has two types of afferent fibers involved in the emetic response: mechanoreceptors, located in the muscular wall of the gut, that are activated by contraction and distension of the gut and chemoreceptors, located in the mucosa of the upper gut, that are sensitive to noxious chemicals. Stimulation of the vagal afferents leads to activation of the CTZ in the area postrema. CTZ can initiate vomiting independent of the vomiting center, is not protected by the blood–brain barrier, and thus can be activated by chemical stimuli received through the blood as well as the cerebrospinal fluid. The CTZ is stimulated by dopamine, serotonin, opioids, and certain anesthetic agents. Gastrointestinal stimulation of mechanoreceptors in the wall of the gut from distention and manipulation results in the release of serotonin.

Several other stimuli can affect the vomiting center including afferents from the oropharynx, mediastinum, peritoneum, and genitalia as well as afferents from the CNS (cerebral cortex, labyrinthine, visual, and vestibular apparatus). The labrinthovestibular center can send input to the vomiting center in response to sudden changes in motion and pressure or initiated by the use of nitrous oxide. Hypotension causes brainstem hypoxia and triggers the vomiting center and can decrease blood flow to the CTZ, which can also induce nausea and vomiting.

PONV encompasses three main symptoms that may occur separately or in combination after surgery: nausea, retching, and vomiting.

Nausea is the subjective sensation of an urge to vomit, in the absence of expulsive muscular movements; when severe, it is associated with increased salivary secretion, vasomotor disturbances, and sweating. Loss of gastric tone, duodenal contractions and the reflux of intestinal contents into the stomach often accompany nausea. The arterial hypertension, that occurs while being nauseated, can complicate efforts to keep the blood pressure within a safe range for a patient after neurosurgery.

Retching follows nausea, and comprises labored spasmodic respiratory movements against a closed glottis with contractions of the abdominal muscles, chest wall, and diaphragm without any expulsion of gastric contents. Retching can occur without vomiting, but normally it generates the pressure gradient that leads to vomiting.

Vomiting is caused by the powerful sustained contraction of the abdominal and chest wall musculature, which is accompanied by the descent of the diaphragm and the opening of the gastric cardia. This is a reflex activity that is not under voluntary control. It results in the rapid and forceful evacuation of stomach contents up to and out of the mouth. During active retching and vomiting (*emesis*), intrabdominal and intra-thoracic pressures increase and traslate into elevated intracranial pressure. Despite the lack of documented cases of intracranial bleeding due to rentching and vomiting, it is reasonable to assume that this is a realistic threat.

Table 73.7 Nausea and
vomiting score

Score	Description
0	No nausea or vomiting
1	Nausea but not vomiting
2	Nausea and retching
3	Nausea and vomiting

Table 73.8 Treatment of
estabished PONV, ≤ 6 h
postoperatively

Prophylaxis: Yes	Prophylaxis: No
Antiemetic different from the drug used for prophylaxis	Low-dose 5-HT3 antagonist: – Ondansetron 1.0 mg – Dolasetron 12.5 mg – Granisetron 0.1 mg – Tropisetron 0.5 mg
• Dexamethasone 2–4 mg	
• Droperidol 0.625 mg[a]	
• Propofol 20 mg[a]	

[a] In neurosurgical patients single dose to avoid sedative effects

Patient Assessment

Periodic assessment of nausea and vomiting should be performed routinely during emergence and recovery, and shoud be part of the "standard" evaluation of neurosurgical patients (Table 73.7).

Intervention/Treatment

There are only few trials on the efficacy of drugs in controlling established PONV in the PACU in adults, and even fewer in children, compared with the multitude of trials on prophylaxis of this complication. Paucity of data particularly exists in the context of neursurgical operations, and we have to rely on the information that is derived from trials in other groups of patients (Table 73.8).

When PONV occurs within 6 h postoperatively, the antiemetic should be chosen from a different therapeutic class than the drugs used for prophylaxis. If no prophylaxis was given, the recommended treatment is a low-dose 5-HT3 antagonist, the only drugs that have been adequately studied for the treatment of existing PONV: ondansetron 1.0 mg, dolasetron12.5 mg (smaller doses have not been studied), granisetron 0.1 mg, and tropisetron 0.5 mg. Studies in adults suggest that ondansetron has greater efficacy than metoclopramide in controlling established PONV.

Alternative treatments for established PONV include dexamethasone, 2–4 mg i.v., or droperidol, 0.625 mg i.v. Propofol, 20 mg as needed, can be considered for rescue therapy in patients still in the PACU and has been found as effective as ondansetron, although its antiemetic effect is probably brief. In neurosurgical patients, however, propofol should be used only after communication with the neurosurgical team, since sedative side effects can alter the neurologic exam.

Beyond 6 h, PONV can be treated with any of the agents used for prophylaxis except dexamethasone, which is longer acting.

Key Points

- Main determinant factors for PONV: patient-associated risk factors, duration and type of anesthesia, postoperative opioids.
- Risk of PONV in a given patient should be established first using established scoring systems.
- Consider acupressure.
- No prophylaxis in minimal risk patients, free from medical sequelae of vomiting.
- Prophylaxis for patients at moderate to high risk for PONV.
- Antiemetic combinations for patients at high risk for PONV.
- Avoid two drugs from the same group (e.g., metoclopramide and domperidone).
- Do not use combinations with antagonistic actions (e.g., cyclizine and metoclopramide, as cyclizine antagonizes the prokinetic effect of metoclopramide).
- Children at moderate or high risk for PONV should receive combination therapy with a 5-HT3 antagonist and a second drug (e.g. dexamethasone).
- Rescue therapy < 6 h post-op: antiemetic chosen from a different therapeutic class than the drugs used for prophylaxis.
- Rescue therapy > 6 h post-op: any of the drugs used for prophylaxis.
- Strategy to reduce baseline risk and the adoption of a multimodal approach will most likely ensure success in the management of PONV.

Suggested Reading

Apfel CC, Laara E, Koivuranta M, et al. A simplified risk score for predicting postoperative nausea and vomiting. Anesthesiology. 1999;91:693–700.

Arnberger M, Stadelmann K, Alischer P, et al. Monitoring of neuromuscular blockade at the P6 acupuncture point reduces the incidence of postoperative nausea and vomiting. Anesthesiology. 2007;107:903–8.

Eberhart LH, Morin AM, Kranke P, et al. Prevention and control of postoperative nausea and vomiting in post-cranioromy patients. Best Pract Res Clin Anaesthesiol. 2007;21:575–93.

Fabling JM, Gan TJ, EI-Moalem HE, et al. A randomized, doubleblinded comparison of ondansetron, droperidol, and placebo for prevention of postoperative nausea and vomiting after supratentorial craniotomy. Anesth Analg. 2000;91:358–61.

Gan TJ, Meyer T, Apfel CC, et al. Consensus guidelines for managing postoperative nausea and vomiting. Anesth Analg. 2003;97:62–7.

Neufeld SM, Newburn-Cook CV. The efficacy of 5-HT3 receptor antagonists for the prevention of postoperative nausea and vomiting after craniotomy: A meta-analysis. J Neurosurg Anesthesiol. 2007;19:10–7.

Chapter 74
The Transport of Neurosurgical Patients

Laurel E. Moore

Neurosurgical intensive care unit (NICU) patients require multiple transports for diagnostic studies and interventions over the course of their hospitalization. While the majority of these transports proceed uneventfully, they are fraught with potential risk, particularly in the setting of a rapidly deteriorating patient. Urgent transports are frequently required at night when staffing numbers and the experience of staff doing the transport may be less than during daytime shifts. Given the potential for patient injury, many institutions are now moving toward the establishment of a team of professionals who provide scheduled and emergent transport and continued care during invasive studies, an entirely new (and yet unrecognized) specialty of transport medicine.

There is very little in the literature regarding the transport of neurosurgical patients per se. There is, however, a growing literature regarding the transport of critically ill patients. This chapter attempts to review this available literature and make recommendations regarding the safe transport of neurosurgical patients.

Overview

Critically ill patients are at increased risk of mortality and morbidity during transport. Complications during transport occur in as many as 70% of transports. These complications range from trivial (pulse oximeter dysfunction) to catastrophic (severe hypotension, need for intubation, accidental extubation, increased intracranial pressure (ICP), and central line displacement affecting administration of inotropes). Respiratory complications can be particularly dangerous. Not surprisingly,

L.E. Moore, MD (✉)
Department of Anesthesiology, University of Michigan Medical School, Ann Arbor, MI, USA
e-mail: laurelmo@med.umich.edu

A.M. Brambrink and J.R. Kirsch (eds.), *Essentials of Neurosurgical Anesthesia & Critical Care*, DOI 10.1007/978-0-387-09562-2_74, © Springer Science+Business Media, LLC 2012

hypoxia during transport is more common in those patients requiring PEEP. Furthermore, in one study of combined medical and surgical ICU patients, hypotension and arrthymias were associated with episodes of inadvertent hypoventilation or hyperventilation with individual changes in $PaCO_2$ as great as 27 mmHg. Clearly this has ramifications for patients with increased ICP. There is evidence that as a group end-tidal CO_2 is well maintained for caretakers hand-ventilating intubated patients. However, variability for individual patients is greater than may be acceptable for patients with abnormal intracranial compliance. Finally, as regards respiratory complications, there is recent evidence that intrahospital transport of intubated patients may place those patients at increased risk for subsequent ventilator-associated pneumonia.

For patient with traumatic brain injury (TBI), pre-hospital secondary injuries (hypotension and particularly hypoxia) are associated with increased mortality and disability. Extrapolation suggests that patients with TBI are particularly sensitive to transport mishaps and particular care must be given to preventing hypoxia and hypotension. In the two studies looking specifically at the intrahospital transport of neurosurgical patients, secondary insults are common. In the first, secondary insults were seen in 51% of transports with the most common insults being arterial hypertension (28%) and intracranial hypertension (44%). Hypoxia (17%) and hypotension (17%) were also common complications of transport. In the second study, ICP increased an average of 27% during transport despite $PaCO_2$s that trended downward. Increases in ICP during transport may be sustained after return to the ICU.

Equipment failures are common during the transport of critically ill patients, occurring in up to 45% of transports. Many of these complications can be quite minor, such as electrocardiogram or pulse oximetry disconnects. Others, however, can be catastrophic such as loss of monitor power mid-transport.

Prevention

Neurosurgical ICU patients require more intrahospital transports than any other group of critically ill patients. Given the risks associated with the transport of our patients, it is imperative that a transport protocol be developed for the safe and consistent transport of neurosurgical patients. A protocol for the routine transport of critically ill patients allows staff to function smoothly during non-routine transports, specifically for emergent transports or the transport of acutely unstable patients. The American College of Critical Care Medicine developed guidelines for inter- and intrahospital transport of critically ill patients in 2004. These have been adapted for the specific needs of neurosurgical patients in this chapter. The "checklist", a simple summary of safety guidelines, has been shown to significantly reduce medical errors and improve outcome. An abbreviated summary of what follows (a transport check list) can be found in Table 74.1. Modified lists for airway equipment and medications can be found in Table 74.2. For this chapter, an attempt has been made to keep the recommended transport supplies practical. The following is a list of considerations to be made prior to the transport of critically ill patients.

Table 74.1 Transport checklist

- Signed consent on chart with patient
- Oxygen cylinder checked and confirmed to have adequate supply
- Monitor fully charged
- Airway kit
- Emergency medications
- Sedatives
- Mask and Ambu bag or transport ventilator with PEEP valve as necessary
- $ETCO_2$ monitor or CO_2 detection kit
- Injection port identified and immediately accessible
- Destination contacted and confirmed ready to receive

1. Does the information to be gained warrant the risk of transport?
   A study looking at the risk/benefit ratio for the transport of general ICU patients demonstrated that information gained from studies resulted in changes in management in only 24% of critically ill patients, while 68% of patients had potentially significant physiologic complications during transport. While these data may not extrapolate well to neurosurgical patients, prior to transport the question must be asked, "Is the potential benefit worth the risk?"

2. Equipment
   (A) Monitor – All ICU patients should continue to receive the same monitoring during transport that they receive in the ICU with the reasonable exception of pulmonary artery or central venous pressure monitoring. At minimum electrocardiogram, blood pressure (either invasive or noninvasive), respiratory rate, and pulse oximetry should be monitored continuously (and documented) for all transports. Continuous end tidal carbon dioxide ($ETCO_2$) monitoring is ideal, although not all transport monitors have this capability. Disposable $ETCO_2$ devices should be available on all transports if continuous $ETCO_2$ monitoring is not available. Patients with abnormal intracranial compliance should continue to have ICP monitored throughout the transport and diagnostic study/procedure, particularly given the frequency of ICP elevation during "road trips." Related to this, patients requiring ICP monitoring should remain whenever possible with the head of bed elevated at 30° with the head in neutral position. Although certain procedures such as CT studies or angiography require the patient to be supine, periods requiring a supine (flat) position should be minimized whenever possible. Finally, monitors with memory capability are ideal for continuous data collection and recovery, and monitor battery should be confirmed to be fully charged (or have a back-up immediately available) prior to initiating transport. Many monitors have combined monitoring/defibrillation capability. When a patient monitor does not have defibrillation capability, the presence of a defibrillator should be confirmed at the destination site.

Table 74.2 Recommended adult transportation supplies

1. *Monitor* capable of monitoring ECG, pulse oximetry, noninvasive blood pressure and at least two pressure channels (e.g., for arterial blood pressure and ICP)
2. *Airway equipment* including
   Appropriate size mask
   Ambu bag with PEEP valve or transport ventilator as appropriate
   Variety of oral airways/nasal trumpets
   Laryngeal mask airways (LMA) in sizes 3, 4, and 5
   Endotracheal tubes (sizes 5.0–8.0 cuffed)
   Stylettes for endotracheal tubes
   Variety of laryngoscopes and blades (e.g., MAC 3 and 4, Miller 2 and 3)
   Portable end-tidal monitor or disposable cartridges
   Bougie or Eschmann stylette
3. *Oxygen tank* (full), consider back-up for prolonged transports with key
4. *Emergency medications* (prefilled syringes when possible and practical)
   Adenosine
   Amiodarone
   Atropine
   Calcium chloride
   Diltiazem
   Diphenhydramine
   Epinephrine
   Esmolol
   Furosemide
   Heparin
   Labetolol
   Lidocaine
   Mannitol
   Naloxone
   Phenylephrine
   Protamine
   Rocuronium
   Succinylcholine
   Vasopressin
5. *Sedative agents* (may set up "transport kit" and obtain immediately pretransport)
   Fentanyl
   Midazolam
   Propofol
   Etomidate
6. *Additional*
   Adequate volume of critical infusions including inotropes
   Consider additional intravenous fluids or IV equipment
   Supply of needles and syringes for medication administration

(B) Airway equipment
  (i)   Oxygen – it is essential to ensure adequate O_2 delivery during transport. To determine whether an oxygen tank will be adequate for a transport the calculation is fairly straightforward. The pressure of a full E cylinder of oxygen is 2,200 psi and the tank contains 660 liters of oxygen. As an ideal gas, the volume of oxygen is proportional to the psi as measured by the pressure gauge. Therefore, if 1,200 psi remains in an oxygen tank, the tank contains:

$$1200 / 2200 = X / 660, X = 360 \text{ liters of oxygen remaining.}$$

If oxygen flow to the patient is 10 liters/minute, then there is oxygen available for 36 minutes of flow. It is reasonable to have oxygen adequate for the anticipated transport plus an additional 15–30 minutes of flow in case of a transport delay. For prolonged transports, a second tank of oxygen is never a bad idea. Oxygen cylinders should be attached to the patient bed with designated tank holders for the safety of the patient and accompanying staff.
  (ii)   A suggested list of airway equipment for transport can be found in Table 74.2. Laryngoscopes and portable $ETCO_2$ monitors should be checked for proper function on a daily basis.

(C) Medications
A list of recommended drugs for the transport of NICU patients is included in Table 74.2. An attempt has been made to tailor this list for neurosurgical patients. It should be adjusted as necessary for patients with additional comorbidities such as significant cardiac disease. Sedation "kits" including scheduled medications such as fentanyl, midazolam, and lorazepam (if the drug of choice for seizures) can be made in advance and stored with other controlled medications until required for urgent transportations. Induction agents such as propofol, sodium thiopental, and etomidate should be included on every transport in case of urgent airway management or management of increased ICP. Certain muscle relaxants including succinylcholine and rocuronium require storage at 40°F or below. There are unpublished data to support that succinylcholine may be kept at room temperature for up to 90 days but manufacturer's recommendations are that succinylcholine not be used after 14–28 days at room temperature (depending on source). Rocuronium may be kept at room temperature for up to 60 days. Expiration dates based on when succinylcholine and rocuronium are removed from cooling should be placed on each vial.

3. Accompanying personnel

   The incidence of transport complications is related to the experience of the personnel accompanying the critically ill patient. Ideally at least three staff should accompany all critically ill patients – at least two with intensive care training (RNs or MDs) and a third individual to help with physically transporting the bed and equipment as directed by the medical staff. Because of critical incidents associated with patient transport, hospitals are increasingly moving toward ICU nurses with additional training in patient transport and sedation who are responsible for the transport of ICU patients. There are currently no data to answer whether the recent development of these "Transport specialists" will reduce the incidence of transport complications in adult ICU patients, but there is evidence in pediatric patients to support this practice. Patient vital signs and clinical care must be charted throughout transport and the procedure/diagnostic study.

4. Patient preparation

   The final element in preparing for an ICU transport is getting the patient ready to travel. Although this component of preparation seems self-evident, there are a few considerations that must be taken with neurosurgical patients.

   (A) Airway – Intubated patients on PEEP are at increased risk for transport. High-grade subarachnoid or severe TBI patients frequently have widened alveolar-arterial gradients for reasons commonly grouped as "neurogenic pulmonary edema," a subject beyond the scope of this chapter. Equipment for providing positive pressure ventilation (e.g., transport ventilator or Ambu bag) with PEEP capability is mandatory for these patients. For patients requiring high levels of PEEP and FIO_2 prior to transport, it may be prudent to hand bag the patient in the ICU for several minutes prior to departure to see how the patient tolerates being removed from the ventilator. Transport ventilators are available at some institutions which vary in technical sophistication. Simple transport ventilators allow patients to receive a constant (high) level of PEEP and defined tidal volumes at constant rates, while more advanced models can deliver respiratory patterns similar to those provided by current ICU ventilators (e.g., LTV1000; PULMONETIC SYSTEMS).

   A key consideration specific to deteriorating neurosurgical patients is whether to intubate prior to transport. Current CT scanners can do a non-contrast CT in mere seconds and thus it is understandable why caretakers frequently argue that airway management can be deferred until CT results are available. This is a dangerous point of view. The decision to intubate under controlled circumstances in the ICU must be determined by the status of the patient and the rate of decline. Unresponsive patients clearly require intubation, if only for airway protection, not to mention the institution of hyperventilation for management of presumed intracranial hypertension. It is the slowly declining marginally responsive patient who may present a dilemma. If the ICU team feels the patient will require sedation to undergo the diagnostic study, it is critical that the airway be controlled to avoid hypercarbia and increasing ICP related to increased cerebral blood flow. Airway management under controlled conditions in the ICU is always preferable to emergent intubation during transport.

(B) Volume status

Hypotension is a common complication of the intrahospital transport of ICU patients. Many of our deteriorating patients receive acute diuretic therapy (for example, mannitol or furosemide) and are being actively dehydrated. However, poor cerebral perfusion pressure is clearly bad for patients with intracranial pathology and if appropriate, small fluid boluses in addition to pressor administration should be considered prior to and during the transport of hypotensive patients. A discussion of fluid therapy for neurosurgical patients is beyond the scope of this chapter, but hypertonic saline or colloids may be considered under these circumstances.

(C) Sedation

Because of their deteriorating neurologic status, neurosurgical patients requiring transport for diagnostic or interventional studies may be unable to cooperate for completion of the procedure. Furthermore, the transport of agitated patients risks complications such as inadvertent extubation or other patient injury. It is therefore recommended that sedation be initiated prior to transport for these patients. Infusions of relatively short-acting sedatives such as propofol or dexmetetomidine are ideal, if the patient can tolerate them hemodynamically. If the patient is hemodynamically unstable, small doses of opiate (fentanyl) and/or benzodiazepines (midazolam) plus paralysis, if necessary, will facilitate completion of the transport and study.

(D) ICP monitoring

Anecdotal experience suggests that complications related to ventricular catheters are common during transport. This is related to both displacement of the catheter during patient transfers and inexperience managing ventricular drains. It is imperative that personnel transporting patients with ventricular drainage systems familiarize themselves with the system and recognize when the patient's drain is closed ("to monitor", no CSF drainage) or open ("to drain"). It is suggested that during transport the catheter be closed to drain but ICP continuously monitored. This is to prevent accidental acute changes in the "pop-off" height (level above tragus at which drainage occurs.) Should ICP increase while the system is closed to drain it should be immediately opened at the original "pop-off" level and CSF allowed to drain. Sterility must be maintained at all times during patient transfers.

(E) General preparation
Finally, prior to departing the ICU, all lines and the endotracheal tube should be checked to ensure that they are well secured. A functioning IV line and port for the administration of medications should be identified and immediately accessible. Adequate volumes of infused medications (such as pressors or sedatives) should also be confirmed. In the case of unstable patients, a call to the receiving end should be made to ensure readiness for the patient.

Crisis Management

The goal of this chapter is the prevention of transport emergencies. Recognition and management of the conditions for which patients are being transported are discussed elsewhere in this textbook. During transport is not the time for clinical intervention and any patient management issues that can be handled in the ICU prior to transport, for example airway management, should be managed under controlled conditions whenever possible. Having said this, a mechanism for contacting immediate help and a knowledge of the location of emergency equipment (e.g., arrest carts) along the transport route is critical in the case of a transport catastrophe.

Key Points

- Complications are common during the transport of critically ill patients
- NICU patients require more transports than other ICU patients
- Standardized preparation for transport may reduce the risk of complications
- Continuation of mechanical ventilation using adequate transport ventilators should be considered in all NICU patients requiring PEEP, or at risk for ICP increase; $ETCO_2$ measurements should be continued during transport
- Risk of complications is related to the experience of accompanying personnel
- In deteriorating neurosurgical patients consider securing the airway prior to transport
- ICP elevation is common during the transport of patients with ICP monitors.

Suggested Reading

Andrews PJD. Secondary insults during intrahospital transport of head-injured patients. Lancet. 1990;335:327–30.

Bekar A. Secondary insults during intrahospital transport of neurosurgical intensive care patients. Neurosurg Rev. 1990;21:98–101.

Papson J. Unexpected events during the intrahospital transport of critically ill patients. Acad Emerg Med. 2007;14:574–7.

Sarren J. Guidelines for the inter- and intrahospital transport of critically ill patients. Crit Care Med. 2004;32:256–62.

Part XIV
Challenges in Neurocritical Care of Neurosurgical Patients

Chapter 75
Altered Mental Status in Neurosurgical Critical Care

Christoph S. Burkhart, Stephan P. Strebel, and Luzius A. Steiner

Overview

Altered level of consciousness is a nonspecific symptom of many complications in neurosurgical patients and may be caused by conditions such as rebleeding of cerebral aneurysms, decompensating brain edema, postoperative hematoma, or seizures. Consciousness can be divided into wakefulness and awareness. The former includes arousal, alertness, and vigilance; and the latter is the sum of cognitive and emotional functions. The anatomical structures, upon which wakefulness and awareness depend, and the signs of dysfunction are shown in Table 75.1. Disorders of wakefulness are always accompanied by impaired awareness. Although the distinction between wakefulness and awareness is important for the understanding of the pathophysiology of altered consciousness, in our experience, the distinction between the two is of limited clinical importance as far as timing and manner of the clinical evaluation of patients with altered levels of consciousness are concerned. However, treatment may differ considerably.

C.S. Burkhart, MD (✉)
Department of Anaesthesia and Intensive Care Medicine,
University of Basel, Basel, Switzerland
e-mail: cburkhart@uhbs.ch

S.P. Strebel, MD
Department of Anaesthesia, University Clinics of Basel, and University Hospital Center
and University of Lausanne, Switzerland

L.A. Steiner, MD, PhD
Department of Anaesthesia, University Hospital Center and University of Lausanne,
Lausanne, Switzerland

A.M. Brambrink and J.R. Kirsch (eds.), *Essentials of Neurosurgical
Anesthesia & Critical Care*, DOI 10.1007/978-0-387-09562-2_75,
© Springer Science+Business Media, LLC 2012

Table 75.1 Anatomy and signs of altered consciousness

	Wakefulness	Awareness
Components	Arousal, alertness, vigilance	Sum of cognitive and emotional functions
Anatomical structures	Ascending reticular activating system (ARAS), descending corticoreticular pathways	Cerebral cortex of both hemispheres, associated white matter tracts, subcortical nuclei, and descending corticofugal systems
Dysfunction	Quantitative disturbance of consciousness • Hypervigilance • Somnolence • Stupor • Coma	Qualitative disturbance of consciousness • Delirium • Persistent vegetative state

Incidence

Overall, neurological complications are reported with an incidence of 3–7% after intracranial procedures, a rate which depends on the investigated patient population. After resection of intra-axial brain tumors, neurological complications have been reported in more than 25% of patients and commonly include motor and sensory deficits as well as coma (2%). Postoperative hematoma occurs in approximately 1% of patients after intracranial surgery, with deceased level of consciousness being the most common clinical symptom (61% of patients with postoperative hematoma).

Elderly patients are particularly at increased risk for postoperative delirium after neurosurgical procedures, especially when preexisting dementia is present.

Epidemiology

Certain patients have an elevated risk for developing neurological complications postoperatively (Table 75.2). Up to 18% of patients have been reported to have postoperatively sustained ICP elevation after supratentorial or infratentorial surgery. The incidence of retraction injuries varies considerably depending on the surgical technique and the duration of retraction.

Etiology (Table 75.3)

Clinical Implications

Rapid diagnosis and treatment of an abnormal level of consciousness is essential. Irreversible brain damage will develop rapidly, within minutes, if the cerebral cortex or other brain areas are not perfused. Generally, patients who are admitted to the

Table 75.2 Most important complications in specific groups of patients; incidence is indicated where available

Operative interventions	Increased risk for
Resection of gliomas	Postoperative seizures, postoperative ICP elevation
Resection of meningioma	Postoperative hematoma, postoperative seizures, postoperative ICP elevation
Surgical procedures for abscess	Postoperative seizures
Evacuation of chronic subdural hematoma	Postoperative seizures
Evacuation of intracerebral hematoma	Postoperative seizures
Surgery for arteriovenous malformations	Postoperative seizures Retraction injury Perforator stroke Normal pressure breakthrough edema
Aneurysmal subarachnoid hemorrhage	Postoperative seizures Retraction injury Perforator stroke
Stenting of symptomatic intracranial stenosis	Perforator stroke (3%)
Skull base surgery	Retraction injuries (10%)
Carotid endarterectomy	Hyperperfusion syndrome (3%)
Repeat surgery	Postoperative ICP elevation
Duration of intracranial surgery >6 h	Postoperative ICP elevation
Large intraoperative blood loss	Postoperative hematoma
Coagulopathy, current use of antiplatelet agents or anticoagulants	Postoperative hematoma

Table 75.3 Etiology of altered level of consciousness

Supra- or infratentorial focal lesions	Diffuse or toxic/metabolic encephalopathies
Postoperative bleeding	Hypoglycemia
Raised ICP	Seizures
Ischemic, embolic, perforator stroke	Electrolyte and osmolality abnormalities
Vasospasm	Hypercapnia
Retraction injury	Hypoxia
Tension pneumocephalus	Drugs/toxins and withdrawal
CSF hypotension	Delirium
Hyperperfusion syndrome	Hypotension
	Renal and hepatic failure

hospital in coma (not postoperative neurosurgical patients) and who do not spontaneously open their eyes within the following 6 h have only a 10% chance of making a good or moderate long-term recovery. After 1 week of coma, the likelihood of a good or moderate recovery is 3%. Such data are not available for the chance of recovery from coma postoperatively following neurosurgical procedures. However, it is reasonable to assume that the chance of making a good recovery decreases with the duration of coma in this group of patients as well.

Anticipated Problems

Delayed diagnosis and treatment of the causes of the altered level of consciousness may lead to significant morbidity or mortality, increased cost, prolonged length of stay in the intensive care unit, and extended overall hospital stay.

Prevention

The management should aim to prevent conditions favoring the development of complications and avoid strategies that interfere with the early detection of changes in the mental status. For example, the use of short-acting anesthetics, early extubation and prevention of unintended hypothermia allow for an early and a more detailed neurological examination. Stable hemodynamics should be achieved. Both, hypo- and hypertension are detrimental. In fact, arterial hypertension during emergence from brain surgery is associated with a higher incidence of postoperative intracranial hemorrhage. Electrolyte, fluid, and metabolic imbalances should be rapidly corrected. In addition, post-craniotomy pain may be significant and should be treated. There is no reason not to use opiates, provided they are carefully titrated and the patient is carefully monitored.

To further reduce the incidence of delirium, risk factors such as sleep deprivation, immobility, dehydration, visual, auditory, and cognitive impairments should be considered and adequately addressed if necessary. Risk factors such as anticholinergic drugs should be eliminated. Drug withdrawal (e.g., benzodiazepines) should be anticipated and avoided if possible by providing adequate substitution. No pharmacological prophylaxis for delirium can be recommended at this time.

Crisis Management

Efficient crisis management of patients presenting with an altered level of consciousness in the intensive care environment aims to identify and treat reversible causes before irreversible brain damage ensues. Thus, even prior to a rapid neurological assessment, measures should be initiated to secure adequate oxygenation and stable hemodynamics (ABCs).

Pathophysiology and Clinical Presentation

Two groups of pathophysiological processes impair consciousness: diffuse or toxic encephalopathies and focal lesions. Diffuse or toxic/metabolic encephalopathies

Table 75.4 Differential diagnosis of altered level of consciousness by clinical presentation in the intensive care unit

Clinical signs	Differential diagnosis	Further steps to consider
Lateralizing signs	Postoperative bleeding Ischemic stroke Perforator stroke Raised ICP Vasospasm Retraction injury Hyperperfusion syndrome	CT, MRI, TCD, angiography, surgical intervention, medically lower ICP, treat vasospasm
Pupillary abnormalities; unilateral vs. bilateral	Postoperative bleeding Ischemic stroke Raised ICP Vasospasm Retraction injury	CT, MRI, TCD, angiography, surgical intervention, medically lower ICP, treat vasospasm
Hypersomnia	Postoperative bleeding Ischemic stroke Perforator stroke	CT, MRI, surgical intervention, EEG
Visual abnormalities	Postoperative bleeding Ischemic stroke Perforator stroke Raised ICP Vasospasm Retraction injury	CT, MRI, TCD, angiography, surgical intervention, medically lower ICP, treat vasospasm
Postural headache	CSF hypotension	Rehydration, surgical intervention
Seizures, convulsions	Postoperative bleeding Ischemic stroke Perforator stroke Raised ICP Retraction injury Tension pneumocephalus Hyperperfusion syndrome	CT, MRI, surgical intervention, EEG, medically lower ICP
Arterial hypertension	Postoperative bleeding Ischemic stroke Perforator stroke Raised ICP Tension pneumocephalus Hyperperfusion syndrome Pain	CT, surgical intervention, lower ICP, analgesics, antihypertensive drugs
Cheyne-stokes respiration	Raised ICP	CT, medically lower ICP, surgical intervention

Precise knowledge of the procedure performed and the associated pathophysiology is essential to indentify the underlying complications and guide further diagnosis and treatment

decrease the function of both hemispheres via hypoxia, ATP-depletion, impaired glucose utilization, or accumulation of cytotoxic metabolites. Focal lesions have a direct or an indirect effect on critical areas of the diencephalon or brainstem that are involved in the maintenance of consciousness. Infratentorial focal lesions directly compromise the ascending reticular activating system (ARAS). Tables 75.4 and 75.5

Table 75.5 Differential diagnosis of altered level of consciousness by clinical presentation of toxic/metabolic encephalopathies

Clinical signs	Differential diagnosis	Further steps to consider
Persistent coma	Non-convulsive epileptic state	CT, MRI, EEG, anticonvulsants
	Intracranial bleeding	
	Stroke	
Small reactive pupils	Opiate overdose	Ventilation, opioid antagonists
Respiratory depression	Opiate overdose	Ventilation, opioid antagonists, CT, MRI
	Intracranial bleeding	
	Stroke	
	Raised ICP	
Inattention, disorganized thinking	Delirium	Reassurance, neuroleptic drugs, correct hypoglycemia
	Hypoglycemia	
Tachycardia	Hypoglycemia	Correct hypoglycemia or hypovolemia, analgesics
	Pain	
	Hypovolemia	
	Withdrawal symptoms	
ECG changes	Electrolyte and osmolality abnormalities	Laboratory analysis, correct electrolytes, treat ischemia, CT
	Myocardial ischemia/infarction	
	Subarachnoid hemorrhage	
Tachypnea	Hypercapnia	Correct hypercapnia and hypoxia, laboratory analysis
	Hypoxia	
	Systemic inflammatory response syndrome	
Sympathetic hyperactivity	Hypercapnia	Correct hypercapnia, laboratory analysis
	Systemic inflammatory response syndrome	
	Alcohol withdrawal	

Precise knowledge of the procedure performed and the associated pathophysiology is essential to indentify the underlying complications and guide further diagnosis and treatment

provide an overview of the clinical findings of focal lesions and toxic/metabolic encephalopathies. The history of the patient and the type of surgery performed will provide crucial insight into the problems that may occur. Unspecific signs include headache, vomiting, restlessness, lethargy, stupor, and tremor.

We suggest that standardization and predefined timing of assessments are crucial to obtain an early diagnosis and allow rapid interventions. Early consultation with neurosurgeons and neurologists is essential.

Patient Assessment (Fig. 75.1)

In patients without focal signs, the decision to perform a CT scan must be based on the patient's history and clinical presentation, and on the judgment of the treating physician. Consider MRI for suspected posterior fossa lesions and early detection of ischemia (diffusion-weighted imaging; DWI). Do not delay imaging while waiting for laboratory results.

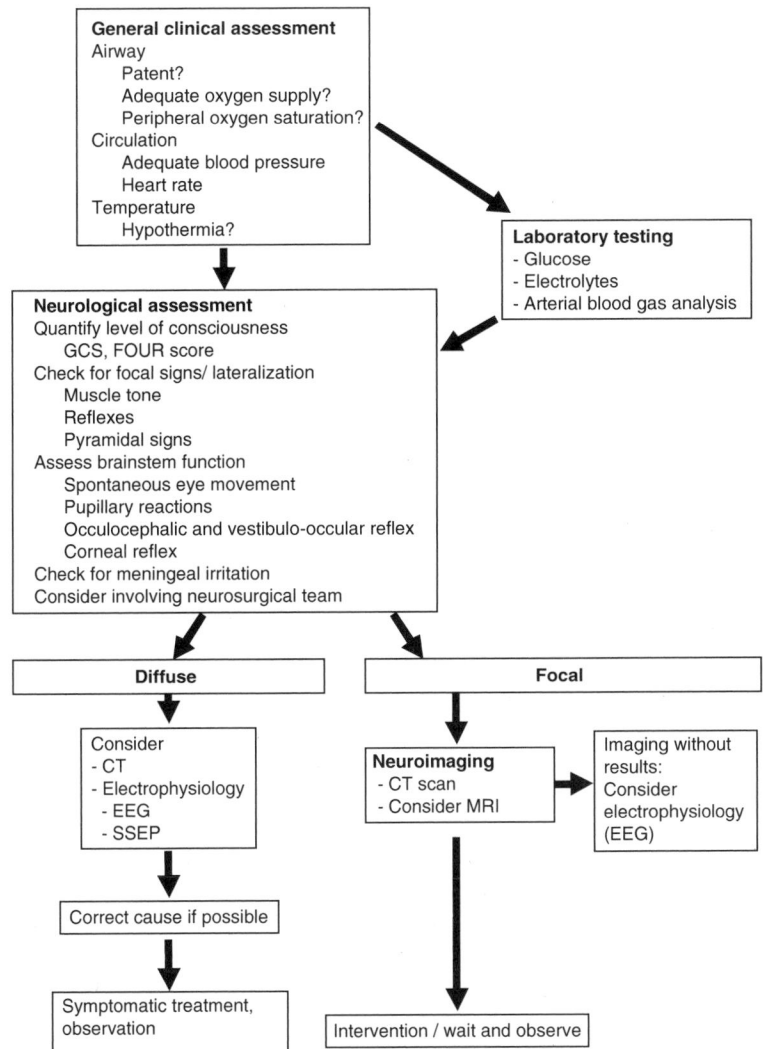

Fig. 75.1 Suggested sequence for the evaluation of patients with a decreasing level of consciousness. *Legend*: EEG electroencephalography, SSEP somatosensory evoked potentials. Hypothermia will influence neurological assessment. Scoring systems: *GCS*: widely used, may not detect subtle neurological changes, does not consider brainstem reflexes. *F*ull *O*utline of *UnR*esponsiveness (FOUR score): includes brainstem reflexes and respiratory patterns, thus, allowing further evaluation of patients with a low GCS (For further information see Wijdicks EF et al. 2005)

Perform EEG in patients with inconspicuous imaging results who remain comatose or with altered levels of consciousness not otherwise explained. Non-convulsive seizures and non-convulsive status epilepticus may be clinically undetectable. If delirium is suspected, use delirium assessment instruments such as the Confusion Assessment Method for the ICU (CAM-ICU) or the Intensive Care Delirium Screening Checklist (ICDSC). Screening for delirium should be performed regularly as part of routine care.

Intervention/Treatment

- Airway management.

  - Ensure adequate oxygen supply
  - Intubation and mechanical ventilation if necessary

- Treat unstable hemodynamics.

  - Correct hypovolemia with crystalloids, colloids, or blood as appropriate
  - Hypotension: vasopressors (e.g., phenylephrine boluses of 50–100 μg i.v. or a norepinephrine infusion)
  - Consider treatment of hypertension (e.g., labetalol boluses of 5–15 mg i.v., esmolol boluses of 10–50 mg i.v., or urapidil boluses of 5–10 mg i.v.)

- Perform surgery if indicated.

  - Early consultation with neurosurgeon
  - CT if appropriate

- Consider antagonists if opioid or benzodiazepine overdose is suspected (naloxone 40–200–400 μg i.v., flumazenil 0.2–0.5 mg i.v., respectively).
- Use specific instruments such as the CAM-ICU or the Intensive Care Delirium Screening Checklist (ICDSC) at regular intervals, i.e. once every shift, to screen for delirium. Consider haloperidol or an atypical antipsychotic drug (off-label use) if delirium is suspected. Elderly patients may be very susceptible to the effects of these drugs. Therefore, treatment is typically started with oral haloperidol at 0.5–1.0 mg every 8 h. Doses may be increased or given intravenously if necessary. Beware: hypotension and prolongation of QT-interval. Atypical antipsychotics (off-label use), e.g., oral quetiapine is typically started at 12.5–25 mg every 12 h. Alternatively, olanzapine (5 mg every 12 h) or risperidone (0.5 mg every 12 h) could be considered.

Key Points

Any change in the level of consciousness may be the first sign of a life-threatening complication.

- Perform regular clinical assessment.
- Perform frequent neurological scoring.
- Careful documentation of observations and scores is crucial.
- If scores are deteriorating (e.g., GCS score is 2 points less than that assessed during the previous scoring) initiate immediate careful examination. Depending on the results, perform further diagnostic tests (e.g., CT scan).
- Develop unit-specific standard operating procedures for patients with an altered or deteriorating level of consciousness.

Suggested Reading

Bassetti C, Aldrich MS. Consciousness, delirium, and coma. In: Albin MS, editor. Textbook of neuroanesthesia: with neurosurgical and neuroscience perspectives. New York: McGraw-Hill Professional; 1996. p. 369–408.

Pfister D, Strebel SP, Steiner LA. Postoperative management of adult central neurosurgical patients: systemic and neuro-monitoring. Best Pract Res Clin Anaesthesiol. 2007;21:449–63.

Wijdicks EF, Bamlet WR, Maramattom BV, Manno EM, McClelland RL. Validation of a new coma scale: The FOUR score. Ann Neurol. 2005;58:585–93.

Chapter 76
Cerebrovascular Vasospasm, Normal Pressure Breakthrough Edema, Posterior Reversible Encephalopathy Syndrome (PRES) in Neurosurgical Critical Care

Syed Arshad and José I. Suarez

Cerebral Vasospasm

Overview

Cerebral vasospasm is one of the leading causes of morbidity and mortality following aneurysmal subarachnoid hemorrhage. It leads to death or permanent neurologic deficits in over 17–40% of SAH patients. Risk factors for vasospasm include thick blood in the basal cisterns determined by head CT scanning, female gender, smoking, cocaine use, hypovolemia, hyponatremia, hypomagnesemia, increased intracranial pressure and systemic inflammatory response syndrome. Factors less robustly linked are a longer duration of unconsciousness following the initial hemorrhage, history of hypertension, and excess weight.

Prevention

To date, there is no evidence from large randomized controlled trials that any therapy is effective for vasospasm prevention. However, some recommended therapies have been used for neuro-protection and are summarized in Table 76.1.

S. Arshad, MD
Department of Neurosurgery, Kaiser Sacramento Medical Center,
University of California, San Francisco, Sacramento, CA, USA

J.I. Suarez, MD (✉)
Department of Neurology, Baylor College of Medicine, Houston, TX, USA
e-mail: jisuarez@bcm.edu

A.M. Brambrink and J.R. Kirsch (eds.), *Essentials of Neurosurgical Anesthesia & Critical Care*, DOI 10.1007/978-0-387-09562-2_76, © Springer Science+Business Media, LLC 2012

Table 76.1 Recommended medical management of patients with subarachnoid hemorrhage

Therapy	Recommendations	Rationale
Calcium antagonist	Administer nimodipine (60 mg PO every 4 h for 21 days)	Neuro-protective cellular effect (good evidence from randomized controlled trials)
Core body temperature	Keep at ≤37.2°C; administer acetaminophen (325–650 mg PO every 4–6 h) and use cooling devices if necessary	Avoid systemic and cerebral metabolic insults (no randomized controlled trials)
Blood pressure	Keep systolic blood pressure at 90–140 mmHg before aneurysm treatment, then allow hypertension to keep systolic blood pressure <200 mmHg	Improving cerebral blood flow (no randomized controlled trials)
Serum glucose	Maintain level at 80–120 mg/dl; use sliding scale or continuous infusion of insulin if necessary	Avoid systemic and cerebral metabolic insults (no randomized controlled trials)
Fluids and hydration	Maintain euvolemia (CVP, 5–8 mmHg)	Improving cerebral blood flow (evidence from randomized controlled trials)
Hyponatremia	With SIADH, restrict fluids; with cerebral salt-wasting syndrome, aggressively replace fluids with 0.9% saline or hypertonic saline solution	Avoid systemic and cerebral metabolic insults
Electrolyte imbalance	Avoid acidosis and hypomagnesemia	Avoid systemic and cerebral metabolic insults
Promising but not yet proven therapies		
Intracisternal thrombolysis (reserved for high-risk patients with subarachnoid hemorrhage)	Postoperative rt-PA 2–4 mg Intraoperative rt-PA 10 mg	Removal of blood clots and decreasing humoral cascade (no randomized controlled trials)
Statin therapy	Pravastatin 40 mg for 14 days Simvastatin 80 mg for 14 days	Biochemical effects (phase III trials ongoing)

Crisis Management

The clinical diagnosis of cerebral vasospasm is made when the patient experiences an altered level of consciousness or a new focal neurologic deficit. Cerebral vasospasm is most likely an inflammatory reaction in the blood-vessel wall and develops between days 4 and 12 after subarachnoid hemorrhage. The best predictor of vasospasm is the amount of blood seen on the initial head CT scan. Angiographic vasospasm is more common, occurring in about two-thirds of patients after aneurismal SAH, than is symptomatic vasospasm, which presents with symptoms of cerebral ischemia in one-third of all patients after SAH.

Table 76.2 summarizes pathophysiology, clinical presentation, diagnostic testing, and medical and interventional strategies.

Table 76.2 Main features of the diagnosis and treatment of cerebral vasospasm

Pathophysiology	In vitro, oxyhemoglobin stimulates the secretion of endothelin-1, inhibits nitric oxide and produces activated oxygen species. These free radicals are believed to play a role in cell membrane lipid peroxidation, possibly mediating the structural changes in the vessel wall
Clinical presentation	Symptoms present between days 4–12 and range from nonspecific, such as excess sleepiness, lethargy, and stupor, to localizing findings such as hemiparesis, language disturbances, visual fields deficits, gaze impairment, and cranial nerve palsies. Need to also evaluate and rule out hydrocephalus, electrolyte disturbances, and seizures
Diagnostic tests	Cerebral angiography is the gold standard for visualizing and studying cerebral arteries
	Transcranial Doppler ultrasonography is performed either daily or every other day to monitor for vasospasm, which is defined as a mean velocity of cerebral blood flow of more than 120 cm per second in a major vessel. Doppler ultrasonography has a sensitivity that is similar to that of cerebral angiography for the detection of narrowed vessels, particularly in the middle cerebral and internal cerebral arteries
Triple-H therapy	Hypervolemia with goal CVP of 8–12 mmHg and or induced hypertension with phenylephrine, norepinephrine, or dopamine (no randomized controlled trials)
Endovascular therapy	Transluminal balloon angioplasty produces a sustained reversal of arterial narrowing. There is a 5% complication rate which includes vessel rupture, occlusion, dissection, and hemorrhagic infarction
	Intra-arterial vasodilators such as nicardipine, verapamil, nimodipine are injected via a micro-catheter at the proximal site of the vasospastic vessel. Nicardipine reverses angiographic vasospasm and significantly reduces mean peak systolic velocities in treated vessels, with no sustained effect on intracranial pressure or cardiovascular function (no randomized controlled trials)

Key Points

- Cerebral vasospasm remains a devastating neurological complication of aneurysmal subarachnoid hemorrhage and is associated with high morbidity and mortality rates.
- Symptoms present between days 4–12 and transcranial Doppler ultrasonography should be performed either daily or every other day to monitor for vasospasm.
- Immediate recognition and management of vasospasm are key in preventing cerebral ischemia.
- Patients should receive Triple-H therapy and undergo endovascular therapy, if vasospasm is suspected.

Posterior Reversible Encephalopathy Syndrome

Overview

Posterior reversible encephalopathy syndrome (PRES) is a clinico-neuroradiological transient condition which is characterized by headache, altered mental status, visual disturbance and selective hyperintensity seen on T2-weighted MRI images over the parieto-occipital white matter. It is associated with conditions summarized in Table 76.3.

Prevention

There are no preventive or neuroprotective strategies for PRES. However, one of the distinctive characteristics of PRES is the reversibility of the clinical and radiological abnormalities once treatment is instituted. Delayed diagnosis and therapy can result in permanent damage to affected brain tissue.

Crisis Management

The exact pathogenesis of PRES syndrome remains incompletely understood but is probably related to failed cerebral autoregulation and endothelial damage resulting in blood–brain barrier breakdown with reversible edema.

It is also important to rule out neurological and systemic diseases that mimic the radiological description of PRES. Table 76.4 summarizes the differential diagnosis of PRES and the key treatment strategies.

Table 76.3 Common causes of PRES

Hypertensive syndromes	Hypertensive encephalopathy, toxemia of pregnancy
Autoimmune diseases	Systemic lupus erythematosus, scleroderma, Wegener's
Immune suppression	Cyclosporine, Tacrolimus, interferon alpha, antiretroviral therapy
Status-post-cancer chemotherapy	Cytarabine, cisplatin, gemcitabine, bevacizumab
Liver and endocrine dysfunctions	Liver failure, primary aldosteronism, pheochromocytoma, hyperparathyroidism
Renal and electrolyte dysfunction	Acute on chronic renal failure, dialysis disequilibrium syndrome, hypercalcemia, hypomagnesemia
Hematological and infection	Hemolytic uremic syndrome, thrombotic thrombocytopenic purpura, porphyria, blood transfusion, erythropoietin therapy, systemic inflammatory response syndrome
Miscellaneous associations	Intravenous immunoglobulin, ephedra overdose, contrast media exposure, tumor lysis syndrome, scorpion poison, digitoxin intoxication, Triple-H therapy

Table 76.4 Differential diagnosis of PRES

Differential diagnosis
Central nervous system vasculitis
Ischemic stroke
Progressive multifocal leukoencephalopathy
Acute-disseminated encephalomyelitis
Infective encephalitis
Cerebral venous thrombosis
Cerebral autosomal dominant arteriopathy with stroke and ischemic leukoencephalopathy
Mitochondrial diseases
Treatment
Rapid correction of blood pressure, Nicardipine (5–15 mg/h) is usually first-line agent
Removal of causative factor (medication and toxin)
Maintenance of hydration
Monitoring of airway and ventilation
Consider insertion of central venous catheter (if cardiac dysfunction is present)
Delivery or cesarean section in pregnant women
Evaluate and treat status epilepticus

Key Points

- PRES is a well-recognized clinico-neuroradiological transient condition.
- Early recognition is important for prompt control of blood pressure or removal of precipitating factor and treatment of status epilepticus.
- Delay in diagnosis and treatment may result in death or in irreversible neurological sequelae.

Normal Perfusion Pressure Breakthrough Edema

Overview

Cerebral arteriovenous malformation obliteration (interventional neuroradiology [INR]) or resection (neurosurgery) is thought to result in hyperemia due to rapid resumption of normal blood flow in the vasodilated vessel. This resumption of pressure causes local capillary breakthrough and leads to uncontrollable cerebral swelling and hemorrhage. This transient circulatory derangement is called normal pressure breakthrough (NPPB) and happens in approximately 10% of cases. Risk factors for this phenomenon are summarized in Table 76.5.

Table 76.5 Clinical and radiological predictors of NPPB

Risk factors and predictors for NPPB
• High-flow AVM with a large venous ampulla
• Postprocedural/postoperative CT showing cerebral swelling and contrast medium leakage
• Extensive preoperative vascular dilation in the brain surrounding the nidus
• Intraoperative increase in local cerebral blood flow around the nidus after temporary clipping of the feeder

Prevention

No randomized studies have been carried out looking at intraoperative prevention of NPPB. However, the following strategies have proved useful.

- Feeder embolization (INR)
- Nidus embolization (INR)
- Intraoperative bleeding control.

Crisis Management

Prior to AVM obliteration, the resistance vessels in the chronically ischemic brain near the AVM are maximally dilated. Immediately after the removal of the AVM, vasomotor tone in these vessels may be overwhelmed by the abrupt increase in blood flow. This hypothesis forms the basis of treatment with fluid restriction, hypotension, and barbiturate therapy. Other strategies include controlled hyperventilation, steroids, and osmotic dehydrating agents to control intracranial pressure elevation. However, to date, there are no randomized controlled trials that have shown any efficacy for managing NPPB edema. Clinical symptoms can vary from migraine-like headaches to seizures and to permanent neurological disability and death. Detection techniques include noninvasive diamox transcranial Doppler ultrasound, postoperative Single-photon emission CT scans, and intraoperative angiogram.

Key Points

- NPPB is responsible for massive hemorrhage and cerebral edema and happens in about 10% of cases of cerebral arteriovenous resection.
- Detection of NPPB is important to prevent further neurological injury. The phenomenon may lasts for several days after surgery and can reoccur when normal blood pressure parameters are restored.
- Preoperative prevention strategies include feeder and nidus embolization. Intraoperative strategies include bleeding control and good microsurgical technique.
- Postoperatively, fluid restriction, hypotension, and barbiturate therapy can be employed.

Suggested Reading

Bartynski W. Posterior reversible encephalopathy syndrome, part 1: Fundamental imaging and clinical features. AJNR Am J Neuroradiol. 2008a;29(6):1036–42.

Bartynski W. Posterior reversible encephalopathy syndrome, part 2: Controversies surrounding pathophysiology of vasogenic edema. AJNR Am J Neuroradiol. 2008b;29(6):1043–9.

Bederson JB, Connolly ES, Batjer HH, Dacey RG, Dion JE, Diringer MN, et al. Guidelines for the management of aneurysmal subarachnoid hemorrhage: A statement for healthcare professionals from a special writing group of the stroke council, American Heart Association. Stroke. 2009 Mar 1;40(3):994–1025.

Chyatte D. Normal pressure perfusion breakthrough after resection of arteriovenous malformation. J Stroke Cerebrovasc Dis. 1997;6(3):130–6.

Hinchey J, Chaves C, Appignani B, Breen J, Pao L, Wang A, et al. A reversible posterior leukoencephalopathy syndrome. N Engl J Med. 1996 Feb 22;334(8):494–500.

Keyrouz S, Diringer M. Clinical review: Prevention and therapy of vasospasm in subarachnoid hemorrhage. Crit Care. 2007;11(4):220.

Kumar S, Kato Y, Sano H, Imizu S, Nagahisa S, Kanno T. Normal perfusion pressure breakthrough in arteriovenous malformation surgery: The concept revisited with a case report. Neurol India. 2004;52:111–5.

Suarez JI, Tarr RW, Selman WR. Aneurysmal subarachnoid hemorrhage. N Engl J Med. 2006 Jan 26;354(4):387–96.

Chapter 77
Sedation, Analgesia, and Neuromuscular Blockade in Neurosurgical Critical Care

Miko Enomoto and Ansgar M. Brambrink

Overview

The essence of this chapter can perhaps be best summarized as: Don't contribute to "ICU Psychosis." In the critical care setting, therapeutic goals include control of pain, relief of anxiety, and facilitation of mechanical ventilation and other necessary medical therapies. In neurocritical care, another important goal is to facilitate repeated neurological examinations. Frequently the use of sedative-hypnotic and analgesic agents, and occasionally neuromuscular blocking agents, are required to achieve the first goals, but their use can be fraught with complications, including interfering with neurological examinations. The most common and serious complications are listed in Table 77.1.

Neurosurgical patients, and critically ill patients in general, often have pain associated with their disease and/or treatment, and often experience altered consciousness. Untreated pain can lead to increased anxiety and a hyperadrenergic state with resulting hemodynamic, immunologic, and neuropsychiatric affects.

Agitation can represent a significant danger to patients and staff. It may contribute to events such as falls, traumatic removal of catheters, patient-ventilator dyssynchrony, and cardiovascular instability. There may be long-term mental health consequences, as well, with the reported incidence of posttraumatic stress disorder (PTSD) in critically ill patients being between 15 and 30%.

M. Enomoto, MD (✉)
Department of Anesthesiology and Perioperative Medicine,
Oregon Health & Science University, Portland, OR, USA
e-mail: enomotot@ohsu.edu.

A.M. Brambrink, MD, PhD
Departments of Anesthesiology and Perioperative Medicine, Neurology and Neurologic Surgery,
Oregon Health & Science University, Portland, OR, USA

A.M. Brambrink and J.R. Kirsch (eds.), *Essentials of Neurosurgical Anesthesia & Critical Care*, DOI 10.1007/978-0-387-09562-2_77,
© Springer Science+Business Media, LLC 2012

Table 77.1 Complications associated with the use of sedation, analgesia, and neuromuscular blockade in neurocritical care patients

Complications
- Respiratory
  - Respiratory depression, hypercapnea, increased ICP
  - Prolonged mechanical ventilation
- Cardiovascular
  - Hypotension, leading to cerebral ischemia
  - Hypertension, leading to increased ICP
- Neurological
  - Oversedation
  - Occult neurological decompensation because of obscured exam
  - Possible worsening of pathophysiology by medications
- Other
  - Delirium
  - Poor pain control due to inadequate analgesia
  - Anxiety and agitation with inadequate sedation
  - Posttraumatic stress disorder (PTSD)
  - Increased hospital length of stay
  - Possible increase in organ failure
  - Medication-related adverse reactions

When treating pain, anxiety, and agitation, or when inducing temporary muscle relaxation, it is important to remember that there are critical differences between the three main categories of medications discussed here. Each needs to be used appropriately. For example, some analgesic agents, especially opioids, have sedative properties, but use of these agents to sedate a patient who does not have pain requires high doses, which contributes to respiratory depression and cognitive dysfunction. On the other hand, analgesics may be useful as primary therapy for agitation due to pain. Useful analgesic agents and advantages and disadvantages to their use in the neurocritical care patient are listed in Table 77.2. Many sedative-hypnotic agents (with a few important exceptions such as ketamine and alpha-2 adrenergic agonists), completely lack analgesic properties and, if used alone, require high doses, often resulting in a comatose patient. By combining a sedative-hypnotic agent with an analgesic agent, it is usually possible to achieve a calm, comfortable patient with lower doses than would be required with either class alone. Useful sedative-hypnotic agents, and advantages and disadvantages to their use in the neurocritical care patient are listed in Table 77.3. Neuromuscular blocking drugs have no sedative or analgesic properties. With the possible exception of the moribund and hypotensive patient, it is never appropriate to treat with a neuromuscular blocking drug without also giving a sedative-hypnotic agent. Useful neuromuscular blocking agents, and advantages and disadvantages to their use in the neurocritical care patient are listed in Table 77.4.

Table 77.2 Analgesic classes of drugs, advantages, and disadvantages in the critically ill neurosurgical patient

Analgesic class	Advantages	Disadvantages
• First generation NSAIDs (non-steroidal anti-inflammatory drugs): ibuprofen, naproxen, flurbiprofen, ketoprofen, indomethacin, etodolac, diclofenac, ketorolac, piroxicam, and phenylbutaxone • COX-2 inhibitors: rofecoxib, celecoxib, meloxicam, nimesulide	• Analgesia without cognitive impairment, respiratory depression, or nausea; opioid sparing • COX-2 inhibitors are associated with less risk of bleeding, but have not been extensively studied in the postoperative neurosurgical patient	• Risk of bleeding (less with COX-2 inhibitors) • Risk of renal dysfunction (increased in elderly and decreased GFR) • Risk of gastric ulcers (less with COX-2 inhibitors) • Risk of cardiovascular events (with long-term use of COX-2 inhibitors, unclear if risk increases with short-term use)
Paracetamol (acetaminophen)	• Effective for control of mild pain • Opioid sparing effect • No increased risk of bleeding or gastric ulcers • No cognitive dysfunction	• Inadequate relief for moderate to severe pain, as a single agent • Risk of hepatic toxicity at high doses
Opioids	• Effective for moderate to severe pain	• Respiratory depression • Cognitive dysfunction/over sedation • Itching • Nausea • Decreased GI motility
NMDA antagonists: ketamine	• Effective for moderate to severe pain; in multi-modal therapy beneficial even at low doses • Anti-nociceptive action (more than analgesic) may be effective in preemptive analgesia • Opioid sparing effect • Less hypotension, decreased need for vasopressor support • Hemodynamic stimulation may be associated with improved cerebral perfusion • Less respiratory depression than seen with equi-analgesic doses of opioids • Experimental studies suggest neuroprotective effects (racemic ketamine) and regenerative effects (S(+)-ketamine)	• Increase ICP in spontaneously ventilating patients (not seen in patients with controlled ventilation and eucapnea) • Animal studies indicate neurotoxicity at high doses in neonatal and elderly brains • Higher doses associated with hallucinations/night terrors • Cardiovascular stimulant, leads to increased myocardial oxygen consumption
Alpha-2 adrenergic agonists: clonidine, dexmedetomidine	• Minimal effect on respiratory drive • Opioid sparing effects • Provide analgesia, sedation and anxiolysis while facilitating neurological examination • Suggested to have cardioprotective effects	• Can be associated with hypotension, hypertension, and bradycardia, especially with loading dose
Anticonvulsants (gabapentin)	• Helpful in the acute treatment of neuropathic pain	• Sedating • Generally not effective enough as sole agent

Table 77.3 Sedative hypnotic classes of drugs, advantages, and disadvantages in the critically ill neurosurgical patient

Drug class	Advantages	Disadvantages
Benzodiazepines: diazepam, lorazepam, midazolam, and others	• Anxiolytic, amnestic, sedative-hypnotic, and anticonvulsant properties • Decrease both, $CMRO_2$ and CBF, but unable to achieve burst suppression • Generally associated with less hemodynamic instability than propofol or barbiturates • Antagonist available (flumazenil)	• Diazepam and lorazepam have very long context-sensitive half-lives • Dose-dependent respiratory depression, synergistic with opioids • Hyperosmolar acidosis with lorazepam (due to propylene glycol diluent) • Hepatic metabolism • Clearance significantly decreases with age
Propofol	• Relatively short context-sensitive half-life; minimally effected by hepatic or renal dysfunction • Decreases equally $CMRO_2$ and CBF, thereby decreasing ICP; putative neuroprotective agent • Does not affect cerebrovascular autoregulation • Effective anticonvulsant • Anti-emetic effect	• Hypotension can lead to reduced CPP • Dose-dependent myocardial depression, decreased systemic vascular resistance • Dose-dependent respiratory depression • Risk for life-threatening propofol-infusion syndrome (increased in neurocritical care patients)
Barbiturates: thiopental, methohexital, thiamylal	• Neuroprotective by decreasing $CMRO_2$ and CBF, thereby decreasing ICP • Thiopental is a potent anticonvulsant at high doses, but methohexital, at therapeutic doses, and thiopental, at low-doses, are epileptogenic	• Long elimination half-life and long context-sensitive half-time • Rely on hepatic and renal metabolism • Decreases CO, BP, and peripheral vascular resistance • Dose-dependent respiratory depression
Alpha-2 adrenergic agonists: clonidine, dexmedetomidine	• Provide sedation, anxiolysis and analgesia without inducing unresponsiveness or coma • Early evidence indicates delirium-relieving effects • Mitigates symptoms of EtOH withdrawal • Minimal effect on respiratory drive • Opioid sparing effects • Facilitate neurological examination • Potentially cardioprotective	• Can be associated with hypotension, hypertension, and bradycardia, especially with loading dose
NMDA Antagonist: ketamine	• Dose-dependent CNS depression leads to dissociative anesthetic state with amnesia and analgesia without inducing coma or loss of protective reflexes • Opioid sparing effect • Less hypotension, decreased need for vasopressor support • Hemodynamic stimulation may be associated with improved cerebral perfusion • Less respiratory depression than seen with equi-sedative doses of barbiturates or propofol • Experimental studies indicate neuroprotective effects (racemic ketamine) and potential regenerative effects (S(+)-ketamine)	• Increases ICP in spontaneously ventilating patients (not seen in patients with controlled ventilation and eucapnea) • Animal studies indicate neurotoxicity at high doses in neonatal and elderly brains • Higher doses associated with hallucinations, night terrors and altered cognition (may precipitate delirium) • Cardiovascular stimulant, leads to increased myocardial oxygen consumption
Inhalational anesthetics	• May be associated with less severe delusional memories and hallucinations (compared to, e.g. midazolam)	• Not commonly used outside the operating room in the USA • Require special equipment • Risk for malignant hyperthermia

Table 77.4 Neuromuscular blocking classes of drugs, advantages, and disadvantages in the critically ill neurosurgical patient

Depolarizing NMB: succinylcholine	• Short acting • Fast onset • Facilitate tracheal intubation	• Increases ICP • Mandates airway management • Infusions can be associated with phase II block • Hyperkalemia; particularly concerning in patients with renal failure, immobile patients, patients with preexisting neuromuscular disease, or paralysis • Risk for malignant hyperthermia
Non-depolarizing NMB: Intermediate-duration agents are the most commonly used for maintenance of NMB in the ICU: atracurium, cisatracurium, rocuronium, vecuronium	• Facilitate tracheal intubation, mechanical ventilation and can be helpful in cases of refractory elevated ICP • Cisatracurium clearance is independent of end organ function (Hoffman-degradation) • Rocuronium is available for rapid sequence induction (RSI) at adequate doses (1.2 mg/kg)	• Use mandates airway management and mechanical ventilation • Risk of critical illness myopathy and polyneuropathy with prolonged use • Increased risk of nosocomial pneumonia • Associated with longer mechanical ventilation, hospital stay • Increased risk of polyneuropathy and increased duration of action in the setting of renal failure make pancuronium a less attractive neuromuscular blocker in the ICU setting

While diagnosis and management of respiratory compromise, hemodynamic instability and other common affects of these agents are well established in current ICU practice, we believe that this is not the case for the undesired effects these drugs have on the mental status of patients. The risk of inducing and/or maintaining confusion, agitation, and delirium with these drugs is concerning, particularly because the intent of their use is to ease pain, anxiety, and restlessness. Patients who require major neurosurgical interventions are at particularly high risk.

Delirium is emerging as an increasingly recognized adverse event. There is mounting evidence that delirium is associated with increased length of ICU stay, increased hospital stay, decreased cognitive function in survivors, and increased mortality. Although the pathophysiology is complex, the use of sedative-hypnotics and analgesics contributes. Identified risk factors for delirium include advanced age, hypertension, severity of illness, preexisting cognitive impairment, sleep deprivation, hypoxia and anoxia, metabolic abnormalities, a history of drug or alcohol abuse, as well as numerous medications (especially those with anticholinergic effects), and multiple psychoactive drugs. Some consider delirium equivalent to CNS or brain dysfunction, with prognostic implications similar to those associated with other organ failure in critical illness. Between 20 and 80% of ICU patients experience delirium, with reported rates varying by severity of illness in the study population and diagnostic methods used.

Prevention

Although the pathophysiology of delirium of critical illness is multifactoral, there is increasing evidence that the following interventions may decrease the incidence and severity of delirium.

- Daily interruption of sedation and analgesic infusions ("sedation vacation")
- Nurse-driven sedation protocols that favor bolus sedation and analgesia rather than continuous infusions, with doses and frequency determined by objective measures
- Frequent assessment of agitation and pain, and titration of sedative and analgesic agents accordingly
- Prioritization of analgesia over sedation
- Use of a validated sedation scale such as the Ramsay sedation scale, the Sedation-Agitation Scale (SAS), or the Richmond Agitation-Sedation Scale (RASS)
- Maintenance of normal sleep–wake and day–night cycles
- Implementation of a period of quiet time during the day
- Frequent orientation
- Presence of family and familiar items (if calming)
- Maintenance of a calm and quiet environment
- Minimizing distracting stimuli (televisions)
- Exposure to natural light

- Prompt treatment of infections and metabolic disturbances and frequent screening for subclinical infections (UTI)
- Providing adequate oxygenation
- Appropriate use of hearing aids and glasses
- Promoting regular daytime voiding
- Avoiding pharmaceutical risk factors such as dopaminergic agents and GABA-agonist agents.

Crisis Management

Pathophysiology and Clinical Presentation

Because of the serious sequelae (increased length of stay and increased mortality), onset of delirium must be seen as a crisis, akin to failure of another organ system (i.e., kidneys). Delirium is defined in the Diagnostic and Statistical Manual of Mental Disorders (DSM)-IV as a disturbance of consciousness and cognition which develops over a short period of time (hours to days) and fluctuates over time. Delirium can be categorized into hyperactive, hypoactive, and mixed deliriums, with pure hypoactive delirium being the most common in critically ill patients, as well as the most difficult to diagnose, mixed delirium being relatively common, and pure hyperactive delirium being relatively rare in this population.

There are multiple hypotheses for the pathogenesis of delirium including neurotransmitter imbalance, with the greatest focus being on an imbalance of dopamine (usually in excess) and acetylcholine (usually deficient); CNS inflammation and impaired oxidative metabolism. In all likelihood, these and other mechanisms contribute. Undoubtedly, the unwanted psychomimetic effects of drugs used for sedation and analgesia in the intensive care environment play a major role in the etiology of delirium.

Patient Assessment

Diagnosis of delirium in the critically ill patient requires assessing every patient's level of consciousness on a regular basis. There are two important components in this evaluation: (1) arousal (sedation) assessment and (2) content (delirium) assessment. Level of consciousness can be assessed using any one of a number of ICU-validated sedation scales [Ramsay scale, SAS, RASS, and Motor Activity Assessment Scale (MAAS)]. Patients who are deeply sedated or comatose (RASS ≤ -4) cannot be evaluated for content. Validated instruments for assessing thought content in critically ill, even ventilated, patients include the Intensive Care Delirium Screening Checklist (ICSDC) and the Confusion Assessment Method for the ICU (CAM-ICU).

In the neurocritical care patient, it is imperative to first rule out treatable and life-threatening causes of altered mental status (e.g., intracranial hemorrhage, cerebral edema, hydrocephalus, cerebral vasospasm, ischemia, seizures, etc.). Vigilance is necessary to identify typical symptoms, which should then trigger the systematic evaluation for potentially treatable causes. In addition to physical examination, appropriate imaging studies or EEG should always be a mainstay of the diagnostic workup in these patients.

Intervention/Treatment

There are no FDA-approved treatments for delirium. The best treatment is prevention. Treatment of acute agitation/hyperactive delirium involves the use of non-pharmacologic and pharmacologic methods to maintain patient safety. In addition to the use of sedative hypnotics (to reduce the immediate danger the patient poses to self or others) and analgesics, the selective use of antipsychotic medications may be an important therapeutic strategy.

Haloperidol (Haldol), a D2 receptor antagonist and typical antipsychotic, is frequently used to treat acute agitation/hyperactive delirium in the critical care setting. However, several significant risks need to be considered, including the risk for extrapyramidal effects, QT prolongation, and malignant neuroleptic syndrome, even with moderate doses. In addition, some experimental data suggest that dopamine- and norepinephrine antagonists may delay neuronal recovery and impair neuronal plasticity. Among persons with traumatic brain injury, typical antipsychotics appear to exacerbate cognitive impairments and may prolong the period of posttraumatic amnesia.

Atypical antipsychotics such as quetiapine (Seroquel), olanzapine (Zyprexa), and risperidone (Risperdal) are being increasingly used in the critical care setting. Quetiapine appears to be as effective as haloperidol for the treatment of delirium in patients who are critically ill (including mechanically ventilated), but tends not to interfere strongly with cerebral dopaminergic function and produces fewer adverse motor effects than haloperidol. These agents may facilitate, or at least not adversely affect, cognition when used for the treatment of posttraumatic delirium.

Treatment of hypoactive delirium, the most common and most difficult to diagnose type of delirium, is difficult. Today's treatments center on the predominate theory that hypoactive delirium is due to excess central serotonin. Atypical antipsychotics, especially rispiradone, which is less sedating, are the most studied therapies so far. Treatment with neurotransmitters (e.g., L-Dopa) is also being explored.

The use of sleep aids and melatonin are currently being studied to determine whether these agents are helpful in decreasing the incidence of hyper- and hypoactive delirium.

Ultimately, the diagnosis of delirium in the neurosurgical patient population remains a challenge, which requires a high index of suspicion and an awareness of the harmful effects of common medications.

Key Points

- Delirium in the critically ill patient is associated with increased morbidity and mortality and needs to be rigorously monitored to not miss the diagnosis.
- Daily sedation and analgesic infusion interruption or the use of nurse-directed sedation protocols decrease ventilator days and ICU length of stay.
- Use analgesics before sedative-hypnotics if the patient appears to have pain.
- Minimize the use of psychoactive medications when possible.
- Most sedatives (with the exception of ketamine, dexmeditomidine, and clonidine) lack analgesic properties.
- With the exception of the treatment of alcohol withdrawal, GABA agonists, especially benzodiazepines, appear to increase the risk of delirium.
- Prolonged neuromuscular blockade conveys significant risk to the patient and is indicated only when other means of treating patient-ventilator dyssynchrony or elevated ICP have failed, or in other rare instances.

Suggested Reading

Arciniegas DB, McAllister TW. Neurobehavioral management of traumatic brain injury in the critical care setting. Crit Care Clin. 2008;24:737–65.

Bergeron N, Dubois MJ, Dumont M, Dial S, Skrobik Y. Intensive care delirium screening checklist: evaluation of a new screening tool. Intensive Care Med. 2001;27:859–64.

de Wit M, Gennings C, Jenvey WI, Epstein SK. Randomized trial comparing daily interruption of sedation and nursing-implemented sedation algorithm in medical intensive care unit patients. Critical Care 2008;12:R70. Available online at: http://ccforum.com/content/12/3/R70.

Girard TD et al. Delirium in the intensive care unit. Critical Care. 2008;12(Suppl3):S3. doi:10.1186/cc6149.

Himmelseher S, Durieux ME. Revising a dogma: Ketamine for patients with neurological injury? Anesth Analg. 2005;101:524–34.

Maldonado JR. Pathoetiological model of delirium: a comprehensive understanding of the neurobiology of delirium and an evidence-based approach to prevention and treatment. Crit Care Clin. 2008;24:789–856.

Ortiz-Cardona J, Bendo AA. Perioperative pain management in the neurosurgical patient. Anesthesiol Clin. 2007;25:655–74.

Riker RR et al. Dexmedetomidine vs midazolam for sedation of critically ill patients: A randomized trial. JAMA. 2009;301(5):489–99.

Sackey PV et al. Short- and long-term follow-up of intensive care unit patients after sedation with isoflurane and midazolam – A pilot study. Crit Care Med. 2008;36(3):801–6.

The Confusion Assessment Method for the ICU (CAM-ICU) training manual (http://wwwicudelirium.org/delirium/CAM-ICU-Training.html).

Chapter 78
Airway and Pulmonary Management in Neurosurgical Critical Care

Edward M. Manno

Airway Management

Overview

Patients at risk for life-threatening deterioration of central nervous system disease are managed in the critical care unit. For example, there are approximately 500,000 traumas per year in the USA with one half of the deaths directly related to head trauma and respective complications. Endotracheal intubations in neurological emergencies are some of the most challenging aspects of airway management.

Management of airways in patients with intracranial hypertension secondary to trauma, intracerebral hemorrhage, subarachnoid hemorrhage, or other space occupying lesions requires a special set of knowledge and skills. The physician managing acute airway emergencies in critically ill patients needs to be familiar with cerebrovascular physiology and the management of intracranial hypertension.

Patients with a Glasgow Coma Score of ≤8 are generally intubated for airway protection. With progressive deterioration in levels of consciousness, there will be a loss of pharyngeal reflexes and muscular tone. Under these circumstances, the tongue will fall posteriorly and the pharyngeal muscles will relax leading to the obstruction of the upper airway. The purpose of elective intubation in this population is to secure the airway to prevent aspiration, maintain adequate oxygenation, and prevent hypercapnia. The practice of electively intubating patients with a GCS ≤8 was supported by a retrospective analysis of the national traumatic coma data base which reported and increase in aspiration rates and worse outcomes in comatose patients that were not immediately intubated.

E.M. Manno, MD FCCM, FAAN, FAHA (✉)
Department of Neurology and Neurological Surgery, Cerebrovascular Center,
Cleveland Clinic, Cleveland, OH, USA
e-mail: MANNOE@ccf.org

A.M. Brambrink and J.R. Kirsch (eds.), *Essentials of Neurosurgical
Anesthesia & Critical Care*, DOI 10.1007/978-0-387-09562-2_78,
© Springer Science+Business Media, LLC 2012

Prevention of Complications

Aspiration Pneumonia

The risk of aspiration is high in patients with significant alteration in level of consciousness. Almost all urgent endotracheal intubations will require rapid sequence intubation with little opportunity to empty the stomach prior to intubation. Cricoid pressure is generally used to prevent regurgitation and aspiration of gastric contents during endotracheal intubation. However, cervical neck injuries may limit the amount of cricoid pressure that can be applied. The cricoid is located at approximately C_4–C_5. If possible, evaluation for the level of injury with a focused neurological exam and neck images should precede endotracheal intubation in patients with a stable airway and good oxygenation (pulse oximetry of greater than 95% on less than 40% inspired oxygen). An esophageal Combi-tube can be placed to help prevent aspiration, if endotracheal intubation cannot be performed safely.

Hypoxia

Hypoxia has been reported in >50% of severe head trauma patients that are not immediately intubated. Hypoxia and hypercapnia will cause cerebral vasodilation and increases in intracranial pressure. The morbidity and mortality of prolonged hypoxia defined as a PaO_2 of <60 mmHg is almost 50%. A functional airway needs to be obtained immediately.

- Clearing the mouth of foreign objects, suctioning and providing a chin lift and jaw thrust to avoid cervical injury can be performed quickly.
- Bag-mask ventilation with high-flow oxygen should be applied as soon as safely possible. In the setting of hypoxia and hypercapnia, bag-mask ventilation may be necessary, even in patients at risk of regurgitation and aspiration.
- All patients with a depressed level of consciousness and the loss of protective airway reflexes should be intubated. The nature and type of neurological injury will dictate what form of intubation should occur.

In general, nasal tracheal intubation is avoided in head trauma due to the possibility of basilar skull fractures. Also patient discomfort may lead to excessive agitation with head and neck movement with possible worsening of hypoxia.

Cervical Neck Injury

Cervical neck injury occurs in about 10% of all severe head trauma and should be assumed in most accidents. Most injuries occur at C_{5-6} and C_{6-7}, however higher lesions can occur. Patients with cervical lesions above C_3 will lose phrenic nerve innervation to the diaphragm and will need immediate intubation. Patients with lesions below C_5 retain diaphragmatic function but will lose the use of their thoracic intercostal muscles. This leads to a form of paradoxical respiration where the abdomen protrudes and the thorax involutes with inspiration. Patients with these injuries will ventilate better in the supine position since this position will push the abdominal contents upwards thus, maximizing diaphragmatic muscle length and optimizing muscle contraction with subsequent air movement. Many if not most of these patients will also require intubation since the patients functional residual capacity will increase as atelectasis progresses. Under these circumstances, an ineffective cough, inadequate chest wall expansion, and incomplete emptying of the lungs can lead to inadequate clearance of secretions and poor gas exchange.

Endotracheal intubation should occur with either fiberoptic bronchoscopy or in conventional technique applying in-line stabilization. In-line stabilization can be performed by an assistant holding the head and neck in alignment from below. Traction from above does not need to be applied and can interfere with the individual performing laryngoscopy. Nasal intubation can be considered but holds the same drawbacks as listed above.

Intracranial Hypertension

Increased intracranial pressure is common in many forms of acute neurological injury. In addition, endotracheal intubation can lead to increased intracranial pressure and subsequent decreases in cerebral perfusion. This response can be attenuated by premedication with intravenous lidocaine or local application of topical anesthesia to airway structures. The use of succinylcholine (1–2 mg/kg) as a paralytic agent to facilitate rapid airway management is common practice. The clinical importance of increased intracranial pressure occurring with the use of succinylcholine appears small. In the balance, the risk of increased intracranial pressure with hypoxia is far greater than the risk of increased intracranial pressure with succinylcholine. Thus succinylcholine should be used for rapid airway management in patients with head injury unless the patient also presents with crush injuries, seizures, prolonged bed rest, or under any circumstance where there may be direct muscle damage due to concerns of the development of life-threatening hyperkalemia. Under these circumstances, Rocuronium may be a better choice as a quick-onset paralytic.

Once an airway is secured hyperventilation can occur to decrease intracranial hypertension through vasoconstriction of cerebral arterioles and a reflex decrease in cerebral blood volume. This effect, however, is relatively short lived and thus other methods of decreasing intracranial hypertension should be initiated as soon as they become available.

Crisis Management

Many issues in airway management in the neurological patient will occur under emergency conditions. Following airway management many patients will need emergent surgery or transfer to an intensive care unit.

Head trauma provides several possible problems. For example, patients with significant facial trauma may not be able to be safely bag mask ventilated. In these circumstances, placement of a Combi-tube or laryngeal mask airway may be needed prior to endotracheal intubation, despite the risk that these patients are at significant risk for regurgitation and aspiration. Fiberscopic intubation after placement of an oral airway is preferred if possible. Cricothyroidotomy may need to be performed, if severe facial trauma precludes any form of endotracheal intubation. This, however, is a technique of last resort since the complication rate is as high as 30% when placed under emergency situations.

Multiple medical issues may also complicate the neurological patient in need of acute airway management. Congestive heart failure, tension pneumothorax, cardiac tamponade, and other chest wall injuries are common in trauma patients. Many patients will be hypovolemic on presentation and will need active fluid resuscitation. Several induction agents administered at the time of intubation may compromise cardiac output and blood pressure. Etomidate may cause less cardiovascular depression than propofol or thiopental and does not compromise cerebral blood flow. However, myoclomus that is often observed after injection of etomidate can be mistaken for seizure activity and confuse the clinical assessment. Vasopressors and atropine need to be available at the time of induction, to facilitate rapid treatment of induction/intubation-induced alteration in hemodynamics. Long-acting paralytic agents are ideally avoided in the neurological patient to allow for serial neurological examinations.

Key Points

- Neurological emergencies present with some of the most difficult airway management issues.
- Patients with a Glasgow Coma score ≤ 8 are intubated for airway protection.
- Outcome after head trauma is directly related to the length of time a patient is hypoxic.
- Cervical neck and facial injuries provide specific challenges to airway management.
- Intracranial hypertension is assumed in most patients with neurological emergencies and needs to be addressed during airway management.

Pulmonary Management

Overview

Pulmonary complications are common after neurological injury. Aspiration can occur at the time of trauma, hemorrhage, or after seizures. Patients treated in intensive care units are at risk for nosocomial pneumonia. Prolonged immobilization in patients with spinal cord injury is associated with increased risk for pulmonary emboli. One study of pulmonary complications in patients with intracerebral hemorrhage reported pneumonia in 20%, pulmonary edema in 8% and rare cases of pulmonary emboli and acute respiratory disease states. Pulmonary complications were related to a Glasgow coma score ≤ 8 and endotracheal intubation. Patients with pulmonary complications had longer length of stays and worse outcomes. Patients with ischemic stroke that require mechanical ventilation have a mortality $> 60\%$.

Prevention of Complications

Nosocomial Pneumonia

Nosocomial pneumonias are prevented through thorough application of pulmonary toilet techniques. The ventilator bundle; a series of maneuvers designed to decrease medical complications should be employed when feasible. Obviously, certain populations (i.e., cervical injuries) may not be immediately amenable to head of bed elevation. Rotation beds for immobilized patients are useful for decreasing pneumonia. Compulsive oral hygiene care with chlorhexidine has been shown to decrease the incidence of nosocomial pneumonias in a medical intensive care unit population but has not been studied directly in a neurological population.

Extubation should occur as soon as feasible. Many patients in a neurological intensive care unit are intubated for airway management (level of consciousness) issues and not for primary pulmonary difficulties. Traditional teaching has required that a patient have a Glasgow Coma Score > 8 prior to extubation. A large retrospective study, however, suggested that maintaining endotracheal intubation based on mental status alone led to an increase in nosocomial pneumonias and worse outcomes. A safety and feasibility trial has recently been completed testing the hypothesis that comatose patients with pulmonary and airway control can be extubated.

Pulmonary Emboli

Prevention of pulmonary emboli in a neurological population can be challenging. Neurological-injured patients are at high risk for the development of deep venous thrombosis. Spinal cord injury and the neurosurgical population is at particular risk.

Available evidence suggests that the early implementation of subcutaneous heparin is useful for the prevention of deep venous thrombosis and can be used safely in a neurosurgical population. Despite this many neurosurgeons have reservations and will not administer anticoagulants to patients who have recently had surgery (or who are planned to have surgery). Sequential compression devices should be used in all patients. When used properly, sequential compression devices decrease the incidence of deep venous thrombosis formation. In high-risk populations (e.g. neurosurgery patients), when possible, both heparin (low-dose or low molecular weight) should be used in combination with sequential compression device stockings. In patients who are at too great a risk for administering heparin, consideration should be given to sequential screening for deep venous thrombosis (Doppler Ultrasound) and with confirmation to placement of an inferior vena cava filter, to prevent the consequences of devastating pulmonary emboli.

Crisis Management

Neurogenic pulmonary edema is common after severe neurological injury. The proposed mechanisms involved include massive sympathetic discharge directly to the contractile elements of the pulmonary endothelium. This leads to the development of a pulmonary exudate. Concurrently, sympathetically mediated cardiac stunning and pulmonary venoconstriction lead to congestive heart failure. The pulmonary edema can be abrupt, severe and present with significant hypoxia. Treatment is largely supportive. Aggressive diuresis is usually necessary. Inotropic or vasopressor support is common. A Swan-Ganz catheter or transesophageal echo evaluation can be useful for directing management. Most neurogenic pulmonary edema will resolve or improve within a few days to a week.

Standard diagnostic methods and treatments of pneumonia and acute respiratory disease states are used in the neurological population. Fluid management may be complicated in acute respiratory disease states since volume depletion is avoided in most neurological disease states. Maintaining euvolemia with hypertonic solutions could be one possible solution.

Key Points

- Pulmonary complications are common after neurological injury and increase length of stay and worsen outcomes.
- Prolonged immobilization places many patients at high risk for deep venous thrombosis and pulmonary emboli. Treatment includes the use of compression stocking and sequential compression devices. Early institution of subcutaneous heparin can be beneficial.
- Aggressive diuresis and support are needed for the management of neurogenic pulmonary edema. Neurogenic pulmonary edema is usually self-limited.

Suggested Reading

Airway References

Albin MS. Textbook of neuroanesthesia. New York: McGraw Hill; 1997.
Luce JM. Cardiopulmonary physiology and management in neurosurgical intensive care. In: Andrews BT, editor. Neurosurgical intensive care. New York: McGraw-Hill; 1993. p. 1–43.

Pulmonary References

Coplin WP, Pierson DJ, Cooley KD, Newell DW, Rubenfeld GD. Implication of extubation delay in brain injured patients meeting extubation criteria. Am J Resp Crit Care Med. 2000;161: 1530–6.
Maramattom BV, Weigand S, Reinalda M, Manno EM, Wijdicks EFM. Pulmonary complications after acute intracerebral hemorrhage. Neurocrit Care. 2006;5:1–5.
Smith WS, Matthay MA. Evidence for a hydrostatic mechanism for neurogenic pulmonary edema. Chest. 1997;111:1326–33.

Chapter 79
Myocardial and Vascular Management in Neurosurgical Critical Care

E. Paige Gerbic and Valerie Sera

Cardiac and hemodynamic dysfunction occurs frequently following acute neurologic injury and are significant cause of morbidity and mortality in neurosurgical intensive care units. Cardiovascular sequela of brain injury includes neurogenic stunned myocardium, arrhythmias, and blood pressure disturbances to name a few. Subarachnoid hemorrhage, intracranial hemorrhage, traumatic brain injury, and stroke are a few examples that have potential to cause neurologically triggered cardiovascular disturbances. Diagnosis of neurogenic cardiovascular effects is facilitated by the common association with major intracranial events. However, patients with cardiac dysfunction following neurologic injury should receive a through workup so as not to miss a primary cardiac origin, such as coronary artery disease. The influence of the nervous system on the heart and hemodynamics has been known for over a century, however, it continues to be incompletely understood today. This chapter focuses predominantly on neurogenic stunned myocardium, arrhythmias, and blood pressure management in the neurosurgical ICU.

Neurogenic Stunned Myocardium

Overview

Stress-induced cardiomyopathy, also called "neurogenic stunned myocardium," "transient left ventricular apical ballooning," "Takotsubo cardiomyopathy," and "broken

V. Sera, MD (✉)
Professor of Anesthesiology and Perioperative Medicine,
Oregon Health & Science University, Portland, OR, USA
e-mail: serav@ohsu.edu

E.P. Gerbic, MD
Columbia Anesthesia Group, Vancouver, WA, USA

A.M. Brambrink and J.R. Kirsch (eds.), *Essentials of Neurosurgical Anesthesia & Critical Care*, DOI 10.1007/978-0-387-09562-2_79,
© Springer Science+Business Media, LLC 2012

heart syndrome," is an increasingly reported syndrome. It is a transient condition and is typically precipitated by intense physiologic stress including that precipitated by brain injury and has even been described in the context of a profound emotional crisis.

Prevention

Prevention is by avoiding the physiologic stress itself. All patients presenting with intracranial pathology should have a 12-lead ECG and cardiac enzyme measurements on admission and telemetry until their neurologic condition has stabilized. A thorough history and physical examination is necessary to identify patients at risk for primary cardiac disease. Awareness of the potential for neurogenic stunned myocardium, especially in those patients presenting with severe neurologic injury, will aid in the prompt search and diagnosis if myocardial stunning occurs.

Diagnosis: The pathogenesis of neurogenic myocardial stunning is not well understood. The clinical presentation is identical to that of an acute MI; however, coronary arteriography shows no critical lesions. It is important to differentiate the two as stunned myocardium is a reversible condition that will resolve completely in about 80% of the patients within days after the initial event, whereas cardiovascular-induced ischemic injury may cause irreversible cardiac dysfunction.

Proposed mechanisms include catecholamine excess, coronary artery spasm, and microcirculatory dysfunction. The ventricular function usually recovers over several days with the treatment of the neurologic insult. Gross examinations of hearts at autopsy that displayed characteristics of stress-induced cardiomyopathy do not show overt pathology in the majority of cases. However, microscopic analysis reviles myofibrillar degeneration, myocytolysis, and inflammatory cell infiltration unevenly distributed throughout the heart, but most dense at the apex and ventricular subendocardial areas.

Characteristics of neurogenic myocardial stunning include:

- Abnormal wall motion involving the cardiac apex and mid-portion with relative sparing of the base, termed "apical ballooning."
- ST-segment elevation or depression, or T-wave changes
- A prolonged QT interval
- Increased cardiac enzymes
- More common in elderly or postmenopausal females
- Precipitated by acute physiologic or emotional stress.

Characteristics that are commonly associated with neurogenic myocardial stunning and not with ischemic acute coronary syndrome (ACS) are: no history of cardiac problems, new onset left ventricular dysfunction, cardiac wall motion abnormalities on echo that do not correlate with the coronary vascular distribution, and cardiac troponin levels <2.8 ng/ml. If there is doubt, then coronary angiography should be performed if feasible.

Crisis Management

Treatment of the underlying neurologic insult will aid in the resolution of myocardial stunning. Patients with significant heart failure and hemodynamic compromise will need inotropic and vasopressive support for a period of time. Early involvement of a cardiologist is recommended.

Key Points

- Onset subsequent to an acute emotional or physiologic stress such as brain injury
- Similar presentation to acute MI, therefore, must differentiate between the two
- Typical echocardiographic appearance of apical ballooning without angiographic critical lesions
- Inotropic and vasopressive support may be necessary
- Complete resolution of the apical wall motion abnormality and depressed cardiac function typically within 48 h after the initial insult and, with successful treatment of neurologic crisis.

Cardiac Arrhythmias

Arrhythmias occur in neurologically injured patients with known cardiac disease as well as in those without. Some arrhythmias are attributable to coronary artery insufficiency or ischemia, but others are due to conduction disturbances that result from the neurological illness itself. The most frequent arrhythmias following brain injury are premature ventricular complexes, sinus arrhythmia, and atrial fibrillation. Other arrhythmias including atrial flutter, ventricular tachycardia, torsades de pointes, ventricular fibrillation, and asystole have been documented as well. SAH patients have arrhythmias about 35–85% of the time. Life-threatening arrhythmias occur in <5% of patients with SAH. As with neurogenic myocardial stunning, resolution of the acute intracranial pathology, e.g., normalization of the ICP, injury generally leads to improvement or resolution of arrhythmias.

Supraventricular Tachycardia/Arrhythmia

Overview

Supraventricular tachycardia (SVT) such as sinus tachycardia, atrial fibrillation, and paroxysmal supraventricular tachycardia (PSVT) are common in all critical care

Table 79.1 Supraventricular arrhythmias crises management

Sinus tachycardia	Analgesia and sedation as appropriate, fluid and electrolyte replacement, resolution of the precipitant
Atrial fibrillation	Determine chronicity – if new onset less than 48 h old then chemical or electrical cardioversion can be instituted. If more than 48 h since onset or undetermined delay cardioversion until anticoagulation can be instituted. Echocardiography to evaluate for clot formation prior to cardioversion. Beta-adrenergic blockers first line – labetolol or esmolol
	Diltiazem and digoxin, if hypotension is a problem
PSVT	Vagal stimulation maneuvers – carotid sinus massage. Adenosine, amiodarone, diltiazem and beta-blockade can all be effective

settings. Sinus tachycardia (HR >100/min) usually represents a physiologic response to pain, stress, hypotension, heart failure, or excessive catecholamine drive.

Atrial fibrillation (A-fib) with or without a rapid ventricular response (RVR) is commonly seen with acute neurologic insults particularly in the elderly. A fair number of patients manifest atrial arrhythmias, mainly atrial fibrillation, within the first few days after stroke. Occasionally, a cardiac arrhythmia will actually be the initial event that provokes brain injury because of clot formation in the heart that embolizes into the brain (ischemic stroke). However, in other cases, the original injury is in the brain, which then is associated with cardiac rhythm disturbances. RVR is often an urgent issue as it can precipitate a demand ischemia of the myocardium or may compromise cardiac function. PSVT is related to a reentry or similar mechanism at the AV node. See Table 79.1 for management.

Prevention

Cardiac monitoring for all ICU patients, adequate pain control, assessment of volume status, adequate sedation, careful assessment of electrolyte balance, and treatment of precipitating cause are paramount to prevention (Table 79.1).

Ventricular Arrhythmias

Overview

Fortunately, ventricular arrhythmias such as ventricular tachycardia, ventricular fibrillation, and torsades de pointes are less common than atrial tachycardias in the neurocritical care unit. These particular arrhythmias, which can be life threatening,

Table 79.2 Ventricular arrhythmia crises management

Ventricular tachycardia (VT)	For significant hemodynamic compromise cardioversion and ACLS guidelines as appropriate
	If hemodynamically stable – amiodarone, then cardioversion
	Polymorphic VT give Magnesium sulfate IV and cardioversion
Ventricular fibrillation (VF)	Early defibrillation according to ACLS guidelines
Torsades de Pointes	Stop all QT prolonging medications, Magnesium sulfate IV, and cardioversion

are likely a cause for sudden death in patients with a significant neurologic insult. Isolated premature ventricular contractions (PVCs) are common and do not require treatment, but if they occur with increasing frequency they may signify elevated ICP and the risk for serious ventricular arrhythmias. Ventricular flutter and fibrillation are more commonly seen in patients with ischemic heart disease. See Table 79.2 for management.

Prevention

All patients with a neurologic injury or insult need cardiac monitoring until the acute phase of the illness has resolved, as prompt treatment will be necessary for ventricular arrhythmias. Monitoring of Q-T intervals is important as a prolonged Q-T places a patient at risk for ventricular ectopy.

Bradycardia

Overview

A HR below 60 bpm is usually the result of sinus node dysfunction or an atrioventricular conduction disturbance. Acute cerebral insults can also produce a vasovagal response. Bradycardia can be seen after carotid angioplasty and stenting procedures from direct and prolonged carotid sinus stimulation as well. Bradycardia in a neuro-critical care patient is a red flag for increased intracranial pressure. The triad of bradycardia, hypertension, and respiratory depression is, of course, termed the "Cushing reflex" and results from acutely increased intracranial pressure. Always consider increased ICP as one of the differential diagnosis for bradycardia and hypertension in the context of neurologic injury. This is of particularly concern, if the disease process is suspected in the posterior fossa.

Crisis Management

Cardiac monitoring and careful assessment of a patient's neurologic exam and ICP monitoring as appropriate is paramount to identify the precipitating causes. Consider anticholinergic drugs such as atropine and glycopyrrolate, and transcutaneous or transvenous pacing in the presence of significant hemodynamic compromise.

Key Points

- Arrhythmias occur in the neurologically injured with and without intrinsic cardiac disease.
- All brain-injured patients need cardiac monitoring until the acute phase of illness has passed.
- SAH patients have arrhythmias about 35% of the time. Life-threatening arrhythmias occur in <5% of patients with SAH.
- Ventricular arrhythmias are less common than supraventricular arrhythmias.
- For life-threatening arrhythmias institute cardioversion and ACLS early
- Chronicity of atrial fibrillation should be determined before cardioversion because of the possibility of mural thrombus and the risk for embolic stroke.
- Bradycardia may be a sign of increased ICP as part of Cushing's triad.

Blood Pressure Disturbances in the Neurocritical Care Unit

The central nervous system (CNS) is susceptible to extremes in blood pressure (BP) fluctuations. Hypertension can be associated with increased risk of bleeding and cerebral edema. Hypotension can be associated with infarcts or global ischemia. Cerebral blood flow (CBF) is relatively constant over a wide range of systemic blood pressures in a healthy brain.

The autoregulation curve is shifted rightward in chronically hypertensive patients (CBF remains stable at higher mean arterial blood pressures (MAP), but becomes flow passive, i.e. is prone to ischemia already at low-normal MAP). This section focuses on blood pressure management in the setting of subarachnoid hemorrhage, intracranial hemorrhage, and ischemic stroke.

Hypertension in SAH

Overview

Blood pressure management in SAH differs according to the presence of an aneurysm, if that aneurysm has been surgically secured, and the presence of additional/residual

Table 79.3 Therapeutic hypertension goals in SAH with vasospasm

Secured aneurysm	Titrate vasopressors to SBP 180–200, DBP 100–120, MAP 120–140
Unsecured Aneurysm	Titrate vasopressors to SBP 160–170, DBP 90–100, MAP 100–120

aneurysms. Hypertension is common immediately following aneurysmal rupture and often reflecting a hyperadrenergic state and/or increased ICP with a Cushing's response. For hypertension in ruptured and unsecured aneurysms, maintaining systolic BPs in a range for adequate perfusion while avoiding rapid and extreme changes in BP is paramount to avoid shear stress on an aneurysm. Shear stress places the patient at risk for rebleeding. Generally systolic BP goals should be between 120 and 160 mmHg, while keeping a cerebral perfusion pressure (CPP) > 70 mmHg to avoid exacerbation of cerebral ischemia. CPP is calculated as MAP – ICP or CVP, whichever is greater, and it ranges normally between 70 and 100 mmHg. After an aneurysm has been secured BP goals should shift in an upward direction due to lessened risk of bleeding and the increased risk of vasospasm. Permissive hypertension is a strategy after an aneurysm is secured to obtain higher perfusion pressures with the goal to prevent further brain ischemia. Arterial hypertension is frequently even induced therapeutically for the treatment of cerebral vasospasm and when applied along with hypervolemia and hemodilution, the concept is termed "Triple-H Therapy." The technique involves the use of vasopressors and IV fluids to achieve a higher than normal MAP and thus augment the CPP. These therapies have the goal of preventing or ameliorating brain ischemia, which is created by cerebral vasospasm.

Prevention

All patients with SAH should have beat to beat blood pressure monitoring via an arterial line in addition to cardiac monitoring. Initial prevention of hypertension in SAH includes initiation of sedation, analgesia, anti-epileptic therapy, and nimodipine (a calcium channel blocker shown to improve outcome in SAH) all of which lower blood pressure.

Crisis Management

Blood pressure management (see Table 79.3) is used in conjunction with ICP control as appropriate (hyperventilation, head of bed elevation >30°, anti-edema therapies, CSF drainage), as well as surgical evaluation for clipping and coiling of aneurysms as determined by a neurosurgeon to prevent further injury.

Table 79.4 Commonly used antihypertensive medications

Drug	Dose
Labetalol	5–10 mg IV q10′ as needed
Enalaprilat	
Hydralazine	0.625–1.250 mg IV q6h as needed
Esmolol	2.5–10 mg (up to 40 mg/dose) IV q4–6 h as needed
Nicardipine	0.25–0.5 mcg/kg load; 50–200 µg/kg/min

Hypertension in Intracerebral Hemorrhage

Overview

Intracerebral hemorrhage (ICH) includes nontraumatic brain injuries with bleeding into the epidural, subdural, subarachnoid, intraventricular, and intraparechymal spaces. There are many causes for nontraumatic ICH. Hypertension is an important cause for ICH and it is of utmost importance to control for the prevention of further bleeding leading to hematoma expansion and poor outcomes. Management of BP is individualized depending on the cause of the ICH. Patient factors such as chronic hypertension, (which shifts the CBF autoregulation curve to the right) age, and time from the hemorrhage are all important factors to consider.

Prevention

All patients, who are at risk for rebleeding after ICH should remain under intensive care surveillance and have beat to beat blood pressure monitoring via an arterial line in addition to cardiac monitoring. Initiation of analgesia and sedation (with close monitoring of neurologic function) as appropriate are initial steps for blood pressure management.

According to the American Heart Association (AHA) guidelines treat for:

- SBP > 230 mmHg or DBP >140×2 readings 5 min apart – sodium nitroprusside
- SBP 180–230 mmHg or DBP 105–140 mmHg or MAP > 130 mmHg × 2 readings 20 min apart – IV labetolol, esmolol, enalaprilat, or nicardipine.

Crisis Management

Goal CPP with ICP monitoring is >70 mmHg.

Blood pressure management is used in conjunction with ICP control (hyperventilation, head of bed elevation >30°, anti-edema therapies) as well as surgical evacuation to prevent further injury. See Table 79.4 for suggestions of antihypertensive medications.

Hypotension in ICH

Overview

Determination of hypotension depends on the patient's history and clinical picture, the presence of elevated ICP, the cause of an ICH. Hypotension is relatively uncommon in ICH.

Prevention

Close monitoring of BP and assessment of a patient's volume status are paramount to the prevention of hypotension which can place a patient at risk for or exacerbation of brain ischemia.

Crisis Management

Treatment with volume replacement is usually first line avoiding hypotonic and glucose-containing solutions. Normal saline and hypertonic saline are the fluids of choice as appropriate. Vasopressors may be indicated.

Hypertension in Ischemic Stroke

Overview

Most ischemic stroke patients become hypertensive after the onset of symptoms in an effort to maintain cerebral perfusion via collaterals. In addition, many affected patients are hypertensive at baseline as one of the risk factors for the disease. Arterial hypertension is permissive in ischemic stroke patients to maintain CPP only limited by the risk of hemorrhagic transformation. If that has occurred judicious blood pressure control is crucial.

Prevention

All patients with ischemic stroke, who are critically ill, should have beat to beat blood pressure monitoring via an arterial line in addition to cardiac monitoring. Consider careful sedation and analgesia, if appropriate with close monitoring of neurologic function.

Crisis Management

According to the AHA recommendations, treatment of hypertension in ischemic stroke should be avoided unless BP is profoundly elevated SBP > 220 mmHg or MAP > 130 mmHg. The recommendation is different in the setting of myocardial ischemia or hemorrhagic transformation to maintain SBP < 170 mmHg. Thrombolytic therapy is a special case and BP management must be much more conservative over the first 24 h after treatment to prevent intracranial hemorrhage (i.e., SBP < 150).

Key Points

- Hypertension is common following SAH, ICH, and ischemic stroke and is secondary to the underlying pathophysiology, a hyperadrenergic state, and increased ICP and need for elevated CPPs.
- Blood pressure management is crucial in SAH to prevent further ischemic damage secondary to rebleeding, increased ICP, and vasospasm.
- Hypertension is an important cause for ICH blood pressure control is paramount to prevent hematoma expansion and poorer outcomes.
- Treatment of hypertension in ischemic stroke should be avoided unless BP is profoundly elevated SBP > 220 mmHg or MAP > 130 mmHg, or IV thrombolytics were given (tight control for 24 h).

Suggested Reading

Banki N. MD: Acute neurocardiogenic injury after subarachnoid hemorrhage. Circulation. 2005; 112:3314–9.

Bhardwaj A, Mirski M, Ulatowski JA: Handbook of Neurocritical Care. Humana press copyright 2004. 999 Riverview Drive, Suite 208 Totowa, New Jersey 07512.

Bybee KA et al. Systematic review: Transient left ventricular apical ballooning: A syndrome that mimics ST –segment elevation myocardial infarction. Ann Intern Med. 2007;141(11):858–65.

Grunsfeld A, Fletcher JJ, Branett RN. Cardiopulmonary complications of brain injury. Curr Neurol Neurosci Rep. 2005a;5:488–93.

Grunsfeld A, Fletcher JJ, Barnett RN. Cardiopulmonary complications of brain injury. Curr Neurol Neurosci Rep. 2005b;5(6):488–93.

Macmillan CSA, Grant IS, Andrews PJD. Pulmonary and cardiac sequelae of subarachnoid hemorrhage: time for active management?

Naval NS, Stevens RD, Mirski MA, Bhardwaj S. Controversies in the management of aneurysmal subarachnoid hemorrhage. Crit Care Med. 2006;34(2):511–24.

Ropper AH. Neurological and neurosurgical intensive care. Fourth Edition. Lippincott Williams and Wilkins. Copyright 2004 227 East Washington Square Philadelphia, PA 19106.

Virani SS, Khan AN, Mendoza CE, Ferreira AC, de Marchena E. Takotsubo Cardiomyopathy, or Broken Heart Syndrome. Division of Cardiology Texas Heart Institute at St. Lukes Episcopal Hospital, Baylor College of Medicine, Houston, Texas 77030.

Chapter 80
Nutrition and Glucose Management in Neurosurgical Critical Care

Michael J. Souter and Arthur M. Lam

Overview

Cognitive and behavioral deficits after brain insult and injury can significantly compromise nutritional status, consequent to the development of nausea, anorexia, vomiting, and feeding intolerance. Over 60% of patients requiring rehabilitation for brain injury demonstrate problems with swallowing, resulting in an incidence of aspiration exceeding 40%.

Acute brain injury. Not surprisingly, acute injury to the brain is associated with significant weight loss (averaging 13 kg), from the time of injury to the start of rehabilitation, with 60% of such patients at less than 90% of their ideal body weight.

Aggressive enteral feeding protocols have been adopted to compensate for this nutritional deficiency, but even under these circumstances, brain injury is associated with nutritional feeding intolerance in up to 55% of cases. The incidence is decreased by the use of continuous enteral feeding as opposed to bolus feeding. Risk factors associated with feeding intolerance in the ICU patient, and particularly after brain injury are listed in Table 80.1.

M.J. Souter, MB, ChB, FRCA
Departments of Anesthesiology and Pain Medicine, Department of Neurological Surgery,
University of Washington School of Medicine, Seattle, WA, USA

A.M. Lam, MD, FRCPC (✉)
Department of Neuroanesthesia and Neurocritical Care,
Swedish Neuroscience Institute, Seattle, WA, USA
e-mail: Arthur.Lam@swedish.org

A.M. Brambrink and J.R. Kirsch (eds.), *Essentials of Neurosurgical Anesthesia & Critical Care*, DOI 10.1007/978-0-387-09562-2_80, © Springer Science+Business Media, LLC 2012

Table 80.1 Risk factors associated with feeding intolerance

General ICU population	Brain injury
Traumatic brain injury (TBI)	TBI
Diabetes mellitus/hyperglycemia	Mechanical ventilation
Sepsis	Paralytics
Narcotics	Increasing age
Sedatives	Ischemic stroke
Catecholamine Infusions	Intracerebral hemorrhage
Gastric residual volumes >100 mL	Abdominal injury
Recumbent position	
Abdominal injury	

Table 80.2 Metabolic responses to brain injury

Increases	Decreases
Cortisol	Albumin
Glucagon	Thyroxine binding protein
Catecholamines	Thyroxine retinol binding prealbumin
O_2 consumption	Serum zinc
CO_2 production	
Acute phase proteins – including fibrinogen and CRP	
Release of calcium from bone	
Urinary calcium excretion	
Urinary zinc excretion	

Feeding intolerance. Subsequent nutritional deficit and hypoproteinemia may further affect fluid and electrolyte balance, as well as complicating healing and pharmacotherapy secondary to altered protein binding/pharmacokinetics. Moreover, intestinal edema from hypoproteinemia, in conjunction with an enteropathy of malnutrition, will diminish the absorption of nutrients.

Feeding intolerance may be further compounded by the development of iatrogenic gastric stasis, ileus, and constipation induced by concurrent pharmacotherapy, as well as by any coincidental abdominal injury in the case of trauma patients.

Gastric acidity. Erosive stress ulceration (Cushing ulcers) is a very real risk, thus protocolized stress bleeding prophylaxis is recommended until feeding is established. However, prophylactic protocols that alter gastric acidity may promote bacterial colonization and increase the risk of aspiration pneumonia. The risk of pneumonia increases with the duration of feeding intolerance and its associated requirement for sustained acid prophylaxis.

Hypermetabolic states. Any primary deficiency in intake is further complicated by the observed hypermetabolic response after brain injury (Table 80.2).

This hypermetabolism results in the induced excessive catabolism of protein, fat, and glycogen stores. Protein breakdown may, in turn, affect oncotic forces determining water distribution, availability of drug-binding sites, and pharmacokinetics, as well as hormonal binding proteins with consequent endocrine effects. All of these preceding considerations are magnified by the concurrent presence of feeding deficiency. Any other increases in metabolic requirements (e.g., fever and seizures) may aggravate a relative nutritional insufficiency.

Enteral vs. parenteral feeding. Controversies exist regarding the initiation of enteral feeding in critically ill patients. Early feeding (day 1) has been considered to be a risk factor for the development of hospital acquired pneumonia, because of the risk of aspiration of gastric contents. However, in brain-injured patients, it has been shown that failure to establish feeding by day 5 is associated with a two to fourfold increase in the risk of death, with a dose–effect relationship between caloric inadequacy and mortality rate, even when controlling for age, hypotension, and intracranial hypertension.

While parenteral feeding had been recommended in the past, recent studies have demonstrated that enteral feeding has been associated with less complications than parenteral feeding, reducing the risk of catheter infection and bacteremia considerably, while preserving intestinal villous architecture. Controversy also exists in the best route of enteral conduit placement. Gastric tubes are easier and quicker to place, but are more susceptible to feeding failure than jejunal tubes because of the development of ileus and obstruction. The latter offer more security in the quality and volume of feeding, but their placement demand more time and expertise, and frequently require radiologic guidance.

The concurrent presence of facial injuries and/or basal skull fracture may compromise the ability to pass the orogastric or nasogastric tube safely, in which case a percutaneous gastrostomy may be required. Given the reduced incidence of feeding intolerance, as well as the reduced risk of sinusitis, oral infection, aspiration, and pneumonia, this is the preferred route for intermediate and long-term enteral feeding. Irrespective of the route used, there are significant known complications associated with their placement and maintenance. Assiduous care should be taken to secure the tube once it is in place, as the disinhibition and/or inability to comprehend and obey commands secondary to brain injury often results in patients dislodging their feeding tubes.

Glycemic control. Glucose intolerance and hyperglycemia are frequently observed in patients with brain injury. Although the hyperglycemia is undoubtedly part of the stress response, its occurrence has been shown to be associated with worse outcome in patients with traumatic brain injury, stroke, and subarachnoid hemorrhage. Moreover, in critically ill patients, tight glycemic control (80–100 mg/dl) was associated with reduced mortality. Thus aggressive insulin treatment regimens have been advocated. This is, however, often achieved at the expense of unacceptably high risk of iatrogenic hypoglycemia. Moreover, patients with traumatic brain injury may develop hyperglycolysis, necessitating an increased demand for glucose. This controversy is summarized below.

Electrolyte derangements may occur as a consequence of injury stress response to systemic trauma, with retention of sodium and water, but increased losses of potassium.

In patients on long-term enteral nutrition, overfeeding can occur resulting in hepatic steatosis, centripetal obesity, and ventilatory insufficiency as a consequence of diaphragmatic embarrassment.

Prevention

Prevention of complications associated with nutritional management is best accomplished by attention to the risk factors above. However, it should be recognized that there is an obligatory catabolism after brain injury that cannot be avoided by any current therapies.

Inclusion of a nutrition specialist in the multidisciplinary ICU team, and the implementation of a protocol to initiate feeding and monitor nutritional progress have been shown to provide useful protection against tissue breakdown and to improve outcome. Regular monitoring and surveillance of both intake and nutritional screen results is a necessary component of daily review to limit and avoid the complications of inadequate, mismatched or excessive feeding.

Crisis Management

Pathophysiology and Clinical Presentation

- Hypercatabolism and malnutrition are unlikely to present as acute crises but can acutely complicate the presentation of other problems.
- Hyperglycemia above 170 mg/dl has been associated with a poor outcome in brain-injured patients, while levels above 140 mg/dl had a worse mortality in a series of critically ill postsurgical patients.
- Conversely both cerebral glycopenia and systemic hypoglycemia have been reported with the introduction of aggressive insulin regimens to attain goals of 80–110 mg/dl. These regimens arose from a single center study on postsurgical patients and have not been demonstrated to result in an improvement in neurological outcome. They have given rise to safety concerns, especially as the reductions in cerebral glucose may occur within a normal range of serum glucose. While hyperglycemia is to be avoided, the translation of an aggressive research-based insulin protocol into general clinical practice has proven difficult. A recent international multicenter trial (NICE-SUGAR) examined aggressive therapy versus controlling glucose to less than 180 mg/dl in a mixed cohort of critically ill patients. There was no demonstrable benefit and increased mortality associated with the use of intensive insulin therapy. Moderate target ranges such as 100–140 mg/dl would appear more prudent.
- Even with conservative insulin regimens, particular care must be taken to maintain continuity of the supply of energy substrate, especially when feeding intolerance develops.

- Refeeding syndrome – some patient populations with preexisting nutritional compromise are more likely to suffer brain injury. These include patients with history of alcohol and/or drug abuse, as well as the elderly and indigent populations. Their protracted malnourishment may reduce body stores of potassium, magnesium, and phosphorous while preserving normal serum concentrations. Energy demands are supplied from fat stores with relative protein sparing and concomitant reduction in insulin secretion. Abrupt restitution of carbohydrate supply induces anabolic restoration of normal intracellular stores. The consequent ionic shift results in an acute reduction of serum phosphate, magnesium, and calcium, with a deficit of adenosine triphosphate and 2,3 DPG. Thiamine is frequently depleted in these patients, contributing to a superimposed encephalopathy. The hypophosphatemia also inhibits sodium and water excretion. The end result is impairment of diaphragmatic/respiratory power, myocardial contractility, oxygen dissociation, and neuromuscular function, the combination of which can be fatal. This can be avoided by careful monitoring and staged institution of feeding to patients with known risk factors.
- Abdominal stasis is a frequent complication seen in patients with brain injury – arising from associated autonomic dysfunction, coincidental abdominal injuries, or as a side effect of the use of narcotics and sedatives. Inauspicious presentation may be followed by progressive intra-abdominal hypertension, diaphragmatic embarrassment, postrenal obstruction, and in severe cases, abdominal compartment syndrome. Attention to the use of prokinetics, stool softeners, and aperients as well as the early recognition of presenting signs and symptoms are key components of care.
- Stress gastric erosion arises commonly within 24 h of brain injury, correlating with the severity of insult, and related etiologically to hypothalamic autonomic activation. It presents with hemorrhage in 17% of cases, with an associated mortality of 50% after bleeding. The incidence in ischemic stroke is relatively low, while spinal cord injury demonstrates an incidence of up to 20%, supporting the concept of vagally mediated hypersecretion. The prophylactic use of H_2-antagonists, proton pump inhibitors, and sucralfate has significantly reduced the development of serious hemorrhage. This is, with the exception of sucralfate, achieved at the expense of associated changes in gastric pH, with consequent colonization by enteric bacterial flora and an increased incidence of pneumonia from the aspiration of infected gastric content. Ventilator-associated pneumonia is seen in up to 45% of patients with TBI. Treatment is largely preventive – by removing prophylactic agents as soon as feeding is established, and simple maintenance of elevation of head of the bed at a 30° angle.
- Diarrhea is a frequent complication of enteric feeding. Possible etiologies include *Clostridium difficile* superinfection, hyperosmolarity of feed, and excess fiber. Hyperosmolarity of feeding is relatively easily prevented with regular appraisal of needs, as is the control of fiber content.

Sixteen percent of patients admitted to rehabilitation after brain injury are already colonized by *C. difficile*, associated chiefly with antibiotic-induced changes in intestinal flora. Typical clinical manifestations of symptomatic infection include diarrhea,

Table 80.3 Suggested nutritional targets for patients after brain injury

Protein	1.5–2.2 g/kg/day
Calories: Harris-Benedict	Women: Basal metabolic rate (BMR) = 655 + (4.35 × weight in lbs) + (4.7 × height in inches) – (4.7 × age)
	Men: BMR = 66 + (6.23 × weight in lbs) + (12.7 × height in inches) – (6.8 × age)
Calories: Mifflin St Jeor	Male: BMR = (10 × weight in kg) + (6.25 × height in centimeters) – (5 × age) + 5
	Female: BMR = (10 × weight in kg) + (6.25 × height in centimeters) – (5 × age) – 161
Lipids	30–40% of calculated caloric requirements
Omega 3:6 ratio	1:2–1:4

abdominal pain, low-grade fever, and leukocytosis. The possible exacerbations include colitis, liver abscess, bacteremia, sepsis, splenic and pancreatic abscesses, peritonitis, small bowel enteritis, and bone and prosthetic joint infection. Treatment is with oral metronidazole and thereafter intravenous vancomycin in resistant cases.

Patient Assessment

A nutritional screen on admission should include physical exam and the assessment of basal metabolic rate. While albumin and prealbumin can be useful trend monitors, they tend to reflect catabolic activity of inflammation rather than nutritional reserve and protein depletion. Trace elements and phosphate levels can be measured on admission, and at regular intervals with the caveat that serum levels may not reflect total body stores as mentioned above.

Indirect calorimetry remains the gold standard of energy requirement assessments. Normal adult requirements are of the order of 2,500 kCal/day. The Harris-Benedict equation has been employed for many years to determine energy requirements but has been shown to underestimate those of brain-injured patients. A conversion factor of 1.4 improves the accuracy of calculation.

The Mifflin St. Jeor equation is currently recommended by the American Diabetic association as providing the most accurate energy calculation in the care of the critically ill, although it remains unproven in the context of brain injury.

Intervention/Treatment

Suggested nutritional goals are listed in Table 80.3.

Branch chain amino acid and glutamine-containing feeds have not been demonstrated as having any more benefit in brain-injured patients than standard protein-containing feeds. Conversely, theoretical concerns on possible conversion of glutamine to glutamate accompanied by its excitatory side effects seem unfounded in reality. One small randomized controlled trial claimed benefit for Probiotic and glutamine mixes, on the basis of improved infection rates and shorter ICU stay although this remains to be duplicated in a larger more convincing study. Omega 3 fatty acids may have advantages in reducing oxidative stress and supporting immune function, while a saturated fat diet (omega 6) reduces neuronal plasticity after brain injury. It remains to be seen whether manipulation of the omega 3:6 ratio will translate to an effect upon outcome. Obviously coexisting renal compromise will require the use of low-protein feed.

The use of anabolic agents, such as growth hormone, has been shown to reduce nitrogen loss and catabolic activity but at the expense of increased mortality in the critically ill. Consequently, their use is not currently recommended.

Key Points

- Nutrition is frequently compromised after brain injury by limited opportunity of intake and significant obligatory catabolism.
- Outcome is adversely affected by nutritional dysfunction.
- Iatrogenic exacerbation of feeding intolerance is common.
- Good nutritional control is best achieved by multidisciplinary input, protocolized care and systematic appraisal.
- Glycemic control can improve outcome but targeting a moderate glucose range appears to be a better strategy for the brain than the use of aggressive insulin therapy for tight control.

Suggested Reading

Cook AM, Peppard A, Magnuson B. Nutrition considerations in traumatic brain injury. Nutr Clin Pract. 2008;23:608–20.

Hartl R, Gerber LM, Ni Q, Ghajar J. Effect of early nutrition on deaths due to severe traumatic brain injury. J Neurosurg. 2008;109:50–6.

Jeremitsky E, Omert LA, Dunham CM, Wilberger J, Rodriguez A. The impact of hyperglycemia on patients with severe brain injury. J Trauma. 2005;58:47–50.

Mackay LE, Morgan AS, Bernstein BA. Swallowing disorders in severe brain injury: risk factors affecting return to oral intake. Arch Phys Med Rehabil. 1999;80:365–71.

Mentec H, Dupont H, Bocchetti M, Cani P, Ponche F, Bleichner G. Upper digestive intolerance during enteral nutrition in critically ill patients: frequency, risk factors, and complications. Crit Care Med. 2001;29:1955–61.

NICE-SUGAR Study Investigators. Intensive versus conventional glucose control in critically ill patients. N Engl J Med. 2009;360(13):1283–97.

Oddo M, Schmidt JM, Carrera E, Badjatia N, Connolly ES, Presciutti M, et al. Impact of tight glycemic control on cerebral glucose metabolism after severe brain injury: a microdialysis study. Crit Care Med. 2008;36:3233–8.

Rhoney DH, Parker Jr D, Formea CM, Yap C, Coplin WM. Tolerability of bolus versus continuous gastric feeding in brain-injured patients. Neurol Res. 2002;24:613–20.

Schlenk F, Graetz D, Nagel A, Schmidt M, Sarrafzadeh AS. Insulin-related decrease in cerebral glucose despite normoglycemia in aneurysmal subarachnoid hemorrhage. Crit Care 2008;12:R9. Epub 24 Jan 2008.

Zygun DA, Zuege DJ, Boiteau PJ, Laupland KB, Henderson EA, Kortbeek JB, et al. Ventilator-associated pneumonia in severe traumatic brain injury. Neurocrit Care. 2006;5:108–14.

Chapter 81
Fluid and Electrolyte Management in Neurosurgical Critical Care

Guillermo Bugedo and Luis Castillo

Overview

Imbalance and dysregulation of the fluid and electrolyte homeostasis are common and of great concern in patients after insults to the central nervous system. Disturbances may occur as a part of the disease process or they may be iatrogenic. The consequences of fluid and electrolyte derangements are frequently life-threatening and are recognized to determine outcome, particularly if unrecognized or persistently severe.

Fluid Management

Prevention

Traumatic brain injury (TBI): Outcome after TBI depends on the magnitude of the initial insult and upon the extend of secondary injuries to the brain that may result if the insult is survived. Systemic hypotension is a major cause of secondary brain injury and should be prevented and treated aggressively. Restoration of normovolemia with isotonic or hypertonic fluids is one essential component of the therapeutic strategy aimed at the restoration of adequate blood pressure, thus ameliorating ischemia and further brain damage.

Fluid management in patients with TBI and brain edema presents many challenges, including preserving adequate cerebral perfusion pressure (CPP), avoiding hypervolemia, and maintaining osmolality.

G. Bugedo, MD (✉) • L. Castillo, MD
Department of Intensive Care Medicine, Faculty of Medicine,
Pontificia Universidad Catolica de Chile, Santiago, Chile
e-mail: gbugedo@gmail.com

A.M. Brambrink and J.R. Kirsch (eds.), *Essentials of Neurosurgical Anesthesia & Critical Care*, DOI 10.1007/978-0-387-09562-2_81, © Springer Science+Business Media, LLC 2012

Some decades ago, hypovolemia and dehydration were widely accepted to decrease brain edema ("keep them dry"), inadvertently producing hypotension and jeopardizing brain perfusion.

Rosner et al., in the mid-1990s, challenged this concept by directing treatment at preserving CPP. Fluid management was aimed at maintaining euvolemia or mild hypervolemia. Isotonic crystalloids, albumin, and packed red blood cells (RBC) were used for the first 24–48 h, to obtain pulmonary artery wedge pressures (PAWP) above 12 mmHg and central venous pressure (CVP) above 8 mmHg, and to mobilize extravascular water into the vascular space, thus decreasing brain edema.

At a similar time, the Lund concept, introduced in Sweden, focused on improving perfusion and oxygenation around contusions (perfusion-targeted goal), and also in reducing intracranial pressure (ICP-targeted goal). For this approach, normovolemia is mandatory, which is accomplished by RBC transfusions to normal hemoglobin (12.5–14.0 g/dl) and albumin to normalize plasma oncotic pressure. This fluid therapy was intended to decrease brain edema and improve microcirculation. Diuretics (but not mannitol) were used to avoid hypervolemia and promote hypernatremia.

Both, the Rosner and the Lund approach require maintenance of normovolemia to avoid hypotension and assure brain perfusion. Careful fluid balance is mostly important to reduce the progressive accumulation of fluids in the extracellular matrix, which can worsen brain edema and increase ICP.

Subarachnoid hemorrhage (SAH) and vasospasm. Cerebral vasospasm is a leading cause of morbidity and mortality after aneurismal SAH. Hypertensive, hypervolemic, and hemodilution ("triple-H") therapy was introduced more than 20 years ago to improve cerebral blood flow in these patients. Several studies described the effectiveness of triple-H therapy for preventing neurologic deficits due to cerebral vasospasm. However, its efficacy has not been proven in randomized controlled clinical trials. Furthermore, triple-H therapy has severe side effects, such as pulmonary edema or arrhythmias, and caution must be taken in older patients or those with cardiovascular diseases. Pulmonary artery catheter, continuous cardiac output monitoring (e.g., PiCCO®), or repeat echocardiography may help orient fluid loading in these patients.

Therapeutic goals for fluid loading should be tailored to CVP and PAWP around 8–12 and 12–16 mmHg, respectively.

Crisis Management

Crystalloids versus Colloids? In patients with TBI both, isotonic crystalloids (Lactated Ringer's solution and 0.9% NaCl) and colloids can be used to achieve normovolemia. However, there is uncertainty about the best choice of fluids due to the lack of adequately powered randomized, controlled trials. Crystalloid-based fluid strategies are favored in trauma-resuscitation protocols, although the clinical evidence is limited. In the recent SAFE study, which compared saline *versus* albumin for fluid resuscitation, in 460 patients with TBI, use of albumin was associated with higher mortality rates than was resuscitation with saline (33.2% vs. 20.4%,

$P=0.003$). Lactated Ringer's solution and 0.9% NaCl can be safely administered in patients with TBI. Hypertonic solutions can also be used to increase plasma osmolality and decrease cerebral edema. Most of these fluid loading protocols are based on physiologic endpoints, assuming that prompt restoration of the blood volume will prevent hypotension and improve the outcome of patients with brain injury.

In patients after SAH, colloids are suggested along isotonic crystalloids to adequate fluid loading (see above). If the patient remains hypotensive and/or neurologic impairment does not improve despite fluid loading, blood pressure support may be achieved with noradrenaline (0.05–0.3 µg/kg/min) to a goal mean arterial pressure (MAP) of 100–130 mmHg.

Optimal hematocrit? Anemia is common in neurocritical care patients and is thought to be associated with worse outcomes by a number of specialists. Although hemoglobin (Hb) concentrations as low as 7 g/dl are well tolerated by most critically ill patients, data from animal and human studies suggest that such a severe degree of anemia may jeopardize cerebral and systemic perfusion, being harmful in the brain-injured patient.

The importance of ischemia in causing secondary brain injury appears to vary for different neurocritical care conditions. For example, cerebral vasospasm and delayed infarction are major causes of morbidity after a ruptured aneurysm. In contrast, the relevance of cerebral ischemia in the pathophysiology of TBI or intracerebral hemorrhage (ICH) is more debated. Beneficial physiologic effects of transfusion have been shown in patients with severe TBI, but whether this practice changes the outcome is under debate.

Electrolyte Disturbances and Management

Hyponatremia

Plasma sodium concentration is the main determinant of plasma osmolality, which regulates the movement of water inside and outside the cells. Thus, hyponatremia (Na <135 mmol/L) is particularly deleterious in the neurologic population, as it will produce or increase brain edema.

Crisis Management

Pathophysiology

Hyponatremia occurs secondary to multiple conditions (Table 81.1 and Fig. 81.1). In the neurocritical care patient, hyponatremia most commonly results of either the syndrome of inappropriate antidiuretic hormone secretion (SIADH) or the cerebral salt wasting syndrome (CSWS). However, hyponatremia may also develop because of excess free water and hypotonic fluids administration. Frequently, hypovolemia may contribute to or perpetuate an hyponatremic state.

Table 81.1 Common causes of hyponatremia in the neuro-surgical patient

Decreased ECF volume
- Extrarenal sodium loss
  - Diarrhea
  - Vomiting
  - Blood loss
  - Excessive sweating
- Renal sodium loss
  - Cerebral salt wasting syndrome
  - Diuretics
  - Osmotic diuresis
  - Adrenal insufficiency

Normal ECF volume
- Syndrome of inappropriate ADH secretion
  - Central nervous system diseases
  - Drugs (carbamazepine)
  - Pulmonary conditions
- Thiazide diuretics
- Adrenal insufficiency
- Hypothyroidism
- Primary polydipsia

Increased ECF volume
- Congestive cardiac failure
- Renal failure
- Cirrhosis

Syndrome of Inappropriate Antidiuretic Hormone Secretion

SIADH is associated with many conditions: neoplasia, nonmalignant lung diseases, drugs and neurologic diseases, including brain tumors, stroke, aneurysmal SAH, traumatic brain injury (TBI), meningitis and encephalitis. Carbamazepine-related hyponatremia might also be relevant in these patients.

Diagnostic criteria for SIADH requires:

- Serum sodium <135 mmol/L
- Serum osmolality <280 mmol/kg
- Urine sodium >20 mmol/L
- Urine osmolality > serum osmolality (usually > 100 mOsm/kg)
- Normal thyroid, adrenal, and renal function
- Absence of peripheral edema or dehydration
- Absence of potassium and acid–base abnormalities.

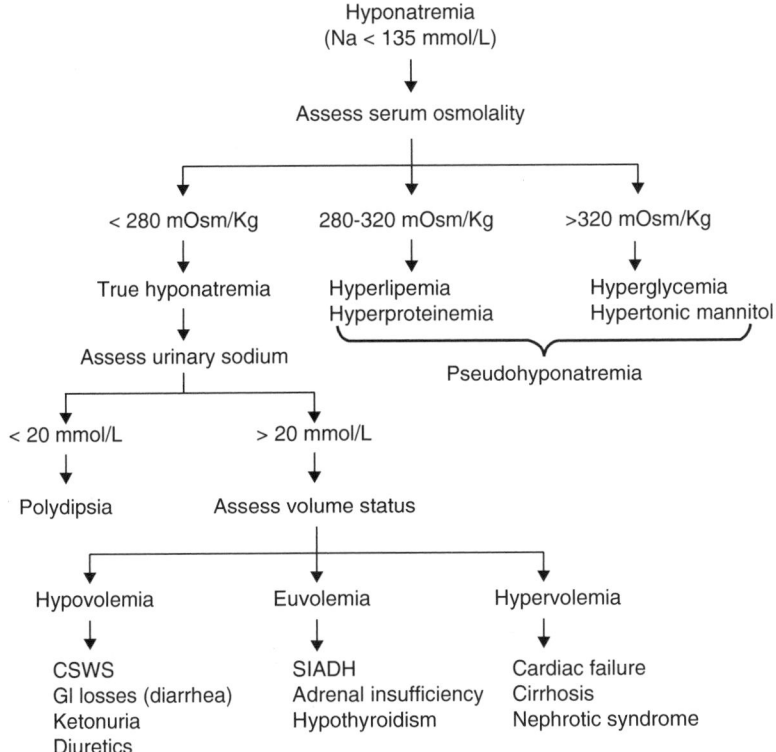

Fig. 81.1 Algorithm for the diagnosis of hyponatremia. *CSWS* cerebral salt wasting syndrome, *GI* gastrointestinal; SIADH, syndrome of inappropriate secretion of antidiuretic hormone

Cerebral Salt Wasting Syndrome

CSWS is characterized by polyuria and marked natriuresis, leading to hyponatremia and hypovolemia. High levels of brain natriuretic peptide (BNP) have been described in patients with SAH and vasospasm. It usually occurs during the first 2 weeks after brain injury and resolves spontaneously after 2–4 weeks.

Biochemical and clinical criteria for CSWS include:

- Serum sodium <135 mmol/L
- Low or normal serum osmolality
- High urine sodium (>50–100 mmol/L)
- Clinical hypovolemia.

The key clinical diagnostic factor in CSWS is the presence of volume depletion and hyponatremia. However, CSWS and SIADH are often difficult to differentiate in the clinical setting and response to treatment may help determine the diagnosis (Table 81.2).

Table 81.2 Clinical features of syndrome of inappropriate antidiuretic hormone (SIADH) and cerebral salt wasting syndrome (CSWS)

	SIADH	CSWS
Extracellular fluid volume	Increased	Normal/decreased
Plasma volume	Increased/normal	Decreased
Salt balance	Positive/equal	Negative
Water balance	Positive/normal	Negative
Preload	Normal/increased	Decreased
Serum sodium	Low	Low
Serum potassium	Normal	Normal/increased
Serum uric acid	Decreased	Normal/decreased
Serum BUN/creatinine	Decreased	Increased
Serum osmolality	Decreased	Decreased
Urine sodium	High	High/very high
Urine osmolality	High	Normal/high
Urine volume	Normal/variable	High

Clinical Presentation and Assessment

Symptoms due to hyponatremia are secondary to its effects on the brain and include headache, anorexia, nausea and vomiting, confusion, and lethargy. Left untreated and as plasmatic sodium drops below 115 mmol/L, hyponatremia may result in seizures, brain edema, apnea, coma, and death.

Hyponatremia is an important comorbidity in the neurosurgical population and may adversely affect outcome. It may be a cause of refractory intracranial hypertension in patients with TBI. In patients with SAH and vasospasm, hyponatremia may increase the frequency and fatality of brain infarction.

Treatment of Hyponatremia

Two basic principles involve the correction of hyponatremia: raising the plasma Na$^+$ at a safe rate and to a safe level, and diagnose and treat the underlying cause.

In patients with severe TBI and increased ICP, reaching an Na$^+$ concentration of 150–155 mmol/L is a common therapeutic goal to decrease brain edema. In these patients, mild hyponatremia (130–135 mmol/L) could be disastrous and should be treated vigorously.

A differentiation must be made if hyponatremia is associated with hypervolemia (suggesting SIADH) or hypovolemia (suggesting CSWS) as treatments are opposed:

1. SIADH is best treated by fluid restriction, while CSWS requires sodium (and fluid) loading. If diagnostic uncertainty exists sodium administration may be attempted before fluid restriction, as hypovolemia may jeopardize adequate brain perfusion and worsen outcome.
2. CSWS: Isotonic fluids, such as normal saline, often in excess of 5 L, may be necessary to restore normal Na and promote volume expansion in patients with

CSWS. Hypertonic solutions, such as 3% sodium chloride/acetate, has been safely used in patients with SAH.

Exogenous mineralocorticoids, such as fludrocortisone (0.1–0.6 mg daily), which induce a positive salt balance, can be safely used in patients with CSWS. Recently, ADH-receptor antagonists ("aquaretics") have been tested and shown effective in SIADH.

Correction of hyponatremia requires frequent measurement of serum sodium levels, and the rate of correction should not exceed 0.5 mEq/L/h to avoid adverse effects associated with rapid serum sodium correction (e.g., pontine myelinolysis). When hypertonic solutions are used in patients with brain edema, sodium levels should be closely monitored, i.e., every 6–8 h.

Hypernatremia and Hyperosmolar Syndromes

Hypernatremia (Na >145 mmol/L) is less frequent but not rare in the neurocritical care patient population in the ICU, both as a result of hypothalamic dysfunction or secondary to treatment with hypertonic saline in patients with brain edema (induced or therapeutic hypernatremia).

Crisis Management

Pathophysiology

Most commonly, hypernatremia may occur due to water loss, inadequate fluid intake, and/or exogenous administration of sodium. Non-induced hypernatremia usually implies a deficit of total body water and denotes a state of hypertonic hyperosmolality causing cellular dehydration.

Hypernatremia-associated mortality has been reported in excess of 50% and often results not from the disorder itself but by inappropriate treatment. Rapid correction of hypernatremia with hypotonic fluids may thus induce osmotic brain edema.

Thirst is the main defense against development of hypernatremia. The hyperosmolar state can be maintained only when access to water or thirst mechanism is impaired, as in patients with altered mental status, intubated patients and those at extremes of age.

Diabetes insipidus (DI) is characterized by complete or partial failure of ADH secretion (central DI) or of renal response to ADH (nephrogenic). Most patients with DI do not develop hypernatremia as their thirst mechanism is intact.

In the context of brain injury, the diagnosis of DI should be suspected in the presence of high urine output associated with hypernatremia:

- High urine volume (> 200 mL/h)
- High serum sodium (>145 mmol/L)
- High serum osmolality (>305 mmol/kg)
- Low urine osmolality (<350 mmol/kg).

The diagnosis of DI is confirmed by response to exogenous ADH.

In neurocritical care patients with brain edema, hypertonic saline (3–7%) is frequently used to induce hypernatremia (Na 145–155 mmol/L) and hyperosmolality and decrease intracranial pressure. In these patients, hypernatremia is associated with an excess of sodium and water. Mannitol can also be used to induce an hyperosmolar state but plasma sodium concentration will move in the opposite direction (Fig. 81.1).

Clinical Presentation and Assessment

Symptoms associated with hypernatremia are nonspecific and secondary to brain involvement and cardiovascular compromise. Anorexia, restlessness, and nausea and vomiting occur early, and may progress to altered mental status, lethargy, or coma. Musculoskeletal symptoms may include twitching, hyperreflexia, ataxia, or tremor.

Treatment of Hypernatremia

In patients with acute hypernatremia, developed on the course of hours, rapid correction of plasma sodium (±1 mmol/L per hour) improves their prognosis. However, rapid correction of hypernatremia of long duration may induce the entrance of water into the cells and induce convulsions and brain edema.

Free water administration by mouth or feeding tube is the preferred route for correcting hypernatremia. If not available, hypotonic fluids, as 5% dextrose or 0.45% sodium chloride, can be safely used intravenously. Extreme care must be taken in the critically ill patient who is at risk for brain edema formation or exacerbation when correcting hypernatremia. Diabetes insipidus is best treated with desmopressin, especially when urinary output > 200–250 mL/h is maintained for 6 h or more.

Hyperkalemia

Potassium is the most abundant cation in the body, being preferentially intracellular. Only 2% of total body potassium is found in the extracellular space, and serum potassium concentration is tightly regulated between 3.5 and 5.0 mmol/L. The large potassium gradient across cell membranes contributes to the excitability of nerve and muscle cells, including myocardium. Thus, disorders of potassium are one of the most common causes of life-threatening arrhythmias.

Table 81.3 Common causes of hyperkalemia	Drugs
	    ACE-inhibitors (e.g., captopril)
	    NSAIDs (e.g., ibuprofen and diclofenac)
	    Beta-blockers (e.g., atenolol)
	    K^+ supplements – e.g., oral or IV replacement
	    K^+ sparing diuretics (e.g., spironolactone)
	Renal diseases
	    Acute and chronic renal failure
	    Type 4 renal tubular acidosis
	    Metabolic acidosis
	Diet
	    Foods with high potassium content
	Endocrine disorders
	    Addison's Disease
	    Hyporeninaemia
	    Insulin deficiency/Hyperglycaemia
	Hematological disorder/massive cell death
	    Tumor lysis syndrome
	    Rhabdomyolysis
	    Massive blood transfusion
	    Massive haemolysis – mechanical cell damage
	Others
	    Hyperkalemic periodic paralysis
	    Pseudo-hyperkalemia
	    Abnormal erythrocytes
	    Thrombocytosis
	    Leucocytosis

ACE angiotensin-converting enzyme, *K^+* potassium, *NSAIDs* nonsteroidal anti-inflammatory drugs, *IV* intravenous

Modified from Alfonzo et al. Resuscitation 2006

Crisis Management

Pathophysiology

Potassium is excreted mainly by the kidney, so hyperkalemia ($K > 5.5$ mmol/L) is most commonly the result of impaired excretion by the kidney, and also can result from increased release from the cells (Table 81.3). Hyperkalemia is a relatively uncommon electrolyte abnormality in neurocritical patients, however, it may occur particularly in those who have coexisting acute or chronic renal failure.

Clinical Presentation and Assessment

The first indicator of hyperkalemia may be the presence of electrocardiographic (ECG) abnormalities or arrhythmias. Progressive ECG changes with potassium levels

Table 81.4 Therapeutic agents for the management of hyperkalemia

Therapy	Dose	Onset (min)	Duration (h)
Calcium chloride	10 mL of 10% IV	1–3	0.5–1
Sodium bicarbonate	1 mmol/kg IV	15–30	Several
Insulin/50% glucose	10 units in 25 g IV	15–30	4–6
Salbutamol	0.5 mg IV/20 mg Neb	15–30	4–6

IV intravenous, *Neb* nebulised
Modified from Alfonzo et al. Resuscitation 2006

include peaked T waves, prolonged PR interval, and flattened P waves. Widened QRS appears when potassium levels are above 8.0 mmol/L, and at this point the patient is at very high risk of cardiac arrest if not treated immediately.

Treatment of Hyperkalemia

There is no standardized treatment for hyperkalemia, and it depends on severity and ECG abnormalities (Table 81.4). Emergency treatment is directed to protect the heart from malignant arrhythmias (calcium and bicarbonate) or shifting potassium into the cells (e.g., hyperventilation [alcalosis], insulin, beta-agonists).

Removal potassium from the body is the definitive treatment of hyperkalemia, and it will often depend on renal function. Loop diuretics (e.g., furosemide) will increase diuresis and potassium excretion and are extensively used along 0.9% saline. If the patient is oligoanuric, dialysis is the indicated treatment. Potassium may also be removed from the body through the GI track following the administration of kayexalate.

Hypokalemia

Crisis Management

Pathophysiology

Hypokalemia ($K < 3.5$ mmol/L) is one of the most common electrolyte abnormalities in ICU patients. It occurs most frequently because of renal and gastrointestinal losses (Table 81.5). Unfortunately, several common therapies in the neurocritical care patient may cause hypokalemia. For example, mannitol, frequently used to treat elevated ICP, has potassium wasting properties. Fludrocortisone is employed in the treatment of hyponatremia in the context of CSWS, and results in renal potassium leakage. Other therapies, such as hyperventilation (alkalosis), steroids, insulin, and salbutamol may also cause hypokalemia by their effect to move potassium from the intravascular to intracellular compartment.

Table 81.5 Common causes of hypokalemia

Increase potassium loss
Drugs: diuretics, mannitol, laxative abuse, liquorice, steroids, fludrocortisone
GI losses: diarrhea, vomiting, ileostomy, intestinal fistula, villous adenoma
Renal: renal tubular disorders, Bartter's syndrome, Liddle's syndrome, Gitelman's syndrome, nephrogenic diabetes insipidous
Endocrine: hyperaldosteronism, Cushing's syndrome, Conn's syndrome
Dialysis: hemodialysis on low potassium dialysate, peritoneal dialysis
Transcellular shift
Insulin/glucose therapy
Beta-adrenergic stimulation (e.g., salbutamol)
Alkalosis
Hypothermia
Hypokalemic periodic paralysis
Decreased potassium intake
Poor dietary intake (less than 1 g/day)
Magnesium depletion (increases renal potassium loss)
Poor dietary intake
Increased magnesium loss

Modified from Alfonzo et al. Resuscitation 2006

Clinical Presentation and Assessment

Moderate to severe hypokalemia induces EKG changes including U waves, T waves flattening, and ST segment alterations. Cardiac arrhythmias are more frequent when combined with other pro-arrhythmic conditions such as ischemia, digitalis toxicity, or magnesium depletion.

In patients with high risk of arrhythmias, such as those with SAH or ischemic stroke, who frequently have coexisting cardiac disease, potassium levels should be closely monitored and replaced as needed.

Treatment of Hypokalemia

Intravenous potassium should be given by continuous infusion at a rate not faster than 10–40 mEq/h. Because of the risk of hyperkalemia, patients should be under continuous ECG monitoring and with serial sampling of potassium levels.

Because of the role of magnesium in transmembrane potassium transport, simultaneous correction of hypomagnesemia is required to correct hypokalemia. Hypokalemia and hypocalcemia can be refractory to replacement therapy in the setting of hypomagnesemia. Therefore, it is common administer magnesium salts (e.g., magnesium sulfate) along with potassium infusion.

Hypomagnesemia

Magnesium is the second most abundant intracellular cation, after potassium. Magnesium acts as a cofactor for many enzymatic reactions involving ATP and regulates the movement of calcium into smooth muscle cells rendering it important for cardiac contractility and vascular tone. Magnesium has been also suggested to have neuroprotective properties. Neuroprotection may be rendered via several mechanisms: Magnesium

- acts as an endogenous calcium channel antagonist
- inhibits excitatory neurotransmitter release (e.g., glutamate)
- acts as a NMDA receptor antagonist
- mediates directly vascular smooth muscle relaxation.

Currently, the therapeutic use of magnesium to provide neuroprotection after ischemic stroke is under investigation.

Magnesium is frequently used as a pharmacological agent for a variety of conditions, usually as an intravenous continuous infusion of 0.5–1 g/h of magnesium sulfate. Magnesium is also a first-line treatment for "torsade-de-pointes" and other cardiac arrhythmias induced by supratherapeutic digitalis.

Crisis Management

Pathophysiology of Hypomagnesemia

Hypomagnesemia (Mg < 1.3 mEq/L) occurs mainly because of renal losses, (e.g., after administration of loop-diuretics) or during CSWS. Clinically, hypomagnesemia is often associated with hypokalemia and hypocalcemia.

Clinical Presentation and Assessment

Hypomagnesemia symptoms include neuromuscular irritability and weakness, muscle spasms, seizures, and coma, as well as cardiac arrhythmias.

Approximately 30% of patients presenting with SAH have coexisting hypomagnesemia upon admission. The relationship between low magnesium levels, SAH, and cardiac arrhythmias remains unclear. Magnesium depletion results in prolonged cardiac cell repolarization and prolonged QT interval on ECG. "Torsade-de-pointes" is frequently associated with hypomagnesemia.

Low magnesium levels reduce the seizure threshold, and magnesium currently is the primary agent used to prevent seizures during preeclampsia.

Treatment of Hypomagnesemia

Magnesium sulfate is usually administered as a slow intravenous infusion up to 10 g/day to correct a magnesium deficit. For an emergency situation, 8–12 mmol (2–3 g) magnesium sulfate can be infused over 1–2 min, followed by 40 mmol (10 g) over the next 5 h. Rapid intravenous administration of magnesium sulfate is often associated with significant nausea and vomiting.

Hypermagnesemia (Mg > 2.0 mEq/L) occurs rarely after therapeutic magnesium infusion, and usually in patients with renal failure. Hypermagnesemia becomes symptomatic at levels > 4 mEq/L. Symptoms progress from hyporeflexia to complete AV heart block, respiratory failure, and cardiac arrest. While not a common problem in neurocritical care patients, hypermagnesemia should be on the differential diagnosis of patients with hyporeflexia.

Hypocalcemia

Calcium is a critical intracellular messenger and regulator of cell function. Calcium is of primary importance in neurocritical care patients due to its central role in neuronal death after central nervous system injury. Cytotoxic intracellular calcium accumulation is mediated via glutamate receptors, voltage-gated calcium channels, and pH-dependent calcium channels. In the context of intensive care management in general, it is important to remember that calcium is also the primary mediator of muscle contraction.

The calcium channel antagonist nimodipine has been shown to reduce the incidence of delayed cerebral ischemia following SAH and is now routinely initiated at hospital admission in affected patients and continued for 21 days. A similar benefit has not been seen in patients after ischemic stroke.

Crisis Management

Pathophysiology

Hypocalcemia (ionized Ca < 1.1 mmol/L) is one of the most frequent electrolyte abnormality in intensive care therapy. Relevant causes include hypoparathyroidism after neck surgery, phenytoin, and phenobarbital therapy, renal failure, and blood transfusion (citrate anticoagulant in packed RBCs binds calcium).

Respiratory alkalosis as a result of hyperventilation (i.e., for the treatment of elevated ICP) results in an increase in protein binding of calcium.

Clinical Presentation and Assessment

Clinical manifestations are related to cardiac and neuromuscular conduction as well as depressed myocardial contractility. Cardiac findings include prolong QT and ST intervals, decreased cardiac output, hypotension, bradycardia, and can progress to ventricular arrhythmias. Neurologic symptoms include parestesias, overall muscular weakness, tetany, and seizures.

Treatment of Hypocalcemia

In symptomatic patients and those with low serum concentrations, calcium may be administered by slow injection of 1 g of calcium chloride. There is no clear evidence that parenteral calcium supplementation impacts the outcome of critically ill patients.

Key Points

- Hypotension is a major cause of preventable secondary brain injury and should be aggressively prevented and treated.
- Fluid substitution to achieve normovolemia with isotonic or hypertonic fluids is essential to restore blood pressure, thus preventing ischemia and further brain damage.
- Isotonic crystalloids are favored in fluid resuscitation protocols, although the clinical evidence is limited.
- RBC transfusions are recommended in patients with increased ICP or those who are at risk for brain ischemia when serum hemoglobin concentrations fall below 8–9 g/dL.
- Sodium is the main determinant of plasma osmolality, which regulates the movement of water inside and outside the cells.
- Sodium disturbances are common and highly detrimental in patients with head injury, and should be avoided or, if present, promptly treated.
- Hyponatremia is associated with water shifts into the cells and therefore may increase brain edema and intracranial pressure.
- When hyponatremia or hypernatremia develops, measurement of urinary sodium, serum, and urine osmolarity and intravascular volume status may help to identify the cause and the appropriate treatment strategy.
- Hypernatremia causes hypertonic hyperosmolality and may occur when hypertonic solutions are used to treat patients with brain edema and intracranial hypertension.
- Close monitoring of plasmatic sodium is required to tailor the desired sodium plasma levels and osmolar state in neurocritical care patients.
- Potassium is excreted mainly by the kidney, and hyperkalemia is most commonly associated with renal failure.
- Therapeutic stimulation of diuresis or dialysis are definitive treatments for hyperkalemia.
- Hypokalemia is one of the most common electrolyte abnormality in ICU patients and occurs frequently because of renal and gastrointestinal losses, frequently secondary to other therapeutic interventions.
- Because of the risk for hyperkalemia, intravenous potassium substitution require continuous ECG monitoring and serial controls of potassium serum levels.

Suggested Reading

Alfonzo AV, Isles C, Geddes C, Deighan C. Potassium disorders – clinical spectrum and emergency management. Resuscitation. 2006;70:10–25.

Ellison DH, Berl T. The syndrome of inappropriate antidiuresis. N Engl J Med. 2007;356: 2064–72.

Fraser JF, Stieg PE. Hyponatremia in the neurosurgical patient: epidemiology, pathophysiology, diagnosis, and management. Neurosurgery. 2006;59:222–9.

Kramer AH, Zygun DA. Anemia and red blood cell transfusion in neurocritical care. Crit Care. 2009;13:R89.

Noronha JL, Matuschak GM. Magnesium in critical illness: metabolism, assessment, and treatment. Intensive Care Med. 2002;28:667–79.

SAFE Study Investigators. Saline or albumin for fluid resuscitation in patients with traumatic brain injury. N Engl J Med. 2007;357:874–84.

Singh S et al. Cerebral salt wasting: truths, fallacies, theories, and challenges. Crit Care Med. 2002;30:2575–9.

Chapter 82
Temperature Management in Neurosurgical Critical Care

Martin H. Dauber

Overview

Experimental evidence and clinical experience demonstrate that there are multiple mechanisms involved in cellular damage following neurological insult. Laboratory experiments since the 1950s demonstrated that there are benefits of mild hypothermia. Since that time hypothermia has been proposed as a valid clinical modality for several neurologic conditions.

Based on experimental and clinical evidence, this overview explores some of the current indications including prevention of elevation of intracranial pressure in the postsurgical and the cerebral hemorrhage patient, as well as use for stroke and central nervous system injury (brain and spinal cord) patients. Brief mention is be made of the postcardiac arrest scenario.

Experimental evidence. During Napoleon's reign Baron de Larrey employed hypothermia both to preserve amputated limbs and to provide numbing effects during battlefield surgery. In 1950, it was demonstrated that mild cerebral hypothermia during and after cardiac arrest improved neurologic outcomes in dog and primate models. Several years later it was shown by Rosomoff and Gilbert that there was a direct relationship between body temperature and both intracranial pressure and brain volume. Several studies proposed that hypothermia afforded beneficial effects in brain tissue because it caused reduced cerebral metabolic rate ($CMRO_2$) and blood flow. These findings were quickly adopted by cardiovascular specialists who employed hypothermia during cardiopulmonary bypass in their efforts to prevent insults to the central nervous system.

M.H. Dauber, MD (✉)
Department of Anesthesia and Critical Care, The University of Chicago Medical Center,
Chicago, Illinois, USA
e-mail: MDauber@dacc.uchicago.edu

A.M. Brambrink and J.R. Kirsch (eds.), *Essentials of Neurosurgical
Anesthesia & Critical Care*, DOI 10.1007/978-0-387-09562-2_82,
© Springer Science+Business Media, LLC 2012

As cerebral metabolism is dependant on temperature, hypothermia reduces oxygen consumption, glucose utilization, and lactate production. It is accepted that every 1°C decrease in temperature from 37° decreases $CMRO_2$ by 6–7%. An increase in brain pH of 0.0161 per degree of temperature decrease also results as a presumably due to the reduction in metabolism. Excitotoxicity, the pathological process by which neurons are damaged and killed, by the neurotransmitters glutamate, dopamine and serotonin is decreased. The calcium-dependant protein kinase C (PKC) translocates to the nerve cell membranes in ischemia, and this destructive process is inhibited by hypothermia.

Cerebral blood flow is also reduced by cold-induced vasoconstriction. This mechanism decreases intracranial volume and therefore, intracranial pressure, especially in traumatic brain injury (TBI). On a microscopic level, the blood–brain barrier (BBB) permeability may be favorably altered by hypothermia. The mechanism is likely due to a decrease in effect of extracellular enzymes that can disrupt the BBB. The effect of hypothermia on the cerebral vasculature, therefore, is an important mechanism for neuroprotection from the increased BBB permeability, vasogenic edema formation, and extravasation of circulating inflammatory mediators seen in ischemic injuries.

Clinical evidence: Although the experimental evidence for the benefits of hypothermia is convincing, there is considerable controversy in the clinical literature regarding the evidence-based medicine indications for the application of therapeutic hypothermia.

Traumatic brain injury: For TBI, many randomized controlled studies have demonstrated widely varying overall mortality, yet have failed to demonstrate statistically significant benefit from hypothermia. A recent meta-analysis of hypothermia treatment for TBI including eight trials with 800 patients, revealed a 20% decrease in mortality and a 25% increase in "good neurologic outcome" relative to the conventional therapy, though these effects were not statistically significant. Patients cooled more than 48 h showed reductions in risk of mortality and more favorable neurologic outcomes. In part, on the basis of this review, Brain Trauma Foundation (BTF)/American Association of Neurological Surgeons (AANS) guidelines task force has issued a (Level III) recommendation for optional and cautious use of hypothermia for adults with TBI.

Spinal cord injury: Although the physiology and anatomy of the spinal cord is in many ways thought of as analogous to brain, there are subtle differences that have impact on our subject. Whereas the brain is rarely exposed to the physician to directly impose hypothermia, during spine and spinal cord surgery, direct application of hypothermia upon damaged or at-risk spinal cord is possible. Spinal cord injury (SCI) can be a devastating injury, and most commonly affects young males. Many treatment modalities including pharmacologic interventions such as steroids, NMDA antagonists, and barbiturates as well as hypothermia have been advocated.

Experimental animal studies done in the 1960s produced promising results supporting hypothermia. Local cooling of the spinal cord was performed with iced saline during surgical decompression. The mechanisms were elucidated in the 1990s when studies demonstrated that early cooling strategies (relative to the timing of the insult) lessened the deleterious effects on the microvasculature and reduce local swelling. Further studies showed better preservation of gray and white matter, and locomotor function in rats when systemic hypothermia was induced 30 min postinjury and maintained for 4 h. Histological studies confirm that these findings of the locomotor benefits to hypothermia in animals.

Clinically spinal cord ischemia can result from trauma, or medical procedures such as aortic cross-clamping. Initial experiments used cool irrigation applied locally during spinal cord exposure, but yielded inconclusive results. More recent attempts at systemic hypothermia have failed to conclusively demonstrate efficacy for hypothermia, due to side effects, primarily shivering. As these consequences can be controlled by medications that lower the shivering threshold, definitive randomized, controlled studies should be available. Case reports in the literature include the 2010 report of a National Football League player who sustained a C3/C4 fracture dislocation and was found to have an A.S.I.A. type A injury. (i.e., complete sensorimotor loss) from which he has recovered nearly fully. The mild hypothermia that was immediately induced while the player was in transport to the hospital, and the passive and active efforts to achieve hypothermia during the first several days are credited with his dramatic improvement.

Postcardiac arrest: In 2002, an advisory statement about therapeutic hypothermia was issued by the Advanced Life Support Task Force of the International Liaison Committee on Resuscitation. Cooling to 32–34°C for 12–24 h was recommended for unconscious adult patients who had return of spontaneous circulation (ROSC) after out-of-hospital cardiac arrest when the initial rhythm is ventricular fibrillation. Two years later the panel stated that hypothermia may also be beneficial for other rhythms as well as in-hospital cardiac arrest. (This author's institution, the University of Chicago, is currently conducting a study of hypothermia for in-hospital cardiac arrest patients with ROSC.) A recent Clinical Practice article highlighted the application of these principals and the clinical difficulties therein. Cardiac arrest outside the hospital is a poorly defined entity in clinical medicine, and though the utilization of hypothermia may improve outcome, it can also confound prognostication.

There is ongoing investigation regarding therapeutic hypothermia for other conditions such as near-drowning, traumatic cardiac arrest, neonatal hypoxia-ischemic encephalopathy, hepatic encephalopathy, ARDS, and a variety of pediatric situations. In each of these scenarios, there is evidence to support the use of hypothermia of a varying degree and for variable durations. Due to the substantial interest in the modality and its potential for benefit in many disease states it is likely to be an area of great research interest in the future.

Ischemic and hemorrhagic stroke: As noted earlier the beneficial effects of hypothermia seen in experimental models of ischemia are the result of many biological effects. There is essentially no effect on infracted tissue, rather any benefits are probably in the penumbra. The imperatives for mechanical ventilation via a secure airway and shivering control has limited the use of hypothermia in stroke patients, though some early reports in spontaneously breathing patients have demonstrated small, and statistically insignificant improvement in mortality. Similar results were obtained when hypothermia was compared with medical management (tissue plasminogen activator). In a prospective study of massive ischemic infarction (>2/3 of one hemisphere), hemicraniectomy with hypothermia showed a tendency toward improved 6 month outcome as compared to hemicraniectomy alone. Many clinical questions currently remain unanswered and are the focus of ongoing trials.

After poor-grade subarachnoid hemorrhage, the addition of hypothermic therapy to barbiturates had no positive long-term effect. The multicenter IHAST (intraoperative hypothermia for aneurysm surgery trial) study failed to show a benefit of intraoperative hypothermia during aneurysm surgery in good-grade subarachnoid hemorrhage patients. Few animal studies and little useful clinical research exist to support the use of hypothermia in intracranial hemorrhage.

Complications of therapeutic hypothermia. Any therapeutic intervention including deliberate hypothermia is associated with its potential complications. The clinician needs to be aware of ways to prevent, recognize, and treat those complications in a timely manner. Patient comfort and tolerance of this intervention is necessary to address during institution of this modality. Several means are available to lower body temperature in a safe and efficient way that may help to prevent or reduce the risk for major complications. "Preventions" presents some of the most common techniques that are in use in neurointensive care units. "Crisis management" discusses adverse effects hypothermia has on cardiovascular function, coagulation and metabolic function, and infectious risk. The section concludes with a protocolized suggestion for achieving therapeutic hypothermia in the neurointensive care unit.

Prevention

There are three basic methods to cool patients in the ICU:

1. Conventional surface cooling and cold fluids
2. Commercial surface cooling devices
3. Intravascular cooling devices
4. Body cavity lavage, extracorporeal circulation, whole-body ice submersion, cooling helmets.

Conventional cooling can begin after neurologic assessment, sedation and placement of a core temperature monitor. Subsequently, to maintain hypothermia ice packs can be placed over the groins, neck, and axillae. Water cooled rubber mattresses can be placed over the patient as placement under patients has caused skin breakdown. Though these relatively simple means are often effective, drawbacks include lack of a feedback loop resulting in a high incidence of overcooling and the concomitant nursing vigilance required to maintain the goal temperature. The rate of cooling is unpredictable with these conventional and widely available methods.

Commercial surface cooling devices such as the Arctic Sun device (Medivance, Louisville, CO) controls the temperature of the water circulating through the ArcticGel Pads via a patient/temperature feedback loop. The patient can be cooled or kept normothermic as the pads which cover approximately 40% of the surface transfer heat from patient. Disadvantages include the purchase cost of the unit and the disposable pads. CoolBlue (Innercool Therapies, San Diego CA) and ThermoWrap (MTRE, Rechovot, Israel) are recently introduced, less-expensive garment-type devices without the gel of the Arctic Sun. As with the Arctic Sun they both have servo units to enhance ease of use and safety. Other similar devices that may cool faster are being tested in animals.

Intravascular cooling devices have the complications associated with placement of very large bore central lines including placement risks, infection, and thrombosis. However, once placed, these catheters can serve the additional functions of a central line. The Celsius Control System (Innercool Therapies) is a servo-controlled system in which water circulates through a (10.7 or 14 Fr) metallic catheter with a textured surface that is placed in the inferior vena cava via a femoral vein. Patients must be immobile during its use to prevent migration of the catheter. There is no infusion or monitoring port on the device so additional central venous access may be necessary.

There has been no direct comparison of the devices or techniques, so each institution needs to compare efficacy and safety in its environment.

Crisis Management

Shivering. Shivering is disturbing to awake patients. It also induces *unfavorable increases* in:

1. overall metabolic rate
2. oxygen consumption
3. work of breathing
4. heart rate
5. myocardial oxygen demand and consumption.

In perioperative patients, hypothermia may lead to additional cardiac morbidity especially in those patients with preexisting cardiac disease. These consequences may be from the hemodynamic and ventilatory responses rather than from the shivering itself. They may be controlled by pharmacologic means including sedatives, opiates, and sympatholytics. Magnesium (2 g intravenously over 1 h) and nondepolarizing relaxants (in patients with controlled ventilation) may also be helpful upon the initiation of hypothermia. Midazolam and meperidine may then be added as needed.

Cardiovascular effects. Hypothermia causes cardiovascular effects that are complex; opposing effects on myocardium and contractility depend upon patient's volume status and presence/degree of sedation. In patients treated to prevent shivering, mild hypothermia will decrease heart rate and increase contractility, but cardiac output will fall as blood pressure increases slightly. The supply–demand balance for myocardial oxygen will thus improve. Deep hypothermia (<30°C), however, will cause a decrease in contractility. Also, diuresis often results with hypothermia and causes hypovolemia through an increase in venous return, increase in atrial natriuretic peptide, and decreased antidiuretic hormone. Nonetheless, with attention to the prevention and treatment of the volume loss, normotension can be maintained.

The increase in venous return will cause mild sinus tachycardia especially in unsedated patients. When temperatures drop below 35.5°C sinus bradycardia results from decreased repolarization of pacemaker cells and gives the ECG findings of prolonged PR and QT intervals and widened QRS complexes. As temperature drops below 28–30°C atrial fibrillation, ventricular tachycardia, or ventricular fibrillation may result. Therefore, temperature below 30°C should be strenuously avoided in the ICU.

Coagulopathy. In the operating room, it is well known that even mild hypothermia can induce coagulopathy from decreased platelet numbers and dysfunction. At temperatures less than 33°C, the synthesis and function of clotting factors in the cascade are affected, at least in vitro. This has not been demonstrated clinically in therapeutic cooling for TBI, cardiac arrest, or stroke patients.

Immunosuppression. The proinflammatory response is inhibited by hypothermia via inhibition of leukocyte migration and phagocytosis, and decreased production of cytokines. The risk for nosocomial infection in hypothermic patients is linked to the duration of the therapy (>24 h are at higher risk) as well as the indication (low risk in cardiac arrest, high risk in stroke patients) for the therapy. Hypothermia may mask the signs of infection, such as fever, C-reactive protein, and WBC counts. An increased workload of the cooling device may be the only clue.

Miscellaneous problems. Other effects of hypothermia include decrease in bowel function and delayed gastric emptying. Serum amylase may increase, but pancreatitis is rare. Other laboratory values changed in hypothermia include:

1. Hyperglycemia
2. Low electrolyte levels
3. Thrombocytopenia
4. Low WBC counts
5. Elevated LFT'S (SGOT and SGPT)
6. Elevated stress hormones (cortisol, epinephrine, and norepinenphrine).

Though there is potential for disruption of many systems throughout the body during therapeutic hypothermia, attention to each of the areas leads to a manageable clinical situation and should rarely be a cause of discontinuation of the intervention.

After identification of a clinical indication for therapeutic hypothermia, a complete neurologic exam must be performed (Fig. 82.1), as it results will be suspect after initiation of therapy. The goal is typically to cool the core to 33°C for 12–24 h.

Thirty to forty milliliter per kilogram of isotonic intravenous fluid at 4°C is administered. This can rapidly decrease core temperature by 3–4°C. Administer sedative agents as tolerated by hemodynamics. Midazolam and meperidine are especially helpful for titratable sedation and decreasing shivering. Maintain serum potassium levels greater than 3.8 mEq/dL. Nondepolarizing neuromuscular blockade can be instituted with vecurounium 0.1 mg/kg or rocuronium 1.0 mg/kg, which are both devoid of cardiovascular side effects or cisatracurium 0.15 mg/kg in patients with

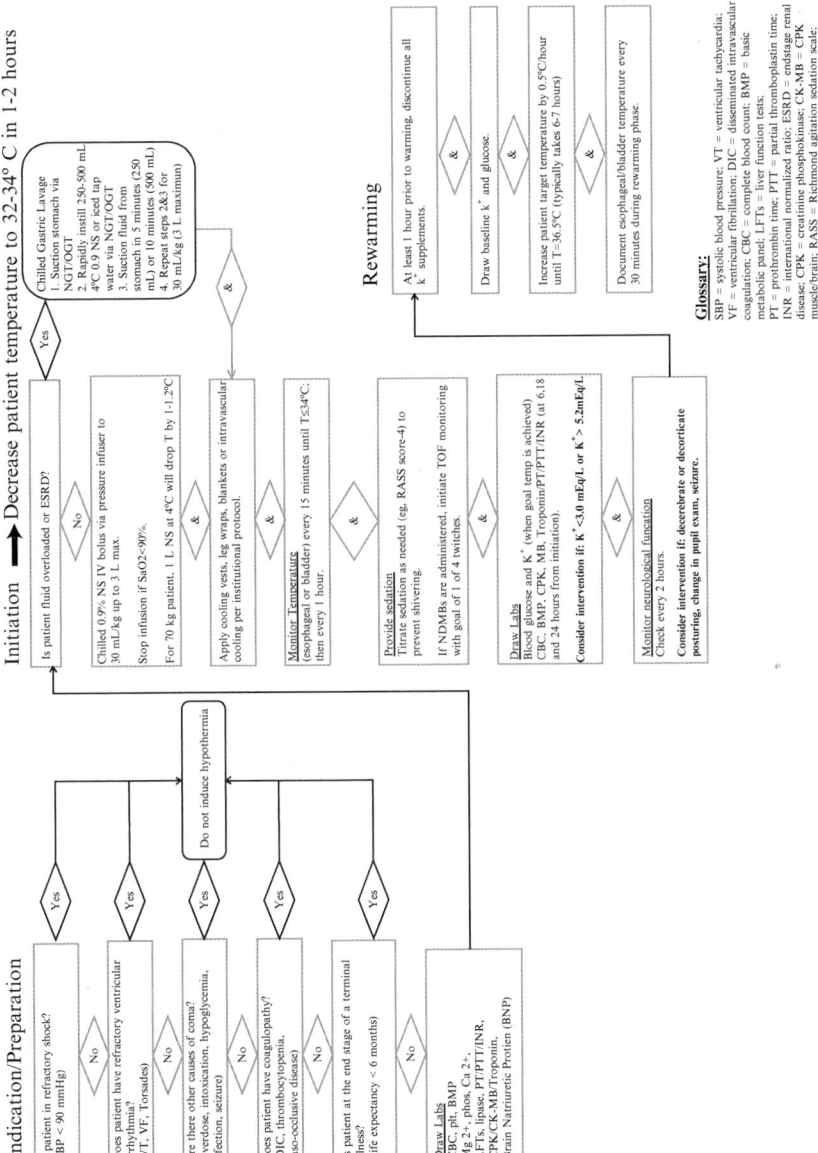

Fig. 82.1 Protocol for therapeutic hypothermia

renal impairment. Full ventilatory support to normalize oxygen and pH levels is almost always required. Blood gases should be managed with the pH stat method during the period of hypotension, as this approach allows the brain to more consistently respond normally to physiologic perturbations.

The serum glucose levels should be tightly controlled in the desired range (<150 mg/dL). The systemic blood pressure should be supported to provide the desired cerebral perfusion pressure (depending upon the indication for hypothermia). Early administration of broad spectrum antibiotics as indicated for suspected infection (e.g., aspiration pneumonia during event/initial resuscitation) should be considered. Attention to the skin to prevent breakdown from the cooling device should be given.

When the decision to begin warming to normothermia has been made, either as a result of presumed success or failure or due to intolerance to the procedures it should be realized that "decooling" should be done at 0.25–0.33°C/h to prevent problems. Hemodynamic instability is common as cutaneous vasodilation occurs and an inflammatory response may begin especially after arrest. The paralytics should be discontinued and their residual effect can be monitored with a peripheral nerve stimulator. Sedation should be weaned slowly during warming. When the patient is ready he/she can be separated from ventilatory support and extubated if appropriate. Shivering can be treated with meperidine or acetaminophen 650 mg. The temperature should not be allowed to increase above 37.5°C for 72 h. At this time, neuroprognostication can be undertaken again.

Key Points

- Significant experimental and clinical data suggest a potential value of therapeutic hypothermia in neurocritical care patients aimed to protect the CNS or prevent deterioration in certain situations including:

  - Postoperative elevated ICP
  - Cerebral hemorrhage complicated by elevated ICP
  - Ischemic stroke
  - Brain and spinal cord injury.

- There are theoretical advantages to the CNS outcomes and these are clinically substantiated in small studies. It is likely that through expanding application of deliberate hypothermia our understanding will be increased and our patients will thereby experience less CNS damage from their underlying diseases.
- Several methods are readily available to cool patients including surface cooling, cool intravenous fluids, body cavity lavage, and extracorporeal circulation. There are also several proprietary devices that can be employed.
- Complications of systemic cooling primarily are related to shivering, which is readily prevented by pharmacologic means. Cardiac, infectious, metabolic, and other systems may be affected, but are rarely reasons to reverse therapeutic hypothermia.

Acknowledgement The author thanks Ms. Amy Cissell in Anesthesiology and Perioperative Medicine at OHSU for designing the hypothermia protocol figure.

Suggested Reading

Seder DB, Van der Kloot TE. Methods of cooling: practical aspects of therapeutic temperature management. Crit Care Med. 2009;37(7):S211–22.

Peterson K, Carson S. Nancy Carney; Hypothermia treatment for traumatic Brain injury: A systematic review and meta-analysis. J Neurotrauma. 2008;25:62–71.

Varon J, Pilar A. Therapeutic hypothermia: past present, and future. Chest. 2008;133(5):1267–74.

Chapter 83
Coagulation Management in Neurosurgical Critical Care

Sarice Bassin and Thomas Bleck

Neurosurgery patients are at extremely high risk for venous thromboembolic complications. The benefits of pharmacologic prevention and treatment of deep vein thrombosis (DVT) and pulmonary embolism (PE) must be weighed against the risk of catastrophic intracranial or perispinal hemorrhage. This section focuses on the two most common coagulation management issues: (1) Thromboembolic disease and (2) Coagulopathy.

Thromboembolic Disease

Overview

Incidence

- Between 6 and 80% – depending on risk factors.
- The incidence of upper extremity DVT (UE-DVT) is unknown in this population, but studies report 20% incidence of pulmonary embolism from UE- DVT.
- Highest rates are for those with multiple risk factors.
- Rate of fatal PE are highest for those with spinal cord injury.

S. Bassin, MD (✉)
Southwest Medical Group Neurology Associates,
PeaceHealth Southwest Medical Center, Vancouver, WA, USA

T. Bleck, MD, FCCM
Departments of Neurosurgery and Anesthesiology, Rush University Medical Center,
Chicago, IL, USA

A.M. Brambrink and J.R. Kirsch (eds.), *Essentials of Neurosurgical Anesthesia & Critical Care*, DOI 10.1007/978-0-387-09562-2_83,
© Springer Science+Business Media, LLC 2012

Risk Factors

- paresis
- immobility
- prolonged surgery
- combined anterior/posterior spinal surgery
- brain tumor
- traumatic brain injury
- central venous catheters (including PICC lines)
- long bone fractures
- spine trauma.

Clinical Implications

- pain
- limb swelling
- chronic venous stasispulmonary embolism
- postthrombotic syndrome.

Prevention

Despite the known benefits of pharmacological prophylaxis, concern for bleeding complications and iatrogenic neurologic injury often limit their use in neurosurgery patients. Studies have shown that chemical prophylaxis is relatively safe for most neurosurgical patients when started 24–72 h after surgery. Chemical prophylaxis started prior to surgery may be associated with a higher rate of hemorrhagic complications. Timing of chemical prophylaxis must be individualized. Mechanical prophylaxis (compression stocking and sequential compression devices) should be started preoperatively or immediately upon entering the OR to decrease the incidence of DVT. The incidence of catheter-related DVT correlates with the size of the catheter (rates are higher with larger caliber catheters). Therefore, practitioners should place the smallest caliber central venous catheter necessary.

Special attention must be paid to patients when epidural/spinal anesthesia or spinal puncture is employed. These patients are at increased risk of developing an epidural or spinal hematoma which may result in permanent neurologic impairment. Chemical anticoagulation should be used with caution in these patients. Risk versus benefit analysis must be fully considered in this patient population.

Options for the prevention of thromboembolic disease are summarized below (Table 83.1).

Table 83.1 Prevention of thromboembolic disease

Prophylactic measure	Mechanism	Dose	Potential adverse effects/CI
Compression stockings	Unknown	Wear daily	Discomfort
Sequential compression device	Unknown; several theories discussed	Use when in bed	Discomfort
Heparin	Activates antithrombin III; inhibits factor Xa	5,000 U SQ bid or tid	Bleeding; HIT
Enoxaparin	LMWH Factor Xa and IIa inhibition	40 mg SQ daily or 30 mg bid (Adjust for patients with CrCl < 30 mL/min)	HIT; Increased risk of bleeding in age > 65 year; <45 kg
Dalteparin	LMWH Factor Xa and IIa inhibition	2,500–5,000 IU SQ daily	Bleeding; HIT
IVC filter	Blocks clot from embolizing to the pulmonary vasculature	Retrievable or permanent	Postthrombotic syndrome; thrombosis of device

LMWH low molecular weight heparin, *HIT* heparin induced thrombocytopenia, *CrCl* creatinine clearance

Crisis Management

DVT may be detected on screening examinations or after extremity pain and swelling is noted. In patients in who anticoagulation is not contraindicated, anticoagulation is the first-line treatment to prevent propagation of clot and PE. If anticoagulation is contraindicated, inferior vena cava (IVC) filter may be considered. However, anticoagulation should be resumed in patients with IVC filters when pharmacologic treatment is no longer a contraindication.

Upper extremity DVT should be treated the same as lower extremity DVT. If a DVT is associated with an indwelling central venous catheter (CVC, e.g., a PICC line), the CVC should be removed if possible.

PE refers to the obstruction of a pulmonary vessel by material that comes from elsewhere in the body. This chapter refers to obstruction due to thrombus. PE is associated with a mortality rate of 30% without treatment; however, accurate diagnosis followed by anticoagulation therapy can significantly reduce the recurrence of PE, and therefore, decrease mortality.

Clinical Presentation-Pulmonary Embolism

- Systolic blood pressure < 90 mmHg or a drop of ≥40 mmHg from baseline (massive PE)
- Hypotension associated with elevated central venous pressure or jugular venous distention

Table 83.2 Assessment of the patient with possible pulmonary embolism

Assessment	Findings	Notes
Electrocardiography	S1Q3T3 Right ventricular strain Incomplete right bundle branch block T-wave inversion	Often nonspecific changes Nondiagnostic
V/Q scan	Mismatch in ventilation and perfusion	Most useful for patients with high probability of PE and high-probability V/Q scan
Ultrasound	Upper or lower extremity Doppler showing filling defect in appropriate clinical setting	If negative, does not rule out PE; if positive, does not rule in PE
D-Dimer	Level < 500 ng/mL by ELISA excludes PE unless the pretest probability is high; <500 ng/mL by latex agglutination excludes PE, if pretest probability is low	Patients with prior events will have higher baseline levels Less sensitive in patients with subsegmental PE
Angiography	Gold standard; Evaluate for filling defect or cutoff in pulmonary vasculature	Invasive study Potential contrast reaction; renal failure
Spiral CT	Evaluate for filling defects in pulmonary vasculature	Potential contrast reaction, renal failure Positive predictive value 96% and 92% for high and intermediate probability cases, respectively

- Acute right ventricular failure
- Tachycardia
- Tachypnea
- Hypoxia/shortness of breath
- Cardiac arrhythmias
- Pleuritic chest pain
- Cough
- Calf or thigh swelling/pain.

Patient Assessment (Table 83.2)

Intervention/Treatment

- Resuscitation

    - Intravenous fluid administration – use with caution in patients with evidence of right heart failure
    - Vasopressors and/or inotropes
    - Supplemental oxygen and/or intubation

- Anticoagulation

  - Should be given after thorough evaluation of bleeding risk
  - Prevents further clot formation, but does not lyse existing clot
  - Heparin titrated to therapeutic aPTT or enoxaparin 1 mg/kg SQ twice daily or enoxaparin 1.5 mg/kg SQ once daily
  - Warfarin titrated to INR 2.0–3.0
  - Treatment recommended for 3–12 months

- Thrombolysis

  - Associated with increased risk of hemorrhage, particularly in patient after surgery and intracranial hemorrhage; relative contraindications need to be considered on a case-by-case basis
  - Persistent hypotension is primary indication
  - Tissue plaminogen activator (tPA) – Administer 100 mg intravenously over 2 h
  - Heparin resumed when the aPTT is less than twice its upper limit of normal and titrated to therapeutic aPTT

- Embolectomy

  - Indicated for persistent hypotension, if thrombolysis fails or is contraindicated

- IVC filter

  - Prevents migration of thrombus from extremities to pulmonary vasculature
  - Indicated when anticoagulation is contraindicated or has failed
  - Does not prevent further clot formation or lyse existing clot
  - Anticoagulation should be started even in patients with filters once bleeding risk deemed acceptable.

Coagulopathy

Overview

Anticoagulants and platelet inhibitors are used with increasing frequency for the treatment of a variety of disorders including atrial fibrillation, thromboembolic disease, and stroke. In addition, bleeding dyscrasias may be seen in primary coagulopathies such as hemophilia, or secondary to liver disease or sepsis. Coagulopathic patients who are suffering from bleeding complications, e.g., intracranial hemorrhage, or need surgical intervention may require acute reversal of coagulopathy.

Incidence

- Warfarin use is associated with a two- to fivefold increase in the rate of intracerebral hemorrhage (ICH).
- Risk of ICH associated with warfarin use increases with age > 75 year, hypertension, history of cerebrovascular disease, and intensity of anticoagulation
- Symptomatic ICH occurs in 6.4% of acute stroke patients treated with alteplace (tPA) at 3 h and 7.9% of those treated up to 4.5 h.
- The incidence of ICH is approximately 2% per year in children with hemophilia.

Risk Factors

- Pharmacologic platelet inhibition
- Anticoagulation
- Fibrinolysis
- Uremia
- Liver failure
- Hemophilia
- Von Willebrand's disease
- Sepsis
- Multi-trauma
- Massive head injury

Crisis Management

Indications for platelet transfusion

- Neurosurgical procedure and platelet count less than 100×10^9/L
- Platelet count greater than 100×10^9/L with platelet dysfunction not responsive to DDAVP or cryoprecipitate
- Consider for bleeding associated with platelet antagonists
- One six-pack of pooled platelet should raise the platelet count by 25×10^9/L.

If urgent hemostasis is needed, the following agents may be used (Table 83.3).

The choice of hemostatic agents depends on the clinical scenario. Determining the cause of the coagulopathy is essential to deciding on the correct treatment plan. Table 83.4 outlines hemostatic options for common drug-induced coagulopathies. Table 83.5 provides hemostatic options for coagulopathies that are due to acquired or congenital coagulopathies.

Table 83.3 Hemostatic agents

Product	Time to normalize coagulopathy	Dose	Side effect	Mechanism and notes
Vitamin K1	At least 6 h for INR normalization; 24 h or longer for full effect	10 mg IV or SQ for 3 days	Anaphylaxis with IV administration	Provides substrate for Vit K-dependent factors II, VII, IX, and X
Fresh frozen plasma	12–32 h for INR normalization	12–20 ml/kg = 1,400 ml = 6 units	Volume overload	Replaces Vitamin K clotting factors
Prothrombin complex concentrate	One hour for INR normalization	25–50 units/kg; first 500–100 IU at 100 IU/min over 10 min, then 25 IU/min	May need repeat dosing if INR 1.2 not met 30 min after infusion	Replaces Factors II VII, IX, and X
Cryoprecipitate	Variable for fibrinogen replacement	30 mg/dL increase in fibrinogen per bag	Volume overload	Replaces fibrinogen, factors VII XIII and vWF
Activated Factor VII	15–30 min	40–80 μg/kg	Risk of thrombosis	Activates extrinsic pathway of coagulation cascade
Protamine sulfate (for reversal of heparinoids)	Neutralizes heparin within 5 min; check aPTT to verify reversal	1 mg per 100 units heparin; 1 mg per 1 mg enoxaparin; 1 mg per 100 IU daltaparin	Hypotension with infusion > 5 mg/min	Disrupts heparin-antithrombin III complex; Anti-factor Xa activity only 60% neutralized
ε-Aminocaproic acid	Variable	150 mg/kg IV bolus followed by 15 mg/kg/h during surgery	Hypotension; thrombosis	Anti-fibrinolytic; competitive inhibitor of plasminogen activation
Tranexamic acid	Variable	10–15 mg/kg IV (optional 1 mg/kg/h for 5–8 h during surgery)	Hypotension, thrombosis	Anti-fibrinolytic; competitive inhibitor of plasminogen activation; 10x more potent in vitro than ε-aminocaproic acid

Table 83.4 Hemostatic options for drug-induced coagulopathy

Drug category (and examples)	Drug mechanism of action	Antidote	Substrate for anti-thrombotic attenuation	Other options	Notes
Platelet antagonist (tirofiban, eptifibatide)	Glycoprotein IIb/IIa receptor	None	Fresh frozen plasma (8 U), platelets transfusion (2U)	Dialysis	
Platelet antagonist (clopidogrel)	ADP receptor inhibition	None	Platelet transfusion (2–10 U)	Methylprednisolone 25 mg IV (10); Desmopressin: 0.3 mcg/kg IV; dilute in 50 ml NS and infuse over 15–30 min	Desmopressin can cause hyponatremia and fluid overload
Anticoagulant (heparin)	Antithrombin III potentiator	Protamine: 1 m per 100 units heparin	None		Hypotension with infusion > 5 mg/min
Anticoagulant enoxaparin, dalteparin	Factor IIa and Xa inhibition	Protamine : 1 mg per 1 mg enoxaparin; 1 mg per 100 IU daltaparin	None		Anti-factor Xa activity 60% neutralized
Fibronolytic (alteplase, reteplase)	Promote plasminogen activation	ε-Aminocaproic acid: 0.1 g/kg bolus + 0.5–1 g/kg infusion Transexamic acid 10–15 mg/kg IV slow infusion	Cryoprecipitate (10 U), fresh frozen plasma (2 U), platelet transfusion (10 U)		Thrombosis; hypotension with rapid medication infusion; Patients with fibrinogen level < 100 mg/dL should receive additional 10 U cryoprecipitate

Table 83.5 Treatment for non-pharmacologic coagulopathy (if active bleeding present or procedure planned)

Disease	Drug and dose	Side effects	Mechanism and notes
Liver disease	Fresh frozen plasma dosed to correct INR	Fluid overload; transfusion reaction	Replaces factors; if used in conjunction with exchange plasmapheresis, may minimize volume overload
	Activated recombinant factor VII 40–80 µg/kg IV	Thrombosis	
	Cryoprecipitate dosed to correct severe hypofibrin-ogenemia (<100 mg/dL)	Fluid overload	Replaces fibrinogen; One bag will raise fibrinogen level by 30 mg/dL
	Vitamin K 10 mg SQ daily for 3 days		
Hemophilia, von Willebrand's disease	For Hemophilia A and von Willebrand's disease type 1:	Hyponatremia; fluid overload	Increases factor VIII and von Willebrand factor
	Desmopressin: 0.3 mcg/kg IV; dilute in 50 ml NS and infuse over 15–30 min	Thrombosis	Can decrease bleeding time without 1 h, but short duration of action (4–6 h)
	Transexamic acid 10–15 mg kg IV slow infusion		Inhibitor of plasmino-gen activation and plasmin
	Factor concentrate (selection and dosing depends on type and severity of specific factor deficiency)		Replaces coagulation factors
Uremia	Desmopressin: 0.3 mcg/kg IV; dilute in 50 ml NS and infuse over 15–30 min	Hyponatremia; fluid overload	Increases factor VIII and von Willebrand factor
	Conjugated estrogens 0.6 mg/kg daily for 5 days		Can decrease bleeding time without 1 h, but short duration of action (4–6 h)
	Erythropoetin 50–100 U/kg IV/SC three times a week		Theorized increase in factor VII, XII, and von Willebrand factor
	Cryoprecipitate dosed to correct severe hypofibrinogenemia (<100 mg/dL)		Unknown, but decreases bleeding time
			One bag will raise fibrinogen level by 30 mg/dL

The treatment of warfarin-associated coagulopathy depends on the severity of the abnormality and the clinical state of the patient. Table 83.6 lists guidelines for the treatment of supratherapeutic INR due to warfarin use.

Table 83.6 American College of Chest Physicians Guidelines for treatment of suprathera-peutic INR due to vitamin K antagonists

Condition	Treatment
INR < 5	Lower or omit next warfarin dose
No significant bleeding	
INR > 5 but < 9	Omit next 1 or 2 warfarin doses
No significant bleeding	Vitamin K 1–2.5 mg PO if increased bleeding risk
INR > 9	Hold warfarin until INR therapeutic
No significant bleeding	Vitamin K 2.5–5.0 mg PO
Any INR	Hold warfarin
Serious bleeding	Vitamin K 10 mg IV
	FFP or PCC or Factor VII
	Repeat Vitamin K q12 h for persistent INR elevation
Any INR	Hold warfarin
Life-threatening bleeding	Vitamin K 10 mg IV
(ICH, SCH, etc.)	FFP or PCC or Factor VII
	Repeat Vitamin K prn

ICH intracerebral hemorrhage, *SCH* spinal cord hematoma, IV infusion at 1 mg/min, *FFP* fresh frozen plasma, *PCC* prothrombin complex concentrate

After successful reversal of pharmacologically induced coagulopathy and further stabilization of the patient practitioners need to start discussing the need, the timing and the dose for reinstitution of anticoagulation treatment, if the underlying medical problem is still present. The current practice varies considerably between clinicians regarding the many patient groups due to the paucity of evidence-based guidelines.

Key Points

- The neurosurgical population is at extremely high risk for both DVT and PE.
- The benefit of chemical prophylaxis and treatment for thromboembolic disease must be weighed again the risk of hemorrhage into the brain or spinal canal.
- Multiple hemostatic agents are available for the treatment of coagulopathy in the setting of bleeding or urgent invasive procedure.
- The treatment of warfarin-associated coagulopathy depends on the clinical state of the patient.

Suggested Reading

Ansell J, Hirsh J, Hylek E, et al. Pharmacology and management of the vitamin K antagonist. Chest. 2008;133:160S–98.

Grove JR, Pevec WC. Venous thrombosis related to peripherally inserted central catheters. J Vasc Interv Radiol. 2000;11(7):837–40.

Hacke W, Kaste M, Gluhmki E, et al. Thrombolysis with alteplace 3 to 4.5 hours after acute ischemic stroke. N Engl J Med. 2008;359:1317.

Hart RG, Tonarelli SB, Pearce LA. Avoiding central nervous system bleeding during antithrombotic therapy: Recent data and ideas. Stroke. 2005;36:1588.

Joffe HV, Kucher N, Tapson V, et al. Upper-extremity deep vein thrombosis a prospective registry of 592 patients. Circulation. 2004;110:1605–11.

Mahdy AM, Webster NR. Perioperative systemic haemostatic agents. Br J Anaesth. 2004;93(6): 842–58.

Nelson MD, Maeder MA, Usner D, et al. Prevalence and incidence of intracranial hemorrhage in a population of children with haemophilia. The hemophilia growth and development study. Haemophilia. 1999 Sep;5(5):306–12.

Pantanowitz L, Kruskall MS, Uhl L. Cryoprecipitate patterns of use. Am J Clin Pathol. 2003; 119(6):874–81.

Qureshi AI, Suri MFK. Acute reversal of clopidogrel-related platelet inhibition using methyl prednisolone in a patient with intracranial hemorrhage. Am J Neuroradiol. 2008;29:e97.

Schroder WS, Gandhi PJ. Emergency management of hemorrhagic complications in the era of glycoprotein IIb/IIIa receptor antagonist, clopidogrel, low molecular weight heparin, and third-generation fibrinolytic agents. Curr Cardiol Rep. 2003;5:310–7.

The National Institute of Neurological Disorders and Stroke rt-PA Stroke Study Group. Tissue plasminogen activator for acute ischemic stroke. N Engl J Med. 1995;333:1581.

Chapter 84
Gastrointestinal Hemorrhage in Neurosurgical Critical Care

Meghan Bost and Kamila Vagnerova

Overview

Upper gastrointestinal bleeding (UGIB) is a common medical condition that results in high patient morbidity and mortality.

Types and Incidence of UGIB in the general population:

- Peptic ulcer disease (PUD) – 55%
- Esophagogastric varices – 14%
- Arteriovenous malformation – 6%
- Mallory–Weiss tears – 5%
- Tumors and erosions – 4%
- Dieulafoy's lesion – 1%
- Other – 11%

Attenuating risk factors for PUD, including prevention of *Helicobacter pylori* infection (*H. pylori*), avoiding nonsteroidal anti-inflammatory drugs (NSAID) and reduction of gastric acid and stress helps to minimize ulcer occurrence and rebleeding rates. Stress-related ulcers are a common cause of acute UGIB in intensive care unit (ICU) patients. There is a paucity of data specific to neurosurgical and neurocritical care patients. Thus much of the information provided in this chapter specific to ICU patients in particular is based on evidence from the general ICU patient population.

M. Bost, MD (✉)
Anesthesia Associates of Medford, Medford, OR, USA
e-mail: megbost@yahoo.com

K. Vagnerova, MD
Department of Anesthesiology and Perioperative Medicine,
Oregon Health & Science University, Portland, OR, USA

A.M. Brambrink and J.R. Kirsch (eds.), *Essentials of Neurosurgical Anesthesia & Critical Care*, DOI 10.1007/978-0-387-09562-2_84,
© Springer Science+Business Media, LLC 2012

Table 84.1 Risk factors in postoperative patients in general and some selected neurosurgical patient populations in particular.

Risk factors in postoperative patients	Incidence of UGIB (%)
Male	6.64
Female	3.40
Age > 50 years	9.88
Age < 50 years	3.35
Adrenocortical hormone therapy	5.46
No adrenocortical hormone therapy	2.13
GCS < 10	17.5
Intracerebral hematoma	15.7
Intraventricular hemorrhage	10.0
Subdural hematoma	6.00
Extradural hematoma	2.94
Tumor of fourth ventricle	15.79
Tumor of brainstem	7.89
Tumor of cerebral hemisphere	5.71
Tumor of sellar hypothalamus	3.74

Two major risk factors for overt GI bleeding:

- Mechanical ventilation >48 h
- Coagulopathy – International Normalized Ratio (INR)>1.5 or platelet count <50,000

Among patients with one or both of these risk factors, almost 4% develop clinically important UGIB compared to 0.1% with neither risk factor.

Additional risk factors for stress ulceration:

- Shock
- Sepsis
- Hepatic failure
- Acute Renal failure
- Multiple trauma
- Burns >35% of total body surface area
- Organ transplantation
- Head trauma
- Spinal trauma
- History of PUD or UGIB

Most UGIB in critically ill is due to gastric or esophageal ulcerations. Stress ulceration can also cause perforation (<1% of surgical ICU patients). However, endoscopy (EGD) performed within 72 h of a major burn or cranial trauma reveals acute mucosal abnormalities in >75% of patients. In isolated head injury, GI tract dysfunction presents early and includes risk of GI bleed. (See Table 84.1 for risk factors in postoperative patients.)

Prevention

Incidence of overt UGIB ranges from 1.5 to 8.5% of all ICU patients but may be as high as 15% if no prophylaxis is used. It is widely accepted that prophylaxis is indicated for ICU patients; however, there is lack of consensus regarding which medications should be used. Antisecretory agents such as H2 receptor antagonists (H2B) or proton pump inhibitors (PPI) decrease the risk of stress-related mucosal damage and UGIB in high-risk patients. Although less commonly used, sucralfate is more effective than no prophylaxis in reducing overt bleeding (see Table 84.2 for recommendations). H2B blockers are still considered the first-line agents; however, thrombocytopenia can develop in neurosurgical patients on H2B. Enteral feeding has

Table 84.2 Common medications used for prophylaxis of stress-related mucosal disease[1]

Medication	Route	Normal renal function	Renal insufficiency	Comments
Histamine₂-receptor antagonists				
Cimetidine	IV	50 mg/h Continuous infusion	If CL_{cr}<30 mL/min: decrease dose to 25 mg/h	For patients requiring a more rapid elevation of gastric pH, continuous infusion may be preceded by a 300-mg loading dose administered as an IV infusion
	po; NG tube	300 mg every 6 h	300 mg every 12 h orally or intravenously has been recommended	Some patients may require higher doses; this should be accomplished by administering 300 mg more frequently, but the daily dose should not exceed 2,400 mg
Famotidine	IV	1.7 mg/h continuous infusion	If CL_{cr}<30 mL/min: 0.85 mg/h by continuous infusion	
	po; NG tube; IV	20 mg every 12 h	If CL_{cr}<30 mL/min: decrease dose to 20 mg once daily	
Sucrose–aluminum complex				
Sucralfate	po; NG tube	1 g every 6 h	Use with caution in severe renal impairment No adjustment necessary	

(continued)

Table 84.2 (continued)

Medication	Route	Normal renal function	Renal insufficiency	Comments
Proton pump inhibitors				
Esomeprazole	po; NG tube; IV	40 mg every day		
Lansoprazole	po; NG tube; IV	15 or 30 mg every day		
Omeprazole	po; NG tube; JT; DT	Two 40-mg doses separated by 6–8 h on the first day, then 20–40 mg daily		
Pantoprazole	po; NG tube; IV	40 mg every day		

IV intravenous, CL_{cr} creatinine clearance, *po* per os (orally), *NG* nasogastric, *JT* jejunal tube, *DT* duodenal tube

proven beneficial due to its ability to improve splanchnic blood flow; however, it has not been proven to reduce GI bleeding per se. In the ICU patients who are receiving enteral nutrition use of oral PPI or H2B is recommended otherwise IV H2B or PPI should be used (Grade 2B). Of note is that the use of H2B and PPI may increase the frequency of nosocomial pneumonia.

Prophylaxis is recommended for ICU patients who exhibit:

- Coagulopathy (platelet count < 50,000 per m^3, INR > 1.5, partial thromboplastin time (PTT) >2 times the control value)
- Mechanical ventilation >48 h
- History of GI ulceration or bleeding within the past year
- Two or more of the following risk factors: sepsis; ICU stay >1 week; occult GIB ≥6 days; glucocorticoid therapy (>250 mg hydrocortisone).

Crisis Management

Most patients with bleeding ulcers can be managed with fluid and blood resuscitation, medical therapy, and endoscopic intervention. *All patients with UGIB require urgent gastroenterology consultation.*

Pathophysiology and Clinical Presentation

The upper GI tract is protected by mucosa. Disruption in this mucosal layer or a significant shift in pH begins the process of ulceration. Ulcerations usually occur in the fundus and body of the stomach but may also develop in the distal esophagus, antrum, or duodenum. They are usually shallow and cause slow bleeding from the superficial capillary beds that rarely lead to hemodynamically significant bleeding. Deeper lesions, usually occurring between the third and seventh ICU day, may erode into the submucosa which may result in injury of larger vessels and massive hemorrhage or even organ perforation.

UGIB commonly presents with melena or hematemesis. Common reasons for UGIB in ICU patients include the following:

- Impaired mucosal protection – Under normal conditions the glycoprotein mucous layer forms a physical barrier to hydrogen ion diffusion and traps bicarbonate but it may be denuded by increased concentrations of refluxed bile salts or uremic toxins common in critically ill. Alternatively, or in addition, mucosal integrity may be compromised due to poor perfusion associated with shock, sepsis, and trauma.
- Hypersecretion of acid – Excessive gastrin stimulation of parietal cells has been detected in patients with head trauma as oppose to be normal or subnormal in most other ICU patients. Gastric acid and pepsin are essential cofactors in the pathogenesis of peptic ulcers. Control of gastric acidity is an essential therapeutic maneuver in active UGIB.
- *Helicobacter pylori* infection – *H. pylori* is a spiral bacterium that infects the superficial gastric mucosa. It may contribute to stress ulceration, but the evidence is limited. It disrupts the mucosal layer, liberating pepsin and hydrogen ions, leaving underlying mucosa more vulnerable. The immune response to *H. pylori* incites an inflammatory reaction that promotes further tissue injury.
- NSAID-induced injury results from both systemic prostaglandin inhibition and local effects. The majority of NSAID-induced ulcers are clinically uncomplicated and asymptomatic. NSAIDs may play a role in nonhealing ulcers.
- Steroids – Systemic steroids frequently used in neurosurgical patient almost double the risk of a new episode of UGIB or perforation. Concomitant use with high doses of NSAIDs has been associated with a 12-fold increased risk for upper GI complications.
- Head injury – GI dysfunction manifests as gastroparesis, ileus, increased intestinal mucosal permeability, and UGIB due to stress ulceration and coagulopathy. Plasma levels of cortisol and age are independent predictors of stress ulcers following acute head injury. There is a relationship between the severity of head injury and the incidence of gastroparesis. Significant gastric intramucosal acidosis occurs commonly in severe head injury. Primary insult to the central nervous system likely results in derangement of splanchnic blood flow secondary to neurohumoral mechanisms.

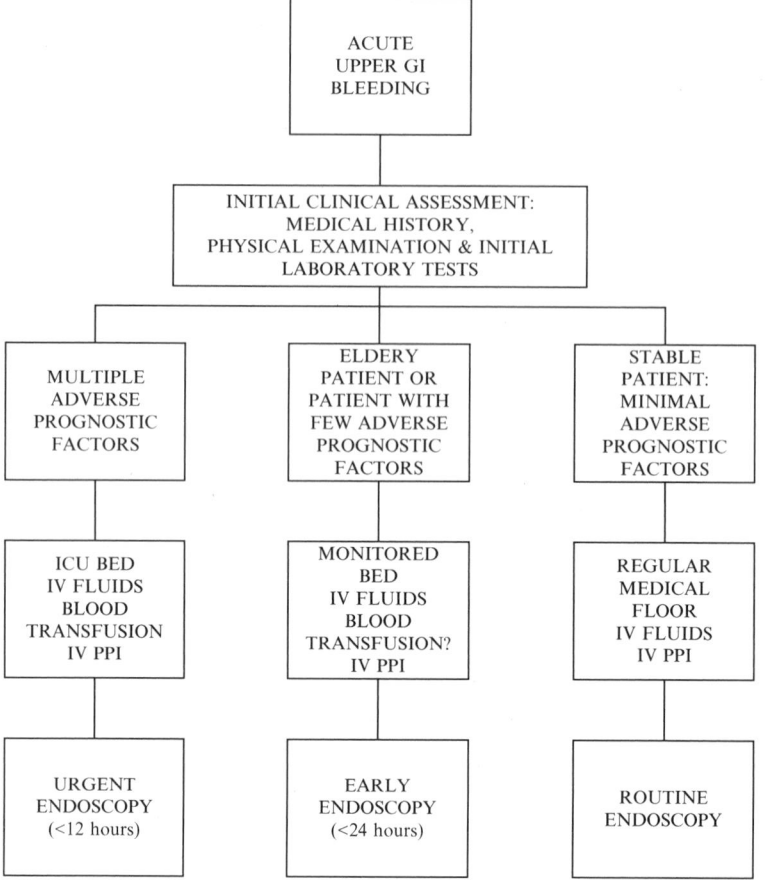

Fig. 84.1 Initial management and triage of patients with UGIB (adapted from Cappell and Friedel 2008)

Patient Assessment

Clinical Assessment

The medical history, physical examination, and initial laboratory values are important for triage decisions, assessing resuscitation requirements, need for further treatment, consults, and prognosis (see Fig. 84.1).

- Medical history

  - Prior GI bleed
  - GI symptoms
  - Gastrotoxic medication, e.g., NSAIDs, *anticoagulants*

- Comorbidities (renal, coronary artery, and peripheral vascular diseases)
- Head injury

• Physical exam and monitoring

- *Hemodynamic stability*

    (a) Tachycardia, thready pulse
    (b) Hypotension, orthostatic hypotension
    (c) Hypoxia

- *Abdominal examination*

    (a) Bowel sounds, abdominal tenderness, ascites

- *Signs of chronic liver disease or portal hypertension*

    (a) Hepatomegaly, splenomegaly
    (b) Palmar erythema, spider angiomata, caput medusa
    (c) Peripheral edema

- *Signs of shock (see vital signs listed above)*

    (a) Cold clammy extremities
    (b) Altered mental status

- *Rectal examination*

    (a) Occult or gross blood

- *Laboratory work-up*

    (a) Complete blood count (CBC), basic metabolic panel (BMP), coagulopathy work-up

Nasogastric aspiration with saline lavage is useful in detecting intragastric blood.

Surgical consultation is recommended for ongoing active or recurrent UGIB, massive bleeding, bleeding associated with significant abdominal pain, acute lower GIB, variceal bleeding, and suspicion for acute abdomen. Patients with severe symptoms, signs of shock, continuing hematochezia, and/or significant comorbidities are critically ill and require aggressive treatment/intervention.

Intervention/Treatment

First, stabilize the patient. Secure IV access (two large-bore IVs) and initiate resuscitation by fluid administration. Start crystalloid infusion to maintain the blood pressure, and send for type and cross-match of several units of packed erythrocytes. Evaluate the patient for airway protection and secure the airway, if needed. Maintain cardiorespiratory support as needed and treat associated conditions, (e.g., sepsis, myocardial infarction, traumatic brain injury). Begin general supportive measures including supplemental oxygen by nasal cannula and cardiac monitoring (e.g., EKG, blood pressure, and pulse oxymetry).

Patients with massive bleeding, active hematemesis, hypoxia, tachypnea, or altered mental status should have airway protection (i.e., endotracheal intubation). Keep the patient NPO for urgent EGD and potential surgery and place a Foley catheter to monitor urine output.

Empiric Pharmacotherapy

PPIs are the initial medical therapy. Currently suggested are omeprazole or lansoprazole; start with an IV bolus of 80 mg and continue IV infusion at 8 mg/h for a total of 72 h. If no signs of rebleeding after 24 h, switch to oral PPI.

Octreotide is used in variceal bleeding. Start with an IV bolus of 50 mcg and continue IV infusion at 50 mcg/h for 3–5 days.

Nonselective beta blockers also help to reduce portal hypertension.

Endoscopy

EGD is a primary diagnostic and therapeutic tool for UGIB. It helps to determine the cause and provides rationale for triage of patients. The most commonly used methods are injection and cautery/thermal techniques, as well as mechanical therapy like endoclips and banding.

Key Points

- Stress ulcer prophylaxis is indicated for patients with

  - Mechanical ventilation>48 h
  - Coagulopathy
  - GI ulceration or bleeding within the past year
  - Two or more of the following: sepsis, ICU>1week, occult GIB>6 days, high-dose steroids

- ICU patients on enteral medications: use oral PPI (Grade 2B)
- ICU patients not on enteral medications: use IV H2B (Grade 2B) or PPI
- Use IV PPI as first-line agent in acute UGIB
- Gastroenterology consult for all GI bleeds

Suggested Reading

Cappell M, Friedel D. Initial management of acute upper gastrointestinal bleeding: from initial evaluation up to gastrointestinal endoscopy. Med Clin N Am. 2008;92:491–509.

Cook DJ, Fuller HD, Guyatt GH, et al. Risk factors for gastrointestinal bleeding in critically ill patients. Canadian Critical Care Trials Group. N Engl J Med. 1994;330(6):377–81.

Cook DJ, Griffith LE, Walter SD, et al. The attributable mortality and length of intensive care unit stay of clinically important gastrointestinal bleeding in critically ill patients. Crit Care. 2001; 5(6):368–75.

Jutabha R, Jensen DM. Management of upper gastrointestinal bleeding in the patient with chronic liver disease. Med Clin North Am. 1996;80(5):1035–68.

Sesler JM. Stress-related Mucosal Disease in the Intensive Care Unit. AACN Adv Crit Care. 2007;18(2):119–28.

Venkatesh B, Towsend S, Boots R. Does splanchnic ischemia occur in isolated neurotrauma? A prospective observational study. Crit Care Med. 1999;27(6):1175–80.

Zheng K, Wu G, Cheng NN, Yao CJ, Zhou LF. [High risk factors of upper gastrointestinal bleeding after neurosurgical procedures]. Chung-Hua i Hsueh Tsa Chih [Chin Med J]. 2005;85(48): 3387–91.

Chapter 85
Intracranial Monitors in Neurosurgical Critical Care

Patricia Harper Petrozza

Over the past decade, intracranial monitoring devices have gained increased acceptance by clinicians. While monitoring devices cannot independently improve outcome, physiologic data are contributed which can be integrated into a therapeutic plan for the individual patient with an acute neurologic illness. Increasingly, anesthesiologists encounter patients with intracranial pressure (ICP) monitors, external ventricular drainage (EVD) devices, and brain tissue oxygen tension (PBO_2) monitors. This chapter will focus on common complications associated with each of these monitors.

Overview

ICP, the pressure within the cranial vault relative to the ambient atmospheric pressure, begins to rise when compensatory mechanisms which control ICP, such as changes in cerebrospinal fluid (CSF) dynamics, cerebral blood flow (CBF), and cerebral blood volume, are exhausted. ICP monitors are most frequently employed in patients at high risk of developing intracranial hypertension; these include patients with severe traumatic brain injury (TBI) who have a Glasgow Coma Scale score ≤8 and an abnormal computed tomographic (CT) scan. ICP monitors may also be useful in patients following subarachnoid (SAH) and intracerebral (ICH) hemorrhage, those with known hydrocephalus or brain edema after large strokes, in the setting of hypoxic brain injury, central nervous system (CNS) infections, and fulminant hepatic failure. In patients with TBI, Brain Trauma Foundation Guidelines recommend that ICP treatment be initiated at an upper threshold of 20–25 mmHg.

P.H. Petrozza, MD (✉)
Department of Anesthesiology, Wake Forest Baptist Medical Center,
Wake Forest Baptist Medical Center, Winston Salem, NC, USA
e-mail: petrozza@wakehealth.edu

A.M. Brambrink and J.R. Kirsch (eds.), *Essentials of Neurosurgical Anesthesia & Critical Care*, DOI 10.1007/978-0-387-09562-2_85, © Springer Science+Business Media, LLC 2012

ICP thresholds are somewhat more moderate in children, while in patients with hydrocephalus, values >15 mmHg are commonly regarded as elevated.

Intraventricular catheters (IVCs) and intraparenchymal sensors are the two methods most commonly utilized to measure ICP. Since they allow direct measurement by insertion of a catheter into one of the lateral ventricles which is then connected to an external pressure transducer, intraventricular catheters are often thought of as the "gold standard." Additionally, these catheters allow therapeutic removal of CSF, and they can be re-zeroed externally.

Intraparenchymal systems for ICP monitoring may be inserted through a support bolt or tunneled subcutaneously through a burr hole. These systems have either a microminiature strain-gauge pressure sensor, side-mounted at the tip (Codman) or a fiberoptic catheter (Camino, Interspace). While intraparenchymal ICP sensors offer a good alternative to IVCs , which may be difficult to place in the setting of advanced brain swelling, their main limitation is a small drift of the zero-line. Neither of the intraparenchymal systems currently allows pressure calibration to be performed in vivo. The systems are zeroed relative to atmospheric pressure during preinsertion calibration, and output is dependent upon zero-drift of the sensor.

Infection

The most significant complications associated with ICP monitoring via external ventricular drainage catheters (EVDs) are infection and hematoma formation. Intraparenchymal catheters have a low infection rate, but may become colonized after 5 days of use. Additionally, the fiber optic system tends to be fragile and may be damaged during routine nursing procedures.

Prevention

EVD-related infections are very common, with a reported incidence between 2 to 27%. The incidence of ventriculitis related to an EVD can be halved by rigid adherence to a standardized protocol during insertion and maintenance. Sampling of CSF and leakage of CSF have been shown to be important factors in the development of infection, while careful attention to site preparation as well as minimizing EVD manipulation may also be important.

The presence of an intraventricular hemorrhage, SAH, cranial bone fracture with CSF leak, craniotomy, systemic infection, and catheter irrigation are risk factors that predispose patients with ventriculostomies to ventriculitis or meningitis. Data on both antibiotic prophylaxis, as well as the effect of the duration of EVD as a risk factor, are controversial. In some studies, the incidence of CSF infection was reduced by the administration of prophylactic antibiotics, but those patients who developed

Fig. 85.1 Cell index

$$\text{Cell Index} = \frac{WBC_{CSF} \, [mm^3] \div RBC_{CSF} \, [mm^3]}{WBC_{BLOOD} \, [mm^3] \div RBC_{BLOOD} \, [mm^3]}$$

infection displayed pathogens which were selectively resistant to antibiotics or opportunistic. Generally, the use of continuous prophylactic antibiotics is discouraged based on the risk of selecting resistant organisms.

Although information in the literature about the relationship of the duration of EVD and the development of ventriculostomy-related infections is mixed, most authors conclude that there is a likely relationship between the duration of EVD and infection. A number of studies directly addressing the duration of catheterization found a significantly increased risk for device-related infection in patients with catheters in place for 5 days or longer, with the peak at days 9–11, and a markedly decreased risk thereafter, despite a population that continued to be at risk. There is little evidence to support the practice of prophylactic catheter exchange at a predetermined interval.

Crisis Management

Pathophysiology and Clinical Presentation

Clinical signs of EVD-related ventriculomeningitis include fever, meningismus, a reduced level of consciousness and photophobia. Muscle rigidity and seizures may also be present. Nosocomial ventricular drainage-related infections are difficult to diagnose because of nonspecific CSF findings, subtle signs of infection, and slow growing and fastidious microorganisms delaying identification of pathogens and appropriate treatment. Typically, three findings in the CSF point to the presence of ventriculitis in susceptible patients:

- Elevated (100–5,000) polymorphonuclear leukocytes.
- Decreased glucose (<40 mg/dL).
- Elevated protein.

Detection of ventriculostomy-related infections in patients with intraventricular hemorrhages has been investigated using the ratio of leukocytes to erythrocytes in CSF divided by leukocytes to erythrocytes in peripheral blood (called the cell index – see Fig. 85.1).

At the time of intraventricular hemorrhage onset, the CSF relationship of leukocytes to erythrocytes should be equal to that in peripheral blood; the cell index should be one. A significant increase of this index is highly indicative of EVD-related ventriculitis in patients with hemorrhagic CSF. The "cell index" has been demonstrated to show a significant rise 3 days before the conventional diagnosis of catheter-related ventriculitis.

In the febrile patient with an EVD in whom ventriculitis is suspected, a CSF sample should be obtained for gram stain and culture. Additionally, peripheral blood culture is necessary.

Intervention and Treatment

Ventriculitis most frequently involves gram-positive organisms; however, if the CSF fluid sample is notably purulent, treatment should be initiated immediately with a broad-spectrum antimicrobial agent that covers resistant gram-positive and gram-negative bacteria. Current recommendations include the use of vancomycin and a cephalosporin with antipseudomonal activity (e.g., cefepime or ceftazidime) or vancomycin with meropenem.

Very often for an optimal response to the treatment of the infection, it is necessary to remove any infected hardware which should be replaced or externalized when appropriate. Some clinicians base their decision about removal of the catheters depending upon the causative organism since coagulase-negative staphylococci tend to respond better to glycopeptide antibiotics while gram-negative bacterial infections are associated with a high frequency of relapse if the catheters are retained.

Key Points

- Complications can be reduced by rigid adherence to a protocol of care.
- Prophylactic antibiotics are discouraged.
- Clinical signs may be subtle.
- CSF analysis and culture are crucial.
- Early broad spectrum treatment should be initiated.

Hemorrhagic Complications

Hemorrhagic complications have been observed following the placement of EVD systems, as well as intraparenchymal catheters, for monitoring ICP. The true incidence of this complication is difficult to assess as parameters for diagnosis vary widely in the literature and most hemorrhages are identified via investigational CT scanning following placement of the monitor. Fortunately, most hemorrhages do not cause significant clinical deterioration. Although rare, fatal intracranial hemorrhages have been reported in both adults and children.

The reported risk of hemorrhage produced by EVDs in adults ranges between 2 and 10%, while the reported incidence of hemorrhagic complications from intraparenchymal monitors ranges from 0 to 10%. Several small studies indicate that the risk of intracranial hemorrhage following placement of both types of monitors is significantly higher in children, although clinically significant hemorrhages in this group of patients are also rare.

Prevention

Classic neurosurgical teaching precludes the placement of either an EVD or intra-parenchymal monitor for ICP in the face of abnormal coagulation parameters and a decreased platelet count. Indeed, in patients with abnormalities in prothrombin (PT) or partial tissue thromboplastin (PTT) or platelet count at the time of placement of an intraparenchymal monitor, a hemorrhage rate of 15% was recorded on follow-up CT scan in patients with coagulation disorders. Clinically insignificant hemorrhages were noted in 2% of patients with normal coagulation studies.

A platelet count of 100,000/mm³ has been recommended as the appropriate trigger for transfusion for neurosurgical procedures. A recent retrospective review of patients with TBI from one center demonstrated that in patients with an INR <1.6, hemorrhagic complications diagnosed with CT scanning following intraparenchymal monitoring were infrequent.

Crisis Management

Serial CT scans (noncontrasted) which are obtained following placement of EVDs may demonstrate an incidence of ICH in as many as 20% of patients. Generally, no surgical intervention is required as long as patients remain neurologically stable without a change in mental status or GCS. In patients where neurologic examination is difficult, serial CT examinations may be necessary to monitor the evolution of the hemorrhage.

Key Points

- Coagulation parameters should be normal before placement of ICP monitors.
- Small hemorrhages are common.
- Serial neurologic examinations may be necessary to monitor for hemorrhage progression.

Brain Tissue Oxygen Pressure

Small flexible microcatheters can be inserted into the brain parenchyma to measure brain tissue oxygen tension in a region of interest. The brain tissue oxygen pressure (PBO₂) value represents the balance between oxygen delivery and oxygen consumption in brain cells, and changes in PBO₂ may reflect pathophysiological alterations.

Two devices are currently available. The Licox (Licox Integra Neurosciences) measures tissue oxygenation through a polarographic technique by means of a Clarke electrode. The Neurotrend device (Neurotrend Johnson and Johnson) used "optimal luminescence" to measure pH, $PBCO_2$, and PBO_2. With both devices, the catheter should be inserted directly into a given region of interest (e.g., a hypoperfused area as determined by CT or MRI perfusion studies), and preferably should pass through gray matter into white matter for optimal value referencing and data comparison. Catheters may be either tunneled after craniotomy or placed through a double- or triple-lumen bolt.

Although literature on these two devices is relatively sparse, complications such as infection or hematoma formation are possible. It is recommended that coagulation parameters, particularly platelet number and function, be normal before insertion of these monitoring probes.

Suggested Reading

Infection

Beer R, Lackner P, Pfausler B, Schmutzhard E. Nosocomial ventriculitis and meningitis in neuro-critical care patients. J Neurol. 2008;255:1617–24.

Bhatia A, Gupta AK. Neuromonitoring in the intensive care unit. I. Intracranial pressure and cerebral blood flow monitoring. Intensive Care Med. 2007a;33:1263–71.

Korinek AM, Reina M, Boch AL, Rivera AO, De Bels D, Puybasset L. Prevention of external ventricular drain–related ventriculitis. Acta Neurochir (Wien). 2005;147:39–45. discussion 45–6.

Stoikes NF, Magnotti LJ, Hodges TM, Weinberg JA, Schroeppel TJ, Savage SA, et al. Impact of intracranial pressure monitor prophylaxis on central nervous system infections and bacterial multi-drug resistance. Surg Infect (Larchmt). 2008;9:503–8.

Ziai WC, Lewin III JJ. Update in the diagnosis and management of central nervous system infections. Neurol Clin. 2008;26:427–68.

Hemorrhage

Anderson RC, Kan P, Klimo P, Brockmeyer DL, Walker ML, Kestle JR. Complications of intracranial pressure monitoring in children with head trauma. J Neurosurg. 2004;101(1 Suppl): 53–8.

Blaha M, Lazar D, Winn RH, Ghatan S. Hemorrhagic complications of intracranial pressure monitors in children. Pediatr Neurosurg. 2003;39:27–31.

Davis JW, Davis IC, Bennink LD, Hysell SE, Curtis BV, Kaups KL, et al. Placement of intracranial pressure monitors: are "normal" coagulation parameters necessary? J Trauma. 2004;57: 1173–7.

Brain Tissue Oxygen

Andrews PJ, Citerio G, Longhi L, Polderman K, Sahuquillo J, Vajkoczy P, et al. NICEM consensus on neurological monitoring in acute neurological disease. Intensive Care Med. 2008;34: 1362–70.

Bhatia A, Gupta AK. Neuromonitoring in the intensive care unit. II. Cerebral oxygenation monitoring and microdialysis. Intensive Care Med. 2007b;33:1322–8.

Pfister D, Strebel SP, Steiner LA. Postoperative management of adult central neurosurgical patients: systemic and neuro-monitoring. Best Pract Res Clin Anaesthesiol. 2007;21:449–63.

Valadka AB, Robertson CS. Surgery of cerebral trauma and associated critical care. Neurosurgery. 2007;61 Suppl 1:203–20. discussion 220–1.

Chapter 86
Central Nervous System Infection in Neurosurgical Critical Care

Mary K. Sturaitis

Overview

Postoperative central nervous system infection is a serious complication with potential disastrous morbidity and mortality, requiring immediate recognition and treatment. Superficial craniotomy wound site infections, while not uncommon, are of significance due to potential contiguous spread to the bone flap or the meninges. Intracranial infection commonly manifests as meningitis, subdural empyema, or brain abscess. In recent large studies the incidence of postneurosurgical infection has been reported from less than 1% to greater than 10% and is dependent on how the data are collected and percentages are calculated.

It is difficult to assign proof that a given factor contributes to infection. Cerebrospinal fluid (CSF) leakage (commonly associated with posterior fossa and transnasal approaches), entry into the paranasal sinuses (clean-contaminated) and the use of external ventricular drainage consistently impact infection risk. Certain general patient characteristics have been associated with an increased risk of surgical infection and include extremes of age, diabetes mellitus, immunocompromised states and malignancy, as well as the presence of concomitant remote site infection such as pneumonia or urinary tract infection. The routine use of prophylactic preoperative antibiotic administration for the prevention of surgical site infection has become common practice in many institutions.

Spinal surgical infections are commonly of the incisional or soft tissue type. The incidence of postoperative intervertebral disc space infection (discitis) or osteomyelitis is less than 1%. Although postoperative spinal epidural abscess is rare, rapid deterioration to paralysis can occur.

M.K. Sturaitis, MD (✉)
Departments of Anesthesiology and Neurosurgery,
Rush University Medical Center, Chicago, IL, USA
e-mail: mary_sturaitis@rush.edu

A.M. Brambrink and J.R. Kirsch (eds.), *Essentials of Neurosurgical Anesthesia & Critical Care*, DOI 10.1007/978-0-387-09562-2_86,
© Springer Science+Business Media, LLC 2012

Prevention

The routine use of prophylactic antibiotics can promote microbial resistance and is not without potential adverse consequences. Antibiotic administration carries the risk of fatal anaphylaxis and allergic reactions; aminoglycosides can cause ototoxicity; hypotension and flushing can be seen with vancomycin.

Most neurosurgical operations are considered clean, and therefore inherently have the lowest risk of developing a surgical site infection. Nevertheless, the potential adverse effects of central nervous system infection accentuate any possible risk.

The efficacy of antimicrobial prophylaxis for clean neurosurgical procedures has been studied over several decades, and has been established in the neurosurgical literature. Current practice mandates coverage against gram-positive cocci, the most common skin contaminants being *Staphylococcus aureus* and *Staphylococcus epidermidis* (methicillin-susceptible). In procedures traversing the paranasal sinuses and that may be complicated by a postoperative CSF leak, *Streptococcus pneumoniae* becomes the common pathogenic species. However, the case for prophylaxis in these *clean-contaminated* (e.g., complex cranial base, transphenoidal) procedures has not been analyzed in the neurosurgical literature, and the assumption for efficacy has extended *primarily from the general surgical literature* (e.g., cholecystectomy, bowel resection) where benefit from preoperative antibiotics has been validated. In neurosurgical patients who have had an extended hospitalization prior to surgery, the incidence of postsurgical infections due to resistant organisms (methicillin-resistant *S. aureus*, vancomycin-resistant *Enterococcus*) and gram-negative organisms rises. Recent evidence has suggested that although perioperative antibiotic prophylaxis is clearly effective for the prevention of incisional infections, it does not appear to prevent postcraniotomy meningitis. The bacteria responsible for meningitis in those patients having received prophylactic antibiotics were predominantly noncutaneous, tended to be resistant to the antibiotic given and had a higher mortality risk, whereas in the patients not having received prophylaxis the microorganisms were cutaneous. Additionally, aseptic meningitis appears to be more frequent in prophylaxis patients.

Of note, the evidence for the timing and duration of prophylactic antibiotic administration also has been derived *primarily from the general surgical literature* where the maximum benefit for elective clean or clean-contaminated procedures was achieved when the drug was given within 30 min but no longer than 2 h of incision. Similarly in well-designed studies of clean cases from other specialties, there has been no additional benefit shown to extending antimicrobial prophylaxis past the operation.

Surgical duration, CSF leakage, and early reoperation are established risk factors for nosocomial meningitis, and preventative operative techniques may help limit this risk exposure.

Maintenance of a physiologic milieu in terms of perfusion, temperature, metabolism, and nutrition is recommended. Data generally is supportive of tight blood glucose management in the range of 80 to 140 mg/dl to prevent systemic infections and possible seeding from remote infection sites. In the setting of neural tissue at

Table 86.1 Prevention of postsurgical infections

Specific indication	Efficacy of prophylactic antibiotics
Placement of CSF shunt	• Efficacy established • ~ 50% reduction in infection rate
Basilar skull fractures with or without CSF leak	• Available data do not support routine use of prophylactic antibiotics
External ventricular drain (EVD)	• Controversial – some studies suggest beneficial effect but no clear evidence • Single dose at time of insertion more common than continued coverage (avoid resistant microorganisms)
	Other preventative measures • No difference in infection rate for ICU vs. operating room insertion • Strict aseptic technique, tunneling of catheter away from insertion site and minimal entry into system (i.e., CSF sampling only when clinically indicated) associated with decreased infection rates • Routine catheter change at specific intervals of no benefit (leave catheter in situ if not infected)

risk, however, overaggressive management causing hypoglycemia can be detrimental. Furthermore, serious hyperglycemia associated with severe CNS infections and poor outcome (e.g., meningitis), may actually be reflective of the severity of the infection.

For additional specific considerations regarding prevention of postsurgical infections see Table 86.1.

Crisis Intervention

Postoperative Meningitis

Pathophysiology and Clinical Presentation

- Incidence of postoperative bacterial meningitis <1% in clean neurosurgical procedures.
- Increased risk associated with CSF shunts, ventricular drainage catheters.
- Common organisms in healthy patients reflective of skin flora; *Staph aureus* (90%); *S. epidermidis*; *proprionobacteri* seen with ventriculoperitoneal shunts.
- Consider gram-negative organisms in patients with extended hospital stays and organisms prevalent to hospital environment.
- Clinical manifestations may overlap with neurological abnormalities expected in the postoperative period.
- Unexplained fevers, headache, altered level of consciousness with or without signs of meningeal irritation.

Patient Assessment

- CNS imaging prior to lumbar puncture in patients who have undergone recent craniotomy.
- CT – expected postsurgical changes in most patients, may show leptomeningeal enhancement.
- MRI – vascular enhancement, associated complications, e.g., sagittal sinus thrombosis.
- *CSF Analysis*

    - Polymorphonuclear leukocytosis >100 cells/mm^3. However, in CSF that is blood contaminated, that is, contains more than a few RBC (e.g., status post traumatic puncture, subarachnoid hemorrhage, etc.), the ratio of leukocytes to erythrocytes in CSF versus whole blood (cell index) should be considered. (Based on CSF analysis alone, a cell ratio of WBC:RBC £ 1:100 indicates that an acute bacterial infection of the CSF is very unlikely; but a CSF WBC:RBC ratio³ 1:100 should trigger further work-up).
    - ↑ protein (nonspecific, present with disruption of blood–brain barrier).
    - ↓ glucose (may be nonspecific, CSF/serum glucose ratio <0.4 suggestive).
    - Gram stain and culture for diagnosis (60 and 80% yield, less with perioperative prophylaxis).

- Initiating antimicrobial therapy prior to obtaining CSF sample should *not* significantly alter CSF WBC count (can see ↑ within 18–36 h) or CSF glucose concentration (return to normal within 3 days).

Aseptic meningitis is a chemical irritation of the meninges from blood introduced into the subarachnoid space at time of surgery and is a diagnosis of exclusion. Patients do not respond to antibiotics but show significant clinical improvement with corticosteroids.

Intervention

- Removal of hardware (e.g., shunts) and other suspicious material (bone flap).
- Empiric antibiotic coverage: gram-positive (Vancomycin) and gram-negative (third-generation cephalosporin, e.g., Cefotaxime, Ceftazidine). Add aminoglycoside if suspect Pseudomonas. Use Vancomycin with Cefepime or Meropenem with resistant strains.
- Efficacy of Vancomycin is hampered by poor CSF penetration. IV Vancomycin at usual dosages can achieve therapeutic concentration in CNS for at least 72 h postoperatively (possibly due to damage to blood–brain barrier that occurs during neurosurgical procedures and lasts for days). Some advocate the administration of intraventricular Vancomycin for EVD-associated staph ventriculitis given these patients may have less blood–brain barrier disruption compared to

postoperatively. Others argue the intraventricular inflammatory reaction in response to the local application is counterproductive.

- Watch for neurologic complications: seizures from focal areas of cortical irritability (e.g., subdural effusion/parenchymal abscess, septic thrombophlebitis); hydrocephalus secondary to inflammatory exudates.

Craniotomy Site or Bone Flap Infection

Pathophysiology and Clinical Presentation

- Associated with surgery of long duration, exposure involving air sinuses, reoperation, prior irradiation, immunosuppressive medical conditions, use of drains/foreign body, scalp devascularization involving the occipital or superior temporal artery.

Patient Assessment

- Fever, local erythema, tenderness, wound dehiscence, ± purulent discharge.

Intervention

- Fluctuance deep to the wound requires surgical drainage and debridement of tissue.
- Treat empirically for *Staphylococcal* infection ± gram-negative.
- Await cultures if patient is not toxic appearing.
- Bone flap is devascularized and consequently more at risk for infection therefore warranting aggressive therapy: removal of bone flap, prolonged systemic antibiotics (4–6 weeks), and followed by cranioplasty when infection eradicated.

Cranial Epidural Abscess and Subdural Empyema

Pathophysiology and Clinical Presentation

- Associated with craniotomy wound site infection, suppuration of paranasal sinuses or foreign body from trauma.
- Epidural abscesses alone may not cause neurologic symptoms, but 10% of epidural abscesses associated with subdural empyema.

- Subdural empyema is a surgical emergency progressing to death if untreated (20% mortality, 30% neurologic morbidity).

Patient Assessment

- Fever, mild mental changes in some patients.
- Lab data are nondiagnostic.
- Epidural abscess seen as lentiform (biconvex) and subdural empyema seen as crescentic on imaging.
- Enhanced MRI can usually differentiate from other subdural collections (effusion, hematoma) – increased signal adjacent to cerebral cortex due to inflammatory edema suggests empyema; MRI may demonstrate complications such as cortical/dural vein thrombosis.

Intervention

- Seizure prophylaxis for subdural empyema.
- Initial empiric IV antibiotic therapy should be broad spectrum.
- Surgical debridement and removal of bone flap.
- Operative cultures positive in 90%; extended IV antibiotics 4–6 weeks.
- Serial imaging following evacuation to monitor for reaccumulation of pus.

Cerebral Abscess

Pathophysiology and Clinical Presentation

- Incidence approximately 0.1% of clean neurosurgical procedures.
- Often associated with abnormal host defenses.
- Solitary lesion from bacteria introduced intracranially at the time of surgery, from trauma, or via contiguous spread from a parameningeal focus.
- Multiple lesions associated with systemic infection and hematogenous spread (grey–white junction, often in MCA artery distribution).

Patient Assessment

- Laboratory findings are generally nondiagnostic.
- Ring enhancing lesion – CT/MRI findings confounded by postoperative changes; steroids may decrease enhancement in early stages.

Intervention

- Nonoperative management considered in early cerebritis stage (without mass effect and with known organism), in cases with multiple small abscesses or abscess in eloquent brain region.
- Most cases require surgical intervention in addition to IV antibiotics (6 weeks).
- Aspiration (open vs. stereotactic, ultrasound guidance).
- Steroids only in cases with severe edema; rapid taper.
- Prophylactic anticonvulsants if near cortex.

Postoperative Spinal Infections (Table 86.2)

Pathophysiology

- Incidence of postoperative spinal infection increases with complexity of procedure: discectomy <1% risk; spinal fusion 1–5% without instrumentation, >6% with instrumentation.
- *S. aureaus* (>50%), many patients with multiple organisms.
- Patient risk factors include advanced age, obesity and diabetes, prolonged hospital bed rest, remote infection.
- Surgical risk factors include prolonged surgery, hardware, use of microscope.
- Spinal epidural abscess after decompression is rare, but rapid neurologic deterioration to paralysis occurs; associated with osteomyelitis; mortality for cervical spinal epidural abscess approaches 18%.

Table 86.2 Postoperative spinal infection

Spinal infection	Clinical presentation	Assessment	Intervention
Wound Infection	• Persistent temperature elevation several days postop • Tenderness, erythema, swelling, drainage	• Gram stain, culture	• Antibiotic therapy • Wound debridement and irrigation for deep tissue or persistent infection despite antibiotic therapy

(continued)

Table 86.2 (continued)

Spinal infection	Clinical presentation	Assessment	Intervention
Discitis	• Typically asymptomatic immediately after surgery • Excruciating back pain or spasms with or without radiation to legs within 2 weeks • Extreme local tenderness and fever	• Spine XR, temperature, WBC with differential is often normal • ↑ESR ↑CRP • CT sensitive early • Bone scan/MRI sensitive but may be falsely positive early in postop period	• Early recognition and treatment to prevent chronic infection • Disc space aspiration (CT-guided) often negative • 4–6 weeks antibiotics until normalization of ESR/CRP • Spinal immobilization • Uncomplicated discitis rarely requires surgery (vs. osteomyelitis requiring surgical intervention)
Spinal epidural abscess	• *Classic triad*: localized back pain, progressive neurologic deficit, fever • *Progression and time course of symptoms uniform*: radicular symptoms within 3 days, followed by weakness within 36 h, paralysis over the next 24 h • Cervical epidural abscesses develop more rapidly and with severe neurologic deficits (smaller epidural space)	• ↑WBC and fever is *absent* in over half of cases • ↑ESR (>75 mm/h) common, nonspecific • MRI can localize	• Emergent spinal decompression • IV antibiotic therapy 4–6 weeks followed by oral therapy

WBC white blood cell count, *ESR* erythrocyte sedimentation rate, *CRP* C-reactive protein

Key Points

- Postoperative neurosurgical infections occur despite best practice. However, the incidence can be minimized. Patients of advanced age, those with diabetes/hyperglycemia or with immunocompromised medical conditions are at higher risk.
- Intracranial subdural empyema is an immediate life-threatening condition; extradural empyema is typically a more subacute condition requiring removal of bone plate.

- Prophylactic antibiotics are clearly beneficial in patients undergoing ventricular peritoneal shunting. Available data do not support routine antibiotic prophylaxis for basilar skull fractures.
- External ventricular drains may be left in place until clear evidence of infection develops. Routine CSF sampling is not indicated. Intraventricular antibiotics may be indicated in certain EVD-related infections.
- Antibiotic coverage should be tailored to prevalent institutional flora.

Suggested Reading

Hoefnagel D, Dammers R, Laak-Poort M, Avezaat CJ. Risk factors for infections related to external ventricular drainage. Acta Neurochir (Wein). 2008;150:209–14.

Korinek A, Baugnon T, Golmard J, et al. Risk factors for adult nosocomial meningitis after craniotomy: role of antibiotic prophylaxis. Neurosurgery. 2006;59:126–33.

McClelland III S, Hall WA. Postoperative central nervous system infection: incidence and associated factors in 2111 neurosurgical procedures. Clin Infect Dis. 2007;45:55–9.

Osenbach RK. Neurosurgical infections. In: Batjer H, Loftus C, editors. Textbook of neurological surgery. Philadelphia, PA: Lippincott-Raven; 2003. p. 3089–267.

Ratilal BO, Costa J, Sampaio C. Antibiotic prophylaxis for preventing meningitis in patients with basilar skull fractures (review). Cochrane Collaboration. 2009;1:1–17.

Wang Q, Zhonghua S, Wang J, et al. Postoperatively administered vancomycin reaches therapeutic concentration in the cerebral spinal fluid of neurosurgical patients. Surg Neurol. 2008;69:126–9.

Zeidman SM, Ducker TB. Infectious complications of spine surgery. In: Benzel EC, editor. Spine surgery: techniques, complication avoidance, and management. Philadelphia, PA: Churchill Livingstone Inc.; 2005. p. 2013–26.

Chapter 87
Antiepileptic Drug Therapy in Neurosurgical Critical Care

Panayiotis N. Varelas and Denise H. Rhoney

There are three postoperative situations when the neuroanesthesiologist may encounter use of antiepileptic drugs (AEDs):

- Prophylactic use after craniotomy for various reasons.
- Continuation of preoperative AEDs (with special subcategories after epilepsy surgery or, if used outside an epilepsy indication, for example, for neuropathic pain/trigeminal neuralgia).
- Initiation of AEDs because of a postoperative seizure or status epilepticus (SE).

Although the older generation of AEDs has more drug interactions with perioperative medications, it is the newer AEDs that bring more uncertainty, due to a less-known (but probably much safer) profile or less familiarity with their use and interactions.

Overview

The prevalence of epilepsy is estimated worldwide at 0.5–2% of the total population. One-fourth to one-third of these epileptic patients may have more than one seizure per month and one-fifth may have medically uncontrolled seizures. On the other hand, many neurosurgical conditions increase the risk for seizures (Table 87.1).

Although the incidence of immediate seizures (within 24 h) after craniotomy is estimated at 3 and 77.5% of those occur within 6 h, the incidence of perioperative

P.N. Varelas, MD, PhD (✉)
Departments of Neurology & Neurosurgery, Henry Ford Hospital, Detroit, MI, USA
e-mail: varelas@neuro.hfh.edu

D.H. Rhoney, Pharm.D, FCCP, FCCM
Department of Pharmacy Practice, Wayne State University,
Eugene Applebaum College of Pharmacy and Health Sciences, Detroit, MI, USA

A.M. Brambrink and J.R. Kirsch (eds.), *Essentials of Neurosurgical Anesthesia & Critical Care*, DOI 10.1007/978-0-387-09562-2_87, © Springer Science+Business Media, LLC 2012

Table 87.1 Risk for seizures after common neurosurgical interventions (modified from Manaka et al.)

	Incidence of postop seizures (%)		Incidence of postop seizures (%)
Arteriovenous malformation	50	Glioma	Biopsy 9
		Metastasis	Resection 20
Intracerebral hematoma	10–20	Suprasellar tumor	5
Cerebral aneurysm	7.5–38	Shunt	22
Meningioma	36	Abscess	92

AED use is unknown. Many of these patients receive AEDs on admission prophylactically and some therapeutically (if they present with a seizure or have a history of seizures). The AEDs used in this situation are those available in an intravenous form. If seizures were diagnosed before the index admission or surgery, the majority of these patients will also be on chronic oral AED management, with various rates of compliance.

Prevention

Medications that have epileptogenic potential should be avoided during the perioperative period in neurosurgical patients. For example, atracurium may decrease the threshold for seizures via accumulation of its metabolite laudanosine and meperidine can also provoke seizures via its metabolite normeperidine and should be used with caution, if at all. In addition, drugs that are associated with seizures in supratherapeutic concentrations (i.e., antibiotics) should have the dosage adjusted for the patient's hepatic or renal impairment in order to minimize the occurrence of seizures.

On the other hand, chronic AED administration may interfere with anesthetic agents during surgery. For example, liver enzyme inducers, like phenytoin, carbamazepine, or phenobarbital reduce the paralytic effect of nondepolarizing neuromuscular blockers. Higher doses of fentanyl may also be required in epileptic patients on AEDs to maintain a comparable depth of analgesia.

Epileptic patients undergoing surgery may not have received their morning AEDs and if those have a short half-life (e.g., valproate, gabapentin, carbamazepine), their levels may drop precipitously and seizures may emerge during the postoperative period. Therefore, a clear list of the home AEDs and the last time that the patient received them is imperative. In patients undergoing intracranial electrode placement the goal is to allow seizures to emerge in order to be recorded. These patients usually are left with fewer AEDs or at decreased doses in the postoperative period intentionally. The neuroanesthesiologist should have a clear understanding of the postoperative plan after discussion with the attending epileptologist or neurosurgeon.

If a serum concentration of the drug is routinely measurable, one should test a trough concentration. For most of AEDs, this corresponds to a level drawn 6–8 h after the most recent dose or a level before the scheduled next dose. Frequently, a mistake is made by not confirming the timing of the last dose and measuring the concentration at its peak phase: it will be artificially high (which may erroneously lead to withholding the next dose or reducing the amount). Seizures may also occur later if this drug drops to subtherapeutic concentrations.

Another cause for confusion is the presence of low albumin in many critically ill or malnourished patients. AEDs highly bound to albumin (phenytoin, valproate) may have low total concentrations in this case, but the free concentration may be adequate. Therefore, free and total AED concentrations should always be measured before adding or withholding an AED that is highly protein bound.

Prophylactic administration of AEDs in patients undergoing craniotomy without previous seizures is not advocated. Despite the presence of cerebral lesions, such as tumors or ischemic stroke, the most recent guidelines do not support prophylactic AED treatment. For head trauma, the guidelines support treatment for up to 1 week to prevent early posttraumatic seizures. For hemorrhagic stroke, the current trend is that they should not be continued for more than 1 week in patients with subarachnoid hemorrhage after securing the cerebral aneurysm and for a brief period (e.g., up to 1 month) after ICH, especially lobar. The physician should, however, individualize the treatment, since specific subgroups of patients may benefit from prophylactic AEDs for longer periods.

If seizures had occurred before or during surgery, however, AEDs should be administered as in any other nonneurosurgical patient presenting with seizures.

Crisis Management

Pathophysiology and Clinical Presentation

Presurgical brain pathology is the most common reason for having preoperative seizures. Two major mechanisms, however, play a role in the development of seizures after craniotomy:

- Free radical generation, mainly due to iron and thrombin from blood components that have leaked in the tissue during surgery.
- Disturbance of ion balance across the cell membranes due to local ischemia or hypoxia.

Additionally, one should not forget that systemic etiologies may also play a role:

- Severe hypoxia–ischemia.
- Drug/substance toxicity or withdrawal.
- Metabolic derangements.
- Systemic infection, including meningitis, ventriculitis, or encephalitis.

The majority of postoperative patients will present with partial seizures, either simple partial (focal motor or sensory phenomena without alteration of consciousness), complex partial (with alteration of consciousness) or partial with secondary generalization (bilateral tonic–clonic convulsions with loss of consciousness). Primary generalized seizures may also occur in an epileptic patient carrying this diagnosis, but pseudoseizures should be considered as low probability in the postoperative period.

The definition of status epilepticus (SE) has evolved over the years and now many experts define it as either a prolonged seizure or multiple seizures in sequence lasting for >5–10 min (without regaining consciousness in-between). A more ominous condition is refractory status epilepticus (RSE), defined as status not controlled after the initial parenteral therapy with the first 2–3 standard "front-line" AEDs or lasting > 1–2 h.

Patient Assessment

- Basic ABCs (establishing a patent airway; assist ventilation as needed; assess and control cardiovascular function). Avoid hyperventilation (unless mandated for other reasons).
- Secure more than one intravenous catheter (peripheral catheters can be easily dislodged or veins blown during convulsions).
- Draw labs for electrolytes, glucose, AED concentrations, ammonia and liver enzymes, toxicology screen, and blood gases. Derangements such as hypoglycemia, hyponatremia, hypocalcemia, hypomagnesemia, hypoxia or hyper- or hypocarbia should be corrected.
- (Initial management of patient is discussed below). After discussion with the attending neurosurgeon or epileptologist, consider a STAT CT of the head to exclude hemorrhage or ischemia.
- Electroencephalogram (EEG), either emergent or continuous, based on the continuation of seizures and the mental status of patient (to exclude ongoing nonconvulsive seizures or SE).

Intervention/Treatment

Patients Already Taking AEDs Before Surgery

The home AEDs should be administered orally at the usual doses in epileptic patients as soon as they are awake enough to swallow or as soon as a bedside swallowing evaluation is completed (because many neurosurgical patients may emerge from surgery with significant new deficits precluding safe oral administration of food and drugs). An alternative, placement of a naso- or orogastric tube and administration of the AEDs is also feasible in the majority of cases.

It is preferable, however, to use AEDs available in parenteral forms in the postoperative period because of potential erratic enteral absorption. Currently, seven major AEDs are available in an intravenous form in the US (Table 87.2). These medications should be used in the IV form to substitute the oral form of the same medication (until the enteral route and absorption is confirmed) or if an extra dose is required to reach therapeutic concentrations rapidly. Additionally, they can be used as a temporary

Table 87.2 Intravenously available AEDs

IV AED	Mechanism of action	Protein binding (%)	$T_{1/2}$ (hours)	Metabolism; elimination	Therapeutic level	Dose
Phenytoin or fosphenytoin	Na+ channel block	90–96	24±12	Hepatic	10–20 µg/ml	L: 18–20 mg/kg IV M: 3–5 mg/kg/day IV[a]
Phenobarbital	Prolongs Cl- channel onductance	20–45	96±12	Hepatic; renal 25%	10–40 µg/ml	L: 20 mg/kg IV M: 2–4 mg/kg/day IV
Pentobarbital	Prolongs Cl- channel conductance	35–40	15–50	Hepatic; renal	10–50 µg/ml	L: 10–15 mg/kg IV M: 0.5–10 mg/kg/h IV to induce burst-suppression on EEG
Thiopental	Prolongs Cl- channel conductance	80	3–6	Hepatic; renal	30–100 µg/ml	L: 50–150 mg IV M: 3–5 mg/kg/h IV
Propofol	Inhibits NMDA receptors; Activates Cl- conductance	95–99	3–12 depending on the duration of gtts	Hepatic; renal	–	L: 1–2 mg/kg IV M: 2–10 mg/kg/h IV
Lorazepam	Increases Cl- channel conductance	90	8–25	Hepatic	–	L: 0.07–0.1 mg/kg IV
Diazepam	Increases Cl- channel conductance	90	24–57	Hepatic		L: 0.15–0.25 mg/kg IV
Midazolam	Increases Cl- channel conductance	94–97	1–5	Hepatic; renal	–	L: 0.1 mg/kg IV M: 0.1–1 mg/kg/h IV
Valproate	Slow Ca++ channel block; Na+ channel block	90	8±2	Hepatic	50–120 µg/ml	L: 10–25 mg/kg IV M: 15–50 mg/kg/day IV
Levetiracetam	Binding to synaptic vesicle protein 2A	<10	7±1	Renal	Not recommended by manufacturer	<65 year old: 500–1,000 mg q 12 h IV >65-year old: 250–500 mg q 12 h IV
Lacosamide	Na+ channel block; binds to collapsin response mediator protein-2 (CRMP-2)	<15	13	Renal	Not recommended by manufacturer	100–200 mg q12 h IV

L loading dose, M maintenance dose

[a]Doses are phenytoin equivalents for fosphenytoin dosing (e.g., fosphenytoin IV: give 18 mg/kg phenytoin equivalents)

alternative to different home AEDs not available parenterally, if an oral/gastric administration is not feasible or enteral absorption is questionable. As a rule of thumb, total IV doses are similar to the total daily oral dose of the same medication, but may be administered at different frequencies. It is important to remember that

- Phenytoin can be administered at a maximum rate of 50 mg/min (in nonemergent situations in 30–60 min for 1 g IV) and is mixed only with normal saline. Since the cardiovascular suppression effects are synergistic with anesthetics, rate of administration should be much slower in the anesthetized patient. Phenytoin also exhibits nonlinear pharmacokinetics, which may lead to supratherapeutic or subtherapeutic concentrations, so a free level (target 1–2 µg/ml) should also be measured. In the absence of IV access, fosphenytoin can be administered IM as phenytoin equivalents (PE, i.e., 1 mg of PE is the same as 1 mg of phenytoin).
- Phenobarbital's sedative effect is minimized after a few weeks and, therefore, in chronic users may not be a problem in the postoperative period.
- The two benzodiazepines, lorazepam, and diazepam are rarely used in chronic AED regimens and their use is limited to management of seizures or SE (*vide infra*).
- Valproate is an excellent drug for primary generalized epilepsies, but one should be careful using it in patients with hepatic failure, thrombocytopenia and pancreatitis, if at all.
- From the newer AEDs, only levetiracetam and lacosamide are available in an IV formulation. These agents are renally eliminated, have minimal interactions with other common medications, and offer advantages in the ease of their use. However, patients with renal impairment will require dosage adjustment. Both agents have complete bioequivalence to the oral dose.

Patients Experiencing a Single Postoperative Generalized Seizure

In this situation, there is usually no time to administer an AED while the patient is convulsing and close observation for a second seizure is required. During this period of time three important diagnostic and therapeutic steps should be undertaken:

(1) Prophylaxis for a second seizure is usually achieved by administering the home AEDs in patients with presurgical epilepsy. If the patient has never experienced seizures before, phenytoin IV (load and continue with the maintenance dose, Table 87.2) or valproate (in phenytoin allergy) or levetiracetam (if allergy to the other two AEDs is suspected or hepatic dysfunction is present) should be administered. Thiamine (100 mg IV) and lorazepam (1–2 mg IV over 3–5 min) are reasonable alternatives for patients with a history of heavy alcohol abuse. These patients are usually not at risk for loss of airway reflexes or catastrophic cardiovascular sequelae. However, use of supplemental oxygen and padding of the bed are recommended.
(2) The diagnostic workup (see above).
(3) If the patients remain encephalopathic or with new unexplained focality in their neurological exam for more than 20–30 min (which is the usual postictal

confusional period), an emergent EEG is also reasonable, to exclude subclinical seizures or interictal activity accounting for the mental status change. Such situation should also result in a careful consideration of the need for an urgent head CT as the seizures could have precipitated postoperative hemorrhage or edema.

Patients Experiencing Multiple Generalized Seizures or SE

This is an emergency and treatment should proceed at a fast pace. The management steps in this situation are similar to those for a single uncomplicated seizure (see above) as far as the diagnostic part (continuous video-EEG monitoring is advocated by many experts; consider STAT head CT). The treatment part is different with focus on ABCs and with benzodiazepines (lorazepam, see Table 87.3) as first-line AEDs.

- Lorazepam is preferable to diazepam, because of lack of active metabolites and redistribution to extracerebral tissues. If these lines of defense fail and seizures continue, the algorithm uses midazolam or general anesthetics.

Table 87.3 Management of multiple seizures or status epilepticus (modified from Varelas and Mirski)

Initial measures
- ABC. Preserve airway and oxygenation by intubation
- Check blood glucose. If less 40–60 mg/dL, give 1 amp DW 50% and recheck in 30–60 min. Give 100 mg thiamine IV
- Check blood count, electrolytes, liver enzymes, toxicology screen, arterial blood gases, and antiepileptic drug concentrations
- Immediately and in parallel with above steps: IV lorazepam 5–10 mg (0.1 mg/kg), diazepam 20–40 mg, or midazolam 5–20 mg over 5 min
- Phenytoin loading dose 20 mg/kg at a maximum rate of 50 mg/min or fosphenytoin 20 mg/kg PE at a maximum rate of 50 mg/min (slower rate when under general anesthesia). Consider Valproic acid IV load 15–20 mg/kg, maintenance 400–600 mg q6 h in phenytoin intolerant patients. Consider IV levetiracetam 1,500 mg bid, if patients are intolerant to phenytoin or valproic
- Continuous video-EEG monitoring, if available; consider STAT head CT

Seizures continue clinically or electrographically

Additional phenytoin or fosphenytoin (IV 5–10 mg/kg or 5–10 mg/kg PE) or valproic acid IV load 15–20 mg/kg

Refractory status (seizures > 60 min):
- Mechanical ventilation. Avoid hyperventilation ($PaCO_2$ 38–45, if intracranial pressure normal)
- Institute 10–20 sec burst-suppression pattern on EEG: propofol 2 mg/kg bolus IV and 100–150 mcg/kg/min infusion or thiopental 3–4 mg/kg bolus IV and 0.3–0.4 mg/kg/min. Alternatively, or if burst-suppression not achieved, use pentobarbital boluses (6–12 mg/kg IV at 0.2–0.4 mg/kg/min) and titrate infusion at 0.25–4.0 mg/kg/h
- Hemodynamic support – fluids, pressors, inotropes
- Consider STAT CT of the head, if not done; the EEG leads must be removed before the CT (to avoid artifacts) and replaced after
- Transfer to the Neuro-ICU
- Once EEG suppressed, continue for 12–24 h and start weaning from general anesthetics

- Midazolam may convey an advantage compared to propofol for seizure control, but if burst-suppression becomes the goal (as in RSE), propofol and, especially, barbiturates are stronger choices.
- Pentobarbital is preferable to phenobarbital because of shorter elimination ($T_{1/2}$ around 24 h vs. 96 h) and in a meta-analysis was more efficacious than midazolam or propofol (albeit with higher risk for hypotension). Blood concentration monitoring is not very helpful in this situation, since there is inconsistent relationship between serum concentration and seizure control.

Key Points

- Home antiepileptics should be administered as earliest as possible in the postoperative period.
- If the patient is unable to swallow or is vomiting, the intravenous form of the home drug should be used. If no IV form is available, load with one of the IV antiepileptics (phenytoin, valproate, or levetiracetam), if the patient had seizures before.
- Craniotomy per se is not a reason for prophylactic antiepileptics.
- If patient has one postop seizure, check trough antiepileptic drug concentrations and, if low, supplement with the IV form. Check STAT glucose and electrolytes. Consider STAT CT of the head and EEG.
- If patient has multiple seizures or enters SE, use the ABC algorithm in parallel with lorazepam up to 0.1 mg/kg IV, load with phenytoin up to 20 mg/kg IV, do a fast diagnostic workup and, if seizures continue, consider general anesthetics with continuous EEG monitoring.

Suggested Reading

Kofke AW, Tempelhoff R, Dasheiff RM. Anesthetic implications of epilepsy, status epilepticus and epilepsy surgery. J Neurosurg Anesthesiol. 1997;9(4):349–72.

Manaka S, Ishijima B, Mayanagi Y. Postoperative seizures: epidemiology, pathology and prophylaxis. Neurol Med Chir (Tokyo). 2003;43:589–600.

Varelas P, Mirski M. Seizures in the adult ICU. J Neurosurg Anesthesiol. 2001;13(2):163–75.

Varelas P, Spanaki M. Management of status epilepticus and critical care seizures. In: Varelas P, editor. Seizures in critical care: a guide to diagnosis and therapeutics. Totowa, NJ: Humana Press; 2004. p. 305–64.

Chapter 88
Withdrawal of Mechanical Ventilation in Neurosurgical Critical Care

Paul Bascom

Overview

Patients arrive in the Neuro ICU critically ill, and their care providers rapidly initiate a variety of measures to sustain life. Commonly, this means placement of an endotracheal tube, and initiation of mechanical ventilation. In the days that follow, further diagnostic testing, or lack of response to treatment, may prompt a discussion with family members about whether to continue these life-sustaining measures. Chapter 91 discusses how to conduct conversations with families in this circumstance. These conversations frequently will conclude with a decision to withdraw life-sustaining measures, such as mechanical ventilation, thus allowing the patient's natural death to occur.

   In the past, some physicians chose to play a very limited role in the procedure. The physician would broadly delegate this responsibility to the nurse and respiratory therapist. A typical set of orders might read: "initiate morphine infusion (titrate to comfort)" and "extubate the patient." The physician would then move on to other responsibilities, leaving the implementation of the orders to the nurse and respiratory therapist. Often, there would be no careful assessment for what might occur upon extubation, nor any specific guidance provided about how to respond as symptoms developed. Such an approach can lead to poor symptom control, increased burdens on staff, and insufficient attention to the experience of the family.

   This chapter seeks to provide some specific guidance to staff in the Neuro ICU caring for patients when life support is withdrawn. Salient points include: remaining present for the key moments of the procedure, involving family and ICU staff in creating a plan for withdrawal, performing a careful assessment before the withdrawal to best anticipate the trajectory after withdrawal, and having sedatives and opiates available in doses that ensure a prompt response to patient symptoms.

P. Bascom, MD, FACP (✉)
Department of Hematology and Oncology, Oregon Health & Science University,
Portland, OR, USA
e-mail: bascomp@ohsu.edu

A.M. Brambrink and J.R. Kirsch (eds.), *Essentials of Neurosurgical Anesthesia & Critical Care*, DOI 10.1007/978-0-387-09562-2_88, © Springer Science+Business Media, LLC 2012

Implications for the Neurosurgical Patient

A poorly planned or poorly implemented withdrawal of life support in the Neuro ICU can result in notable physical suffering for the patient. Though some patients with catastrophic illnesses or injuries will be deeply comatose and insensate, others will have some retained awareness, and will experience distress when symptoms remain uncontrolled. Families as well may suffer, as they witness uncontrolled agitation or respiratory distress in their loved one, even if the patient is deeply comatose. Families may carry memories of their loved one's uncomfortable dying for many years. Alternatively, when withdrawal of life support is carried out with skill and compassion, not only will patients benefit, but their families may be able to move into their grieving with a sense of gratitude for a painless and comfortable dying.

Concerns and Risks

Patients in the Neuro ICU may have specific characteristics that distinguish them from patients in a general medical or surgical ICU. Patients in medical and surgical ICUs more often have multiorgan failure. As such these patients have very little physiological reserve. Withdrawal of mechanical ventilation, often accompanied by discontinuation of pressor medications, usually leads to prompt cardiopulmonary collapse. There may be few visible symptoms, as respiratory capacity and drive are quite limited, and cognition impaired by encephalopathy.

In contrast, many patients with isolated catastrophic brain injuries and illnesses will have substantial, and even excellent, cardiopulmonary function. This means that the trajectory toward dying in these patients can be quite variable. A study in 1999 found a median survival after extubation of 7.5 h, with a range of 10 min to 11 days. Agonal or labored breathing occurred in 59% of patients.

In general, three broad trajectories can be expected:

- Near Apnea with minimal respiratory effort. These patients will die quickly with a minimum of signs or symptoms.
- Excellent retained ventilatory function, even after discontinuation of mechanical ventilation. These patients may breathe quite comfortably after extubation, and may have a prolonged trajectory, with survival measured in days to a few weeks, with death intervening from dehydration or respiratory infection.
- Some retained ventilatory function and effort, but with progressive dyspnea and respiratory distress in the hours following extubation. This may be due to respiratory muscle fatigue, increased upper airway resistance due to decreased level of consciousness, or retained secretions. These patients may linger for several hours, and will require frequent assessment, and alteration of the treatment regimen for tachypnea and labored breathing. Rarely, extubation may lead to immediate severe upper airway obstruction. This is the most challenging patient, as extubation may lead to stridorous breathing and severe respiratory distress.

Table 88.1 Sample order set to guide withdrawal of mechanical ventilation

Do not resuscitate, do not intubate (if not already noted in chart)

Attending signature_____

Note written in chart documenting discussions with family leading to change in goals of care to comfort

Nursing interventions

☐ Implement standards of nursing care for end of life/comfort care discontinue vital signs, I/Os, monitoring except as needed to assess patient comfort/prognosis. Remove NG tube, sequential compression devices, extra IV sites

Respiratory therapy interventions

1. Spontaneous breathing trial (SBT) to assess prognosis and potential symptoms. Goal: CPAP 5/5; no change in FiO2
2. Record symptoms and rapid shallow breathing index (RSBI/Tobin Index)
3. Resume prior vent settings as soon as patient is symptomatic or unstable

MD orders

☐ Discontinue all medications, IV fluids, and tube feeds except those medication such as vasopressors that sustain life moment to moment

Medication principles for vent withdrawal

1. Provide frequent boluses as necessary to control symptoms
2. If already on analgesics and sedatives maintain continuous infusion at current level
3. No change in continuous infusion until patient stable and trachea extubated

Opiate (choose one only)

☐ Morphine 5–10 mg IV q 15″ as needed (prn) for pain/dyspnea RR >20

☐ Hydromorphone 1–2 mg IV q 15″ prn pain/dyspnea RR >20

☐ Fentanyl 50–100 mcg IV q 15″ prn pain/dyspnea RR >20

Sedative (choose one only)

☐ Lorazepam 1–2 mg q 20″ IV prn distress

☐ Midazolam 1–2 mg q 15″ IV prn distress

☐ Propofol 20–40 mg q 5″ IV prn distress

Procedure – begin upon confirmation from family that is ready to proceed

1. Discontinue pressors – if indicated. If death likely upon discontinuation of pressors, await imminent cardiac death before ventilator withdrawal
2. Wean mechanical ventilation to CPAP and room air
   (a) If earlier SBT uneventful proceed directly to tracheal extubation
   (b) If symptomatic for respiratory distress during SBT, then wean pressure support to CPAP over 20–30 min, administering bolus opiate and/or sedative with each decrease in ventilator support to maintain calm respirations
3. Discontinue ventilator and extubate trachea (unless patient has tracheostomy)
   (a) Proceed only if symptoms controlled on CPAP
   (b) Monitor carefully for upper airway obstruction

Key Points

- *Remain present*. Optimal coordination of withdrawal of mechanical ventilation occurs when the physician remains present and involved during the key portions of the process. Patients with impending death may generate strong emotional reactions for the ICU physician. These emotions, along with the pressure of other critically ill patients may lead physicians to distance themselves from the process. The physician who remains present will not only ensure a good outcome, but will be able to witness and receive the gratitude of the family for their loved one's safe and peaceful dying.
- *Care for the family*. Create a setting conducive to family presence in the room. Encourage families to bring in photos, music, or other mementos of their loved one. Extraneous medical devices, that is, SCDs, monitoring devices, etc., should be removed. Those families with specific religious beliefs or practices may incorporate those rituals into their time at the bedside. Often, the pace and timing of a withdrawal will be dictated by family concerns or preferences. Withdrawals may be delayed so that families can gather at the bedside for the death. Time at the bedside can be spent eliciting reminiscences of the loved one, as a way of transitioning families toward their time of grief. Families will benefit from specific guidance about what to expect as the withdrawal proceeds. Some family members will prefer to remain at the bedside throughout the process. Others will prefer to remain in the waiting room until stable breathing and symptom control are achieved. Others will choose to leave the building and ask to be notified by phone when the death occurs. Such preferences should be solicited and respected. Their perception of their loved one's distress should be sought, as perhaps the best "gold standard" of the patient's suffering. Frequent updates should be provided as the withdrawal proceeds. A physician's calm presence in the room as extubation proceeds will help reassure families that symptoms will be promptly assessed and alleviated.
- *Work closely and collaboratively with the other members of the ICU staff*. The nurses and respiratory therapists will be most effective when they have the opportunity to participate in the creation of a plan for withdrawal of mechanical ventilation. Table 88.1 has specific examples of orders to guide nursing staff and respiratory therapists. Some staff members will be highly experienced and skilled, while others may be inexperienced and caring for a dying patient for one of the first times in their career. A well-functioning interdisciplinary team has the flexibility to assess and adjust to the skills and capabilities of the other team members.
- *Perform a spontaneous breathing trial*. This brief trial provides valuable information both for families and for the team implementing the withdrawal. For example, if there is near complete apnea, then families can be advised that the death will occur quickly. The nurse will know that minimal

sedatives or opiates will be needed for control of tachypnea. In contrast, if the trial shows excellent ventilatory function, then families can be advised well in advance that dying may be prolonged. In such a circumstance the family should expect a transfer out of the intensive care unit to a hospital ward, nursing home, hospice facility, or even home. When the breathing trial provokes significant agitation and tachypnea, the trial helps anticipate the level of symptoms during weaning. Many patients may appear unresponsive while receiving intermittent mandatory ventilation, yet may become agitated upon receiving the stimulation to breath.

- *Wean ventilator support as guided by results of spontaneous breathing trial*. Those patients with symptoms noted on spontaneous breathing trial will need gradual decrease in ventilator support over 20–30 min. There is no specific right way to decrease this support. One method is to switch to pressure support (PS) mode, which allows the patients underlying respiratory drive to emerge. Frequent boluses of sedative and opiate medication are administered to control symptoms. As PS is diminished, then demands on the respiratory system increase, and further boluses are given. Once respiratory drive and effort are controlled (RR < 20 and calm) at PS of 0, then extubation can proceed. This whole process need not take more than 15–30 min. For those patients with near complete apnea or excellent ventilator function on spontaneous breathing trial, extubation can occur directly, without any weaning.

- *Extubate with attention to upper airway and body positioning*. There are no specific data to guide whether to remove the endotracheal tube. However, leaving the endotracheal tube in place may unnecessarily prolong the dying process, and families may miss the chance to see their loved one's last moments free of medical devices. Removal of the endotracheal tube is usually well tolerated. At times, the removal of the endotracheal tube will cause a significant increase in upper airway resistance. In these cases, an excellent spontaneous breathing trial will be misleading. These patient upon extubation develop notable respiratory distress or, at a minimum, noisy breathing. The sudden respiratory distress in this circumstance requires prompt administration of additional opiates or sedatives. Noisy breathing may resolve with changes in body position. Some practitioners recommend routine use of steroids (to decrease airway edema) and anticholinergics (to decrease airway secretions) prior to extubation.

- *Provide frequent boluses of sedatives and/or opiates for relief of distressing symptoms*. Continuous infusion are useful for maintaining symptom control, but not for immediate symptom relief. Some initial starting doses are noted in Table 88.1. These doses can be increased by 50–100%, when the initial doses are ineffective. Those patients already receiving continuous infusions of opiates and/or sedatives may need starting bolus doses equal to their continuous rate. Opiates are used primarily for control of respiratory distress, and sedatives for generalized agitation, though these agents may be more effective in combination. Analgesics and sedatives should be administered according to the patient's level of symptoms. For example, medication might be administered until respiratory rate is under 20 min and there is an absence of grimacing or labored breathing. Studies have confirmed that there is no risk of hastening death when opiates are titrated in this fashion. Paradoxically, effective control of respiratory rate may delay respiratory muscle fatigue and time to death. Families, at times, may express distress as their loved one lingers quietly near death. This distress can be acknowledged, even as families are informed that increasing medication with the goal of hastening death is not permitted. Once symptoms are controlled no further bolus medication need be administered, and a continuous infusion should be administered at 25–50% of the total bolus dose required to achieve symptom control. Morphine infusion dosages usually range from 2–20 mg/h.

- *Provide bereavement support.* Kind and empathetic words, such as "You all have demonstrated how much you care for your loved one in making this difficult decision," "He (or she) must have been a remarkable person," or "This is such a sad time for all of you" will be help families feel supported as they enter their time of grief. This can be a time also for the team to gather together and share memories they have of the patient, and express gratitude for the opportunity to care for patients and families in such an emotional and difficult time.
- *Prepare if prolonged survival is expected.* Some patients will survive days after extubation. These patients often will be discharged from the ICU. Options for care outside the ICU may include hospital ward, inpatient hospice unit, or even the patient's home, in certain circumstances. Transfers of care must be well coordinated to insure continuity of symptom control and complete understanding of goals of care and family needs by the accepting medical team. Careful and ongoing assessments of prognosis will ensure that transfers happen only when justified by expected duration of life.

Suggested Reading

Chan JD, Treece PD, Engelberg RA, Crowley L, Rubenfeld GD, Steinberg KP, et al. Narcotic and benzodiazepine use after withdrawal of life support: association with time to death? Chest. 2004;126:286–93.

Kompanje EJ, van der Hoven B, Bakker J. Anticipation of distress after discontinuation of mechanical ventilation in the ICU at the end of life. Intensive Care Med. 2008;34:1593–9.

Mayer AM, Kossoff SB. Withdrawal of life support in the neurological intensive care unit. Neurology. 1999;52:1602–9.

Chapter 89
Brain Death in Neurosurgical Critical Care

Amit Prakash and Basil Matta

Overview

Up until the mid-twentieth century, circulatory cessation was used to determine death. Thereafter, the advent of medical technology especially our ability to mechanically ventilate patients with severe brain injury, long after cessation of brain function, required medical communities to review the definition and understanding of death.

Brain death is best defined as absence of clinical brain functions when the primary etiology is known and demonstrably irreversible. The three cardinal findings in brain death are coma, absence of brain stem reflexes, and apnea. However, the term "brain death" can be confusing because many believe that brain-dead patients are dead because they have irreversibly lost the higher brain functions of consciousness and cognition, which falls into the category of persistent vegetative state.

The diagnosis of death has major implications not only for the family but also on our ability in recent times to support organ transplantation.

Whole brain death formulation codified as, "an individual who has sustained irreversible cessation of all functions of the entire brain, including the brainstem, is dead," by the Uniform Determination of Death Act 1993 is the accepted norm in USA, Canada, and most parts of EU. It mandates ancillary testing to confirm the diagnosis.

In 1976 the Conference of Medical Royal Colleges in the UK, published a document emphasizing the importance of brain stem death. The brainstem formulation of brain death was formally adopted in the UK in 1995. The Academy of Royal Colleges published a Code of Practice in 2008, which builds upon the earlier Code published in 1998. It provides rigorous criteria for confirming death in clinical settings where confirmation of death by brainstem testing is appropriate.

A. Prakash, MD, FRCA (✉)
Department of Anesthesia, Toronto Western Hospital, Toronto, ON, Canada

B. Matta, MD, FRCA
Department of Emergency and Perioperative Care,
Cambridge University Hospitals, Cambridge, UK

A.M. Brambrink and J.R. Kirsch (eds.), *Essentials of Neurosurgical
Anesthesia & Critical Care*, DOI 10.1007/978-0-387-09562-2_89,
© Springer Science+Business Media, LLC 2012

Implications for the Neurosurgical Patient

The effects of cerebral edema in a fixed-volume container such as the skull are well known. The initial etiology can be intracranial or extracranial. The consequent rise in intracranial pressure opposes cerebral perfusion pressure and limits cerebral oxygen delivery. This in turn contributes toward the secondary brain injury that neuro-critical care aims to limit.

Ultimately, a significantly raised intracranial pressure will cause brainstem death by causing coning – the brainstem is forced through the foramen magnum.

Besides a reduced level of consciousness, severe brain injury may be associated with localizing signs as well as disturbance of both homeostasis and autonomic function. Cranial nerve affections can be correlated with the site of injury: anterior fossa (I–VI), middle fossa (VII, VIII), and posterior fossa (IX, X). Early uncal herniation caused by the expansion of the proximate lesion can produce false localizing signs such as VI nerve palsy and stretching of III cranial nerve over the tentorium cerebelli is associated with pupillary constriction followed by dilatation. Cardiovascular changes occur as the cardio respiratory centers are affected. The classic Cushing's reflex of systemic hypertension and compensatory bradycardia may be observed; however, there may be tachycardia or other dysrrhythmias. Eventually, brainstem death leads to hypotension and tachycardia. Diabetes insipidus may be preexistent and indicates a compromised hypothalamic–pituitary axis. In late stages, control of temperature homeostasis is lost, and persistent hypothermia ensues.

Diagnosis of Brainstem Death

In the UK, clinical testing must be undertaken by two physicians who have been fully registered for more than 5 years, are competent in the procedure, and independent of the transplant team. At least one should be a consultant. Testing should be undertaken by the doctors together and must be successful on two occasions in total. The legal time of death for documentation is when the first set of tests was completed. The legal ramification determining brain death varies between countries and states around the world.

Preconditions

All of the following conditions must be fulfilled before clinical testing is undertaken

- The etiology of irreversible brain damage must be known. In most cases this is obvious but when the primary event was prolonged circulatory insufficiency or cerebral hypoxia, it may take longer to establish the diagnosis and to be confident of the prognosis.

- The patient must be irreversibly comatose, unresponsive and apneic, and being artificially ventilated.
- There should be no consideration that the state is due to centrally depressant drugs. The action of narcotics, tranquilizers, and hypnotic agents can be prolonged due to hypothermia or renal/hepatic failure. If drug assays are available it is recommended that testing to assess for brain death should not be undertaken if, for example, thiopentone level is >5 mg/L or midazolam level is >10 µg/L. If opioids or benzodiazepines are thought to be contributing to the coma, specific antagonists such as naloxone or flumazenil (Anexate©) should be used. In other circumstances, residual sedative effects must be predicted according to pharmacokinetic principles.
- The core temperature should be greater than 34°C at the time of testing.
- Potentially reversible circulatory, metabolic and endocrine disturbances must have been excluded as the cause of the continuation of unconsciousness.

  - The mean arterial pressure should be consistently >60 mmHg with maintenance of normocarbia and avoidance of hypoxia, acidemia or alkalemia ($PaCO2 < 6.0$ KPa, $PaO2 > 10$ KPa and pH 7.35–7.45).
  - Sodium levels above 160 mmol/L and below 115 mmol/L can be associated with unresponsiveness.
  - Serum potassium concentration above 2 mmol/L and significant weakness is unlikely unless levels of magnesium and phosphate are <0.5 or >3.0 mmol/L, respectively.
  - Severe hypoglycemia with glucose levels below 3.0 mmol/L (=54 mg/dL) and significant hyperglycemia with levels above 20 mmol/L (=360 mg/dL) can itself be associated with coma and stupor and should be corrected.
  - Thyroid storm, myxedema, and addisonian crisis may be associated with severe neuromuscular weakness or coma. These conditions are extremely rare; however, if there is any clinical reason to expect these disturbances then appropriate hormonal assays should be undertaken.

- Neuromuscular blocking agents and other drugs must have been excluded as the cause of respiratory inadequacy or failure (simple twitch monitor testing is helpful for differential diagnosis).
- An underlying high cervical spine injury and associated cord injury can rarely cause apnea and invalidates the apnea test.

Brainstem Testing

The brain stem often fails from the rostral to caudal direction and therefore it is logical to undertake testing in the same manner.

Pupillary reflexes: The pupillary light reflex involves cranial nerves II and III and localizes to midbrain. The pupils should be nonreactive to both direct and consensual light reflex. Fixed dilated pupils occur due to cervical sympathetic innervation, midsized pupils due to midbrain damage and pinpoint pupils are indicative of damage to descending sympathetic fibers as a result of damage to pons. The size of the pupils only provides an indication of the site of brainstem involvement and is not crucial for testing brain stem death.

Oculocephalic reflex: It involves cranial nerves III, VI, and VIII and interneurons within the midbrain and pons. Before performing this test the physician must rule out cervical fracture or instability. On head movement toward right or left, the eyes remain "fixed" on a point in an intact patient. In the brain-dead patient, the eyes move with the head, hence the name "dolls eye" reflex.

Corneal reflex: The reflex tests the V, VII, and III cranial nerves and localizes entirely to the pons. In the intact patient, touching the cornea with a cotton swab causes eyelid closure. The eye rotates upward, demonstrating the cranial nerve III component, known as "bell's phenomenon."

Oculovestibular reflex: The oculovestibular reflex tests cranial nerves III, VI, VIII, and IV. It involves the entire pons and midbrain. The following are steps to perform the test: Elevate the head 30°C. Irrigate tympanic membrane with 50-cc iced water or saline. Wait 1 min for response. Repeat test on the other side after waiting 5 min. If the *oculovestibular reflex* is intact using cold water as stimulus, the eyes tonically deviate toward the side of the stimulus immediately followed by a fast recoil toward the contralateral side (apparent nystagmus). In the brain stem dead patient this response is absent.

Gag and cough reflexes: They require a functioning medulla and test cranial nerves IX and X. The cough reflex is easily tested by stimulation of carina by suction through the endotracheal tube. The gag reflex can be elicited by stimulating the posterior pharynx with a tongue blade. Both reflexes should be absent in brain stem death.

Apnea testing: This final test aims to demonstrate the failure of medullary centers to drive ventilation. Apnea test should be the last brain stem reflex to be tested. The objective is to stimulate the medulla while avoiding hypoxia and hemodynamic compromise associated with acidosis secondary to hypercarbia. After ensuring pre-oxygenation for 10 min a blood gas is performed to confirm baseline $PaCO_2$ and SaO_2. With oxygen saturation greater than 95% the ventilatior is disconnected inducing apnea for a period of time to achieve $ETCO_2$ above 6 KPa (=45 mmHg). A repeat arterial blood gases is used to confirm that the $PaCO_2$ is at least 6 KPa and the pH is less than 7.40. An oxygen flow rate of 2–5 L/min via an endotracheal catheter or in difficult cases CPAP may be used to maintain oxygenation till this state is attained. Apnea is continued for a further 5 min after a $PaCO_2$ of 6 KPa (=45 mmHg) has been achieved. If there is no spontaneous respiratory response, a presumption of absence of respiratory activity is made. A further blood gas can be done to confirm that the $PaCO_2$ has risen by 0.5 KPa (=4 mmHg) from the initial 45 mmHg baseline.

Ancillary Testing

Confirmatory tests are essential when doubt exists about the clinical findings, conditions preclude an apnea challenge, or suspicion of confounding conditions exists. These are routinely undertaken in parts of the world where the whole brain death concept is applicable.

EEG: It must be noted that the mere presence of EEG activity does not preclude the diagnosis of brain death, and reversible causes such as barbiturate poisoning may result in an isoelectric EEG in a living patient. A result of no activity greater than 2 µV at a sensitivity of 2 µV/mm with the filter set at 0.1 or 0.3 s and 70 Hz over a 30-min time span supports the diagnosis of brain death.

Cerebral angiography is the gold standard for diagnosis of brain death and conclusively proves the absence of cerebral perfusion. The absence of intracerebral filling detected above the entry level of the carotid or vertebral artery in the skull *confirms* the diagnosis of brain death. The study requires that the patient be transported to the neuroradiology suite and can take several hours.

Technetium nuclear medicine scan: As with the cerebral angiogram, it is a positive test that *confirms* the diagnosis of brain death by demonstrating failure of uptake in the brain consistent with absent cerebral perfusion.

Other techniques include CT and MR angiography and transcranial Doppler studies.

Controversies

Despite numerous publications there is a paucity of evidence-based literature to support many current practices related to brain death determination. Definitions of brain death vary around the world and so does physician expertise specified to be qualified for testing. Many guidelines explicitly exclude transplant physicians from brain death determination process. Clinical assessment criteria, however, are similar in all guidelines except for subtle differences notably:

- North American guidelines (vary between states) recommend an apneic threshold $PaCO_2 \geq 60$ mm of Hg and some also require an acidemic $pH < 7.28$.
- Oculocephalic or doll's eye reflex is not required by the UK code for brain death determination.
- Many guidelines (including UK) incorporate specific core temperature thresholds for clinical determination of brain death, but recommended thresholds range from 32.2 to 36.0°C without clear evidence base for any of these limits.

Where full examination is restricted by the nature of the injuries, it is generally, but not uniformly, recommended that ancillary diagnostic testing be performed.

Conclusion

Care of the brainstem dead patient is subsequently dictated by the presence and wishes of the next of kin and the potential for organ and/or tissue donation. If donation is not an option, ventilatory support can be withdrawn at a time acceptable to all parties. Brain death testing is subject to strict controls and although variability exists these reflect the indigenous social beliefs of different populations.

Key Points

- The definition of brain death varies in different parts of the world with whole brain death requiring ancillary testing being the norm in USA, Canada, and most of Europe with the exception of UK where clinical brain stem death is legally and medically accepted.
- Strict adherence to the criteria for brain death diagnosis should be followed according to the region and institution.
- The diagnosis of brain death is primarily clinical. However, ancillary tests are performed when the clinical criteria cannot be applied reliably or are legally applicable.
- Attentive care of the brain-dead organ donor should be undertaken to preserve organ viability.

Suggested Reading

A code of practice for the diagnosis and confirmation of death. London: Academy of Medical Royal Colleges; 2008.

Baron L, Shemie SD, et al. Brief review: history, concept and controversies in the neurological determination of death. Can J Anaesth. 2006;53(6):602–8.

Lang CJG, Heckmann JG. Apnea testing for the diagnosis of brain death. Acta Neurol Scand. 2005;112:358–69.

Morenski JD, Oro JJ, et al. Determination of death by neurological criteria. J Intensive Care Med. 2003;18(4):211–21.

Smith M. Physiologic changes during brain stem death – lessons for management of the organ donor. J Heart Lung Transplant. 2004;23:S217–22.

Wijdicks EFM. The diagnosis of brain death. N Engl J Med. 2001;344:1215–21.

Young GB, Shemie SD, et al. Brief review: the role of ancillary tests in the neurological determination of death. Can J Anaesth. 2006;53(6):620–7.

Chapter 90
Organ Donation in Neurosurgical Critical Care

Pamela A. Lipsett

Introduction

Advances in the science of immunology and transplantation have made organ donation a culturally and socially accepted practice. However, in spite of advances in patient selection and pretransplantation management, the imbalance between the number of patients on the waiting lists for organ donation and the number of available organs for transplantation continues to widen. According to the United Network for Organ Sharing (UNOS), as of April 2009 over 101,643 patients are on the waiting list for organ donation, with only 1,170 donors having given the gift of life to 2,357 transplanted patients so far this year. This paper will discuss the current possibilities for organ donation and the ICU care of the potential organ donor, as well as a systems-based approach to the development of institutional protocols for organ donation.

Incidence and Epidemiology

In the USA and Canada the majority of organ donation involves patients after brain death, while living related and unrelated donors account for nearly 40% and donation after cardiac death (DCD) accounts for about 7% of all donors [1]. With improved donor management the number of donors over age 50 years has increased more than 135% in recent years. Currently, up to one-fourth of all deaths occur in intensive care units (ICUs) with patients dying according to either cardiac or neurological criteria (brain death). While many of the ICU deaths are related to respiratory failure or pneumonia, many patients die after withdrawal of life-sustaining measures. Up to

P.A. Lipsett, MD, FACS, FCCM (✉)
Department of Surgery, Johns Hopkins University School of Medicine, Baltimore, MD, USA
e-mail: plipsett@jhmi.edu

A.M. Brambrink and J.R. Kirsch (eds.), *Essentials of Neurosurgical Anesthesia & Critical Care*, DOI 10.1007/978-0-387-09562-2_90,
© Springer Science+Business Media, LLC 2012

61% of deaths that occur in a neurological ICU may be related to withdrawal of support due to predicted poor prognosis for recovery and patient wishes. Given that many deaths occur in hospital intensive care units, strategies for improving the donation process have been focused in the ICU and have proven to be successful in facilitating organ donation. The strategies include aggressive donor management (ADM) and the use of an in-house coordinator (IHC) for organ donation.

In contradistinction to a decade ago, the most common mechanism of death for those who die and donate their organs is now intracranial hemorrhage or stroke (40%), followed by head trauma (35%), and cerebral anoxia (22%).This change in the manner of death from traumatic brain injury in younger and healthier patients, to those who are older with cerebrovascular disease with ischemic stroke or anoxic injury has important implications for the ICU care team caring for the potential organ donor.

Pathophysiology of Brain Death and Medical Management of the Potential Donor

Alterations and instability in the virtually all organ systems can be expected as part of the physiological changes that occur as or after brain death occurs. In the early stages of brain death there is a loss of blood pressure regulation and sympathetic tone. As cerebral ischemia progresses toward the brainstem, a "catecholamine storm" can arise and a severe increase in systemic vascular resistance (SVR) and blood pressure occurs. This quickly subsides and a decrease in SVR, vasodilatation, increase in capillary permeability, and intravascular hypovolemia and hypotension result. The primary goal of management of the potential donor is to maintain adequate blood pressure through the use of volume expansion, either crystalloids or colloids, institution dependent (Table 90.1). More than 80% of patients will require some form of vasocative support. During this time period, ongoing aggressive medical management of the patient is critical to maintain optimal conditions for organ procurement and transplantation and ensure good graft function and quality of life for the recipient. Standard patient monitoring includes blood pressure measurement, cardiac monitoring, and measurement of urine output and central venous pressures. While still controversial, many authors suggest that a pulmonary artery catheter (PAC) should be utilized to monitor hemodynamics and to guide and balance fluid administration. The primary goal of management of the potential donor is to maintain adequate blood pressure through the use of volume expansion. Often additional vasocative agents are needed. Clinical trial evidence cannot guide us firmly with respect to the best vasoactive or inotropic agents to use in patients with hypotension and/or depressed cardiac contractility. As noted above, first and foremost, the clinician must ensure that the patient is well hydrated, recognizing that maximal hydration is beneficial for renal transplantation, but worsens pulmonary transplantation. Dopamine has been typically a frontline agent for inotropic support, though it has not been shown to be superior to any alternative agent. The use of catecholamines

Table 90.1 Goals of organ donor management

Overall goals of organ donor management
Mean arterial pressure > 70 mmHg
Vasoactive agent requirement: ≤ 10 mcg/kg/min (dopamine, dobutamine)
Urinary output ≥ 1.0 ml/kg/h
Left ventricular ejection fraction > 45%

Volume goals
Pulmonary capillary wedge pressure 8–12 mmHg
Central venous pressure 6–8 mmHg
Action: Fluids (crystalloids or colloids) and/or diuretics

Cardiac performance
Cardiac index > 2.4 l/min
Left ventricular stroke work index ≥ 15 g meters/cm^3/beat
Urine output ≥ 1.0 ml/kg/h
Action: Ionotropic agents (dopamine, dobutamine, or epinephrine)

Resistance
Mean arterial pressure > 70 mmHg
Systemic vascular resistance 800–1,200 dynes sec cm^{-3}
Action: Vasopressors (Norepinephrine, epinephrine, vasopressin)

Endocrine failure
Hormonal replacement

Drug	Bolus dose	Continuous infusion
Triiodothyronine	4.0 μg	3.0 μg/h
or		
Thyroxine	20 μg	10 μg/h
and		
Methylprednisolone	15 mg/kg	Repeat in 24 h
Vasopressin	1 U	0.5–4.0 U/h
Insulin	10 U (50% dextrose)	Maintain glucose between 80 and 150 mg/dl (minimum insulin rate, 1 U/h)

has been shown to promote long-term graft survival and a lower incidence of kidney rejection; however, some clinicians find the vasoconstrictive properties of these drugs harmful in that they may lead to organ ischemia. Vasopressin has been suggested for its catecholamine-sparing effects as initial therapy for hemodynamic support and the treatment of diabetes insipidus. Echocardiography is done early on to assess potential cardiac donation, and focal wall motion abnormalities. Somewhat surprisingly the use of a PAC and hormonal replacement with T3 has resulted in dramatic improvement and reversibility in cardiac function. Dobutamine stress echocardiography is used to identify dobutamine-responsive individuals who may go on to successful cardiac donation. Coronary angiography is used in selected individuals.

More than 90% of individuals will have abnormalities in the posterior pituitary function, with low or undetectable levels of vasopressin. Hormones controlled by the anterior pituitary are seen at variable levels (thyroxine, human growth hormone, adrenocorticotropic hormone, thyroid-stimulating hormone). All patients should have vasopressin replaced. 1-desamino-8-D-arginine vasopressin (desmopressin; DDAVP) is highly selective for the V2 receptor which mediates renal medulla antidiuretic effects and has little vasopressor activity. It is best used in patients without hemodynamic instability while vasopressin in doses less than 0.04 units/min can be used in patients with both diabetes insipidus and hemodynamic instability.

As might be expected by common management strategies and the pathophysiology of brain death, electrolyte abnormalities are common in the dying patient with neurological injury. Hypernatremia may be used as a therapeutic strategy to treat the patient with elevated intracranial pressure. However, the clinician must be able to recognize and treat the patient who transitions to diabetes insipidus. Diabetes insipidus causes polyuria (1–2 l/h), dehydration, hypernatremia, and other electrolyte abnormalities (hypokalemia, hypomagnesemia, hyopcalcemia, and hypophosphatemia). Careful monitoring of urine output is essential and routine electrolyte monitoring is important. Monitoring donor sodium levels and correcting hypernatremia are critical for successful liver transplantation because high serum sodium levels (>155 mEq/L) in the donor can lead to primary graft nonfunction.

The American Society of Transplantation and American Society of Transplant Surgeons endorsed the use of the Critical Pathway after recommending that hormonal resuscitation (HR) be made an integral part of the protocol (Table 90.1). From the UNOS database use of this protocol resulted in the patient being more likely to be a renal (+7.3%), heart (+4.7%), liver (+4.9%), lung (+2.8%), and pancreas (+6.0%) donors.

Identifying patients who are eligible for pulmonary donation is a significant challenge, with less than 20% of all donors able to donate lungs. The best strategy for pulmonary management appears to include: performing ventilator recruitment maneuvers, restricting fluid administration, administering diuretics, and implementing techniques for preventing aspiration, as well as ensuring that the patient does not have a pulmonary infection. Thus therapeutic aspiration by bronchoscopy is considered useful for all potential donors. Steroids as above, and maintaining of a central venous pressure of 4–6 mmHg is considered optimal for pulmonary donation.

The liver, as an allograft, is fairly resistant to the immune factors which can cause immediate posttransplantation problems. As noted above, serum sodium should be maintained at levels less than 155 mEq/L. In addition, outcomes appear best if the central venous pressure of the donor is in the range of 8–10 mmHg, PEEP is kept as low as possible and nutrition is provided to restore glycogen in the liver.

Outcomes of Aggressive Donor Management

ADM protocols have been shown to reduce incidence of cardiovascular death before consideration of organ donation, and improve organ recovery and function in the recipient. In addition to the aggressive management noted above, identification of potential donors, and by using a clear facilitated process of the declaration of brain death, additional patients may be eligible for organ donation. The success of these programs is attributed to early aggressive management of the potential donor, education of the staff, a collaborative relationship with the Organ Procurement Organization (OPO), and guidelines of a standardized protocol.

Identification and Process Management for the Potential Organ Donor

The identification of potential donors in the ICU is a multidisciplinary effort that should originate from identifying a high-risk patient population from the admitting diagnosis (traumatic brain injury, respiratory arrest, cardiac arrest, stroke, drug overdose, intraventricular hemorrhage) (Fig. 90.1). Accurate documentation of the presence or absence of central nervous system reflexes is critical when brain death is imminent and when explaining poor prognoses to families. The critical care nurse and the respiratory therapist are often the first members of the ICU team to detect a

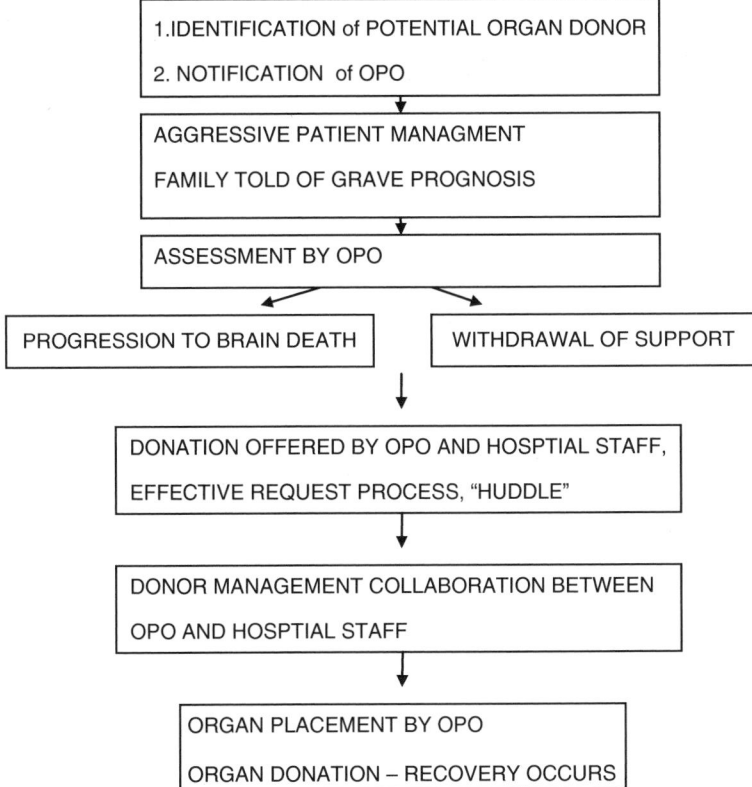

Fig. 90.1 Organ donation process

change in the level of consciousness and loss of neurologic exam and notification of providers who can rapidly begin brain death testing should follow. Thus, timely initiation of brain death testing is imperative, as cardiac instability often follows.

While this chapter has focused on the clinical aspects of the medical management of the potential organ donor, communication and support of the family during the discussion of grave prognosis and brain death testing is essential. Consent for organ donation is the biggest impediment to organ donation, and the family's understanding of the death of the patient, and the initial interaction with the team requesting consent has been shown to influence the probability of consent. The time period between identification of a grave medical prognosis and ultimate death allows the family time to consider the imminent death of the patient while the medical team maintains the dying patient in the best medical condition. Discussion of organ donation should be seen as a routine part of end-of-life process and every patient and family must have the opportunity to consider organ donation.

In the USA, regulations state that the person requesting organ donation be specifically trained to perform this function and training and role delineation of the members of the multidisciplinary team help alleviate stress during the request for donation. A collaborative approach with the Organ Procurement Organization staff and hospital staff is considered best practice for informing the family of a patient's death. Effective requesting is a term maximized by the Organ Donation Breakthrough Collaborative and begins with the "huddle." The huddle a short, timely, coordinated exchange between hospital and OPO staff which establishes an effective request process that meets the needs of the family. An effective request includes the following components: the right person making the request, the right timing of the request, the right family, staff (including OPO) present for the request, and the right place for the request to occur. When death is imminent and the family understands the prognosis, the hospital and OPO staff, working collaboratively, can introduce organ donation as a possibility and provide information to assist the family in understanding what to expect.

One best practice is the implementation of the IHC. The IHC typically assists and facilitates the donation process by donor surveillance, timely referral, education, family support and consent, donor management, and hospital/family follow-up. The IHC improves the donation process, consent rates, and conversion rates for donation through early and frequent interaction with families of potential donors and ICU staff.

Organ Donation After Cardiac Death

Organ DCD significantly contributes to the numbers of successful organ transfers, and protocols development in appropriate hospitals is expected by the joint commission to further increase this opportunity for patients and families involved. A patient may be considered a candidate for DCD when the patient does not meet the criteria for brain death and the decision has been made to withdraw active life-sustaining medical support. Other patients who could be considered for DCD are patients with nonrecoverable and irreversible neurologic injury resulting in ventilator dependency but not fulfilling brain death criteria, end-stage musculoskeletal disease, high spinal cord injury and some pulmonary diseases. In all cases, the patient or family should have made the decision to withdraw life-sustaining therapy. When this decision to withdraw support has been made, but before the therapies have been withdrawn, an assessment should be made in conjunction with the local OPO and the ICU team, about whether the patient would be a candidate for organ DCD. No predetermined assumptions about the candidacy of the patient should be made by the ICU team. The needs and respect of the patient and family at the time of withdrawal of life-sustaining therapy should be at the forefront of all decisions made about care, processes, and protocols. Importantly, the candidacy of the patient for organ donation will depend on an assessment of whether death would occur within a predefined period of time (usually 1–1.5 h). This time limit is used to preserve the ultimate function of the transplanted organ due to ischemia and reperfusion injury that occurs in DCD.

Legal consent for donation of organs after cardiac death should include all donor-related procedures (placement of lines, administration of drugs such as heparin, withdrawal of the endotracheal tube and termination of medication for blood pressure support). No donor-related procedures or medication administration should occur without consent. In some cases, the medical examiner or coroner must provide clearance before the staff can proceed for DCD.

Hospital protocols will vary as to where withdrawal of support will occur. While it is ideal for a patient to be transferred to the operating room or near the operating room for withdrawal of support and DCD, the needs of the family should be paramount in the development of protocols and the family should have the option to be present (or not) with the patient at the time of withdrawal of support and death. If the family wants to be with the patient at time of death, the family support team must prepare them for what they will see and that they will need to leave the room shortly after death occurs so that organ donation procedures can occur. The psychosocial needs of the family must be addressed and members skilled in providing this support should be available on site.

In DCD, members of the transplant recovery team are not allowed to be present in the operating room with the potential donor at the time of withdrawal of support nor are these personnel allowed to participate in the guidance or administration of end-of-life care or declaration of death. The Ethics Committee of the Society of Critical Care Medicine (SCCM) recommends that physicians who are part of the transplant team or who will be responsible for care of an identified recipient may not determine cardiac death. In DCD deaths, only one physician is required to certify death because objective data from an arterial line transducer can confirm the physical exam findings. Once cardio-respiratory function has ceased, the patient is pronounced dead based on cardiopulmonary criteria in the usual fashion by the attending physician or designee and the time of death is established. If death does not occur within the established timeframe after withdrawal of life support (usually a 90-min time period; in about 20% of cases), organ donation is not an option any longer and protocols for continued end-of-life care and notification of the family need to be followed. The family must be aware of the fact that donation may not be possible and the hospital system should have a well-established process for aftercare in the event that death does not occur.

When cardiopulmonary function is absent, typically a predetermined time must elapse for the declaration of death, and recovery of organs for donation. This time period is to ensure that reanimation cannot occur, but keeps the needs of the transplanted organ and benefit of successful donation balanced. The Institute of Medicine guideline suggests 5 min but individual policies may vary from 2 to 5 min. The consensus of the Ethics Committee of SCCM states that no less than 2 min is acceptable and no more than five is necessary. As soon as declaration of death is determined by the declaring physician, the organ recovery team can begin. All OPOs and transplant centers must develop and comply with protocols for organ recovery according to the Organ Procurement and Transplantation Network for Organ Sharing (OPTN/UNOS) standards which were established in 2007.

Designations and Advanced Directives

The Uniform Anatomical Gift Act created the power for individuals to donate organs, eyes, and tissues. In 2006, this was revised to enable OPO's access to the registries or Motor Vehicle Administration records to determine individuals' preferences. Occasionally, the ICU team may be faced with managing a situation where the patient has made the decision to be a donor by driver's license designation, donor registry or advance directive, yet the family may wish to override this decision. Although there are well-established legal and ethical guidelines substantiating the right of a patient to determine their wishes for organ donation, a family may still override or refusal to consent for donation (against the wishes or previous designations by the potential donor; research showed a 20% incidence). Factors that influence hospital and OPO's hesitancy to follow the patient's legal and ethical right to be an organ donor include the "dissonance" produced by family refusal, and the real or imagined threat of adverse publicity. Health-care providers within the OPO and the hospitals are obligated to maintain the patient's autonomy, even after death when the wishes of the patient are clearly known. A conflict can occur if the patient does not clearly discuss their desire to be an organ donor with their family member or decision-maker.

Summary

The development of clear protocols and aggressive clinical management of potential donors with the use of specialized personnel for identification and management of donors is key to successful organ donation. Best practices for Organ Donation have been identified by the *Collaborative* and should be employed in protocol development and in the verification of practice. Institutional commitment is critical to the success of organ donation protocols, and retention and recruitment of dedicated professionals to care for these potential donors. Ongoing training of the intensive care staff, the inclusion of donation as part of the end-of-life decision making and commitment to the donation process with a multidisciplinary team approach to standardize donor management in the ICU will narrow the gap between the supply and demand for organ donation.

Suggested Reading

Angel LF, Levine DJ, Restrepo MI, et al. Impact of a lung transplantation donor-management protocol on lung donation and recipient outcomes. Am J Respir Crit Care Med. 2006;174(6): 710–6. Epub 2006 Jun 23.

Christmas AB, Burris GW, Bogart TA, Sing RF. Organ donation: family member's NOT honoring patient wishes. J Trauma. 2008;65:1095–7.

Howard DH, Siminoff LA, McBride V, et al. Does quality improvement work? Evaluation of the organ donation breakthrough collaborative. Health Serv Res. 2007;42(6 Pt 1):2160–73.

Kutsogiannis DJ, Pagliarello G, Doig C, et al. Medical management to optimize donor organ potential: review of the literature. Can J Anaesth. 2006;53:820–30.

Salim A, Brown C, Inaba K, et al. Improving consent rates for organ donation: the effect of in house coordinator program. J Trauma. 2007;62:1411–5.

Shah VR. Aggressive management of multiorgan donor. Transplant Proc. 2008;40(4):1087–90.

Steinbrook R. Organ donation after cardiac death. N Engl J Med. 2007;357:209–13.

United Network for Organ Sharing: Organ Donation and Transplantation. http://www.unos.org/donation/index.php?topic=data, Accessed, October 11, 2011.

Varelas PN, Abdelhak T, Hacein-Bey L. Withdrawal of life-sustaining therapies and brain death in the intensive care unit. Semin Neurol. 2008;28(5):726–35. Epub 2008 Dec 29.

Wood KE, Coursin DB. Intensivists and organ donor management. Curr Opin Anaesthesiol. 2007; 20:97–9.

Chapter 91
Interaction with Family and Friends in Neurosurgical Critical Care

Amy E. Guthrie, Robert Hugo Richardson, and Mary Denise Smith

Overview

Quality medical care requires clinicians to have expertise in many areas of practice; one essential area is communication with patients, families, and surrogates. This expertise is especially important when the patient is critically ill in an intensive care unit (ICU), where information exchange occurs more commonly with families and surrogates. Communication challenges in the ICU are greater because critically ill patients frequently are unable to speak for themselves and the clinician is dependent on surrogate decision-makers, friends, or family members, to understand the patient's goals and values regarding life and health care. Evidence shows that skillful communication with family members contributes to higher patient and family satisfaction, while also improving efficiency of the clinicians' time and efficacy of treatment.

Clinician–family communication is crucial in developing a care partnership to improve outcomes for patients and families in the ICU. Communication patterns in the ICU consist of two major processes:

1. Informal – day-to-day contact with family members in response to questions and changes in the patient's condition.

A.E. Guthrie, MSN, CNS, ACHPN (✉)
Oregon Health & Science University, Portland, OR, USA
e-mail: guthriea@ohsu.edu

R.H. Richardson, MD
Departments of Pulmonary and Critical Care Medicine,
General Medicine and Geriatrics, Oregon Health & Science University,
Portland, OR, USA

M.D. Smith, RN, MSN, CNS
Departments of Internal Medicine and Palliative Medicine, Oregon Health & Sciences
University, Portland, OR, USA

A.M. Brambrink and J.R. Kirsch (eds.), *Essentials of Neurosurgical Anesthesia & Critical Care*, DOI 10.1007/978-0-387-09562-2_91, © Springer Science+Business Media, LLC 2012

2. Formal – planned family conferences attended by multiple family members, medical specialties, and an interdisciplinary health-care team.

Health-care providers can maximize family contacts, information exchange, and consensus building if a trusting relationship is built early in the patient's hospitalization and the family feels supported and valued.

Implications for the Neurosurgical Patient

Communication and decision-making with the critically ill patient is most often limited due to severity of illness and compromised cognitive function. Since clinicians rely on family members when the patient is incapacitated, building a relationship with them requires special attention. Because family members have a tendency to support each other at times of health-care crisis, many family members may influence decision-making even though one person is listed on the advance directive or considered legal next of kin. Building rapport with the family presents a unique challenge to the health-care team and awareness of the patient and each family member's influence on decision-making can allow for greater success in consensus building.

Building Rapport

There are many aspects to the care of the critically ill patient that can work to challenge the traditional clinician–patient relationship. Time pressures, lack of continuity, and technology all add to the difficulty of relationship building. Because the ICU team often meets the family for the first time as a result of the patient's severe illness, there is little time to establish the trust necessary to make major treatment decisions. Clinicians should work to initiate contact with the family early in the hospitalization by making an effort to meet them on the day of admission and remaining available for daily informal contact. Providing a private meeting place can help the health-care team in building trust; however, many informal contacts occur at the bedside and are most effective using the five-step approach identified by the mnemonic V.A.L.U.E.

- Value and appreciate the family's input.
- Acknowledge the family's emotional needs.
- Listen actively to what the family is saying.
- Understand by asking questions about the patient.
- Elicit questions from family members.

Information can best be elicited by asking open-ended questions that allow the family to describe what is important to the patient and how the family has been affected by the current condition of their loved one.

Initially, focus on common goals and discuss routine aspects of care before introducing more emotionally charged information. Listen for the family's perspective on the patient's illness and goals of care, allowing the family to do most of the talking during each meeting time. With each family contact, continue to emphasize mutual goals and values.

As interaction with family members increases, acknowledge the stress of having a loved one in the hospital and assess their readiness to come to terms with the patient's illness. Utilize chaplains, social workers, and palliative care specialists to meet the additional needs of the family.

Finally, build consensus with the family and health-care team members by identifying points of agreement with broad goals and specific therapies. Building consensus may require multiple family contacts establishing continuous and open communication with easy access to the health-care team.

Communication

There is evidence that family members of critically ill patients who survive the ICU hospitalization are less satisfied with communication from ICU clinicians than family members of patients who do not survive. Regardless of outcome, skillful communication with family members can reduce emotional stress caused by the uncertainty of critical illness. In addition, families report clinician communication skills as being equally important as clinical expertise.

There are many opportunities for informal clinician–family contacts in the ICU; however, a more formal meeting known as a Family Conference conducted within 72 h of admission has been associated with reduced length of ICU stay and a favorable family experience. Improved patient and family outcomes have been associated with consistent communication by all health-care members and following Family Conference guidelines listed in Table 91.1.

Table 91.1 Family conference

Preparation
• Identify all family members planning to attend the meeting
• Capacity fluctuates, consider including the patient in the meeting when appropriate
• "Preconference"/Provider conference
– Coordinate health-care team
– Discuss goals of meeting with health-care team
– Establish a unified medical opinion among health-care providers participating in the meeting to provide a consistent message
– Identify a meeting leader among the health-care team
• Arrange a private, quiet location with seating for all
• Limit distractions: plan for enough time to reduce interruptions
• Turn off pagers if possible

(continued)

Table 91.1 (continued)

Open the meeting

- Introduce all attendees
  - Establish and recognize appointed surrogate decision maker or next of kin, while addressing the importance of each family member's input
  - Assess family perception in the role of decision-maker along with influences affecting that role
- Establish and communicate overall goal of the meeting
  - Allow for flexibility as the family may desire to change the original goal(s) for the meeting
- Inform the family that the meeting will allow them to speak for the patient, as the patient would communicate for him/herself
- Spend more time listening to the family and less time talking

Elicit family understanding

- Inquire about the family's understanding of the patient's illness and current course of treatment
- Review medical information
  - Diagnosis and prognosis
  - Current treatment plan
  - Recommended changes to treatment plan

Elicit family values and goals

- Multiple perspectives may be represented
- Understand ethnic and cultural influences on communication styles, family relationships, medical treatments, and end-of-life care
- Explore the family's knowledge of the patient's perspective on health and illness
  - What would be acceptable outcomes for the patient?
- Explore the family's perspective on health and illness
- Assist the family to compare and contrast the perspectives if necessary

Discuss decisions that need to be made

- Establish a common understanding of the medical issues and probable outcomes
- Remind the family that decisions rely on an exchange of medical information and their understanding of the patient's values and desires for medical care
  - Using substituted judgment and best interests standards
  - Seek consensus

Close the meeting

- Offer a brief summary of what was discussed
- Ask for final questions
- Express appreciation for the family's willingness to work with the health-care team to provide a plan closest to what the patient would have requested
- Acknowledge the difficulty of living with uncertainty as the family cares and speaks for a critically ill loved one using empathic statements
- Make a clear follow-up plan, including plans for the next meeting and how to contact the health-care team

Follow-up

- Document the meeting in the medical record. Record a summary of the information exchange, observations of the family, and plan
- Follow up with family to reassess information processing and understanding
- Arrange for emotional, spiritual, and social service team members to provide additional opportunities to listen to the family and respond to new questions

Concerns and Risks

Family Members as Surrogate Decision-Makers

Building consensus, while making treatment decisions for the incapacitated patient, represents an ethical challenge in clinical care. High-quality shared decision-making is a process with many important components and requires more than a simple agreement to allow family members to be involved in the process.

In a truly shared decision, physicians and families mutually influence the other, each potentially ending up with a different perspective and a different understanding than either would have reached alone. Shared decision-making promotes establishment of an environment of mutual influence and helps to eliminate power imbalances.

Shared decision-making relies on the standard of Substituted Judgment to make treatment decisions that the patient would have made if he or she were capacitated. This standard extends autonomy allowing the patient's preferences and values to guide medical care during times of incapacity.

- Does the family have a recent advance directive document? The written directives may have been completed at a time of health. It is important to share information with the family regarding the patient's change in health, expected outcomes, and prognosis.
- Can the family recall previous conversations when the patient clearly stated treatment preferences in similar situations and similar expected outcomes?
- Did the patient ever express an opinion regarding life-sustaining medical treatment of other loved ones or controversial medical cases in the news?

The stress, sorrow, and uncertainty that family members experience while caring for a loved one in a critical condition can cloud accurate accounts of previous conversations and influence their evaluation of the patient's best interests. For that reason, it is important to acknowledge the physical, emotional, spiritual, and financial support of the family as complete care for the ICU patient. Since decision-making in the ICU is more frequently a process, and not an event, an interdisciplinary team is extremely helpful. Interdisciplinary team members should represent medicine, nursing, social services, chaplaincy, and ancillary therapies. Palliative Care specialists are clinicians representing multiple disciplines with advanced training in communication skills and grief support that can assist family members as they understand the meaning and realize the impact of the medical information received.

When sufficient evidence is lacking to identify the patient's preferences and values, health-care providers can encourage family members to use the Best Interests standard, which directs them to make decisions based on what they perceive to be in the patient's best interests. Questions to address when exploring Best Interest:

- Is there evidence the current treatment is causing the patient to suffer?
- Do the benefits of the treatment outweigh the burdens?

If consensus is not easily attained, points of conflict can be renegotiated by exploring the values and influences of the individuals in disagreement. If needed, discussions can be deferred to a later time; timed treatment trials can be offered; and if all else fails, it is acceptable to agree to disagree.

Grief Support

Families make decisions for loved ones in a time of uncertainty and loss based on long-standing family behavioral patterns. There is evidence that family caregivers experience loss through emotional strain, financial hardship, and physical health risks even if the patient is expected to survive the ICU stay. When family caregivers are expected to speak for the patient, they also struggle with internal emotional tension between their own emotional reaction to the experience and the desire to make the right decision for the patient. That tension may also originate from a difference of values and health-care goals from those of the patient. Ethical and legal models recognizing the surrogate decision-maker as only a spokesperson overlooks the emotional needs of that family member and underestimates the influence that the fear of "giving up" on a loved one has on decision-making. Providing an interdisciplinary team with advanced skill in grief counseling can provide family members with emotional support and a framework for future grief work. Sensitivity to how the family will grieve the experience of the hospital stay and the patient's last days will incorporate individualized patient–family care, increase family satisfaction with care, and establish a foundation of healing through the bereavement process.

Key Points
    Cultivate a clinician–family relationship building practice by:

- Initiating contact with family members upon admission to the unit.
- Utilizing an interdisciplinary health-care team for additional support and continuity.
- Organizing a family conference within 72 h of admission to the unit and at regular intervals thereafter.
- Planning to listen more to the family and speaking less.
- Acknowledging family emotions and stressors using empathic statements.
- Scheduling continuous and consistent communication with the patient and/ or family.
- Providing the family a route for easy access to team members familiar with prior meetings and the treatment plan.

Suggested Reading

Abbott K, Sago J, Breen C, Abernethy A, Tulsky J. Families looking back: one year after discussion of withdrawal or withholding of life-sustaining support. Crit Care Med. 2001;29(1):197–201.

Curtis JR, White D. Practical guidance for evidence-based ICU family conferences. Chest. 2008; 134:835–43.

Goldstein N, Back A, Morrison S. Titrating guidance: a model to guide physicians in assisting patients and family members who are facing complex decisions. Arch Intern Med. 2008;168(16): 1733–9.

Hanson J. Shared decision-making: have we missed the obvious? Arch Intern Med. 2008;168(13): 1368–70.

Maukisch L, Dugdale D, Dodson S, Epstein R. Relationship, communication, and efficiency in the medical encounter: creating a model from a literature review. Arch Intern Med. 2008;168(13): 1387–95.

Quill T, Holloway R, Shah M, Caprio T, Storey P. Recommendations for conducting a family meeting when the patient is unable to participate. In: Quill T, Holloway R, Shah M, Caprio T, Storey P, editors. Primer of palliative care. 4th ed. Glenview, IL: American Academy of Hospice and Palliative Medicine; 2004. p. 112–3.

Shalowitz D, Garrett-Mayer E, Wendler D. The accuracy of surrogate decision makers. Arch Intern Med. 2006;166:493–7.

White D, Braddock C, Bereknyei S, Curtis JR. Toward shared decision making at the end of life in intensive care units: opportunities for improvement. Arch Intern Med. 2007;167:461–7.

Index

A.M. Brambrink and J.R. Kirsch (eds.), *Essentials of Neurosurgical Anesthesia & Critical Care*, DOI 10.1007/978-0-387-09562-2,
© Springer Science+Business Media, LLC 2012